Natural Pathogens of Laboratory Animals
Their Effects on Research

Natural Pathogens of Laboratory Animals
Their Effects on Research

David G. Baker
Division of Laboratory Animal Medicine
School of Veterinary Medicine
Louisiana State University
Baton Rouge, Louisiana

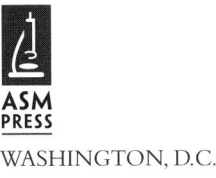

WASHINGTON, D.C.

Cover photos: (Top left) Multilabel confocal microscopy demonstrating infection of macrophages and multinucleated giant cells by simian immunodeficiency virus (SIV) in the lung of a rhesus macaque with AIDS. Macrophages are labeled with HAM56 and appear green. SIV nucleic acid is detected by fluorescent in situ hybridization and appears red. Where the two labels overlap, the addition of red and green results in yellow. Cell nuclei are labeled with ToPro3 and appear blue. The image was generated by Juan Borda and provided by Xavier Alvarez, Confocal Microscopy Core Facility, Tulane National Primate Research Center, Covington, La. (Top center) A coenurus of *Taenia serialis* removed from the subcutaneous tissues of a rabbit. This is a light microscopic image of a protoscolex cut in coronal section and stained with hematoxylin and eosin. Photographed by Dan Paulsen, Department of Pathobiological Sciences, School of Veterinary Medicine, Louisiana State University, Baton Rouge. (Top right) Two unembryonated eggs of the rodent pinworm, *Aspiculuris tetraptera*. Eggs were recovered from fresh mouse feces. (Middle left) Mouse hepatitis virus-infected NCTC1469 cells stained with anti-sialodacryoadenitis virus antisera and FITC-labelled anti-rat antisera. Image provided by Susan Compton, Serological and Virological Diagnostics, Section of Comparative Medicine, Yale University School of Medicine, New Haven, Conn. (Middle center) *Pneumocystis carinii* in lung tissue of a mouse. Stained with Gomori-methanamine-silver. Stained section provided by Cheryl Crowder and photographed by Dan Paulsen. (Middle right) *Clostridium piliforme* in the liver of a mouse with Tyzzer's disease. Warthin-Starry stain. (Lower left) Large trophozoite and smaller cyst of *Entamoeba histolytica* from a nonhuman primate fecal sample. Stained with iron-hematoxylin. Photographed by Dan Paulsen. (Lower center) Electron microscopy image of simian hemorrhagic fever virus grown in MA104 cells. Image provided by Elmer Godeny, Department of Pathobiological Sciences, School of Veterinary Medicine, Louisiana State University, Baton Rouge. (Lower right) Microfilaria of *Dirofilaria immitis* recovered from the blood of a dog. Giemsa-stained slide photographed by Dan Paulsen.

Copyright © 2003   ASM Press
American Society for Microbiology
1752 N St., N.W.
Washington, DC 20036-2904

Library of Congress Cataloging-in-Publication Data

Baker, David G., 1956-
Natural pathogens of laboratory animals: their effects on research / David G. Baker.
    p. cm.
Includes bibliographical references and index.
    ISBN 1-55581-266-X
1. Laboratory animals—Diseases.   2. Communicable diseases in animals.   3. Pathogenic microorganisms.   4. Laboratory animals—Diseases—Research.   5. Communicable diseases in animals—Research.   6. Pathogenic microorganisms—Research.   I. Title.

SF996.5.B35 2003
636.088′5—dc21

2003045109

All Rights Reserved
Printed in the United States of America

Address editorial correspondence to ASM Press, 1752 N St., N.W., Washington, DC 20036-2904, U.S.A.

Send orders to: ASM Press, P.O. Box 605, Herndon, VA 20172, U.S.A.
Phone: 800-546-2416; 703-661-1593
Fax: 703-661-1501
E-mail: books@asmusa.org
Online: www.asmpress.org

*To my mentors, colleagues, and friends,
Laurel J. Gershwin and Dale L. Brooks.*

CONTENTS

Preface / xi

INTRODUCTION / 1
Historical Perspective / 1
Infection versus Disease / 2
Scope of the Text / 2
References / 3

Chapter 1
ANIMAL HOUSING AND PATHOGEN SURVEILLANCE / 5
Animal Housing / 5
Pathogen Surveillance / 12
References / 16

Chapter 2
PATHOGENS OF RATS AND MICE / 19
Introduction / 19
Viruses / 19
  Adenoviruses / 19
  Cytomegalovirus / 21
  Ectromelia virus / 22
  H-1 virus / 23
  Kilham rat virus / 24
  Lactate dehydrogenase-elevating virus / 25
  Lymphocytic choriomeningitis virus / 27
  Minute virus of mice / 28
  Mouse hepatitis virus / 29
  Mouse mammary tumor virus / 31
  Mouse parvovirus-1 / 32
  Mouse rotavirus / 32
  Mouse thymic virus / 34
  Pneumonia virus of mice / 34
  Rat rotavirus-like agent / 35
  Reovirus-3 / 36
  Sendai virus / 37
  Sialodacryoadenitis virus / 38
  Theiler's murine encephalomyelitis virus / 39

Bacteria / 40
  Cilia-associated respiratory bacillus / 40
  Citrobacter rodentium / 41
  Clostridium piliforme / 42
  Corynebacterium kutscheri / 43
  Corynebacterium spp. in athymic mice / 44
  Helicobacter spp. / 45
  Klebsiella pneumoniae / 47
  Mycoplasma pulmonis / 48
  Pasteurella pneumotropica / 49
  Pseudomonas aeruginosa / 51
  Salmonella enterica / 52
  Staphylococcus aureus / 54
  Streptococcus pneumoniae / 55

Fungi / 56
   Pneumocystis carinii / 56

Parasites / 57
   Acariasis (mite infestation) / 57
   Encephalitozoon cuniculi / 58
   Giardia muris / 59
   Oxyurids (pinworms) / 60
   Spironucleus muris / 61

References / 64

Chapter 3
PATHOGENS OF GERBILS / 109

Introduction / 109

Bacteria / 109
   Clostridium piliforme / 109
   Staphylococcus aureus / 110

Parasites / 111
   Oxyurids (Pinworms) / 111

References / 113

Chapter 4
PATHOGENS OF HAMSTERS / 115

Introduction / 115

Viruses / 116
   Lymphocytic choriomeningitis virus / 116
   Pneumonia virus of mice / 117
   Sendai virus / 117

Bacteria / 118
   Clostridium piliforme / 118
   Lawsonia intracellularis / 119
   Staphylococcus aureus / 120

Parasites / 121
   Demodex spp. / 121
   Oxyurids (pinworms) / 123

References / 123

Chapter 5
PATHOGENS OF GUINEA PIGS / 129

Introduction / 129

Viruses / 129
   Cytomegalovirus / 129
   Lymphocytic choriomeningitis virus / 130

Bacteria / 131
   Bordetella bronchiseptica / 131
   Chlamydophila psittaci / 132
   Streptococcus pneumoniae / 133
   Streptococcus zooepidemicus / 134

Parasites / 135
   Cryptosporidium wrairi / 135
   Eimeria caviae / 136
   Trixacarus caviae / 137

References / 138

Chapter 6
PATHOGENS OF RABBITS / 147

Introduction / 147

Viruses / 147
   Adenovirus / 147
   Cottontail rabbit papillomavirus / 148
   Lapine parvovirus / 149
   Myxoma virus / 149
   Pleural effusion disease virus / 151
   Rabbit enteric coronavirus / 151
   Rabbit hemorrhagic disease virus / 152
   Rabbit oral papillomavirus / 153
   Rotavirus / 154

Bacteria / 155
   Bordetella bronchiseptica / 155
   Cilia-associated respiratory bacillus / 155
   Clostridium piliforme / 156
   Clostridium spiroforme / 157
   Francisella tularensis / 158
   Listeria monocytogenes / 159
   Pasteurella multocida / 160
   Staphylococcus aureus / 161
   Treponema paraluis-cuniculi / 162

Fungi / 163
   Dermatomycosis / 163

Parasites / 164
   Cheyletiella parasitivorax / 164
   Cryptosporidium parvum / 164
   Encephalitozoon cuniculi / 165
   Hepatic coccidiosis / 167
   Intestinal coccidiosis / 168
   Passalurus ambiguus / 169
   Psoroptes cuniculi / 169
   Sarcoptes scabiei / 170

References / 172

Chapter 7
PATHOGENS OF FERRETS / 193
Introduction / 193
Viruses / 193
Human influenza virus / 193
Rotavirus / 194
Rabies virus / 195
Canine distemper virus / 196
Parvovirus / 197
Bacteria / 198
Helicobacter mustelae / 198
Lawsonia intracellularis / 199
Parasites / 200
Fleas / 200
Dirofilaria immitis (heartworm) / 201
References / 202

Chapter 8
PATHOGENS OF CATS / 207
Introduction / 207
Viruses / 207
Feline calicivirus / 207
Feline coronavirus / 209
Feline herpesvirus type 1 / 210
Feline immunodeficiency virus / 212
Feline leukemia virus / 214
Feline parvovirus / 216
Bacteria / 217
Chlamydophila felis / 217
Fungi / 219
Dermatomycosis / 219
Parasites / 221
Fleas / 221
Intestinal nematodes / 222
References / 224

Chapter 9
PATHOGENS OF DOGS / 239
Introduction / 239
Viruses / 240
Canine adenoviruses / 240
Canine coronavirus / 242
Canine distemper virus / 243
Parainfluenza virus type 2 / 244
Parvovirus / 246
Bacteria / 248
Bordetella bronchiseptica / 248
Brucella canis / 249
Campylobacter jejuni / 251
Fungi / 252
Dermatomycosis / 252
Malassezia pachydermatis / 254
Parasites / 255
Demodex canis / 255
Dirofilaria immitis (heartworm) / 257
Fleas / 259
Intestinal nematodes / 260
Intestinal protozoa / 262
References / 265

Chapter 10
PATHOGENS OF SWINE / 281
Introduction / 281
Viruses / 282
Encephalomyocarditis virus / 282
Hemagglutinating encephalomyelitis virus / 283
Porcine circovirus / 284
Porcine enteroviruses / 286
Porcine parvovirus / 287
Porcine reproductive and respiratory syndrome virus / 289
Porcine rotavirus / 291
Swine herpesvirus (pseudorabies) / 293
Swine influenza virus / 295
Transmissible gastroenteritis virus / 297
Porcine respiratory coronavirus / 298
Bacteria / 299
Actinobacillus pleuropneumoniae / 299
Bordetella bronchiseptica / 300
Clostridium perfringens type C / 302
Erysipelothrix rhusiopathiae / 304
Haemophilus parasuis / 305
Lawsonia intracellularis / 307
Leptospira spp. / 308
Mycoplasma hyopneumoniae / 310
Pasteurella multocida / 311
Streptococcus suis / 313
Parasites / 315
Ascaris suum / 315
Isospora suis / 316
Sarcoptes scabiei var. *suis* / 318
References / 320

Chapter 11
PATHOGENS OF NONHUMAN PRIMATES / 341
Introduction / 341
Viruses / 342
    Hepatitis B virus / *342*
    Herpesvirus / *343*
    Respiratory syncytial virus / *345*
    Rotavirus / *346*
    Simian hemorrhagic fever virus / *347*
    Simian immunodeficiency viruses / *348*
    Simian retrovirus type D / *351*
    Simian T-cell leukemia virus / *352*
    Simian virus 40 / *354*
Bacteria / 355
    Campylobacter spp. / *355*
    Shigella flexneri / *357*
    Streptococcus pneumoniae / *359*
Parasites / 360
    Balantidium coli / *360*
    Entamoeba histolytica / *361*
    Strongyloides spp. / *363*
References / 366

INDEX / 377

PREFACE

Laboratory animals often serve as the essential building blocks with which advances in biomedical research are made. During the last century, it became obvious to many that the validity and value of research findings derived from the use of animals were directly dependent upon their physiologic health and uniformity. Considerable resources were thus devoted to improving and standardizing the health and care of laboratory animals, with tremendous results. The improvements continue to this day. While these improvements are most evident for laboratory rodents, new approaches to animal husbandry developed for these species have to some extent benefited larger species as well.

In addition to environmental, nutritional, genetic, and social influences, pathogen status has emerged as an important influence on host physiology. Improvements in animal husbandry and care have greatly reduced the number and scope of pathogens found in the modern laboratory animal facility. For example, pathogens requiring multiple hosts for the completion of life cycles have been eradicated as modern housing systems and commercial diets greatly limit the availability of unwanted host species. Likewise, those pathogens causing overt clinical disease drew the most attention and so were largely eliminated. Yet we are left with those natural pathogens of laboratory animals that are directly transmitted from host to host and that, for the most part, cause few if any clinical signs in otherwise healthy animals. So why worry about these? The purpose of this book is to inform laboratory animal veterinarians, animal caretakers, research scientists, and others about how natural pathogens of laboratory animals can and do alter host physiology and, in so doing, compromise research findings.

The text opens with a historical perspective on changes in the general awareness of laboratory animal pathogens. Next follows an overview of the important distinction between infection and disease. The first formal chapter provides brief descriptions of housing systems for pathogen exclusion or containment and then a brief description of approaches to pathogen surveillance. The body of the text includes sequential chapters on the natural pathogens of rats and mice, gerbils, hamsters, guinea pigs, rabbits, ferrets, cats, dogs, swine, and nonhuman primates. For each pathogen, there is a description of the agent, epidemiology, clinical signs, pathology, interference with research, and methods of diagnosis and control. Each description concludes with a convenient table indicating the organ systems affected by each pathogen and, finally, a reference list.

Anyone seeking to write a text like this faces the difficult task of determining which pathogens to include and which to consider too uncommon or unlikely for inclusion. This author faced such a dilemma. I apologize in advance to the helpful reviewers who suggested additional pathogens that were not ultimately included. I assure you that your input was not ignored. The pathogens covered were considered by this author to be the most relevant. Also, the need to have all information as current as possible necessitated drawing the line somewhere so that the text could be published. Concerning review of earlier drafts, the author acknowledges a debt of gratitude to the colleagues who helped in this way. Your constructive criticisms and suggestions for improvement are greatly appreciated.

I express my sincere thanks to Laurel J. Gershwin, Norman F. Baker, Ming M. Wong, Yuan Chun Zee, Dwight C. Hirsh, Ernst L. Biberstein, Dale L. Brooks, and other faculty of the University of California, Davis. Together, these mentors and friends patiently laid the foundations of my knowledge in microbiology, immunology, pathology, and laboratory animal science. This text could not have been written, at least by this author, without that foundation. I also thank the administration of the School of Veterinary Medicine, Louisiana State University, Baton Rouge, for allowing and encouraging me to write this text. The author also acknowledges the helpful assistance of Sue Loubiere and the library staff of the School of Veterinary Medicine. Lastly, I deeply thank my wife, Brenda, and my children, Anne, Martin, and Michael, for their unwavering support.

DAVID G. BAKER

INTRODUCTION

HISTORICAL PERSPECTIVE

Weisbroth (25), in an excellent review of the historical struggle against pathogens of laboratory rodents, divides the last 100+ years of research involving laboratory animals roughly into three periods. The first, from 1880 to 1950, was the period of domestication, during which many rodent species became much used research subjects. Many of these original stocks harbored a variety of natural, or indigenous, pathogens. However, during this period many improvements were made in sanitation, nutrition, environmental control, and other aspects of animal husbandry. The result was a great reduction in the range and prevalence of pathogens found in laboratory animals. The second period, from 1960 to 1985, was the period of gnotobiotic derivation, when cesarean rederivation was exploited as a means of replacing infected stock with uninfected offspring. In this procedure, full-term fetuses are removed from an infected dam and transferred to a germ-free environment and foster care. This procedure was very successful in eliminating pathogens not transmitted in utero. Weisbroth describes the third period, from 1980 to 1996, as the period of eradication of the indigenous murine viruses. In this period additional pathogens dropped from the scene or were found less and less often. These reductions were accomplished through serologic testing of animals for antibodies to specific pathogens, and subsequent elimination or cesarean rederivation of antibody-positive colonies, in addition to continued advances in animal husbandry methods. Pathogen prevalence studies have been and continue to be conducted (11, 14). Examination of these and previous publications confirm the steady decline in the range and extent of microbiologic contamination in laboratory colonies.

To put things another way, someone has summarized the advances in laboratory animal disease control in the following way: At the beginning of the last century, an investigator might have said, "I can't do my experiment today because my rats are all dead." At the midpoint of the last century an investigator might have said, "I can't do my experiment today because my rats are all sick," while today, an investigator might say, "I can't do my experiment today because my rats are antibody positive." Surely there has been a steady increase in awareness of the varied and generally unwanted effects of natural pathogens in laboratory animals, and ever greater efforts to exclude pathogens from research animals. Only when laboratory animals are free of pathogens that alter host physiology can valid experimental data be generated and interpreted.

INFECTION VERSUS DISEASE

When interpreting the microbiologic status of laboratory animals, it must be understood that infection is not synonymous with disease (14). In fact, few agents found in laboratory animals today cause overt, clinical disease, or do so rarely. Infection simply indicates the presence of microbes, which may be pathogens, opportunists, or commensals, the last two of which are most numerous. However, one must ask, at what point does an infection alter host physiology despite a lack of overt clinical signs? Is there truly such a thing as a "subclinical" infection from a research perspective, where host physiology is not affected in any manner whatsoever? These questions are impossible to answer with certainty, given the current state of information. Specific studies would have to be designed and conducted to answer these questions directly, and these types of studies have not been done. It is hoped that investigators will appreciate that, although infection is not synonymous with disease, overt disease need not be present for microorganisms to affect their research. Animals that appear normal and healthy may be unsuitable as research subjects because of the unobservable but significant local or systemic effects of viruses, bacteria, fungi, and parasites with which they may be infected or infested. On the other hand, this is not to imply that all animals harboring any microbe whatsoever are therefore unsuitable for use in research. There is clearly considerable variability in microbial virulence, as well as in the degree to which hosts respond to infectious agents. Response to infectious agents is part of phenotype, and naturally differs according to genotype. The point is merely made to illustrate that, given the current state of knowledge, it is difficult if not impossible to know when a microbe "crosses the line" between commensal and pathogen, despite a lack of clinical disease. For these and other reasons, interpretation of microbiology and serology reports should be done with the assistance of a veterinarian trained in laboratory animal medicine. Such a professional can assist the investigator in determining the significance of the organisms reported.

As accrediting and funding bodies increase scrutiny of the pathogen status, and by inference, the experimental suitability of the animals utilized in sponsored research, investigators will also want to work with a laboratory animal veterinarian or animal facility manager to ensure that laboratory animals are obtained from reputable, pathogen-free sources and are maintained under conditions that preclude, as much as possible, the introduction of pathogens. It is far better to prevent the introduction of pathogens than to have to account for their presence when interpreting experimental results. At this point it is appropriate to mention another valid reason for preventing pathogen entry into an animal facility. In some cases the drugs used to clear pathogens will themselves alter host physiology and interfere with research. For example, parasiticides with proven immune-modulating activity include ivermectin (4), levamisole (22), and thiabendazole (24). In addition to immune modulation, levamisole is known to affect host physiology in numerous ways (3, 5, 6, 8, 10, 12, 16, 18, 21, 23). Other antiparasitic drugs with known physiologic effects on vertebrate hosts include chlorpyrifos, which decreases brain acetylcholinesterase activity (15); fenbendazole, which causes subtle changes in behavioral performances in young rats (2); albendazole, which is embryotoxic in rats, induces liver drug-metabolizing enzymes (20), and delays rat brain microtubule assembly (19); and the avermectins, which possess anxiolytic effects (7), are selectively cytostatic against tumor cells (9), and cause developmental neurotoxicity (17, 26). Similar examples can be found among other antimicrobial compounds.

SCOPE OF THE TEXT

This text is intended to inform clinical and other research scientists, laboratory animal veterinarians, and students of laboratory animal medicine of known or potential effects of natural pathogens of laboratory animals on host physiology, and subsequently on research efforts utilizing those laboratory animal species. Efforts have been made to include what this author considers the most common and/or important infectious agents currently found in laboratory animals. It is not intended to include pathogens that were historically prevalent and important but are no longer so, or are only very rarely found in modern animal facilities. Also, known differences in the genetics, physiology, and responses of commonly used transgenic and/or inbred animals have been noted where appropriate. However, given the vast and growing number of such animals, particularly mice, extensive coverage of transgenic and/or inbred animals is beyond the scope of this text. Thorough coverage of this important subject would require a text by itself. In addition, efforts have been made to include as much information as possible from natural outbreaks of disease, but a considerable amount of information has also been included from experimental infections when the conditions of infection, e.g., route and dose, were compatible with those of natural infections. Some information has been included from in vitro studies when that information seemed relevant. Information from infections induced by abnormal routes of infection has been, for the most part, excluded.

This text is essentially an expansion of an earlier work (1), and is intended to add current information to the excellent body of similar literature concerning rats and mice (13, 14), and to bring together in one text comparable information on the pathogens of other laboratory animal species. Coverage is not intended to be exhaustive, but to provide the biomedical research community with enough information to determine whether a particular pathogen in question is likely to affect the outcome of intended or ongoing research. For the reader seeking information on the pathogenesis of infectious diseases in general, or additional information concerning the biology and pathophysiology of these and more obscure pathogens, several excellent texts and reviews on these subjects are available.

The reader may notice that considerably more information is presented on the effects of natural pathogens of rats and mice, compared with those of other laboratory animals covered in the text. This reflects the disparity between what is known about the pathogens of these species. Rats and mice have achieved a level of use in biomedical research unparalleled by other species. Consequently, far greater efforts have been made to identify effects of pathogens in rats and mice. In addition, many of these infections serve as useful models of human infections or disease mechanisms and have therefore been more extensively studied than those of other host species, with the occasional exception of particular diseases of nonhuman primates.

REFERENCES

1. **Baker, D. G.** 1998. Natural pathogens of laboratory mice, rats, and rabbits and their effects on research. *Clin. Microbiol. Rev.* **11**:231–266.
2. **Barron, S., B. J. Baseheart, T. M. Segar, T. Deveraux, and J. A. Willford.** 2000. The behavioral teratogenic potential of fenbendazole: a medication for pinworm infestation. *Neurotoxicol. Teratol.* **22**:871–877.
3. **Basi, N. S., M. George, and R. H. Pointer.** 1994. Regulation of glycogen synthase activity in isolated rat adipocytes by levamisole. *Life Sci.* **54**:1027–1034.
4. **Blakley, B. R., and C. G. Rousseaux.** 1991. Effect of ivermectin on the immune response in mice. *Am. J. Vet. Res.* **52**:593–595.
5. **Brunner, C. J., and C. C. Muscoplat.** 1980. Immunomodulatory effects of levamisole. *J. Am. Vet. Med. Assoc.* **176**:1159–1162.
6. **Cetinkaya, Z., H. Ulger, M. A. Akkus, O. Dogru, C. Cifter, M. Z. Doymaz, and L. H. Ozercan.** 2002. Influence of some substances on bacterial translocation in the rat. *World J. Surg.* **26**:9–12.
7. **de Souza Spinosa, H., M. Gerenutti, and M. M. Bernardi.** 2000. Anxiolytic and anticonvulsant properties of doramectin in rats: behavioral and neurochemistric evaluations. *Comp. Biochem. Physiol. C Toxicol. Pharmacol.* **127**:359–366.
8. **de Waard, J. W., B. M. de Man, T. Wobbes, C. J. van der Linden, and T. Hendriks.** 1998.

Inhibition of fibroblast collagen synthesis and proliferation by levamisole and 5-fluorouracil. *Eur. J. Cancer* **34:**162–167.

9. **Driniaev, V. A., V. A. Mosin, E. B. Krugliak, T. S. Sterlina, A. V. Viktorov, V. G. Tsyganova, A. F. Korystova, A. S. Grichenko, K. I. Zenchenko, and L. M. Kokoz.** 2001. Selective cytostatic and cytotoxic effects of avermectins. *Antibiot. Khimioter.* **46:**13–16.

10. **Evangelista, S., C. A. Maggi, and A. Meli.** 1984. The effect of levamisole on gastric ulcers induced in the rat by anti-inflammatory and necrotizing agents. *J. Pharm. Pharmacol.* **36:**270–272.

11. **Giglioli, R., J. K. Sakurada, L. A. G. Andrade, V. Kraft, B. Meyer, and H. A. Rangel.** 1996. Virus infection in rat and mouse colonies reared in Brazilian animal facilities. *Lab. Anim. Sci.* **46:**582–584.

12. **Klein, B.Y., I. Gal, and D. Segal.** 1993. Studies of the levamisole inhibitory effect on rat stromal-cell commitment to mineralization. *J. Cell. Biochem.* **53:**114–121.

13. **Lussier, G.** 1988. Potential detrimental effects of rodent viral infections on long-term experiments. *Vet. Res. Commun.* **12:**199–217.

14. **National Research Council.** 1991. *Infectious Diseases of Mice and Rats: a Report of the Institute of Laboratory Animal Resources Committee on Infectious Diseases of Mice and Rats.* National Academy Press, Washington, D.C.

15. **Pence, B. C., D. S. Demick, B. C. Richard, and F. Buddingh.** 1991. The efficacy and safety of Chlorpyrifos (Dursban™) for control of *Myobia musculi* infestation in mice. *Lab. Anim. Sci.* **41:**139–142.

16. **Pinto, A., R. Sorrentino, and L. Sorrentino.** 1990. Levamisole inhibits in vivo rat platelet aggregation by a release of prostacycline-like factor. *Gen. Pharmacol.* **21:**255–259.

17. **Poul, J. M.** 1988. Effects of perinatal ivermectin exposure on behavioral development of rats. *Neurotoxicol. Teratol.* **10:**267–272.

18. **Schinetti, M. L., A. Mazzini, R. Greco, and A. Bertelli.** 1984. Inhibiting effect of levamisole on superoxide production from rat mast cells. *Pharmacol. Res. Commun.* **16:**101–107.

19. **Solana, H. D., M. T. Teruel, R. Najle, C. E. Lanusse, and J. A. Rodriguez.** 1998. The anthelmintic albendazole affects in vivo the dynamics and the detyrosination-tyrosination cycle of rat brain microtubules. *Acta Physiol. Pharmacol. Ther. Latinoam.* **48:**199–205.

20. **Souhaili-el Amri, H., X. Fargetton, E. Benoit, M. Totis, and A. M. Batt.** 1988. Inducing effect of albendazole on rat liver drug-metabolizing enzymes and metabolite pharmacokinetics. *Toxicol. Appl. Pharmacol.* **92:**141–149.

21. **Thomaskutty, K. G., N. S. Basi, M. L. McKenzie, and R. H. Pointer.** 1993. Regulation of pyruvate dehydrogenase activity in rat fat pads and isolated hepatocytes by levamisole. *Pharmacol. Res.* **27:**263–271.

22. **Trabert, U., M. Rosenthal, and W. Muller.** 1976. The effect of levamisole on adjuvant arthritis in the rat. *J. Rheumatol.* **3:**165–174.

23. **Utsumi, E., A. Yamamoto, T. Kawaratani, T. Sakane, M. Hashida, and H. Sezaki.** 1987. Enhanced gastrointestinal absorption of drugs in rats pretreated with the synthetic immunomodulator, levamisole. *J. Pharm. Pharmacol.* **39:**307–309.

24. **Van Arman, G. G., and W. C. Campbell.** 1975. Anti-inflammatory activity of thiabendazole and its relation to parasitic disease. *Texas Rep. Biol. Med.* **33:**303–311.

25. **Weisbroth, S. H.** 1979. Bacterial and mycotic diseases, p. 193–241. *In* H. J. Baker, J. R. Lindsey, and S. H. Weisbroth (ed.), *The Laboratory Rat*, vol. I. Academic Press, New York, N.Y.

26. **Wise, L. D., R. L. Allen, C. M. Hoe, D. R. Verbeke, and R. J. Gerson.** 1997. Developmental neurotoxicity evaluation of the avermectin pesticide, emamectin benzoate, in Sprague-Dawley rats. *Neurotoxicol. Teratol.* **19:**315–326.

ANIMAL HOUSING AND PATHOGEN SURVEILLANCE

ANIMAL HOUSING

In the past 40 years, remarkable progress has been made in laboratory animal housing systems, both conceptually and technically. These advances have in large part been responsible for the precipitous drop in the prevalence of pathogens of laboratory animals, particularly among laboratory rodent populations. Housing improvements have also reduced the difficulty of housing animals with less than fully functional immune systems, and have, in fact, facilitated the development of these valuable research animals. Animal housing is itself a broad topic. Complete coverage of this important topic may be found in other excellent sources, and the interested reader is referred to them (1, 3, 4, 7, 8, 9, 12). This text will provide investigators with a brief overview of common housing options available for pathogen exclusion or containment. Additional information may be obtained from the sources listed above, as well as from the local laboratory animal veterinarian. It should be noted that pathogen exclusion and containment represent two aspects to be considered when selecting the most appropriate housing for research animals. Environmental and host factors may also greatly affect host physiology, behavior, animal accessibility, the general well-being of the animal subjects, and ultimately, the validity of research data.

The modern animal facility incorporates a wide range of housing paradigms to meet the varied needs of animal research. These include the concepts of conventional, barrier, and isolation housing systems. Conventional housing relies on good husbandry and close adherence to standard operating procedures. The objective is to maintain animals in good health by providing a clean housing environment that is safeguarded from pathogen entry. This end is reached by such practices as examination of preshipment health records, quarantine, postentry physical or visual examinations, personal hygiene by animal care personnel, and routine health monitoring. Limited restrictions are placed on personnel entering the facility. Conventional animal caging is open to the room or animal holding area, and does not employ protection at the cage, rack, or room level (Fig. 1). Therefore, animals housed in a conventional manner cannot be assumed to be pathogen-free. In fact, it should be assumed that conventional colonies harbor one or more enzootic pathogen(s), until demonstrated otherwise through appropriate diagnostic testing. Conventional housing is adequate in facilities without a history of serious disease outbreaks, where animals are obtained from reputable

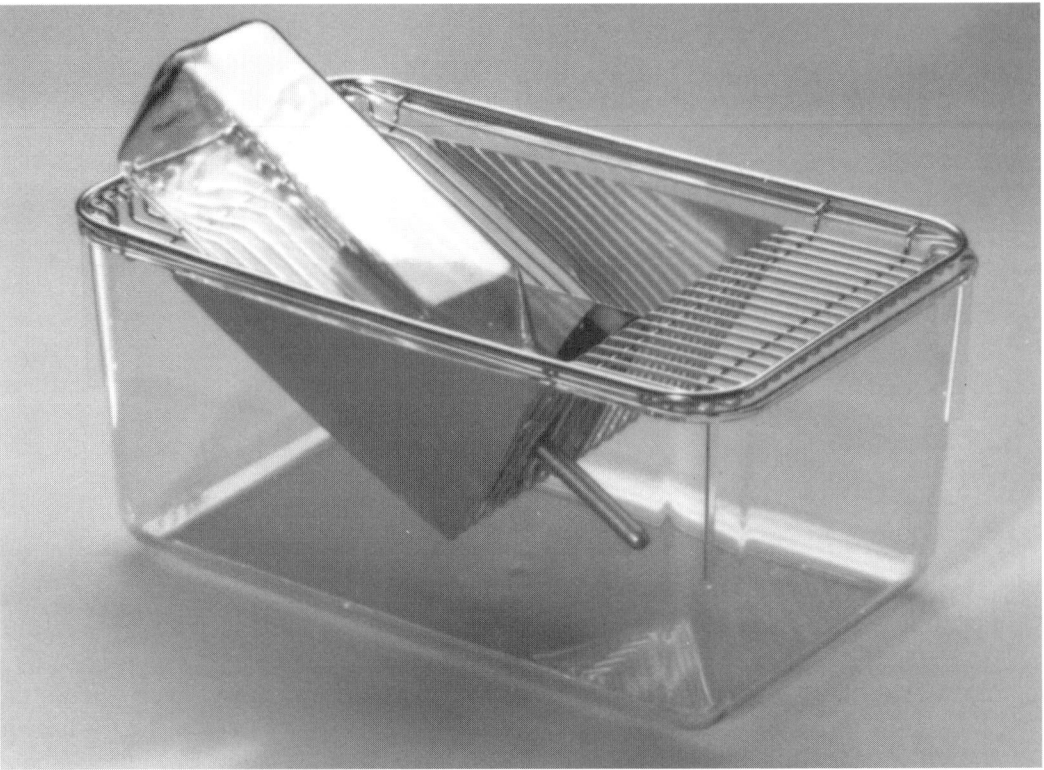

FIGURE 1 Conventional small mouse cage with lid and bottle. (Courtesy of Lab Products, Inc., Seaford, Del.)

sources, and where limited numbers of personnel are moving through the facility.

Barrier (pathogen exclusion) and containment housing systems rely on a complete program that incorporates equipment, standard operating procedures, and engineering standards to provide adequate exclusion or containment of pathogens, respectively. For barrier housing, some structural modification at the equipment, at the cage, rack, room, and/or building level, is incorporated to protect animals from adventitious infection. In addition, there are standard operating procedures that, when followed, preclude the spread of pathogens. These are more stringent than for conventional housing, and include stocking with specific-pathogen-free (SPF) animals, rigorous management of the physical plant, and health surveillance (12). Finally, engineering practices address the need for air filtration and directional airflow. The complexity of the system usually reflects the level of protection required. Determinants of protection needed include the microbiologic environment that the animals must live in or pass through, the value of the animals, and the potential outcomes of contamination. The potential outcomes of contamination are generally more severe in animals lacking a fully competent immune system. For this reason, more stringent protection is usually employed when housing immune-deficient animals (8). It should be noted that SPF does not mean that animals are not infected with any pathogens. It only means that they are not infected with pathogens for which they have been tested and found negative. It should also be noted that animals previously certified as SPF may no longer be so if there is a "break" in barrier practices. For example, transporting SPF animals from a barrier facility to a laboratory, whether across the building or the country, without maintaining barrier-level protection, negates their SPF status, until such status is once again "earned" through retesting and validation. Containment housing, also called isolation housing, is essentially a form of barrier housing, and is therefore in many ways conceptually similar to barrier (pathogen exclusion) housing in design and procedures. However, it is specifically employed to prevent egress and spread of infection from the research animals to other animals, or to humans in the case of zoonotic agents (those pathogens capable of spread from animals to humans). Containment housing may be used only during postarrival quarantine, or on a continual basis. As with barrier housing, the complexity of containment housing often depends on the virulence of the pathogen under study. Zoonotic agents are classified accordingly, as requiring Animal Biosafety Levels 1 to 4 (ABSL-1 to -4) housing; ABSL-4 housing is most stringent and protective (1). Most animal facilities are capable of creating ABSL-2 space, often out of conventional housing areas. This can usually be accomplished by incorporating additional and appropriate personal protective equipment, standard operating procedures that address the zoonotic nature of the pathogen, and changes in the physical plant that ensure proper airflow, biosecurity, and disinfection capabilities. Larger institutions often have ABSL-3 capabilities, but these require more stringent engineering standards, and so may necessitate new construction or considerable renovation of conventionally used space. The main difference between ABSL-2 and ABSL-3 is that ABSL-3 pathogens are more easily transmitted by aerosol, cause more severe illness in people, and require more sophisticated physical plant engineering, especially relative to human respiratory protection.

As the risk of infectious disease increases, pathogen exclusion or containment can be exercised at several levels. All of these illustrate the barrier concept, whether used to exclude or contain pathogens. For example, protection at the cage level may include the use of microisolation cages that incorporate filter tops or bonnets. These are fiber products that are incorporated into the cage lid, or fit over the cage lid (Fig. 2). These additions are useful for preventing gross contamination, and for exclusion or containment of pathogens that are not highly contagious. These devices are also useful for temporarily covering rodent cages when animals must be transported outside of the animal facility. A disadvantage to the use of filter tops or bonnets is the reduced visibility of the animals. As a result, daily examination of animals may require additional caretaker time and effort. Additional protection at the cage level is achieved with the use of another form of microisolation cage, the individually ventilated cage (Fig. 3). These systems are commonly used for housing rats and mice, and have been developed for other species as well. The placement of filters and/or direction of airflow determines whether air is high-efficiency particulate air (HEPA) filtered before entering the cage for pathogen exclusion, or is HEPA filtered as exhaust for pathogen containment. Individually ventilated caging is highly effective at preventing introduction or spread of infection, especially when combined with protection at additional levels, such as at the room or facility level. The disadvantages of individually ventilated caging include somewhat reduced visibility of the animals and high purchase cost.

Protection at the level of the cage rack or shelving unit may be achieved in several ways. All of these share the common theme of providing a "room within a room," where the cage rack or shelf essentially becomes a small "room" that is contained within the larger, standard animal room. HEPA-filtered air is blown or drawn over the caging. The cubicle is one form of such housing (Fig. 4). Cubicles allow some degree of flexibility as to the animal species housed, although the most common units are limited by design to housing

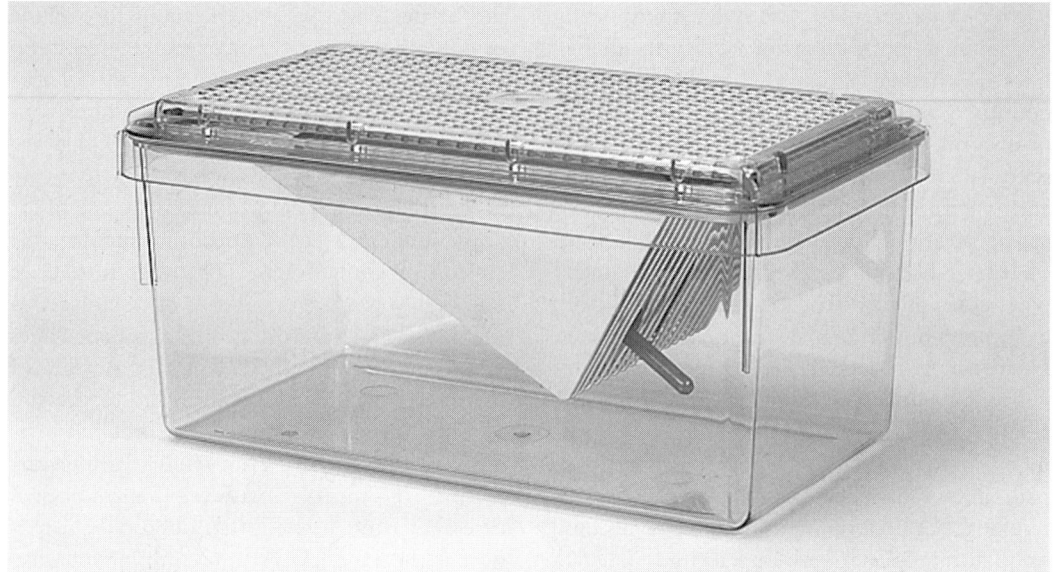

FIGURE 2 Static Micro-Isolator cage with filter top. (Courtesy of Lab Products, Inc.)

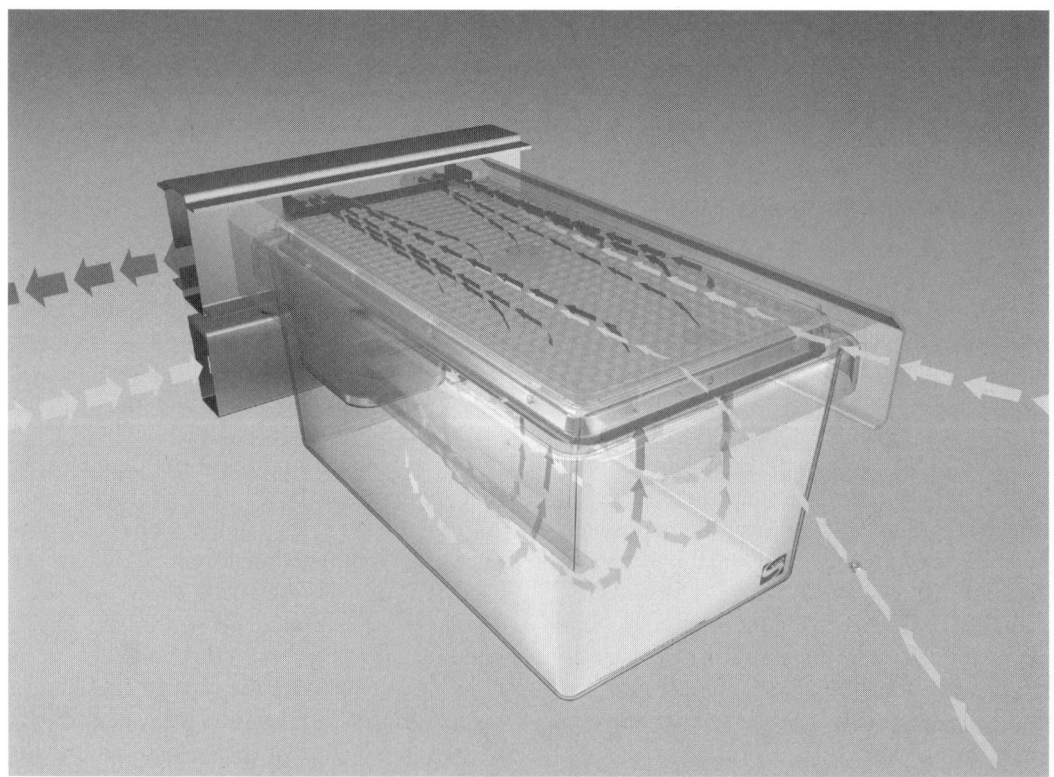

FIGURE 3 Ventilated Micro-Isolator cage. (Courtesy of Lab Products, Inc.)

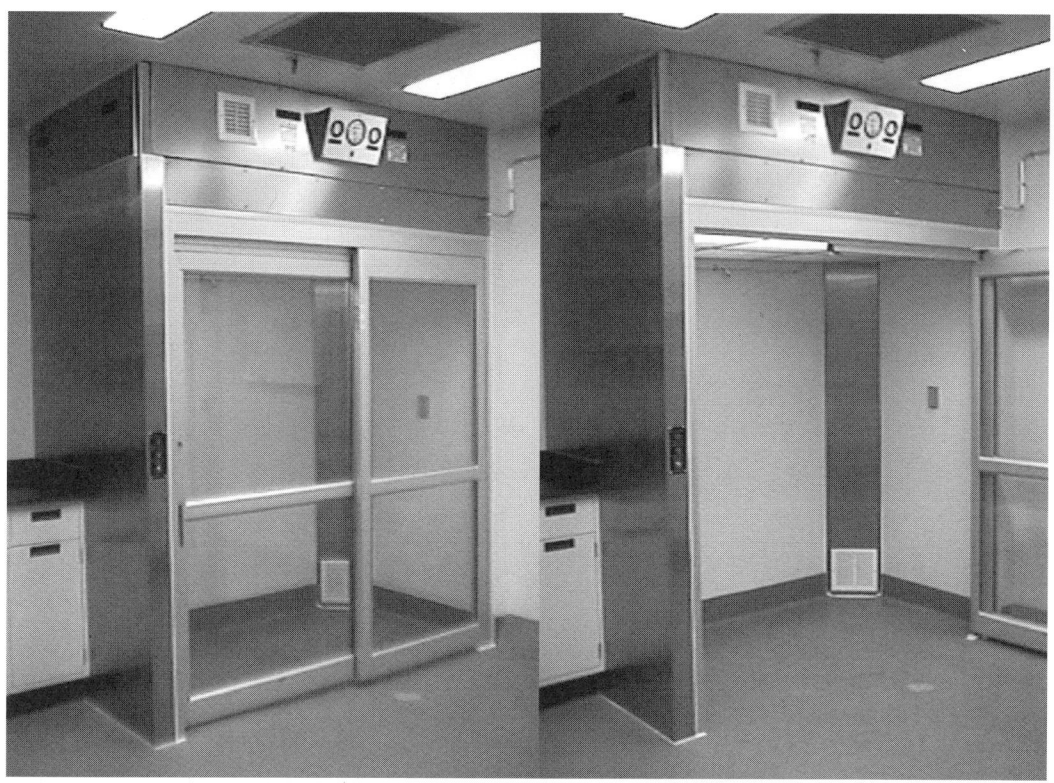

FIGURE 4 Built-in cubicles. (Courtesy of Lab Products, Inc.)

rodents. Larger units are available for housing larger animals. An additional advantage is the ability to build several cubicles into one animal room, allowing for separated housing of animals from different sources, or in use on different projects, without the need to utilize different animal rooms. While cubicles offer these advantages, they also present numerous challenges. First, once cubicles are built into a room, the room cannot be used to accommodate other housing arrangements. Second, cubicles are expensive to build and maintain. Last, because each cubicle has a dedicated heating, ventilation, and air-conditioning (HVAC) system, yet are all in a common animal room, it can be extremely difficult to balance the airflow for each unit. A superior form of protection at the rack or shelf level involves the use of freestanding cubicles (Fig. 5). These are known by various names (e.g., isolators), but are essentially mobile units into which a cage rack is rolled. Most of these can be set to blow filtered air over a rack of cages, or to filter potentially "dirty" air before release into the animal room or exhaust system. These units have several advantages over built-in cubicles, including reduced cost, better visibility, and most important, retention of space flexibility within the animal room. Since no permanent alterations need be performed on the animal room, the freestanding cubicle can be removed after conclusion of the study, and the room can be used to house other animal species. Racks of animal cages can also be protected from pathogen exposure by housing them in a germ-free isolator (Fig. 6). These units are commercially available with rigid, semirigid, or flexible film construction. Isolators are expensive and cumbersome to work with, but they do an excellent job of pre-

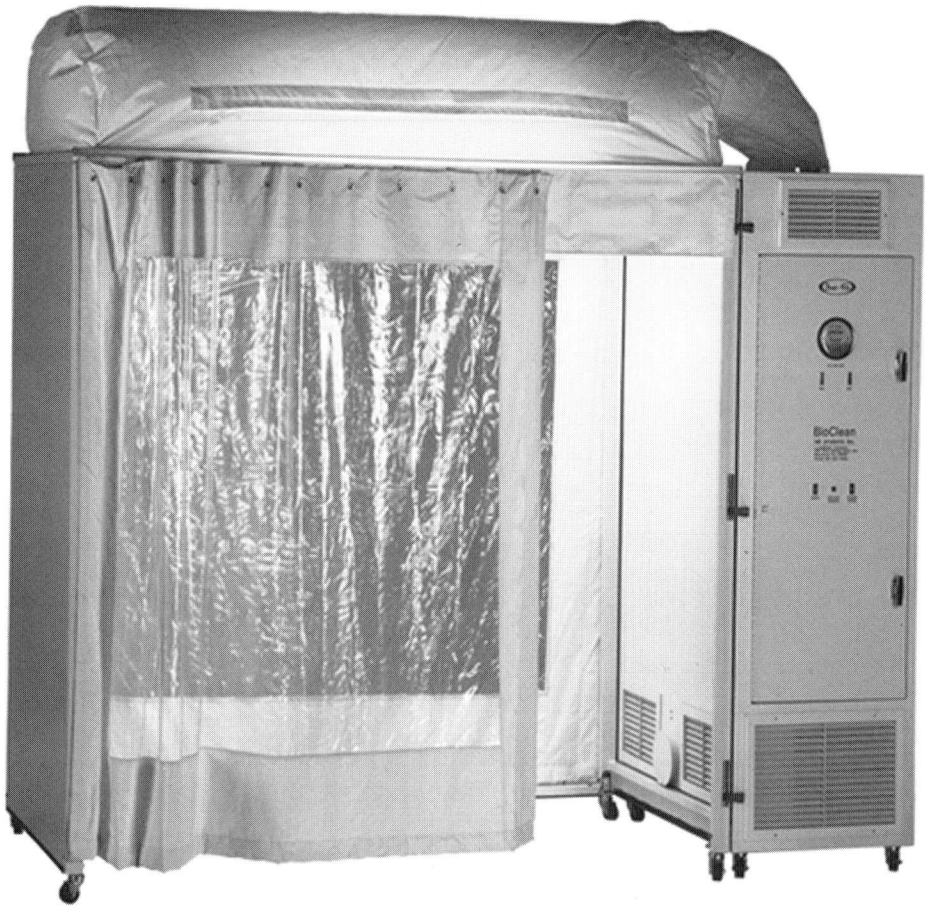

FIGURE 5 Mobile freestanding cubicle. (Courtesy of Lab Products, Inc.)

venting pathogen exposure. Lastly, groups of animal cages may be protected from pathogen exposure, or more commonly, used to contain pathogens, by locating them inside biological safety cabinets (1). These are designed in different "classes," each with specific features and capabilities depending on the level of air filtration required and the structural features of the facility available for exhausting air from the units. Some units exhaust HEPA-filtered air back into the animal room, while others are vented to the outside. Class II units are most commonly used to house animals. Other, more specialized types of isolators are also available, and are described elsewhere (3).

Protection can also be achieved at the room level, through the use of mass air displacement "clean" (MADC) rooms (Fig. 7). These are rooms in which HEPA-filtered air enters the room through small orifices in the ceiling and flows downward in a laminar pattern. This system may be used for housing animals, but it is used more often in rooms where pathogen transmission must be prevented, as in surgery suites. With the development of freestanding cubicles, construction of MADC rooms for animal housing is seldom warranted.

Lastly, a partial substitute, or preferably, an adjunct to the approaches presented above, is the use of personal protection or "tyvek" suits. These protect the wearer, and may be equipped with a dedicated air source for maximum protection. Positively pressurized HEPA-filtered respirator suits are generally

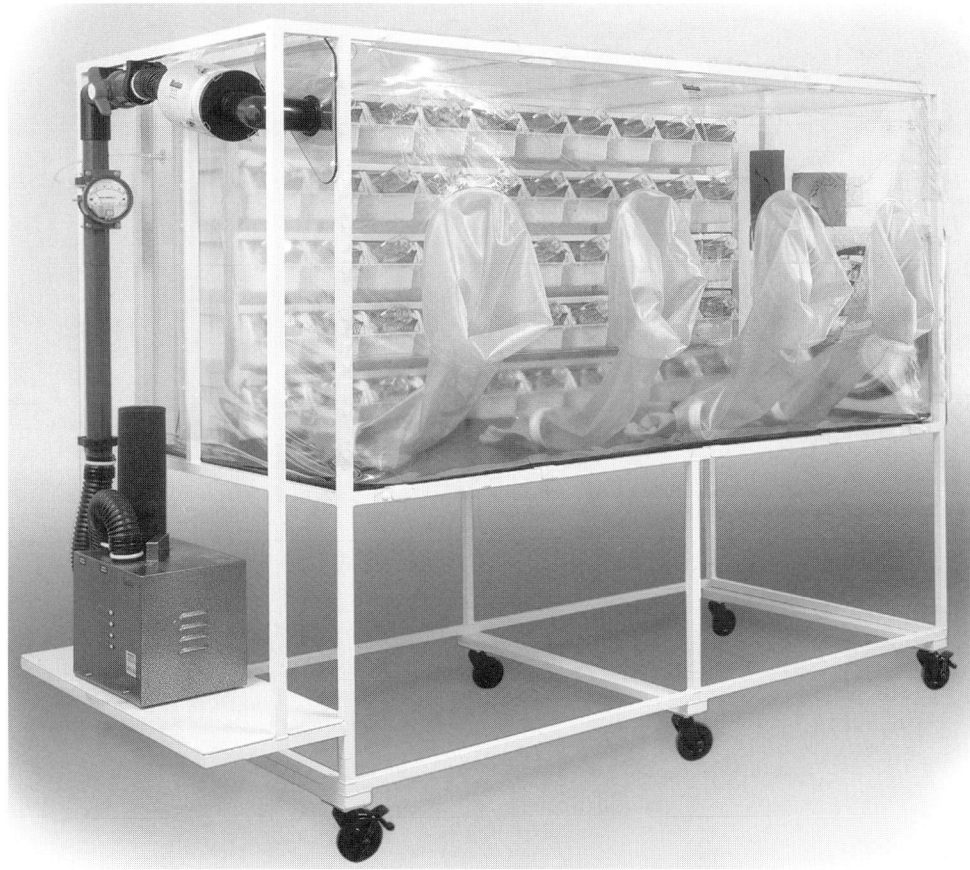

FIGURE 6 Germfree isolator. (Courtesy of Harlan, Indianapolis, Ind.)

only used in ABSL-4 facilities, while those that offer static protection are commonly used in barrier or lower level containment facilities. At higher ABSL levels (3 and 4), it is standard practice to combine personal protective equipment with physical plant engineering for maximal protection.

Relatively fewer housing options are available for nonrodent species. Specialized, microbiologically secure housing for nonrodent species are usually custom designed to fit the specific research needs of the institution. The obvious elimination of flexibility in space usage is acceptable because these housing systems are intended to be dedicated pathogen containment facilities. Because of the cost of such units, they are uncommonly built. However, much can be accomplished by simply isolating research animals away from people and other animals, and adhering to strict protocols of sanitation and personal protection. Cats, dogs, and other small- to medium-sized mammals are usually housed in movable cages, because these are easily disinfected and restrict the physical area to which animals are exposed. However, when pathogen considerations allow, socially compatible animals do well when housed free in rooms, with multiple resting sites placed at different vertical levels. Noisy and relatively dirty species such as dogs and pigs should be housed away from other animals and from people. Long-term dog housing that allows for pathogen exclusion or containment is complicated by the legal mandate to provide opportunities for dogs to exercise. Nonhuman primates are often

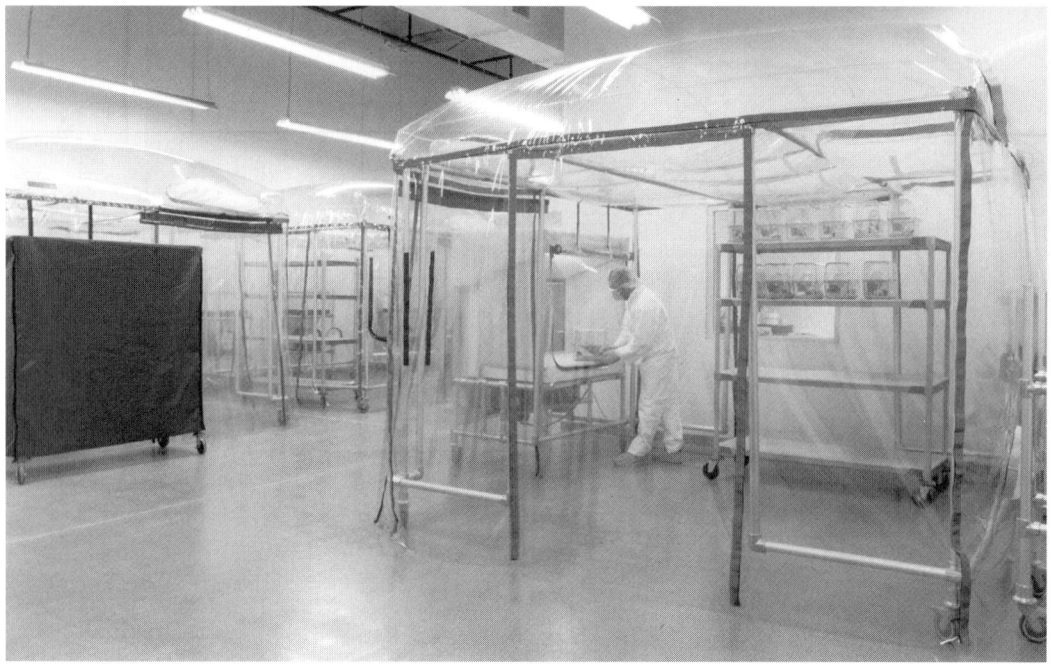

FIGURE 7 Multiple freestanding positive-pressure clean rooms with negative-pressure airflow option. Portable changing station docked to side of clean room; clean materials delivered in covered rack at far left. (Courtesy of bioBubble, Inc., Fort Collins, Colo.)

housed in an ABSL-2 facility because of their relatively high prevalence of infection with a variety of zoonotic agents, potential negative outcome of animal escape, amount of noise they generate, and concern for public perceptions. An additional consideration for housing rabbits, dogs, cats, pigs, and nonhuman primates is the desire and/or need to provide environmental enrichment. Objects used to accomplish this important task must be easily sanitizable.

PATHOGEN SURVEILLANCE

Pathogen surveillance is an important component of animal research. As the body of this text shows, data derived from animal subjects may be altered by unwanted pathogens. Unless one tests for pathogens, one will never know what potential effects those present may have on the research data. Many investigators fail to appreciate this point, and resent the added cost associated with pathogen surveillance. However, in this author's view, it is money well spent. The old adage, "an ounce of prevention is worth a pound of cure," certainly holds true where pathogen surveillance is concerned. The reader is warned that there is little consensus on which pathogens should be monitored. The purpose of this text is not to seek to resolve this issue, since the breadth of pathogen surveillance is influenced by source of research animals, species housed, history of disease in the facility, intended research use of the animals, and the availability of financial resources, among other factors. Instead, an overview of health surveillance systems will be presented to provide investigators with a knowledge base on which to build discussion with the laboratory animal veterinarian. The laboratory animal veterinarian is an excellent source of information concerning pathogen surveillance, diagnostic methodologies, and appropriate responses when pathogens are detected. In addition, several excellent publications are available which describe health surveillance systems in detail, and the reader interested in additional information is referred to those sources (10, 11, 12, 13, 18).

Research animal health surveillance begins with adequate diagnostic resources. The first component of the process is the astute animal caretaker or other personnel who observes the animals on a frequent basis. The value of adequately training animal personnel to recognize signs of disease cannot be overstated. Thereafter, more formal diagnostic resources are utilized. One of the most essential resources is the diagnostic laboratory. It is ideal if such a laboratory can be incorporated in the "in-house" services of the animal facility. In general, this will greatly speed the diagnostic process. A diagnostic laboratory is often not possible because of the high labor costs associated with adequate staffing of such a service, but when possible, it should be requested and encouraged by investigators. Whether an in-house or external laboratory is utilized, diagnostic services should include animal receiving, clinical examination, ante mortem sample collection, euthanasia, necropsy, anatomic and clinical pathology, bacteriology, parasitology, mycology, virology, and serology capabilities.

Traditional methods of pathogen detection have included serologic, microbiologic, and pathologic methods. These have proven very useful for detecting the present or past infections. Microbiologic approaches detect existing infections, assuming that the most appropriate samples are collected, and that they are processed correctly. A disadvantage to microbiologic diagnosis is the long culture time required for some organisms. Also, not all pathogens can be cultured. Serologic methods that detect microbial antigens are useful for demonstrating current infections. These methods are highly sensitive but are not easily performed in-house unless done so routinely. Serologic methods that detect pathogen-specific antibodies only indicate exposure, and not necessarily continued infection. One must then rely on increasing titers to determine whether the infection is current or historical. Also, immune-deficient animals often do not mount immune responses adequate for detection of infection. Serologic tests have nonetheless been the mainstay of pathogen detection for many years. A variation on traditional serologic testing is the mouse, rat, or hamster antibody production tests (MAP, RAP, HAP). These involve injecting transplantable tumors, hybridomas, cell culture lines, and other biological materials into SPF mice or rats, and testing for antibodies to a spectrum of pathogens. However, these tests have been largely replaced by more direct molecular methods. Histologic examination of necropsy specimens can be extremely useful in those cases where infection results in the development of pathologic lesions. However, tissues must be promptly fixed or frozen after death of the animal, and many commonly encountered pathogens cause few lesions, yet may still alter host physiology. Recent advances in molecular biology have facilitated the application of these methods to the diagnosis of research animal pathogens. Among the most significant has been the development of PCR assay technology. This approach is rapidly replacing traditional methods of pathogen detection. It is important to keep abreast of new opportunities to incorporate PCR assay into the health surveillance program. PCR assays are relatively simple to set up and perform. In addition, most institutions already possess the instrumentation required to perform them. Therefore, this very powerful diagnostic test can often be performed in-house, when circumstances warrant, such as for the derivation of *Helicobacter*-free mice and rats (16). One diagnostic application of PCR technology is the infectious microbe PCR amplification test (IMPACT) conducted by the Research Animal Diagnostic Laboratory, University of Missouri-Columbia. This application is useful for testing transplantable tumors, hybridomas, cell culture lines, and other biological materials. Modifications of the now standard PCR assay, including reverse transcriptase (RT)-PCR, solid-phase enzyme-linked PCR, TaqMan quantitative PCR, competitive RT-PCR, multiplex PCR, random primed PCR, inverse PCR, nested PCR, and *in situ* PCR further enhance molecular diagnostic capabilities (6). In addition to PCR technology, other molecular amplification technologies that have, or are likely to prove useful in diagnostics include the ligase chain reaction, self-sustaining sequence replication, solid- and liquid-phase nucleic acid hybridization, and microarray technology (6).

When establishing an animal health surveillance program, the issue of sample selection arises. Sample selection includes questions of which animals to evaluate, how many to evaluate, and how often to evaluate. Ideally, resources would be available to sample animals according to published guidelines and formulae (2, 12). Surveillance programs would address the scientific objectives of the research program. Unfortunately, adequate resources are often not available, and the laboratory animal professional must arrive at a system that offers maximal protection with minimal cost. This requires selective pathogen testing.

A number of sampling strategies have been developed for animal health surveillance. These will be described briefly. But first, some general information about health surveillance is offered. It should be recalled that the goal of health surveillance is the detection of at least one infected animal. In general, it is not necessary to determine the infection status of every individual. Also, when selecting the animals to be sampled, several considerations should be recalled. For example, juvenile animals are more likely to harbor greater parasite burdens and show more marked pathologic changes following infection with viral pathogens. On the other hand, young adult or retired breeder animals are superior for detecting active antibody responses, without interference from passively acquired maternal antibodies (12). Lastly, in mice, as animals age beyond about 12 weeks, the serum of some strains becomes "sticky" and nonspecifically adheres to assay wells. This results in frequent false-positive test results. This necessitates confirmation of findings by an alternative diagnostic method, thereby increasing costs and delaying final determination of infection status.

At an absolute minimum, health records should be obtained and examined before shipment of the animals, or at the time animals are delivered to the research facility. It should be obvious that health records are historical, and only reflect the pathogen status of the animals at the time of testing. The animals received may have become infected after the last testing, or may have been infected while in transit or on arrival at the new facility. Therefore, animals arriving with "clean" health records should be quarantined, observed, and preferably retested before release into the general population. There is disagreement concerning the timing of subsequent retesting after arrival. This author recommends testing 2–3 weeks after arrival, rather than immediately upon arrival. One of the most direct sampling strategies involves testing of principal, that is, experimental, animals. This may not always be possible because the sampling procedure often necessitates the euthanasia of the animal, or subjects the animal to stresses not experienced by the remaining principal animals, thereby potentially introducing physiologic variability. A variant of this approach is the sampling of "extra" animals shipped along with the principals. While this approach adds expense, it does allow for the testing of animals that have had opportunities for pathogen exposure most like those of the principal animals. A more common strategy is the use of sentinel animals. These are animals that are placed in the same room (usually) or primary enclosure (cage, pen, etc.) as the principal animals, and are sampled in their place. Sentinel animals should be selected for immune responsiveness, susceptibility to pathogens of interest, and ease of identification.

Efforts are under way to develop international standards for microbiologic monitoring of laboratory rodents (17, 19). This author recognizes the increase in global movement of animals and therefore sees much merit in these efforts. However, there will always remain the need to accommodate local experience and the scientific needs of the research at hand, when developing pathogen-screening profiles. To carry this concept further, specific colonies within an institution may at times require different testing strategies, each tailored for the scientific needs of the research.

While these systems have been thoroughly described for rodent (12) and nonhuman primate (5) species, little comparable information is available for health monitoring of larger animal species. In most cases, larger principal animals can be bled repeatedly or have fecal samples collected without disrupting research, and so can be monitored directly, without the need for sentinels or euthanasia of principal animals. Guidelines are lacking for health surveillance of species such as cats, dogs, and many other larger, mammalian species. In these cases, health surveillance strategies should be based on the planned use of the animals, and be arrived at through agreement between the laboratory animal veterinarian and scientific investigator. For example, a vaccination and health-monitoring program might be customized for cats intended for use in viral research. In this way, specific vaccinations will protect against infection without interfering with serologic tests or with desired susceptibilities to other viruses. Health surveillance would be directed toward detecting infection with other pathogens that might compromise the cats as research subjects. Such a customized approach to health maintenance can only be achieved through open communication between the veterinarian and investigator.

As a general rule, the expected prevalence of the agents in question will greatly influence the sample size. Pathogens expected to be highly prevalent will require the sampling of fewer animals to detect infection. This is because, with the testing of each successive animal, the probability of obtaining another negative test result diminishes. In contrast, when prevalence rates are expected to be low, many animals may need to be sampled before one can be confident that infections have not been missed. Such a situation might exist in an animal room where filter tops are used because, when used properly, filter tops slow the spread of infection. Prevalence-based sampling principles are more easily applied to populations >100 animals (2). For smaller populations potentially infected with a pathogen expected to be prevalent in only a few animals, there may not be a sufficient number of animals to sacrifice and test to be confident that infections have not been missed. On the other hand, if the pathogen is even moderately prevalent, the probability of detecting it with each successive sampling increases greatly in a small population compared with a larger population, because with each sampling, one is sampling a greater percentage of the remaining animals. For routine health surveillance, infection rates of roughly 50% are assumed. However, in the author's experience, this assumption is erroneous. Some of the problems inherent in sampling small populations may be overcome by exposing clean sentinel animals to bedding from all other cages. However, dirty bedding transfer is not uniformly effective in transmitting pathogens (14). Another means of more thoroughly sampling small populations is, where possible, to pool samples for PCR assay. However, not all PCR assays have been validated for pooled samples. An example of where this is feasible is the PCR assay of mouse feces for *Helicobacter* spp. DNA. Up to 10 fecal pellets can be combined for one PCR assay.

The frequency of testing should be determined by the likelihood of contamination (15). Most laboratory animal programs function this way intuitively. Animals received from sources considered to be a high risk for enzootic infections, or those with a history of "dirty" animals, are observed more closely, contained more stringently, and tested more frequently. Likewise, one might naturally test animals in quarantine more frequently than animals in a barrier facility with essentially no contact with the outside world, because contamination is much more likely in quarantine (15). Otto and Tolwani have recently described in more formal terms a risk-based health-monitoring program focused on testing of incoming animals, but conceptually applicable to wider usage within the facility (14). This system considers the likelihood of infection when establishing housing and testing programs.

In summary, animal-housing systems and husbandry practices have improved tremendously during the past several decades. While this is particularly true for rodent housing, significant advances have also occurred in the housing of larger species. Despite these improvements, unwanted pathogens remain a threat to the research program, and in the case of zoonotic agents, to human health. Therefore, animal health surveillance programs continue to be important and fundamental components of the research effort. While useful guidelines exist for health monitoring of rodent and primate species, optimal health-monitoring programs must be tailored to some degree to institutional needs and experiences. Program development should be a joint effort by the laboratory animal veterinarian and the scientific investigators.

REFERENCES

1. **Centers for Disease Control and Prevention-National Institutes of Health.** 1999. *Biosafety in Microbiological and Biomedical Laboratories*, 4th ed. U.S. Department of Health and Human Services, Public Health Service, Centers for Disease Control and Prevention, and National Institutes of Health, stock no. 017-040-00547-4. U.S. Government Printing Office, Washington, D.C.
2. **Clifford, C. B.** 2001. Samples, sample selection, and statistics: living with uncertainty. *Lab. Anim.* **30:**26–31.
3. **Clough, G.** 1999. The animal house: design, equipment and environmental control, p. 97–134. *In* T. F. Poole (ed.), *The UFAW Handbook on the Care and Management of Laboratory Animals*, 7th ed. Blackwell Science Ltd., Oxford, England.
4. **Federation of Animal Science Societies.** 1999. *Guide for the Care and Use of Agricultural Animals in Agricultural Research and Teaching.* Savoy, Ill.
5. **Federation of European Laboratory Animal Science Associations.** 1999. Health monitoring of non-human primate colonies. Recommendations of the Federation of European Laboratory Animal Science Associations (FELASA) Working Group on non-human primate health accepted by the FELASA Board of Management, 21 November 1998. *Lab. Anim.* **33:**S1:3–S1:18.
6. **Feldman, S. H.** 2001. Diagnostic molecular microbiology in laboratory animal health monitoring and surveillance programs. *Lab. Anim.* **30:**34–41.
7. **Hessler, J. R., and S. L. Leary.** 2002. Design and management of animal facilities, p. 909–953. *In* J. G. Fox, L. C. Anderson, F. M. Loew, and F. W. Quimby (ed.), *Laboratory Animal Medicine*, 2nd ed. Academic Press, San Diego, Calif.
8. **Institute of Laboratory Animal Resources.** 1989. *Immunodeficient Rodents. A Guide to Their Immunobiology, Husbandry, and Use.* Institute of Laboratory Animal Resources, Commission on Life Sciences, National Research Council. National Academy Press, Washington, D.C.
9. **Institute of Laboratory Animal Resources.** 1996. *Guide for the Care and Use of Laboratory Animals.* Institute of Laboratory Animal Resources, Commission on Life Sciences, National Research Council. National Academy Press, Washington, D.C.
10. **Koszdin, K. L., and R. F. DiGiacomo.** 2002. Outbreak: detection and investigation. *Contemp. Top. Lab. Anim. Sci.* **41:**18–27.
11. **Laber-Laird, K., and M. Proctor.** 1993. An example of a rodent health monitoring program. *Lab. Anim.* **22:**24–32.
12. **National Research Council.** 1991. *Infectious Diseases of Mice and Rats: a Report of the Institute of Laboratory Animal Resources Committee on Infectious Diseases of Mice and Rats.* National Academy Press, Washington, D.C.
13. **Nicklas, W., P. Baneux, R. Boot, T. Decelle, A. A. Deeny, M. Fumanelli, and B. Illgen-Wilcke.** 2002. Recommendations for the health monitoring of rodent and rabbit colonies in breeding and experimental units. *Lab. Anim.* **36:**20–42.
14. **Otto, G., and R. J. Tolwani.** 2002. Use of microisolator caging in a risk-based mouse import and quarantine program: a retrospective study. *Contemp. Top. Lab. Anim. Sci.* **41:**20–27.
15. **Selwyn, M. R., and W. R. Shek.** 1994. Sample sizes and frequency of testing for health monitoring in barrier rooms and isolators. *Contemp. Top. Lab. Anim. Sci.* **33:**56–60.

16. **Singletary, K. B., C. A. Kloster, and D. G. Baker.** Optimal age at fostering for derivation of *Helicobacter hepaticus*-free mice. *Comp. Med.*, in press.
17. **Smith, A. L.** 2000. Experts address international standards for rodent quality. *Comp. Med.* **50:**233.
18. **Weisbroth, S. H., R. Peters, L. K. Riley, and W. Shek.** 1998. Microbiological assessment of laboratory rats and mice. *ILAR J.* **39:**272–290.
19. **Weisbroth, S., and E. Poe.** 2000. Global harmonization of laboratory rodent health surveillance standards. *Lab. Anim.* **29:**43–47.

PATHOGENS OF RATS AND MICE

2

INTRODUCTION

It is impossible to adequately define the role that rats and mice have played in biomedical research. It is clear that rats and mice have held a central position in the advancement of biomedical science. It is critically important to protect this scientific resource from corruption caused by infectious diseases. The observation that infectious diseases of laboratory rats and mice have been on the decline for decades (1) could lead one to a general sense of complacency regarding the plethora of pathogens to which these animals are susceptible. However, as pointed out by Stephen W. Barthold at a recent meeting of the American Association for Laboratory Animal Science, the development of literally thousands of new strains of mice and rats, many with less than fully competent immune systems, has been accompanied by the reappearance of pathogens thought to have disappeared. Additionally, pathogens thought not to affect host physiology may in fact effect some alteration, with adverse consequences to otherwise excellent research. These findings have come with the advent of molecular approaches to research, where cellular and subcellular investigations may be influenced by subtle changes brought on by infectious agents. For example, induction of cytokines by natural pathogens may be detected in molecularly based immunologic research, but not attributed to the offending organism, leading to erroneous conclusions about the outcome of a particular experiment. Therefore, this chapter presents a wide, although certainly not exhaustive, scope of natural pathogens of laboratory rats and mice, and their effects on host physiology.

VIRUSES

Adenoviruses

Agent

Mouse adenoviruses are double-stranded (ds) DNA viruses of the family *Adenoviridae*. Two strains have been reported: MAd-1 (formerly FL-1) and MAd-2 (formerly K87). These are likely distinct species (9).

Epidemiology

Natural infections in the mouse, the principal host, have been reported only rarely. Infections in rats have been suspected on the basis of serologic and morphologic studies (18). Transmission of both strains is by direct contact. MAd-1 has a systemic distribution pattern and may be shed in the urine for up to 2 years (23). The mechanism of viral persistence is currently unknown. Persistence of MAd-1 cannot be explained by the model of reduced class I major histocompatibility complex (MHC)-associated antigen presentation proposed for human adenoviruses (15). MAd-2 may be shed in the feces for 3 weeks in immunocompetent mice (11) and for at least 6 months in athymic mice (22).

Clinical signs

Clinical signs have never been observed during natural infection with either viral strain. However, clinical signs have been observed in a mouse stock- or strain-dependent manner following experimental infection with MAd-1. At the extremes, SJL/J and C57BL/6 mice are highly susceptible, while C3H/HeJ and BALB/c mice are more resistant to development of clinical disease (4, 8, 20). Susceptible mice showed symptoms of acute central nervous system (CNS) disease, including tremors, seizures, ataxia, paralysis, and death (7, 8, 14, 20, 23). In contrast to MAd-1, experimental infection with MAd-2 causes no clinical signs.

Pathology

MAd-1 infection has a striking tropism for the vascular endothelium of the CNS and spleen, as well as for cells of the monocyte/macrophage lineage. Interestingly, development of clinical disease occurs more readily in susceptible versus resistant mouse strains, yet there are only modest differences in pathologic changes (20). Susceptibility to infection is determined by the ability of the virus to replicate within vascular endothelium (4), while susceptibility to disease appears to be determined by Th1/Th2 immune response potential, as displayed by cytokine responses (5, 20). Light microscopic examination of CNS tissue revealed petechial hemorrhages, edema, neovascularization, and mild inflammation in the brain and spinal cord (8). Recruitment of inflammatory cells may be associated with expression of a MAd-1 early region 3 protein, gp11K (2). In other reports, pathologic lesions were most prominent in the kidneys, heart, spleen, adrenal glands, pancreas, liver, and intestines (1, 7, 10, 12, 16). These are tissues in which virus is also known to localize following intranasal infection and hematogenous spread (13, 19, 20). In contrast to MAd-1, infection with MAd-2 is localized to the intestine and results in pathologic changes that are limited to intranuclear inclusions in crypt and villous cells of the small intestine. These are in fact pathognomonic for MAd-2 infection (21). Immunity to adenovirus is primarily humoral, restricted to the immunoglobulin G subclass 2a (IgG2a) isotype, and is independent of gamma interferon (IFN-γ) (17, 20).

Interference with research

While pathologic lesions have not been observed in mice naturally infected with adenoviruses, reports of pathologic changes observed in experimental infections suggest that MAd-1 may confound research involving several organ systems, including the cardiovascular, nervous, renal, lymphoreticular, endocrine, and hematopoietic systems. In addition to pathologic changes, MAd-1 infection has been shown to alter chemokine profiles in the spleen and CNS (3) and to stimulate interleukin 11 (IL-11) production in airway stromal cells (6). The enterohepatic system may be the only system directly affected by MAd-2, and this only experimentally. Differences in formation of pathologic lesions in natural versus experimental infection are particularly evident in mouse adenovirus infections, and highlight the need to include histologic evaluation of research animals into the experimental design of all studies. It is likely that on occasion natural infection of mice with adenovirus may be discovered, yet histologic assessment of tissues will suggest that viral infection has not compromised the research at hand. In these cases, data derived from adenovirus-infected mice should remain valid.

Diagnosis and control

Diagnosis of mouse adenovirus infection is accomplished by serology, specifically, indirect immunofluorescence assay. There is no treatment for adenovirus infection. Because adenoviruses persist in the host for long periods, infected mice should be culled, or rederived by cesarean rederivation or embryo transfer. Prevention of infection is by purchase of virus-free animals from reputable sources, and protection from infection during transport.

Cytomegalovirus

Agent
Cytomegaloviruses are dsDNA viruses of the family *Herpesviridae,* subfamily Betaherpesvirinae. Multiple natural and experimental strains of mouse cytomegalovirus (MCMV) differing in virulence have been reported (3, 13).

Epidemiology
MCMV is commonly found in wild mice (11), with the striated duct cells of submandibular salivary glands serving as the site of persistent infection (22). Prevalence in laboratory colonies is low, although survey results are affected by the screening method. Transmission is by contact with infectious saliva, tears, and urine, although vertical transmission may also occur (43).

Clinical signs
Natural infections of immunocompetent mice with MCMV are asymptomatic. However, subtle signs associated with myocarditis and/or CNS involvement may not yet have been adequately investigated.

Pathology
Pathogenesis of MCMV infection is influenced by a variety of host factors, with newborn and immunocompromised mice more susceptible than adult immunocompetent mice (10, 28). BALB/c and A/J mice are more susceptible to infection than C57BL/10 and CBA/CaH mouse strains, and BALB/c mice are more susceptible to persistent MCMV hepatitis and hepatic oval cell formation than are C57BL/6 mice (5). However, Dangler and coworkers (9) reported that C57BL/6 mice infected with MCMV more readily develop inflammatory lesions affecting the ascending aorta and pulmonary artery than do BALB/c mice, while Olver and Price (31) reported some kinetic and functional differences in liver-infiltrating leukocytes in infected BALB/c versus C57BL/6 mice. Clearly, there are organ-specific mechanisms for the control of MCMV in addition to overall mouse strain effects (42). To further complicate matters, multiple natural and experimental strains of MCMV differing in virulence have been reported (3, 13). In addition to the salivary glands, latent infections can occur in many organs and tissues, including kidney, prostate, pancreas, testicles, heart, liver, lung, spleen, neurons of the cerebral cortex and hippocampus, and cells of the myeloid lineage, and are directly correlated with the extent of viral replication during acute infection (7, 26, 32, 35, 43). Pathologic changes are limited to varying degrees of autoimmune myocarditis (11), and intranuclear inclusions in enlarged (cytomegalic) salivary gland cells (32), which also occur experimentally (12). In addition, experimental infection results in adrenalitis without compromise of adrenal function (36). Athymic mice develop focal pneumonitis (39). There is considerable literature on the murine immune response to MCMV. Immunity involves both humoral and cell-mediated components. Natural killer (NK) cells (24), α/β and γ/δ (29) T cells, macrophages (16), IFN-γ (29), and IL-12 (34) have critical roles in controlling MCMV replication. In this regard, susceptibility to MCMV is also associated with the presence of an activating NK cell receptor of the C-type lectin superfamily (25). The humoral immune response is dependent upon persistence of virus in salivary gland cells (22).

Interference with research
Natural MCMV infection has not been shown to interfere with research results. In this author's view, however, further evaluation of CNS and myocardial functions should be performed. In contrast, experimental infection may alter a variety of host physiologic functions, including antibody (20) and interferon production, MHC class I (45) and class II (37)

restricted antigen presentation, NK cell accumulation (8), brain neuronal migration (40), lymphocyte proliferation (20), cytotoxic lymphocyte responses, and allogeneic skin graft rejection. In addition, MCMV blocks hepatitis B replication (6) and increases expression of the gp49B inhibitory receptor on NK cells (44); IFN-γ, tumor necrosis factor (TNF), IL-1α, IL-6 (with resulting increase in circulating glucocorticoids), IL-10 (37), and IL-12 production (38); hepatic oval cell formation (5); and apoptosis of hematopoietic progenitor cells leading to myelosuppression (27). MCMV infection is also associated with decreased fecundity; thrombocytopenia, exacerbation of normal cardiac calcification in BALB/c mice, formation of anti-cardiac autoantibodies (30), increased susceptibility to opportunistic infections, and induced reactivation of dormant *Toxoplasma gondii* infection (14). Lastly, MCMV alters cholesterol profiles in mice in a manner compatible with human arterial plaque development (1), and cytomegaloviruses (CMVs) have recently been recognized as having superantigen activity (18).

Natural cases of rat cytomegalovirus (RCMV) have been reported in wild, but not in laboratory rats (4). The biology and pathophysiology of experimental RCMV infection is similar to that of MCMV infection. Experimental RCMV infection has been reported to alter macrophage function, response to sheep erythrocytes, and peripheral lymphocyte subset populations; exacerbate development of collagen-induced arthritis (15); induce vascular wall inflammation (23); accelerate graft rejection (21); enhance collagen synthesis, smooth muscle cell proliferation, and intimal thickening of rat aortic allografts (19); and induce interstitial lung disease in allogeneic bone marrow transplant recipient rats independent of acute graft-versus-host response (41).

Mice and rats are commonly used as models of human CMV infection (2), and CMV particles and promoters have been used in gene vector research (17). Natural infection of these and other laboratory mice and rats could confound research through alteration of cardiovascular, endocrine, enterohepatic, and respiratory function and/or cytoarchitecture.

Diagnosis
Diagnosis of CMV is by serology, and more recently, by PCR (33). There is no treatment for CMV infection. Because CMVs are not readily transmitted between cages, use of cage filters and rigid adherence to sterile cage-changing methods will help contain the pathogen to a specific locale within the facility (28). Depopulation of seropositive animals can be used as a means of eliminating the infection from the colony.

Ectromelia virus

Agent
Ectromelia virus is a dsDNA virus in the family *Poxviridae*, and is the causative agent of mousepox. For background information, the reader is referred to Fenner's very interesting review of the biology and pathogenesis of ectromelia virus (6).

Epidemiology
Mice are the natural hosts. Rats may be transiently infected only experimentally (13). Reports of natural infection in laboratory mice have become rare in the United States but continue to be common in Europe. However, clinical mousepox was recently reported in mice from two facilities in the United States (5, 10). The mice had been injected with contaminated, imported, pooled, and commercially marketed mouse serum. Serologic surveys conducted in the United States occasionally reveal seropositive mice, further confirming that the agent is present, and serving as a reminder that the disease poses a continual threat to research colonies (10). Global movement of animals and/or tissues presents opportunities for introduction of the virus into clean animal facilities. Once present, transmission is primarily by direct contact and fomites, with skin abrasions serving as portals of entry.

Clinical signs
Resistance to mousepox varies among mouse strains and depends on multiple genes (2). The C57BL/6 and C57BL/10 strains are highly resistant and generally do not show signs of infection (13). In contrast, C3H, BALB/c, and DBA/2 are among the strains most commonly showing signs of disease. In these mice, clinical signs are evident in nearly all mice within the colony and consist of foot swelling, pocks, lethargy, depression, and sudden death (13).

Pathology
Following entry through broken skin, the virus replicates locally in skin and lymph nodes prior to mild, primary viremia and spread to the liver and spleen. Massive replication in macrophages of these organs results in a greater secondary viremia. Virus then localizes in many tissues, but most prominently in the skin, conjunctiva, and lymph nodes (6). Pathologic changes include massive splenic, lymph node, thymic, and hepatic necrosis; small intestinal mucosal erosions; and cytoplasmic inclusions in the skin and liver. Distal portions of the tail and limbs may necrose and slough, giving rise to the name ectromelia (13). While virus persists for several months in the spleens of infected mice, virus is shed in the feces for only about 3 weeks (13). Immune clearance of the virus is absolutely dependent on the effector functions of $CD8^+$ T cells, while NK cells (4), $CD4^+$ T cells, and macrophages are necessary for the generation of an optimal response (7, 15, 19). Ectromelia virus-specific cytotoxic T cells home to sites of viral replication (9) and effect protection largely due to granzymes and perforin, key constituents of cytolytic vesicles (12). In addition, nitric oxide, produced by liver, lung, and spleen cells, is important in innate resistance (8).

Interference with research
Multiple strains of ectromelia virus exist; the Moscow strain is the most virulent. Virulence seems to depend on the presence of a poxvirus protein with a CHC_4 ("RING") zinc finger motif (16). Recently, several other ectromelia virus-encoded proteins have been found to potentially influence virulence through binding of specific host cytolytic inducer and effector molecules (3, 17). For example, ectromelia expresses a soluble IFN-γ receptor homolog capable of inhibiting the antiviral activities of IFN-γ (11). In addition, ectromelia virus p13 protein, bearing homology to the mammalian IL-18 binding protein, binds to IL-18, thereby inhibiting IFN-γ and NK cell cytotoxicity (1, 18). Natural infection of laboratory mice with ectromelia virus would usually warrant immediate euthanasia of all affected or potentially affected mice. This would, of course, severely compromise most research efforts involving mice. In particular, studies involving the dermal, enterohepatic, hematopoietic, and lymphoreticular systems would be most adversely affected.

Diagnosis
Diagnosis of ectromelia infection is by observation of clinical signs, or by enzyme-linked immunosorbent assay (ELISA). A PCR assay has been developed recently (14). There is no effective treatment for mouse pox. Because of the seriousness of this disease, control is best achieved by depopulation. Small, valuable colonies may be quarantined, with cessation of breeding. Alternatively, vaccination with vaccinia virus has been shown to facilitate elimination of the pathogen (6). Because intrauterine transmission has been documented (6), cesarean rederivation is not a useful method of virus elimination. However, to the author's knowledge, embryo transfer has not been evaluated. Prevention of entry into the facility is through serologic screening of incoming mice, and by laboratory evaluation of tumor and cell culture lines prior to admission to the facility.

H-1 virus

Agent
H-1 virus (Toolan's H-1 virus) is a single-stranded DNA (ssDNA) virus of the family *Parvoviridae*. The interested reader is referred

to the excellent review of rodent parvovirus infections by Jacoby and colleagues (4). Relatively little is known of the natural biology of H-1 virus, although that situation is changing because H-1 virus is studied as a model for the biology of the parvoviruses. H-1 virus has also been studied as a model for experimentally produced malformations in the CNS and skeletal system of rats (6).

Epidemiology
Seroprevalence of the infection varies, but is generally decreasing as husbandry practices improve (5, 12). The significance of the virus is low in rats, the presumed natural host, since natural infection does not cause obvious clinical disease. Transmission is by exposure to infectious urine, feces, nasal secretions, and milk.

Clinical signs
Natural infection with H-1 virus does not cause disease in adult animals, but like other parvoviruses, may cause intrauterine loss of fetal rat pups (4).

Pathology
Despite the mostly asymptomatic nature of H-1 virus infection, pathologic changes have been observed in the developing livers and cerebellums of experimentally infected rats. These lesions result from the propensity of parvoviruses to infect replicating cells, wherein they are lytic (4). Similar cell pathology has been observed in regenerating livers following partial hepatectomy (9). Lastly, in tumor cell culture systems, cell death is due to induction of apoptosis and necrotic cell death (8).

Interference with research
Potential research-altering effects of H-1 virus include hepatocellular necrosis in rats exposed to pathogens or chemicals causing liver injury (6); reduction of the incidence of *Yersinia*-associated arthritis (3), although in that study other copathogens may also have been present; alteration of lipid metabolism (10); induction of a caspase-3-dependent apoptosis activation pathway in the cerebellum (7); and inhibition of human tumor cell growth in mice (2, 11). Natural infection of laboratory rats could alter studies of fetal development, lipid metabolism, infectious diseases, and tumor formation. Contamination of cell cultures could alter a variety of studies utilizing those cultures.

Diagnosis and control
Diagnosis of infection has historically been by ELISA. More recently, a PCR assay has been developed (1). There is no treatment for H-1 virus infection. Prevention is by screening incoming animals, transplantable tumors, cell lines, and virus stocks prior to entry into the facility. Eradication of the pathogen is best accomplished by total or partial depopulation, although cesarean rederivation may also be used (6).

Kilham rat virus

Agent
Kilham rat virus (KRV) is another ssDNA virus of the family *Parvoviridae*. More is known of the natural biology of KRV than of the H-1 virus.

Epidemiology
The rat is the only known natural host of KRV (7). Natural transmission occurs by direct contact with infectious urine, feces, nasal secretions, and milk; or by contact with contaminated fomites. Experimentally, KRV may pass by transplacental transmission. Parvoviruses are stable in the environment, and so may remain infective outside of the host for long periods. In addition, transplantable tumors and cell cultures may be infected (9).

Clinical signs
Clinical signs of infection are rarely observed, and are highly dependent on age at infection (7). Susceptibility is greatest in utero or within the first few days of life. In utero infections most often result in neonatal loss. Infections

contracted later may result in signs ranging from those associated with neurologic, hepatic, and vascular disease in newborns, to sudden death in rats infected as adults (3, 7).

Pathology
Like other parvoviruses, KRV infects actively replicating cells and results in cell lysis and tissue destruction, which explains the predominance of lesions during fetal development and neonatal life. Infection may persist for varying times, depending on age at infection, and in general, is longer the earlier in life the infection occurs (7). Athymic rats may excrete virus indefinitely (5). Lesions are associated with endothelium; may occur in multiple organs, including the CNS, lymphoreticular, hematopoietic, gastrointestinal, and reproductive systems; and consist of focal necrosis, hemorrhage, and infarction (1, 7). KRV is known to induce autoimmune diabetes in rats, which results from a breakdown in the finely tuned balance of the Th1-like $CD45RC^+CD4^+$ and Th2-like $CDRC^-CD4^+$ T cells, resulting in the selective activation of beta cell-cytotoxic effector T cells (2). Immunity is primarily humoral, although T cells appear to be important for clearing of the virus. Experimentally, the effectiveness of humoral immunity depends on having antibodies present prior to or at the time of infection (7).

Interference with research
Infection of laboratory rats has been reported to result in teratogenesis, suppression of leukemia development due to Moloney virus, alteration of lymphocyte responses (7, 8), induction of cytokine production (1), acute autoimmune type I diabetes due to macrophage and T-cell activity (2), and alteration of lipid metabolism (10). Lastly, KRV may alter leukocyte adhesion to rat aortic endothelium (4) and may reduce the incidence of *Yersinia*-associated arthritis (6), although in those studies other copathogens may also have been present. KRV could profoundly interfere with research involving a variety of body systems, especially if infection occurred during fetal development. Potentially affected systems include the vascular, nervous, lymphoreticular, hematopoietic, gastrointestinal, and reproductive systems.

Diagnosis and control
Diagnosis of KRV infection is generally accomplished by serology-based assays such as ELISA, although more recently, PCR assays have also been used (7). There is no treatment for KRV infection. Eradication of the virus is best accomplished by elimination of the colony followed by restocking with clean animals, or by testing and elimination of seropositive animals. Tumor lines and cell cultures should be tested and certified free of infection prior to admission to the animal facility.

Lactate dehydrogenase-elevating virus

Agent
Lactate dehydrogenase-elevating virus (LDV) is a single-stranded RNA (ssRNA) virus of the family *Arteriviridae*. Neuropathogenic and nonneuropathogenic quasi species, strains, or variants exist (8), and may in fact coexist in many virus stocks (4).

Epidemiology
Mice and mouse cell cultures are the only hosts (19). Rats are not susceptible. The major importance of LDV is as a contaminant of transplantable tumors and of inocula of other infectious agents serially passaged in mice (27, 28). Transmission is by transplantation of contaminated tumors, cells, or serum; but may also occur by direct contact, bite wounds, and transplacental or transmammary passage (31). Given the short period in which viral shedding occurs, these latter routes are of lesser importance.

Clinical signs
Clinical signs are limited to neurologic disorders in aging or otherwise immunosuppressed mice of selected strains. Affected strains possess N-tropic ecotropic murine leukemia virus

proviruses and are homozygous at the Fv-1n locus (23). In general, however, there are no clinical signs of infection.

Pathology
Pathologic changes have not been described in natural infections. Most of what is known of the pathogenesis of LDV derives from experimentally induced infections. Following infection, virus replicates within macrophages. These transport the virus to a variety of organs, including the liver, spleen, lymph nodes, and testes. Lesions are observed in these sites and infection is maintained by the continual generation of LDV-permissive macrophages and other cells (2). Where CNS infection occurs, replication is generally transient and limited to the leptomeninges, although in mouse strains susceptible to paralytic infection, extensive cytocidal infection occurs in the anterior horn neurons (1). LDV causes persistent viremia, which induces antiviral antibodies and, eventually, circulating antigen-IgG antibody complexes (15). These may cause a mild membranous glomerulonephritis (26). In CBA/Ht, but not BALB/c mice, LDV induces autoantibody formation against a wide range of cryptic epitopes (9), in some cases through molecular mimicry (18). Experimental immune suppression of mice, followed by infection with LDV, results in autoimmune, age-dependent poliomyelitis and respiratory failure (29). This is a useful model for study of neurodegenerative diseases, but it is not likely to be relevant to natural LDV infection.

Immune response to LDV infection is primarily cellular (6, 24), with a transient increase in IL-12 production one of the earliest immune indicators (5). However, cellular immune responses are apparently too slow to control the rapid rate of virus replication, and therefore, infection persists (30). In addition, LDV infection induces IgG2a antibody production (21). Antibodies may neutralize neuropathogenic, but not nonneuropathogenic quasi species (3). The ability to establish persistent infections is virus strain dependent and likely associated with the number of N- glycosylation sites on the short ectodomain of the primary envelope glycoprotein, VP-3P, which may be part of the attachment site for the LDV receptor on permissive cells (3).

Interference with research
LDV alters several physiologic functions. These include transient increases in cytokine and cell receptor activities; transient depression of cellular immunity (7); altered humoral immunity (10); increased (or suppressed) tumor growth (both spontaneous and transplanted), prolonged survival of allografts, altered immunity to copathogens, increases in several serum enzymes (26); decreased binding of asparaginase to monocytes (25); suppressed streptozotocin-induced insulinitis (12), altered neutrophil migration (13); B-lymphocyte polyclonal activation leading to hypergammaglobulinemia (9); development of autoantibodies (22); altered superoxide anion production by macrophages (16); inhibited contact sensitivity to 2,4-dinitrofluorobenzene (14); and abrogated increases in intercellular adhesion molecule 1 (ICAM-1) and leukocyte function-associated antigen 1 (LFA-1) expression associated with the development of glomerulonephritis seen in NZB × NZW F_1 mice (17). Clearly, infection of laboratory mice with LDV could seriously alter research results, including studies involving the enterohepatic, hematopoietic, lymphoreticular, nervous, and urinary systems, without any outward evidence of infection. Other studies are likely to be affected, through indirect association with affected organ systems.

Diagnosis and control
The diagnostic hallmark of LDV infection is elevation of serum lactate dehydrogenase (LDH), which occurs because of reduced clearing of one LDH isozyme (26). Other serum enzymes are also elevated, although not to the same extent. Infection of transplantable tumor lines may be diagnosed by PCR (11); however, it is imperative to determine that inhibitory factors do not cause false-negative results (20). There is no treatment for LDV

infection. Rather, viral persistence justifies eradication of infection by elimination of the colony. This pathogen highlights the importance of testing mouse cell lines prior to admission into the animal facility.

Lymphocytic choriomeningitis virus

Agent
Lymphocytic choriomeningitis virus (LCMV) is a noncytopathic ssRNA virus of the family *Arenaviridae*. The primary importance of LCMV is as an occasionally serious zoonosis (2, 9) and as a contaminant of transplantable tumors and cultured cell lines (20).

Epidemiology
Natural infection of mice with LCMV is uncommon (17). Only mice and hamsters are known to transmit the infection, although rats and many other mammals (and chickens) are also susceptible (19). Along with implantation of infected tumors, transmission is by exposure of mucous membranes and broken skin to infectious urine, saliva, and milk, and possibly by ingestion (25). In addition, both transovarian and transuterine transmission occur in mice (19).

Clinical signs
Patterns of infection differ depending on host and pathogen factors, including mouse strain and age, dose and route of inoculation, and virus strain (18, 19). A typical clinical pattern is the persistent tolerant infection, which follows in utero or neonatal infection. Clinical signs include initial growth retardation and eventual immune complex glomerulonephritis (ICG) accompanied by emaciation, ruffled fur, hunched posture, ascites, and occasional death (19).

Pathology
Persistent tolerant infection occurs due to selective clonal exhaustion of antigen-specific $CD8^+$ T cells (22). Infection is characterized by persistent infection of T-helper lymphocytes, viremia, and lifelong viral shedding. Pathologic features of this pattern, including ICG, stem in part from unabated B-cell activity, including production of pathologic amounts of anti-LCMV antibodies, lymphoid hyperplasia, and perivascular lymphocyte accumulation (19). In contrast, T-cell activity is diminished. Eventually immune tolerance breaks down resulting in chronic illness with widespread lymphocytic infiltration and vasculitis (24). A second clinical pattern is that of the nontolerant infection. This pattern occurs with acute infection of postneonatal mice. Viremia occurs without viral shedding. It was originally believed that infected mice either die or eliminate the virus, frequently without showing signs of disease (19). More recently, it has been demonstrated that virus or viral antigen may persist in "immune" adult mice (6). Pathologic features of this pattern may include necrotizing hepatitis (12) and generalized lymphoid depletion (24). Lymphocytic choriomeningitis is generally only seen following experimental intracerebral inoculation and is not a feature of natural infection (24).

Eventual clearance of the infection requires T-cells (14), particularly those secreting the Th1-associated cytokines (1, 29) or expressing the class I receptor Ly49G2 (23). Additional immune effector components include NK cells (27), IL-12 (21), and cells utilizing perforin-dependent mechanisms (15). Intestinal intraepithelial lymphocytes are activated (28), and virus-specific antibody is also induced (26).

Interference with research
Several investigators have reported effects of LCMV on research; however, nearly all of this information comes from experimental infections (19). LCMV has been shown to alter synaptic plasticity and cognitive functions (8); abolish experimental hepatitis B infections (13); increase serum levels and/or expression of ICAM-1 and other endothelial adhesion molecules (5); cause hepatitis (12), bone marrow aplasia (3), and hemolytic anemia (16); alter behavior (11); alter immune reactivities (4, 10); alter cytokine gene expression (7); in-

hibit tumor induction by polyomavirus; delay rejection of skin and tumor allografts; increase susceptibility to other pathogens, bacterial endotoxin, and radiation; and alter the time course of naturally occurring diabetes (19). Natural infection of laboratory mice would jeopardize human health and interfere with a variety of research endeavors, especially those involving the lymphoreticular, vascular, enterohepatic, hematopoietic, nervous, and urinary systems.

Diagnosis and control
LCMV infection can be diagnosed serologically. There is no treatment for LCMV infection. Because of the persistent and zoonotic nature of the infection, eradication of the pathogen requires depopulation of the affected colony. Transplantable tissues should be tested prior to entering the animal colony.

Minute virus of mice

Agents
Minute virus of mice (MVM) is an ssDNA virus of the family *Parvoviridae* and therefore shares many biological features with other murine parvoviruses such as mouse parvovirus-1,
H-1 virus, and KRV.

Epidemiology
Like other parvoviruses, MVM is extremely contagious. Prevalence has historically been high but appears to be declining with improvements in husbandry practices (14). Transmission is primarily by exposure to infectious feces and urine, but MVM may also be transmitted on fomites and by exposure to nasal secretions. In addition, MVM may be found as a contaminant of transplantable tumors, virus stocks, and cell culture ingredients (9). Multiple strains have been described. The best studied are MVM(p), the prototype strain, and MVM(I), an immunosuppressive strain (1, 8). MVM(I) grows lytically in mouse T lymphocytes whereas MVM(p) infects fibroblasts.

Recently, segments of the MVM(I) genome required for lytic viral growth were identified (4).

Clinical signs
MVM causes an acute, self-limiting infection, with infant mice more susceptible to infection than adult mice (6). Also, mouse strains differ in susceptibility to infection with MVM (7). Regardless, there are usually no clinical signs associated with MVM infection.

Pathology
Natural infection of mice with MVM causes no pathologic changes. Lesions can be induced experimentally if infection occurs during fetal development or shortly after birth. In these cases, damage occurs in multiple organs, including the brain, liver, intestine, kidney (3, 10). It remains to be determined whether similar lesions develop during natural infection. Immunity is humoral, and is not cross-protective for other parvoviral infections (5).

Interference with research
MVM(I) infection results in T-lymphocyte lysis, altered B- and T-lymphocyte activities, and myelosuppression; while MVM(p) suppresses growth of ascites tumors (8, 12, 13). Clearly, natural infection of laboratory mice with MVM will interfere with research involving the hematopoietic and lymphoreticular systems.

Diagnosis
Diagnosis of MVM infection is best accomplished using ELISA and PCR assay. Results must be considered within the context of mouse strain and age, as these variables influence length of time to seroconversion, as well as results of PCR assay (2). There is no treatment for MVM infection. MVM may be eradicated from infected colonies by cesarean rederivation or embryo transfer. However, elimination of the colony and restocking with uninfected animals may be more practical. Cell cultures and/or ingredients used in cell

culture should be tested for the presence of MVM prior to use in the animal facility (11).

Mouse hepatitis virus

Agent
Mouse hepatitis virus (MHV) is likely the most important pathogen of laboratory mice. Rats may also become infected but only as sucklings and only under experimental conditions (53). MHV is an ssRNA virus of the family *Coronaviridae*.

Epidemiology
MHV is extremely contagious and is transmitted by aerosol, direct contact, and fomites, and experimentally, by transplantable tumors and transplacental passage (22, 39). Infection remains common in many animal facilities (68).

Clinical signs
Most infections follow one of three clinical patterns (38). First, enzootic (subclinical) infection, commonly seen in breeding colonies, occurs when infection is endemic in the colony and is maintained only by the continual arrival of susceptible animals (newborns). No carrier state exists, although in one study viral RNA was detected in the liver up to 60 days after infection (26). Also, some unusual strains of transgenic mice may remain persistently infected (47). Adults are asymptomatic and their young become asymptomatically infected by the time passively transferred maternal immunity wanes at weaning. Second, epizootic (clinical) infection occurs less commonly, when the pathogen is introduced to a naive colony. Adult infections are usually asymptomatic. Clinical signs depend on virus and mouse strains and are most evident in infant mice, but typically include diarrhea, poor growth, and death. As the infection becomes established in the colony, the epizootic pattern is replaced by the enzootic pattern. Third, immunodeficient mice, such as athymic (*nu/nu*) mice, develop a wasting syndrome characterized by severe generalized disease and eventual death (57).

Pathology
Susceptibility, tissue tropism, clinical signs, and pathologic lesions are dependent on several host (1, 4, 41, 51, 61, 69), environmental (6), and pathogen (46) factors. To date, nearly 30 strains or isolates of MHV have been described, with others still being added (66). Most strains have been classified as either respiratory or enterotropic; however, an outbreak of a highly hepatotropic strain of MHV was reported from a breeding colony of nude mice in Taiwan (34). More recently, a variant "MHV OBLV" with tropism for the olfactory bulb was also described (49). Immune pressure may result in viral mutations, leading to the development of additional strains (45). The presence or absence of the MHV viral receptor, a glycoprotein in the carcinoembryonic antigen family of the Ig superfamily, may determine tissue tropism (17). Respiratory (polytropic) strains establish in the nasal mucosa, descend to the lungs, and disseminate hematogenously throughout the body (2) or ascend along neurons to the CNS (43). Intestinal involvement is usually absent. Polytropic strains include MHV-1, MHV-2, MHV-3, A59, S, JHM, and others. Enterotropic strains may also become established in the nasal mucosa or in the intestinal tract but disseminate only locally to the liver, abdominal lymph nodes, and in some cases, to the CNS (19). Pulmonary involvement is uncommon. Enterotropic strains include LIVIM, MHV-D, MHV-Y, and others (19). While polytropic strains have historically been considered more common, this is no longer the case (19). Lesions are present for only 7 to 10 days following infection, are dependent on strain of virus, and are characterized by multifocal necrosis and multinucleate syncytial giant cell formation. The latter may be associated with fragmentation and rearrangement of the Golgi apparatus (32). Lesions seen with polytropic strains may be observed in the olfactory mucosa, brain, lungs,

and liver. Concerning the latter, hepatic necrosis seems to be due to induction of procoagulant production by hepatic endothelial and Kupffer cells (11). In the CNS, nitric oxide appears to promote apoptosis (8). Lesions are generally, although not always, confined to the intestinal tract following infection with enterotropic strains. Lesions caused by either strain tend to be more severe and widespread in immunocompromised mice. Immunity to MHV is primarily but not entirely cell mediated; is partially protective between closely related virus strains; and is known to involve $CD4^+$ and $CD8^+$ T lymphocytes (29, 30, 64), macrophages (63), NK cells (20, 21, 48), IFN-γ-inducible protein 10 (12), and interferon-γ (59). T cells appear to have a role in accelerating CNS inflammation in MHV-induced demyelinating encephalomyelitis (18, 44). The role of antibody in viral clearance varies by viral strain and organ system affected. For example, antibody is required for clearance of MHV strain A59 from the CNS but not from the liver (36).

Interference with research
Numerous reports document effects of natural or experimental infection with MHV on host physiology and research. In immunocompetent mice, reported effects include depletion of LDV-permissive and other macrophages (3, 13); microcytic anemia and changes in ferrokinetics; alterations in the function and surface antigens of lymphocytes and other immune cells (9,10, 15, 25, 28, 31, 54); number of hepatic sinusoidal endothelial cell fenestrae (50), incidence of diabetes mellitus in nonobese diabetic mice (65), apoptosis-induced thymic atrophy (16, 33), hepatic uptake of injected iron (58), susceptibility, resistance, or pathogenicity of copathogens (14, 56, 60), hepatic enzyme activity; and induction of procoagulant by hepatic cells (11), and serum α-fetoprotein and antiretinal autoantibodies (23). In immunocompromised mice, reported effects include necrotic changes in several organs, including liver, lung, spleen, intestine, brain, lymph nodes, and bone marrow; differentiation of cells bearing T-lymphocyte markers; altered serum enzyme activities, bilirubin concentration, and antibody responses to sheep erythrocytes; enhanced phagocytic activity of macrophages; rejection of xenograft tumors; impaired liver regeneration; and hepatosplenic myelopoiesis (24, 38). Clearly, natural infection of laboratory mice with MHV may affect a plethora of scientific studies and seriously compromise the value of such animals as research subjects. Organ systems likely to be involved include the enterohepatic, hematopoietic, lymphoreticular, nervous, and respiratory systems.

Diagnosis and control
Diagnosis of MHV is routinely accomplished by ELISA and/or histopathology. To these has been added PCR assay of fecal pellets, tissues, and biological materials (5, 67). Like pathologic lesions, viral excretion is transient, having ceased by 27 days postinfection in one report (7). For this reason, some have advocated using PCR assay of colon samples from nude mice exposed to potentially contaminated bedding (62). Infected mouse colonies may be rederived by embryo transfer (37, 52) or cesarean rederivation, or by temporary cessation of breeding, with subsequent generation and testing of litters (38). Concerning the latter, it should not be assumed that all transgenic mice follow the same pattern of acute infection followed by virus clearing (47). Static filter-top caging, combined with automatic watering systems slow the spread of MHV within a contaminated animal room (35). Transplantable tumors may be rendered free of MHV by implantation in nude rats (55). Embryonic stem cells are susceptible to infection with MHV (27), although prevalence appears to be low (40). Given the extremely contagious nature and pathologic potential of MHV, serologic screening of new animals prior to and a few weeks after arrival at the animal facility is essential for exclusion of MHV. Animals should be transported in filter-

topped plastic shipping containers, because these have been shown to preclude infection of mice by MHV (42).

Mouse mammary tumor virus

Agent
Mouse mammary tumor virus (MMTV) is an ssRNA type B retrovirus of the family *Retroviridae*. At least four major variants of the virus have been identified in laboratory mice, including MMTV-S ("standard"), MMTV-L ("low oncogenic"), MMTV-P ("pregnancy"), and MMTV-O ("overlooked") (11). More recently, additional variants, including MMTV-SW and MMTV-C4 have been described (17).

Epidemiology
Nearly all mice are infected with some variant of MMTV (2). Like many other retroviruses, MMTV may be an endogenous component of the host genome, and therefore, to some extent defines the mouse as a species. However, mechanisms of transmission differ among the major variants. MMTV-O is endogenous to the genome of most mice, MMTV-S is transmitted by milk, MMTV-L is transmitted by germ cells, and MMTV-P is transmitted through both milk and germ cells (16). T cells are needed for transmission of milk-borne MMTV from the gut to the mammary gland (21). These routes of transmission indicate that horizontal spread of infection within the facility is not of concern. The variants also differ in oncogenicity, with MMTV-S and MMTV-P being highly oncogenic, and MMTV-L and MMTV-O less so (16). Depending on the mouse strain and virus variant, MMTV may be expressed in mammary and many other tissues (20), including lymphoid tissues (9, 15), or may exist as a provirus in the DNA of the host (19).

Clinical signs
Clinical signs of infection are generally limited to mammary tumors, which may arise several months after infection. Distant metastases can also occur with subsequent organ compromise.

Pathology
B cells and immature dendritic cells are the primary targets of infection for MMTV (18). Productive retroviral infection of B cells requires vigorous T-cell stimulation through the virally encoded superantigen (sag). Most viral-induced tumors are adenocarcinomas (16). While the mechanism of tumor induction is unknown, it is thought that MMTV induces hyperplastic nodules, which eventually become neoplastic. MMTV may integrate into and disrupt the Tpl-2/cot proto-oncogene (6). Various hormones (4), carcinogens (16), diet (7), and transforming growth factor α (TGF-α) (14) may accelerate the development of tumors. Infected mice develop both cellular and humoral immune responses to MMTV (11).

Interference with research
Several reports indicate that not only MMTV, but also the MMTV sag, affect host physiology. MMTV has been shown to affect T-cell (10, 24) and B-cell (5) responses, activate NK cells through sag-dependent and -independent pathways (8), lower the amount of prolactin required to elicit α-lactalbumin production from mammary epithelial cells (3), and even affect body odor (23). The sag is expressed on lymphocytes (22); binds MHC class II molecules; stimulates $CD4^+$ T cells, potentially to anergy, by interaction with the V β domain of the T-cell receptor (TCR) (1); activates B cells, leading to cell division and differentiation (5); is involved in the transmission of milk-borne MMTV from virus-infected milk in the gut to the target mammary gland tissue (22); may initiate or aggravate graft-versus-host disease (12); has the ability to destroy a large portion of $CD4^+$ T cells (24), and may act as an oncogene in certain mouse mammary epithelial cells (13). MMTV is used as a model for viral carcinogenesis. Natural infection of

laboratory mice with MMTV will interfere with studies involving the endocrine, hematopoietic, and lymphoreticular systems, as well as with carcinogenesis studies, and studies in which life span is measured.

Diagnosis and control
MMTV can be diagnosed using a variety of molecular, immunologic, and phenotypic methods, and is best performed by a specialized diagnostic laboratory. Elimination of the pathogen is essentially impossible for most variants of MMTV. MMTV-S-infected mice can be rederived by fostering on uninfected mice. In contrast, eradication is not a viable option for the endogenous or germ-line transmitted MMTV variants.

Mouse parvovirus-1

Agent
Mouse parvovirus-1 (MPV-1), formerly known as "orphan" parvovirus, is an ssDNA virus of the family *Parvoviridae*. Three isolates (MPV-1a, MPV-1b, and MPV-1c) of one serotype have been reported (4).

Epidemiology
MPV-1 is a recently recognized and very important pathogen of laboratory mice. Prevalence of infection is declining as awareness of the pathogen grows and diagnostic tests improve (11). Like other parvoviruses, MPV-1 requires actively dividing or differentiating cells for survival. Virus is excreted by urinary, fecal, and perhaps respiratory routes (10). Transmission is therefore most likely and primarily direct, although extensive transmission studies have yet to be conducted (10). Transmission may also occur following experimental exposure to selected, infected T-cell lines (6).

Clinical signs
Natural infections of mice are generally asymptomatic and apathogenic, even for neonatal and immunocompromised mice (10).

Pathology
In immunocompetent mice, viral replication occurs in the pancreas, small intestine, lymphoid organs, and liver of mice of virtually any age, and may persist for several weeks (9, 10). Viral replication is more widespread in immunodeficient mice (10). MPV-1 shares some antigenic cross-reactivity with minute virus of mice, another rodent parvovirus, due to two highly conserved nonstructural proteins (1). However, humoral immunity to either MPV-1 or MVM is not cross-protective (3).

Interference with research
MPV-1 has been shown to affect processes linked to cell proliferation. Reported effects include direct modulation and dysfunction of T lymphocytes and altered patterns of rejection of tumor and skin allografts (7). It is anticipated that additional effects will be reported as more studies are conducted on this important virus. Natural infection with MPV-1 would compromise studies involving the enterohepatic and lymphoreticular systems.

Diagnosis and control
MPV-1 can be diagnosed by immunohistochemistry, ELISA, indirect immunofluorescence assay (IFA), and more recently, by PCR, in situ hybridization, and mouse antibody production (MAP) testing (5, 8, 9). However, it should be noted that age at infection and/or mouse strain may profoundly affect serologic, as well as PCR diagnostic efficiency (2). There is no treatment for MPV-1 infection. MPV-1 persists in vivo because of the continual availability of actively dividing or differentiating cells. Therefore, elimination from the colony is best accomplished by depopulation or rederivation. All mice and rats should be certified free of all parvoviruses prior to entry into the animal facility.

Mouse rotavirus

Agent
Mouse rotavirus, formerly known as epizootic diarrhea of infant mice (EDIM), is a dsRNA

virus of the family *Reoviridae*. Mouse rotavirus is a member of the group A rotaviruses, which are known to infect a variety of vertebrate hosts, including humans. Multiple strains of mouse rotavirus have been identified (4, 12).

Epidemiology
Mouse rotavirus is highly contagious. Infection is acquired through exposure to contaminated airborne dust and bedding, and through contact with infected mice. There is no evidence of transplacental transmission. Mice are most susceptible from birth to about 2 weeks of age, possibly because of transient features of intestinal enterocytes (23). Virus is shed in the feces for up to about 10 days postinfection. It remains uncertain whether a carrier state, with persistent, low-level fecal virus shedding, may exist.

Clinical signs
Disease caused by mouse rotavirus is commonly diagnosed in young laboratory mice with diarrhea. Clinical signs generally are seen only in mice infected within the first 2 weeks of life, and include watery, mustard-colored stool, lethargy, and distended abdomen.

Pathology
Infection and pathologic changes progress from proximal to distal intestine. Apical villous enterocytes are primarily affected, while crypt cells are largely spared (15). Affected enterocytes may be vacuolated and contain pyknotic nuclei. Malabsorption and osmotic diarrhea with overgrowth of *Escherichia coli* may contribute to the clinicopathologic pattern (26). Athymic (*nu/nu*) mice are no more susceptible to rotavirus disease than are normal mice (7). In contrast, severe combined immunodeficient (*scid/scid*) mice are more severely affected (27). Rotavirus may bind to mouse intestinal cells by a subset of sialylated glycoconjugates, that is, glycoproteins containing O-linked sialic acid moieties (33), consistent with the observation that intestinal mucins inhibit rotavirus infection and may represent a barrier to infection (5). Viral attachment or entry is sufficient to induce diarrhea (29). In vitro studies suggest that the rotavirus nonstructural protein NSP4 mobilizes Ca^{2+} in human intestinal cells, and these ionic changes are at least partially responsible for, but are not critical to, diarrhea induction (1, 11, 22). Recent findings also suggest a potential role for the enteric nervous system in induction of diarrhea (16).

Immunity to rotavirus infection in mice is contributed by the activities of several effector components, including nonantibody inhibitors (2), antibodies (3, 20, 32), antigen-presenting cells (10), and T lymphocytes (9, 18, 19). Protection may be related to the intestinal replication properties of the virus rather than to specific immunogenic properties of specific viral proteins (17).

Interference with research
Rotavirus has been shown to alter host physiology in many ways and may therefore confound research. Infected mice are more susceptible to pathologic effects of copathogens (24) and have alterations in intestinal physiology (6, 13), including altered oxidative/antioxidative profiles indicative of oxidative stress (30), and reduced amino acid uptake in the small intestine (14). In addition, infection may alter results of dietary and nutritional studies (21, 25, 28). The rotavirus-infected mouse serves as a model of human rotavirus diarrhea, which is responsible for the deaths of approximately 800,000 children per year (8). Natural infection of laboratory mice with rotavirus would confound such research efforts, and may interfere with other studies involving the enterohepatic system, and possibly the nervous system.

Diagnosis and control
Mouse rotavirus can be diagnosed by ELISA and other serologic tests, and by PCR. Recently, molecular and immunologic methods have been developed for detecting rotavirus in formalin-fixed tissues (31). There is no treatment for rotavirus infection. Cessation of breeding should allow the infection to clear

from isolated breeding mice, with subsequent resumption of breeding and testing of offspring. However, cesarean rederivation and embryo transfer may be more practical in some instances. The highly contagious nature of the virus warrants the strictest attention to husbandry practices, to minimize potential for transmission, if isolation and cessation of breeding are used to eradicate the pathogen from the colony. It is essential that mice be tested and demonstrated free of rotavirus prior to admission into the animal facility.

Mouse thymic virus

Agent
Mouse thymic virus (MTV) is a dsDNA virus in the family *Herpesviridae*. Relatively little is known of MTV due to the inability to culture the virus in vitro.

Epidemiology
Transmission appears to be by contact (6), and possibly transmammary passage (4).

Clinical signs
Natural infections are subclinical.

Pathology
Pathologic changes are limited to transient lymphoid necrosis of the thymus, lymph nodes, and spleen of neonatal mice, followed by a diffuse granulomatous response with giant cells, which eventually resolves (7). The thymus is most severely affected, especially lymphocytes, epithelial reticular cells, macrophages, and lymphoepithelial cell complexes (thymic nurse cells). $CD4^+8^+$ and $CD4^+8^-$ lymphocytes have been found to be selectively lysed by MTV (1). Both T-helper and T-cytotoxic lymphocytes may be involved (2). The virus also infects and persists in salivary glands.

Interference with research
MTV infection has been shown to reduce T-cell responsiveness to concanavalin A (ConA) and phytohemagglutinin (PHA) and to reduce graft-versus-host response (3). Natural infection of laboratory mice would confound research involving the hematopoietic and lymphoreticular systems. Salivary involvement might also affect studies involving the enterohepatic system, since food consumption, mastication, and digestion could be affected.

Diagnosis and control
MTV is best diagnosed by ELISA. Inoculation of neonatal mice with salivary gland homogenates from suspect neonatal mice, or with other suspect tissues, followed by examination of the thymuses, lymph nodes, and spleens of recipients, has also proven efficacious (5). There is no treatment for MRV infection. Given the lack of viral persistence, isolation of infected mice with temporary cessation of breeding followed by repopulation by seronegative offspring, should allow successful eradication of MTV from a colony.

Pneumonia virus of mice

Agent
Pneumonia virus of mice (PVM) is an ssRNA virus of the family *Paramyxoviridae*, genus *Pneumovirus*. Seroprevalence remains high in some rodent colonies (7, 13). Multiple strains exist, and differ in pathogenicity based on F- and G-glycoprotein sequences as well as other features (5, 9).

Epidemiology
Transmission is by aerosol and contact exposure to the respiratory tract.

Clinical signs
Viral strains differ in their ability to cause clinical signs. Experimentally, strain J3666 is highly pathogenic, and causes respiratory distress and death in mice. In contrast, the tissue-passaged strain 15 rarely causes more than transiently ruffled fur (5). Active natural infections are short lived and generally without clinical signs in euthymic mice and rats, and there is no carrier state (1, 8). In contrast, athymic mice (*nu/nu*) develop chronic pneumonia and wasting, and die (10).

Pathology
Pathologic lesions have not been reported in naturally infected mice or rats. Experimental intranasal infections of mice have resulted in mild rhinitis and interstitial pneumonia (2). Susceptibility of mice and rats may be increased by local and systemic stressors. Immune responsiveness is host strain dependent (12). Experimentally infected athymic mice develop persistent interstitial pneumonia (3). Eosinophils are rapidly recruited to the lungs of BALB/c mice infected with PVM, resulting in granulocytic bronchiolitis. Recruitment appears to be in response to release of the chemokine macrophage inflammatory protein-1-α (MIP-1-α) (4). Once in the lung, eosinophils release ribonucleases that inactivate the virus (11). In this and many other ways, mouse infection with PVM is similar to respiratory syncytial virus (RSV) of humans, another pneumovirus.

Interference with research
While natural PVM infections appear to be of little consequence in immunocompetent rodents, PVM infection could alter pulmonary cytoarchitecture and interfere with immunologic studies (6). Like RSV, PVM is known to alter gene expression, resulting in production of proinflammatory cytokines, adhesion molecules, elements that are related to the apoptosis response, and others (5). Natural infection of athymic mice results in death and would therefore confound studies using such animals.

Diagnosis and control
Diagnosis of PVM is based on serologic evidence of infection in previously seronegative colonies. There is no treatment for PVM infection. Control measures include cessation of breeding, combined with active spreading of the pathogen throughout an infected colony, to hasten extinction of the infection. Alternatively, cesarean rederivation and embryo transfer to clean recipient females are useful methods of eradicating the pathogen. Prevention is based on purchase of virus-free animals from reputable vendors.

Rat rotavirus-like agent

Agent
Rat rotavirus-like agent (RVLA), like mouse rotavirus, is a dsRNA virus in the family *Reoviridae*. Unlike mouse rotavirus, however, RVLA has been tentatively classified as a group B rotavirus (5). The natural hosts of RVLA include rats and humans. It has yet to be grown in culture.

Epidemiology
Transmission is likely by direct contact with contaminated feces, fomites, human contact, and possibly airborne spread of contaminated dust and bedding (1).

Clinical signs
Clinical signs are seen in rats 1 to 11 days of age and consist of poor growth, diarrhea, and perianal dermatitis (4). These signs led to the designation "infectious diarrhea of infant rats" (IDIR).

Pathology
Pathologic changes noted in rats infected with RVLA include watery, discolored proximal small intestinal contents; villous atrophy, and epithelial necrosis; increased crypt depth; and syncytial cell formation (3, 4). RVLA infection results in a net secretory state for water and impaired sodium absorption (2, 3). Relatively little is known about immune mechanisms in RVLA infection, but it is likely that similarities exist with immunity to mouse rotavirus infection. In addition to acquired immunity, intestinal mucins may inhibit rotavirus replication, and may be dependent on specific mucin–viral interactions (6).

Interference with research
Natural infection of rats with RVLA would likely confound studies involving the enterohepatic system.

Diagnosis and control
Diagnosis of RVLA infection is somewhat complicated by the relative paucity of diagnostic assays for RVLA. However, ELISA is

likely most reliable. It is assumed that PCR assays will soon be available as well. Guidelines for control of RVLA are currently lacking. However, since humans may serve as sources of infection for laboratory rats, animal caretakers should be instructed in personal hygiene and the use of personal protective clothing as a means of minimizing transmission to colony rats.

Reovirus-3

Agent
Mammalian reoviruses are grouped into serotypes 1, 2, and 3. Reovirus-3 is the most pathogenic reovirus of laboratory rodents (3). Reovirus-3 is a dsRNA virus in the family *Reoviridae*. The primary importance of reovirus-3 is as a contaminant of transplantable tumors and cell lines (19).

Epidemiology
Transmission is thought to be primarily by direct contact. However, Barthold and coworkers (3) demonstrated that transmission of virus to cagemates or mothers of infected infants did not occur, indicating low contagiousness.

Clinical signs
The preponderance of literature on the effects of reovirus-3 concerns experimental infections. Effects of natural infections as well as relevant findings from experimental infections are reviewed here. Natural infection with reovirus-3 is nearly always asymptomatic. Cook reported the following clinical signs in first litters of mice infected with reovirus-3: stunting, diarrhea, oily coats, abdominal alopecia, and jaundice (5).

Pathology
Pathologic changes associated with reovirus-3 infection consist of enlarged, black gall bladders; hepatic necrosis with syncytial giant cell formation; and yellow kidneys (5, 11, 17). Experimentally inoculated mice have a wider scope of organ involvement (3, 21). Immunity to reovirus infection is primarily humoral (2, 6, 28) but also involves T lymphocytes (6, 8, 14, 30). Protective antibodies may act at least partially by inhibiting internalization and intracellular proteolytic uncoating of the virion (29). Athymic (*nu/nu*) mice are no more susceptible to disease than are immunocompetent mice (23).

Interference with research
Reported effects of natural infection with reovirus-3 are limited to lysis of transplantable ascites tumors (4, 18). Experimentally, reovirus-3 has also been shown to reduce pulmonary clearance of *Staphylococcus aureus* (12); suppress pulmonary carcinogenesis (27); inhibit cellular DNA synthesis and induce apoptosis (20); cause pulmonary neutrophil influx, increased levels of chemokine mRNA expression (9), and acute myocarditis (24); induce murine NK cell cytotoxicity (1), TNF-α (10), and IL-1α (7); synergize with chemotherapeutic agents to cause the rejection of various murine tumors (26); and enhance tumor-specific immunity (13, 22). Mice, and to a lesser extent rats, infected with reoviruses are commonly used as models of human acute and chronic hepatitis, chronic biliary obstruction, extrahepatic biliary atresia, pancreatitis, lymphoma (25), otitis (15), and pneumonia (16). Reovirus-3 illustrates the need to include gross and histopathologic evaluations in research studies. The paucity of literature on physiologic effects of natural reovirus-3 infection suggests that reovirus-3 should not compromise research. However, the reports describing physiologic changes associated with experimental infection suggests otherwise. If the physiologic effects observed following experimental infection also occur naturally, infection of laboratory rodents could compromise studies involving the cardiovascular, dermal, enterohepatic, hematopoietic, lymphoreticular, and urinary systems. It remains to be determined to what extent natural infection compromises studies involving these organ systems.

Diagnosis and control
ELISA-based tests are considered the standard for diagnosis of reovirus-3 infection. It is cer-

tain that PCR methodology will also assume a prominent role in diagnosis, particularly in the evaluation of transplantable tumors and cell lines. There is no treatment for reovirus-3 infection. Affected colonies should be eliminated, or rederived by cesarean rederivation or embryo transfer. Prevention is based on purchase of virus-free animals from reputable vendors.

Sendai virus

Agent
Sendai virus (SV) is one of the most important pathogens infecting laboratory mice and rats. Hamsters may also be infected, although asymptomatically. SV is an ssRNA virus of the family *Paramyxoviridae,* genus *Paramyxovirus* and species *parainfluenza 1.* Multiple strains have been described (33).

Epidemiology
SV is extremely contagious, and transmission is by contact and aerosol infection of the respiratory tract (10, 29). There are considerable host strain differences in susceptibility to SV among both rats and mice. Among rat strains, LEW and Brown Norway (BN) rats are more susceptible than F344 rats (22, 37). Among mouse strains, 129/J and DBA strains are among the most susceptible, and the SJL/J and C57BL/6J among the most resistant (13, 26, 27, 29).

Clinical signs
While natural infection of rats with SV is generally asymptomatic, with only minor effects on reproduction and growth of pups (24), pulmonary cytoarchitectural changes do occur (38). Natural infections of mice present as enzootic or epizootic infections. Enzootic infections are those endemic to a colony, where the constant supply of susceptible animals maintains the infection. Mice are infected shortly after weaning as maternal antibody levels wane. Affected animals show few clinical signs. Since there is no carrier state, cessation of breeding eventually results in elimination of the infection, although antibody titers remain in previously infected animals. Epizootic infections occur on first introduction of the virus to a colony. Clinical signs may include teeth chattering, dyspnea, prolonged gestation, poor growth, and death of young mice (29). Where breeding is occurring, the enzootic pattern eventually takes over.

Pathology
Because of virus strain differences, as well as host strain differences in susceptibility to SV, pathologic lesions vary in severity. SV produces a number of virulence factors. Among the most important is the highly conserved cysteine-rich zinc-binding V protein (12). In addition, SV contains HN protein with hemagglutinating and neuraminidase activities; F glycoprotein with cell fusion, cell entry, and hemolytic activities; nonstructural proteins with self-protective properties; and others (9, 42). The hallmark of SV infection is transient hypertrophy, necrosis, and repair of airway epithelium as the virus descends the respiratory tract. Repair of airway epithelium results in epithelial hyperplasia, squamous metaplasia, and syncytial cell formation. Proximally, SV causes laryngotracheitis with regionally dependent influx of immune cells (16). On reaching the lungs, focal interstitial pneumonia occurs with inflammatory and hyperplastic changes most severe around terminal bronchioles, in contrast to infection with *Mycoplasma pulmonis,* which affects more proximal airways. The lungs appear focally reddened, in part due to ICAM-1-mediated recruitment of inflammatory cells (40). Viral replication occurs in the respiratory tract for only about 1 week postinfection, so lesions resolve quickly and eventually consist only of loose peribronchiolar and perivascular lymphocyte cuffing. Lesions are more severe and varied when additional pathogens such as *M. pulmonis* are present. Chronic pulmonary dysfunction in previously infected rats appears to be modulated by IFN-γ (38). Aged and immunodeficient mice and rats infected with SV develop a severe form of pneumonia, with viral clearance delayed (15, 31). There is a considerable volume of literature on immune responses to

SV (14, 28). Immunity to SV is both cell- and antibody-mediated (23, 43, 45). Interestingly, viral mutation may be accelerated by oxidative stress associated with the host response to the pathogen (1).

Interference with research
SV has been shown to affect rodents in many ways. Reported effects include modulation of the endothelin receptor-effector systems in mouse but not rat tracheal smooth muscle (19); interference with early embryonic development and fetal growth (21); blockage of INF-α signaling to signal transducers and activators of transcription (STATs) (20); alterations of macrophage (7, 32), NK, and T- and B-cell function (3, 6, 8, 17); cytokine and chemokine production (5, 11, 44); bronchiolar mast cell populations (37); pulmonary hypersensitivity (4, 39); isograft rejection (41); airway physiology (35, 47, 48); response to transplantable tumors (25) and lung allografts (46); neoplastic response to carcinogens (30); apoptosis rates (2); and wound healing (18). Recently, SV has been used experimentally as a gene vector (34). Natural infection of laboratory rodents would compromise studies involving the lymphoreticular, reproductive, and respiratory systems.

Diagnosis and control
Diagnosis of SV is by serology and histologic evidence of pulmonary infection. More recently, PCR assays have been developed. These will likely assume an increasing role in diagnosis of SV. There is no treatment for SV infection. Control is by depopulation, cesarean or embryo transfer rederivation, or cessation of breeding with forced spread of the infection throughout the affected colony. It is essential that incoming animals arrive with a documented history of freedom from SV infection. Of great interest is the recent report of experimentally induced SV infection in nonhuman primates (36). This, coupled with reports from the 1950s, of SV isolations from humans, suggests that SV may eventually be shown to be zoonotic. Until the issue is resolved, animal-care personnel and scientific staff are advised to protect themselves from exposure to SV.

Sialodacryoadenitis virus

Agent
Sialodacryoadenitis virus (SDAV) is an ssRNA virus of the family *Coronaviridae*. Multiple strains have been identified. These differ in pathogenicity and tissue tropism.

Epidemiology
SDAV is a common, important, and highly contagious pathogen of laboratory rats. Transmission is by direct contact and fomites (7). Infant mice, but not adult immunocompetent or severe combined immunodeficient (SCID) mice are susceptible to experimental infection (1, 13). Natural infection of mice has not been reported. SDAV infections follow patterns similar to those of MHV, another coronavirus. Enzootic infection occurs in breeding colonies and is sustained only by the continual introduction of susceptible hosts (newborns). Epizootic infection occurs when the virus enters a susceptible population. In these cases, outbreak of disease is explosive and complete.

Clinical signs
Clinical signs are mild or unapparent in enzootic infections. Suckling rats develop transient conjunctivitis. Weanlings and most adults are asymptomatic (5). Female rats may show periparturient signs of conjunctivitis and exophthalmos. Clinical signs of epizootic infection are again transient, may occur in rats of any age, may vary in severity, and may include cervical edema, sneezing, photophobia, conjunctivitis, nasal and ocular discharge, porphyrin staining, exophthalmos, and corneal ulceration and keratoconus (5, 9).

Pathology
Multiple strains of SDAV exist (6), and tissue tropisms differ somewhat among strains (9). SDAV has a tissue tropism for tubuloalveolar glands of the serous or mixed serous-mucous

types (9). Therefore, inflammatory changes consisting primarily of diffuse necrosis are seen in the lacrimal (including the Harderian) glands, and submandibular and orbital salivary glands (18). Secondary damage may occur to structures of the eye. Cervical lymph nodes and the thymus may also be mildly necrotic. Some strains of SDAV affect the respiratory tract, where pathologic changes may include patchy necrotizing rhinitis, tracheitis, bronchitis, and bronchiolitis, with multifocal pneumonitis (2, 19). SDAV causes more severe respiratory tract lesions in LEW rats than in F344 rats (8). Virus is present in tissues for only about 1 week, until humoral immunity develops. There is no carrier state, so clinical signs and pathologic changes are transient. In athymic rats infection is more severe, is persistent, and may be fatal (4).

Interference with research
SDAV has been shown to alter estrous cycles, increase embryonic and postnatal mortality (17), cause depletion of epidermal growth factor in submaxillary salivary glands (12), cause anorexia and weight loss (11, 16), and reduce IL-1 production by alveolar macrophages (3). In addition, SDAV potentiates lesions caused by *M. pulmonis* (14, 15), though not by altering pulmonary clearance or intrapulmonary killing (10). Natural infections of laboratory rats with SDAV would be expected to interfere with studies involving the dermal, enterohepatic, lymphoreticular, reproductive, and respiratory systems; and interfere with growth of infected rats.

Diagnosis and control
Diagnosis is based on gross clinical signs, histolopathologic lesions, ELISA, and more recently, PCR (20). There is no treatment for SDAV infection. Control is by cessation of breeding, and rapid and forced distribution of the virus throughout the entire colony, if it is likely that all animal rooms have been exposed. After an outbreak and following seroconversion of all animals except newly introduced sentinels, the breeding program can resume. Prevention is based on procurement of virus-free rats. The highly infectious nature of SDAV justifies exclusion of nonessential personnel from the animal facility, and restricting movement of personnel within the animal facility.

Theiler's murine encephalomyelitis virus

Agent
Theiler's murine encephalomyelitis virus (TMEV) is an ssRNA virus of the family *Picornaviridae*. Multiple strains exist, and are classified according to pathogenic features, which themselves appear to be rooted in viral structural differences. For example, the more virulent GDVII strain produces acute polioencephalomyelitis in mice, while the DA and BeAn strains may cause autoimmune demyelination, with virus persisting largely in astrocytes in the CNS white matter (28).

Epidemiology
Infection of *Mus musculus,* the natural host of TMEV, appears to be common globally (10). Despite this, TMEV has been reported infrequently in laboratory mice, and even less often in rats. Its primary importance is as a model of poliomyelitis, multiple sclerosis, and virus-induced demyelinating disease (26). Infection is not highly contagious. Because the virus naturally infects the intestinal mucosa, transmission is primarily fecal-oral. Viral shedding occurs for roughly 2 months (15). In addition, transplacental transmission has been documented (1), and mouse and rat cell cultures may be infected.

Clinical signs
No clinical signs of infection have been reported during natural infection of mice with TMEV. In contrast, experimental infection with virulent strains results in unilateral or bilateral flaccid paralysis of the hind limbs, and rarely, other neurologic signs (5, 21). It is uncertain whether clinical signs ever develop in natural infections.

Pathology

In some mice, viremia may disseminate virus from the intestine to many tissues, including the liver, spleen, and CNS, spreading by axonal transport (11). Following dissemination, pathologic changes may be seen in the spinal cord and brain, and consist of poliomyelitis with necrosis, nonsuppurative meningitis, microgliosis, perivasculitis, neuronophagia of ventral horn cells (19), and autoimmune demyelination mediated by T lymphocytes (24), TNF-α (6), and IL-1 (22). Mouse strains differ in susceptibility to demyelinating disease (2, 3, 16, 18). Viral persistence in the CNS is virus strain dependent (17). In addition, clearing of the virus depends on involvement of virus-specific cytotoxic T lymphocytes (7), and is modulated by cytokines IL-2 (9), IL-4, and IL-10 (13). Intraperitoneal inoculation may result in acute myositis that progresses to a chronic inflammatory muscle disease that may be immune mediated (4).

Interference with research

Natural infection of mice has reportedly caused spontaneous demyelinating myelopathy in aging laboratory mice (8). Other physiologic changes include virus strain-dependent induction of apoptosis in the CNS (27), electrophysiologic abnormalities and spinal cord atrophy (12), and induction of cytokine (23), chemokine (20), and eicosanoid (14) expression in the CNS. Infection with TMEV could compromise studies involving the enterohepatic, lymphoreticular, musculoskeletal, and nervous systems.

Diagnosis and control

Diagnosis of TMEV has traditionally been accomplished by serologic methods, including hemagglutination inhibition and ELISA. More recently, these methods have been augmented by molecular-based methods such as RT-PCR (25). Likewise, serology-based methods, such as the MAP test, used to detect contamination of biological materials, will certainly be augmented or replaced by molecular methods. There is no treatment for TMEV infection.

Once the virus has been found in a colony, TMEV-free mice or rats may be produced by foster nursing newborns onto TMEV-negative mothers, selecting TMEV-negative pups, or cesarean rederivation (15). Prevention is through purchase of virus-free animals.

BACTERIA

Cilia-associated respiratory bacillus

Agent

Cilia-associated respiratory (CAR) bacillus is a relatively recently identified pathogen of wild and laboratory rats, and to a lesser extent, mice and rabbits; and experimentally, guinea pigs and hamsters (1, 18). CAR bacillus is a gram-negative, filamentous rod of uncertain classification. Analyses of small-subunit ribosomal RNA sequences indicate that rat-origin CAR bacillus may be closely related to *Flavobacterium ferrugineum* and *Flexibacter sancti* (7). CAR bacillus isolates of rat and rabbit origins differ in antigenic profile (6), may be distinct strains and, in mice, isolates of rat origin may be more virulent than those of rabbit origin (3). Rat strains such as F-344, LEW, and SD do not seem to differ in susceptibility to CAR bacillus disease. However, bacterial isolates differ in virulence in rats (16).

Epidemiology

Transmission is likely by contact exposure to respiratory tract secretions (12).

Clinical signs

Current information suggests that CAR bacillus is usually a copathogen (2), most prominently of *M. pulmonis* in rats, and that CAR bacillus exacerbates lesions of murine respiratory mycoplasmosis (MRM) (5). However, primary infection of rats with CAR bacillus has been reported (14). The clinical signs following natural CAR bacillus infection that have been reported for rats are similar to those of severe MRM (see discussion of *M. pulmonis*), and include hunched posture, lethargy, rough coat, and periocular porphyrin staining (11, 15).

Pathology
Lesions of CAR bacillus infection in rats are also similar to those of MRM, and the reader is referred to that section for a full description. In addition, CAR bacillus infection also produces severe bronchiolectasis, pulmonary abscesses, and atelectasis of entire lung lobes (11, 15). These lesions are due mainly to accumulation of pus in the airways. Large numbers of CAR bacilli can be observed between cilia on respiratory epithelial surfaces and cause the ciliated border to appear dense. Lesions may also be found on epithelial surfaces in nasal passages, larynx, trachea, and middle ears (15). In BALB/c mice, pulmonary lesions consist of mild mucosal hyperplasia and a lymphocytic response, followed by macrophage and neutrophilic infiltration (9). Lesions were observed in mice of the ICR strain experimentally infected with CAR bacillus (18), and lesions compatible with CAR bacillus infection have been reported in C57BL/6J-*ob/ob* mice, although these latter mice may have also been infected with SV and/or PVM (5). In this regard, others have found isolates of CAR bacillus to be contaminated with *M. pulmonis* (17). Immunity appears to be primarily humoral, consisting of IgM and IgG3 antibody responses, which are nevertheless ineffective (8). In this regard, there is local accumulation of B and double-negative lymphocytes (likely $\gamma\delta$ T cells), and later macrophages and neutrophils. This immune response is principally responsible for pathology associated with CAR bacillus infection, and is typical of extracellular bacterial pathogens expressing T-cell-independent polysaccharide antigens (9).

Interference with research
Information is generally lacking concerning effects of natural CAR bacillus infection on rats and mice. Kendall and coworkers (8, 10) demonstrated increases in cytokine production in CAR bacillus-infected mice. It is likely that CAR bacillus infection would contribute to the morbidity and mortality associated with MRM, and could compromise studies involving the respiratory and lymphoreticular systems.

Diagnosis and control
Diagnosis of CAR bacillus infection is by serology and by silver staining of histologic sections. More recently, PCR assays have been developed (4). Control measures have yet to be fully determined. There is no completely effective therapy for eradicating CAR bacillus from a rat colony. However, cesarean rederivation has been suggested (15), while others have suggested the use of sulfamerazine for clearing CAR bacillus from mice, allowing that mycoplasmas, which may also be present, are resistant to sulfonamides (13). Prevention of infection is through purchase of pathogen-free animals from reputable vendors, followed by husbandry practices that preclude opportunity for infection.

Citrobacter rodentium

Agent
Citrobacter rodentium (17), formerly *Citrobacter freundii* biotype 4280, is the etiologic agent of transmissible murine colonic hyperplasia (11). *C. rodentium* is a gram-negative, facultatively anaerobic rod. It appears that all isolates are identical; that is, members of the species are clonal (10).

Epidemiology
The prevalence of *C. rodentium* in laboratory mice is largely unknown. Transmission is by direct contact (4) or by contaminated food or bedding. *C. rodentium* is generally considered an opportunistic pathogen. For example, use of antibiotics effective primarily against gram-negative rods may allow for an overgrowth of *C. rodentium* in the mouse intestine (20). Rats are not susceptible to infection (2).

Clinical signs
Clinical signs, when present, are nonspecific, and may include ruffled coat, weight loss, de-

pression, stunting, perianal fecal staining, and rectal prolapse (14). Nursing mice are most susceptible. Strain differences in susceptibility exist, with C3H/HeJ mice more susceptible than DBA/2J, NIHS (Swiss), or C57BL/6J mice (3). Infection is transient; there is no carrier state.

Pathology
The hallmark pathologic lesion of *C. rodentium* infection is colonic hyperplasia. In general, the descending colon is most affected. However, the entire colon and cecum may be involved, with crypt elongation, mucosal inflammation, crypt abscesses, occasional erosions and ulcers, and with healing, goblet cell hyperplasia (1, 14). Transient colonization of the mouse small intestinal mucosa, followed by colonization of the large bowel, is dependent on the presence of the chromosomal eae gene (16) encoded in the pathogenicity island called the locus of enterocyte effacement (LEE) (5). Once colonization has occurred, *C. rodentium* causes the formation of attaching and effacing (A/E) lesions. Outer membrane proteins, known as intimins, are required for formation of the A/E lesions (6). Immunity is primarily humoral, and is largely directed toward intimin and other antigens encoded by the LEE (7). In addition, experimentally infected mice develop a strong Th1 response, with induction of IL-12, INF-γ, and TNF-α (8, 18). In fact, lymphocytes appear to contribute to the pathologic changes associated with infection (19).

Interference with research
Reported effects on research are relatively few. Infection with *C. rodentium* is known to promote tumorigenesis (2, 15). Following experimental infection, Th1 cytokine production is induced (8), while others report that lysates of *C. rodentium* directly inhibit cytokine production by murine lymphoid cells from multiple sites (13). Lastly, *C. rodentium* was implicated in diminished fecundity and immune competence in a colony of T-cell receptor transgenic mice (12). In that study, however, the authors could not say with certainty that *C. rodentium* was causative. These reports describe changes in host physiology that may have an impact on specific research studies involving the enterohepatic, reproductive, and lymphoreticular systems. *C. rodentium* is used as a model of A/E lesions in vivo and in intestinal disease of humans.

Diagnosis and control
Diagnosis of *C. rodentium* infection has been by culture and biotyping of isolates obtained from blood, spleen, and colon, or by ELISA. More recently, highly sensitive PCR assays have been developed (9). These will likely increase in use as automation of molecular diagnostic procedures proceeds. Losses may be minimized during outbreaks by use of antibiotics as a means of preserving valuable mouse strains, in preparation for embryo transfer or cesarean rederivation (8). Prevention is through purchase of pathogen-free animals from reputable sources.

Clostridium piliforme

Agent
Clostridium piliforme (2), formerly *Bacillus piliformis,* is the causative agent of Tyzzer's disease. *C. piliforme* is a gram-negative, filamentous, endospore-forming bacterium.

Epidemiology
Prevalence remains high in some laboratory rodent colonies (1, 9). Possible explanations for this include the moderately contagious nature of the organism and a wide range of susceptible and naturally infected host species (5). However, concerning the latter, Franklin and coworkers (3) have suggested that both cross-infective isolates and more host-specific isolates may exist. With this in mind, transmission is thought to be by ingestion of infectious endospores in contaminated food or bedding, although transplacental infection also occurs (4). Inadequate sterilization of feed or bedding components may facilitate the entry of the pathogen into an otherwise well-

managed rodent colony. Mouse strains differ in susceptibility to infection with *C. piliforme*. For example, DBA/2 are susceptible, while C57BL/6 are resistant (16). Also, mice deficient in IgM production are reportedly more susceptible than fully immune competent mouse strains, or mice deficient only in T-cell function (17).

Clinical signs
Most infections are subclinical. Various host and environmental stressors may precipitate clinical disease. Clinical signs occur most commonly in suckling and weanling rodents, and may include sudden death, watery diarrhea, lethargy, and ruffled fur (11). However, experimental manipulations have been reported to provoke or exacerbate clinical disease caused by *C. piliforme* (11).

Pathology
Pathologic changes involve three main phases. These include the establishment of infection in the ileum and cecum, the ascension of the pathogen to the liver via the portal circulation, and hematogenous spread to other tissues such as the myocardium. This triad of organ involvement is the hallmark of Tyzzer's disease. In mice, affected intestine is thickened, edematous, and hyperemic. Necrotic foci develop in the affected intestine, liver, and myocardium. Lesions are similar in rats except that megaloileitis is a common finding (8). As previously noted, Waggie and coworkers (17) demonstrated that B-cell- but not T-cell-deficient mice were more susceptible and concluded that immunity to *C. piliforme* was therefore primarily humoral. More recently, neutrophils, NK cells, IL-6, and IL-12 have been shown to mediate the course of infection (14, 15, 16). Lastly, others have demonstrated increased susceptibility to a toxigenic isolate of *C. piliforme* in nude mice, and have concluded that T cells may also have a role in immunity to Tyzzer's disease (9), while acknowledging that the cytotoxin produced by the isolate may have contributed to the severity of clinical disease and lesions. Athymic (*nu/nu*) rats have also been shown to be highly susceptible (12).

Interference with research
Effects on research include increased mortality, alteration of the pharmacokinetics of warfarin and trimethoprim (6), and alteration of the activity of hepatic transaminases (11). In addition, experimental infection may result in cytokine induction, including IL-6, IL-12, IFN-γ, and TNF-α (13, 14, 15). Natural infection of laboratory mice and rats could severely alter the findings of studies involving the cardiovascular, enterohepatic, and lymphoreticular systems.

Diagnosis and control
Diagnosis of *C. piliforme* infection is routinely accomplished by ELISA (10), although PCR-based assays have been developed more recently (7). The organism cannot be cultured on artificial media. In addition, *C. piliforme* may be visualized in histologic section, or other biological materials, using silver staining. While antibiotic usage can lessen morbidity and mortality in the face of an outbreak, elimination of the pathogen is by termination of the colony, caesarean rederivation, or embryo transfer. Prevention of infection is through purchase of pathogen-free animals from reputable sources. Lastly, immunocompromised persons should be especially careful when working with *C. piliforme*-infected animals, since *C. piliforme* may infect these persons and cause serious disease.

Corynebacterium kutscheri

Agent
Corynebacterium kutscheri is a gram-positive bacillus that infects both mice and rats.

Epidemiology
Transmission is fecal-oral. The oral cavity and large intestine most commonly serve as reservoir sites for a latent carrier stage (1, 2, 4).

Clinical signs

Natural infections are usually subclinical (1, 2, 4) and are only revealed with the immunosuppressive effects of certain drugs, experimental manipulations, or other infectious agents (9). Clinical signs in rats, when present, usually include dyspnea with abnormal lung sounds, weight loss, humped posture, and anorexia.

Pathology

Hematogenous spread occurs in both species, and accounts for abscess formation in various organs. In rats, abscesses commonly develop in the lungs and extend to the pleura, while in mice abscesses more often occur in the kidneys and liver (10, 11). Strain differences in colonization sites (1, 2) and susceptibility have been reported. C57BL/6 and B10.BR/SgSn mice are among the more resistant strains while Swiss, BALB/cCr, and A/J are among the more susceptible strains (3, 5). Strain susceptibility may reflect differences in efficiency of mononuclear phagocytes, or cytokine responses (7). In addition, male ICR mice more commonly developed infections, and had greater bacterial loads, following experimental inoculation, than did females (8). The underlying mechanisms of these sex differences are unknown.

Interference with research

Experimental procedures that immunosuppress rats or mice may result in the unwanted development of active *C. kutscheri* infection, which could compromise a variety of studies, especially those of the enterohepatic, respiratory, and urinary systems.

Diagnosis and control

Diagnosis of *C. kutscheri* infection can be challenging. Several approaches have been reported, but none with universal success. Diagnosis of subclinical infections has been accomplished with cortisone challenge, followed by the tube agglutination test for a rise in titer (9). More recently, Amao and coworkers described a method of recovery and culture of *C. kutscheri* from the oral cavities of subclinically infected rats (1). Traditionally, diagnosis of clinical infections is best approached using culture of the organism; examination of gram or Giemsa stained tissue imprints, or methenamine silver-stained tissue sections; and examination of tissue sections for characteristic pathologic lesions (9). PCR-based methods allow for rapid and consistent identification of infection and will likely supplant traditional test methods. There is no entirely successful therapy to eradicate *C. kutscheri*. Cesarean rederivation followed by barrier containment is the accepted means of eliminating the pathogen from an animal colony (9). It should be noted, however, that there is one report of potential vertical transmission (6). Prevention is through purchase of pathogen-free animals from reputable sources.

Corynebacterium spp. in athymic mice

Agent

Corynebacteria are gram-positive, diphtheroid bacilli. Reports of hyperkeratosis in nude mice naturally infected with *Corynebacterium* spp. have occasionally appeared in the literature (6, 7). In the report by Richter and coworkers (6) the pathogen isolated was similar to *Corynebacterium pseudodiphtheriticum,* while in more recent reports the pathogen was most like, or was identified as, *Corynebacterium bovis,* based on biochemical profiles and 16S rRNA gene sequence (1, 2, 7).

Epidemiology

The prevalence of *Corynebacterium* sp. infections in nude mice is unknown but appears to be increasing. Whether this is due to a real increase in prevalence or simply increased awareness of the condition is also unknown. Transmission occurs by direct contact and by contaminated bedding and gloves (1). Once present, infection spreads extremely rapidly through an animal colony (7). Little is known about other aspects of the biology and epidemiology of *C. bovis,* such as the role of potential reservoir hosts, including humans; resistance of the organism in the environment; and the most common modes of entry into animal facilities.

Clinical signs
Clinical signs have most commonly been reported in athymic mice, and have included flaking of the skin, primarily along the dorsum, and, in some animals, pruritus.

Pathology
Pathologic changes include orthokeratotic hyperkeratosis and follicular keratosis; marked acanthosis; and mild neutrophilic, macrophage, and mast cell infiltration (1, 6, 7). Morbidity frequently reaches 100%, while mortality remains low, with spontaneous regression of signs a frequent occurrence. Infections in haired mice have also been reported, with or without clinical signs (4, 5, 8).

Interference with research
Documented effects of *Corynebacterium* sp. on research are thus far limited. Field and coworkers (3) reported decreased tumor growth and enhanced toxicity of chemotherapeutic agents in nude mice with coryneform hyperkeratosis. Mice naturally infected with this pathogen would be unsuitable for dermatologic, and possibly other, research projects.

Diagnosis and control
Currently, diagnosis is based on culture and evaluation of biochemical characteristics. Histologic features alone are inadequate for establishing a diagnosis, since other pathogens may cause dermatitis in mice (7). Recently, a PCR assay has successfully detected as few as 3 viable organisms (2). Elimination of the affected colony, with strict attention to disinfection procedures (7), appears to be the best approach to eradicating the pathogen. Because haired (including SCID) mice may serve as asymptomatic reservoirs of infection for nude mice, these mice should not be housed with athymic mice without prior testing.

Helicobacter spp.

Agents
The genus *Helicobacter* contains an ever-increasing number of recently identified, gram-negative, spiral, microaerophilic, gastrointestinal system pathogens known to infect mammals (11). Species naturally infecting mice and/or rats include a number of lesser known *Helicobacter* spp., such as *H. bilis,* which is associated with multifocal chronic hepatitis, and is isolated from the liver, bile, and lower intestine of aged, inbred mice (14, 41) and immunodeficient rats (21); *H. muridarum* from the intestinal mucosa of rats and mice (26); *H. rodentium* (39, 40), *"Flexispira rappini"* (5, 37), *H. ganmani* (36), and *H. typhlonius* (16) from the intestinal tracts of mice; and *H. trogontum,* recently isolated from the colonic mucosa of Wistar and Holtzman rats (33). However, *H. hepaticus,* a pathogen of mice, is undoubtedly the most prominent of the murine *Helicobacter* spp., and is responsible for the most lesions. Therefore, this review will focus on *H. hepaticus.*

Epidemiology
The prevalence of *H. hepaticus* is mostly unknown. Following initial reports, many animal facilities were evaluated for *H. hepaticus* and found contaminated (18, 38). Since then, rederivation efforts have somewhat reduced the number of contaminated facilities. Susceptibility among mouse strains appears to be multigenic (22, 44). Transmission is by direct fecal-oral contact, or by fomites. A recent report indicates that *H. hepaticus* may contaminate transplantable tumors unless the material is cryopreserved (17). Rats are also commonly found infected with *Helicobacter* spp.

Clinical signs
Clinical signs of *H. hepaticus* infection are absent in immunocompetent mice, but include

rectal prolapse, hemorrhagic diarrhea, and decreased weight gain in immunodeficient mice (42, 46). Clinical signs are rarely observed following infection with other *Helicobacter* spp.

Pathology
Mouse strains differ in susceptibility to infection and pathologic lesions. For example, A/JCr mice more readily develop *H. hepaticus*-induced hepatitis and have lower cecal bacterial burdens, while C57BL/6 mice experience just the opposite (51). *H. hepaticus* selectively and persistently colonizes the bile canaliculi and cecal and colonic mucosae (10). Cytolethal distending toxin appears to be one of the most significant virulence factors in hepatitis and enterocolitis caused by *H. hepaticus* (53). Pathologic changes include chronic, active hepatitis, possibly of autoimmune etiology (47); occasional enterocolitis; progressive typhlitis; colitis; and hepatocellular neoplasms induced by as yet undelineated nongenotoxic mechanisms (3, 9, 12, 15, 27). Immunity is primarily humoral (34). Mice seroconvert 2 weeks after inoculation (29). Cellular responses occur, and some may contribute to pathologic changes (2, 25). For example, SCID mice develop inflammatory bowel disease within 5-6 weeks following infection with *H. muridarum* and receipt of T cells (23). In contrast, the transcription factor NF-κB inhibits development of colitis (8).

Interference with research
H. hepaticus has been associated with hepatic carcinomas (6), possibly due to alterations in enzymes associated with production of reactive oxygen species (4). The presence of *H. hepaticus* may also alter rates of cell proliferation and apoptosis in male, but not female mice (35). Others have reported elevations in serum levels of alanine aminotransferase (48). *H. hepaticus* serves as a model for *H. pylori*-induced chronic gastritis, gastric ulcers, and gastric adenocarcinoma (12). It should not be assumed that all mouse strain and *Helicobacter* spp. combinations will present similarly. For example, *H. bilis* infection accelerates development of colitis in multiple drug resistance-deficient ($mdr1a)^{-/-}$ mice, while *H. hepaticus* delays development (30), yet the two *Helicobacter* species behave similar to one another in SCID and A/J mice (42). Humans with *H. pylori* gastritis have higher local leptin concentrations in the gastric corpus (1). It is not known whether similar changes occur in rodents infected with gastric helicobacters. Natural infection of laboratory mice with *H. hepaticus*, and possibly other *Helicobacter* spp., have been shown to confound carcinogenicity research (20), and could alter research involving other aspects of the enterohepatic system.

Diagnosis and control
A number of authors have published guidelines on diagnostic detection of rodent Helicobacters, and on the procurement of *Helicobacter*-free animals (49, 52). Diagnosis may be accomplished using a variety of methods, including serology (28), fecal or tissue PCR (7, 32), histologic examination of silver-stained tissues, and less commonly, fecal culture. Fecal or tissue PCR appears to be most reliable (13, 31, 52), and is therefore rapidly becoming the diagnostic method of choice. A recent report indicated that *Helicobacter* spp. may be shed inconsistently in the feces (24), somewhat complicating detection by fecal PCR. More recently, a PCR-denaturing gradient gel electrophoresis technique has been developed for detecting and speciating Helicobacters colonizing the lower bowel of laboratory mice (19). Monitoring of sentinel animals after exposure to soiled cage bedding will generally reveal room contamination (52), although in the author's experience, *Helicobacter* spp. are not highly contagious and spread slowly among animals within a room. These features facilitate eradication efforts. *Helicobacter* infections have been eliminated from mouse and rat colonies through antibiotic administration, embryo transfer, or cesarean rederivation. More recently, however, mouse colonies have been easily rederived free of *H. hepaticus* by neonatal transfer of mouse pups onto uninfected foster dams (45). Neo-

natal transfer must be done before the pups reach 1 day of age to prevent infection (43). This method is also useful for rederiving *Helicobacter*-free rats (43). Use of microisolator caging, disinfected forceps to transfer animals, and the opening of only one cage at a time will facilitate containment or exclusion efforts (50).

Klebsiella pneumoniae

Agent
Klebsiella pneumoniae is a gram-negative bacterium typically inhabiting the intestinal tract of rats, mice, and numerous other animals. Reports of clinical disease in immunocompetent rodents are rare (7, 11, 15, 24) and *K. pneumoniae* is therefore considered an opportunistic pathogen (20).

Epidemiology
The prevalence of infection with *K. pneumoniae* in rodent colonies is high and may increase with antibiotic treatment used to eliminate other bacteria (10). Transmission is primarily fecal-oral, with aerosol transmission less effective (1).

Clinical signs
When present, clinical signs in mice most commonly include dyspnea, sneezing, cervical lymphadenopathy, inappetance, hunched posture, and rough hair coat (7, 24), and in rats include cervical and inguinal abscesses (11, 15). Clinical signs in immunocompromised rodents are generally more severe. Some transgenic mice, including the apoE$^{-/-}$ mouse, experience greater mortality, and have greater outgrowth of bacteria from their organs, indicating impaired immune response to *K. pneumoniae* (6).

Pathology
Following infection, hematogenous spread allows for focal abscessation in any organ. In the lungs of mice, this results in granulomatous pneumonia (31). The majority of clinical *K. pneumoniae* isolates produce a high-molecular-weight capsular polysaccharide, which is one of the dominant virulence factors (35). Immunity is age related (32) and consists initially of recruitment of macrophages and neutrophils. This immune response pattern is typical of extracellular bacterial pathogens expressing T-cell-independent polysaccharide antigens (23, 35). Immune components include TNF and TNF-α-mediated mast cell chemoattraction (17), which may be influenced by macrophage inflammatory protein-2 (8); INF-γ (34); IL-1 (30), IL-6 (27), IL-8 (29), IL-12 (8), and other cytokines; ICAM-1 (22); the acute-phase protein α_1-acid glycoprotein (α_1-AGP) (13); leukotrienes (19), chemokines (25, 26); neutrophil (14) and macrophage (22) activity; and production of defensins (16). The immune response is moderated by IL-10 (36).

Interference with research
Rats and/or mice experimentally infected with, or exposed to products from *K. pneumoniae*, serve as models of pneumonia (4), endotoxemia (21, 28), sepsis (5, 12), cystitis and pyelonephritis (3), antibiotic pharmacokinetics (9), host resistance (18), riboflavin metabolism (2), and human phacoantigenic uveitis (33). In addition to the physiologic changes which may accompany the above-mentioned clinical scenarios, infection has been shown to lower plasma thyroxine levels (2), and activate the hypothalamus-pituitary-adrenal axis (27). Natural primary or opportunistic infection of laboratory mice and rats could interfere with studies involving several organ systems, but most notably the endocrine, enterohepatic, hematopoietic, lymphoreticular, respiratory, and urinary systems.

Diagnosis and control
Diagnosis of *K. pneumoniae* infection is routinely accomplished by culture followed by examination of typical colony morphology, gram-staining characteristics, and biochemical tests. Control is generally not practiced, since epizootics are rare. Nearly all infections present as individual cases, and most are diagnosed postmortem. Prevention of disease centers

around sound hygienic practices and maintenance of a low-stress environment for the laboratory animals.

Mycoplasma pulmonis

Agent
Mycoplasma pulmonis is, without question, one of the most important pathogens infecting laboratory rats and mice, and is the cause of MRM. *M. pulmonis* lacks a cell wall and has membrane-associated hemolytic activity (24).

Epidemiology
Prevalence rates can be high within animal facilities (45), and *M. pulmonis* can contaminate isolates of CAR bacillus (37). Transmission is primarily intrauterine and by aerosol (15, 42). The organism readily establishes infection by colonizing the nasopharynx and middle ears (9).

Clinical signs
Infection is initially asymptomatic, causing some to consider *M. pulmonis* a commensal under ideal conditions (28). Clinical signs typically follow chronic infection and include "snuffling" in rats and "chattering" in mice; dyspnea; weight loss; hunched posture; lethargy; and in rats, periocular and perinasal porphyrin staining (28). Mice may be asymptomatic while bearing significant pulmonary lesions.

Pathology
M. pulmonis preferentially colonizes the luminal surfaces of respiratory epithelium lining the proximal airways. This characteristic gave rise to the earlier designation "proximal airway disease" (28). Pathologic effects vary, depending on a variety of host, organismal, and environmental factors (6, 7, 11, 17, 19, 23, 28, 38, 39, 47). Regarding host factors, the most resistant mouse strains include those derived from Th1 dominant C57BL mice (5), while Th2 dominant BALB/c and C3H mice are more susceptible (14, 43). Differences in susceptibility are also related to the mycoplasmal killing ability of alveolar macrophages (14), as well as differences in T-cell subset dominance (43). Male mice tend to develop more severe pulmonary lesions (47). Grossly, the lungs appear focally consolidated and airways contain a highly viscous exudate. Microscopically, the spectrum of pathologic changes includes rhinitis, otitis media, laryngitis, tracheitis, suppurative bronchitis, bronchiectasis, pulmonary abscesses, and alveolitis (30). *M. pulmonis* is both chemoattractive and mitogenic for rat lymphocytes and induces hyperplasia of bronchus-associated lymphoid tissue (27, 35), which is a histologic hallmark of MRM in rats. The severity of airway disease may be influenced by profiles of cytokine production (12), by interactions with sensory nerve fibers (2), and by alveolar macrophage viability (10). Immunodeficient mice are equally susceptible to pneumonia and death when compared with immunocompetent mice, and may develop severe arthritis following infection with *M. pulmonis* (36). Genital mycoplasmosis also occurs, and is particularly severe in SD rats (31). Time of infection plays a major role in determination of pregnancy outcome and spread of infection from the genital tract to the respiratory tract, with pregestational infection an important factor in subsequent gestational transmission (3).

Host defense in respiratory mycoplasmosis consists of both innate and acquired components (4). In mice, innate immunity represents the primary line of pulmonary antimycoplasmal defense. Pulmonary surfactant protein A mediates killing of mycoplasmas by alveolar macrophages through peroxynitrite generation (13). Typical of extracellular bacterial pathogens, humoral immunity plays the major acquired role in defense against systemic infection, while cellular immunity is minimally contributory, and exacerbates pulmonary lesions (4, 6). In fact, both humoral and cellular immunity are ultimately incompetent in controlling mycoplasma infection. There are significant perturbations in $CD4^+$ and $CD8^+$ T-cell populations in both the peripheral blood and thymus, with a general shift from a Th1 to a Th2 response that is ineffective. This state of immune incompetence allows *M. pulmonis* to survive chronically (33). In rats, cellular immunity, primarily through CD4$^+$ T cells, marginally controls infection but again also causes immunopathology (18). While cellular immunity is more active in the lungs, antibody responses occur in the spleen. Regarding the latter, humoral responsiveness is age related, with older animals mounting a more pronounced, though delayed, antibody response (41).

Interference with research
M. pulmonis may disseminate widely throughout the host and therefore may alter experimental results in numerous ways. Most effects appear to be centered on the respiratory system. Effects include alterations in pulmonary carcinogen response, electrogenic ion transport (21), decreased ciliary function, altered microvascular endothelial cell morphology and function (26), and altered airway innervation (29). Neurogenic inflammation is increased (8). Concerning the latter, *M. pulmonis* infection induces respiratory tract angiogenesis and remodeling, with angiogenic blood vessels abnormally sensitive to substance P released from tracheal sensory nerves. These changes induce leakage of plasma by neurokinin-1 receptors (1, 22). In addition to these, *M. pulmonis* induces profound alterations in immune function. These include altered cytokine and chemokine production, reduced delayed hypersensitivity responses, T-cell subset changes, increased total lymphocyte and neutrophil counts, increased splenic weight, diminished antibody response to sheep erythrocytes, reduced phagocytic capability, and decreased colloidal carbon clearance (32, 33, 34, 40). On a more systemic level, *M. pulmonis* intensifies the accumulation of some antibiotics that usually accumulate in the lung, specifically the macrolide tilmicosin (25); induces chronic arthritis in Fas ligand-defective mice (16); and lowers reproductive efficiency (31). Natural infection of laboratory rats and mice could seriously impair research efforts investigating a variety of body systems, primarily the cardiovascular, hematopoietic, lymphoreticular, musculoskeletal, nervous, reproductive, and respiratory systems; and could compromise pharmacokinetic studies.

Diagnosis and control
Diagnosis of MRM has for many years been primarily serologic. Bacteriological culture of the mycoplasmas is unreliable for diagnosis and requires extended culture periods. More recently, nested PCR has been found to be useful (37). Histopathology reveals typical lesions and is therefore a valuable adjunct. Control is through preventing entry of infected animals into the facility. This should include testing of transplantable tumor lines (48). Once *M. pulmonis* is found in a facility, depopulation and cleanup are effective at eliminating the pathogen. Cesarean rederivation may also be effective, if dams are used which have repeatedly been demonstrated to be seronegative. The placental membranes from donor females should be tested, either by culture or PCR, since transplacental transmission is common (42). Antibiotic administration prior to rederivation may increase the success of those efforts, but will not by itself eradicate the infection (44). Experimentally, vaccination with DNA encoding *M. pulmonis* antigens may facilitate clearing of infection, but is unlikely to be widely practical (20). Mice and rats from other than commercial vendors are commonly infected with *M. pulmonis* (46). Prior to receiving animals from any source, but particularly from noncommercial sources, the receiving institution should request and critically evaluate recent health surveillance records. Also, animals from such sources should be quarantined and retested prior to release into the general animal population.

Pasteurella pneumotropica

Agent
Pasteurella pneumotropica is a gram-negative, nonhemolytic bacterium. Multiple biotypes have been reported (2, 12).

Epidemiology
The prevalence of *P. pneumotropica* is unknown but anecdotally appears to be very

high. *P. pneumotropica* is frequently isolated from several sites on and within healthy rats and mice and is therefore considered an opportunistic pathogen. Most commonly, these sites include the upper respiratory tract, intestines, and vagina (15, 18). Transmission is by direct contact with feces, saliva, and reproductive tract secretions, as well as fomites (20). *P. pneumotropica* has also been found as a contaminant of transplantable tumors (17).

Clinical signs
While most species of rodents may harbor the organism, reports of natural outbreaks are rare and are often, although not always, limited to rats and immune-compromised mice (1, 3). When apparent, clinical disease most commonly involves the orbits and presents as ophthalmitis and conjunctivitis (1). Infections involving other areas of the skin and adnexal structures also occur, including abscesses, otitis media, mastitis, and infections of the reproductive tract (8, 9, 11, 18). McGinn and coworkers (14) reported otitis media in CBA/J mice used in hearing research. *P. pneumotropica* was isolated from infected otic bullae. Similar findings in outbred mice were previously reported (10). However, in neither report was the primary pathogen unequivocally established. In this regard, *P. pneumotropica* has often been observed as a secondary pathogen or copathogen with *Pneumocystis carinii* (13), KRV (5), and others.

Pathology
Following infection, *P. pneumotropica* colonizes primarily the upper respiratory tract. In most cases, no pathologic lesions are noted (4). Immune suppression facilitates establishment of the pathogen in the lungs, with lesion development characterized by diffuse, suppurative, interstitial pneumonia (9). Lesions developing at mucocutaneous junctions are often purulent, with a pronounced neutrophilic component (8). Typical of infection with extracellular bacterial pathogens, immunity is primarily humoral. In this regard, mice deficient in MHC class II antigens are more susceptible to infection than wild-type mice (6).

Interference with research
Natural infection of laboratory rodents with *P. pneumotropica* could compromise research involving the dermal, enterohepatic, reproductive, and respiratory systems, and could confound other studies if the general health of the animals was compromised. It is known that several members of the *Haemophilus–Actinobacillus–Pasteurella* group of bacteria share the general property of being resistant to cellular defense mechanisms (7). This occurs through a variety of means, including the presence of an antiphagocytic capsule, active insult to phagocytes, and alteration of leukocyte and macrophage function (7). Therefore, it is possible that *P. pneumotropica* may also interfere with studies involving the lymphoreticular system.

Diagnosis and control
Diagnosis is established by culturing the organism, preferably following enrichment (16). More recently, PCR of nasopharyngeal swab specimens has been shown to be more sensitive than culture (19, 23). To legitimately ascribe clinical significance to *P. pneumotropica* one must determine that other pathogens were not involved. Where *P. pneumotropica* must be excluded from the colony, the use of acidified or chlorinated water, along with other "barrier" husbandry procedures, will usually prevent exposure. However, it is difficult to eradicate many opportunistic pathogens from even well-managed rodent colonies. *P. pneumotropica* is known to survive for up to 120 min on mouse hair, and for <30 min on laboratory coat fabric (20). In vitro fertilization, followed by embryo transfer, has been used to rederive mice free of *P. pneumotropica* (21). Others have reported the elimination of *P. pneumotropica* from asymptomatic mice after 14 days of oral or parenteral administration of enrofloxacin at 25.5 and 85.0 mg/kg body weight (9, 22).

Pseudomonas aeruginosa

Agent
Pseudomonas aeruginosa is a gram-negative rod that usually inhabits the nasopharynx, oropharynx, and lower digestive tract of many vertebrate species.

Epidemiology
The primary importance of *P. aeruginosa* is as an opportunistic pathogen, and as a model for numerous human medical conditions. *P. aeruginosa* is commonly found in soil, organic waste, and as a normal skin inhabitant and is frequently cultured from facility water systems. Active exclusion of the organism from the animal facility is achievable but costly. Transmission is by contact with contaminated water, feed, bedding, and infected rodents and humans (49).

Clinical signs
Clinical signs are generally not observed in immune-competent hosts. Some immune-compromised mice and rats may develop hunched posture, apathy, dullness, shortness of breath, ruffled coat, emaciation, circling movements around their longitudinal axis, oblique head posture, and die (5, 15).

Pathology
Following exposure, *P. aeruginosa* colonizes the upper respiratory and lower intestinal tracts of rodents. The host response to *P. aeruginosa* infection varies among inbred mouse strains and is determined by differences in host inflammatory responses (27, 38). For example, from most resistant to most susceptible, relative to lung infection, inbred mouse strains include: C3H/HeN > BALB/c > DBA/2 and C57BL/6 (26, 29, 38, 46). Pathologic lesions develop as a result of invasion of deep tissues, resulting in hematogenous spread of the bacteria to multiple organs. Entry into the vascular system may be facilitated by pseudomonal proteases and bradykinin generated in infectious foci (37). Pathologic lesions are found in affected tissues and consist of multifocal necrosis, abscessation, and suppuration. Lesions are often most severe in the lungs (33). Vegetative lesions may be found on heart valves of animals with infected indwelling vascular catheters (33). In addition, strains of *P. aeruginosa* differ widely in virulence (9). Bacterial flagellae (21); pyoverdin and pyochelin, which may compete directly with transferrin for iron (24, 45); pyocyanin (43); elastase (47); porins (4); and potent exotoxins (11, 14, 32, 48) play major roles in determining virulence. Most prominent among the exotoxins is exotoxin A, a superantigen (25, 35). In addition, *P. aeruginosa* exotoxin A may act synergistically with endotoxins and enterotoxins from other pathogens to cause TNF-α-mediated hepatotoxicity (42).

Much of what is known of the cell biology of *P. aeruginosa* infections comes from experimentally induced infections. Studies of immune responses to *P. aeruginosa* present evidence for both humoral (34) and cellular (7, 44) contributions to immunity, which is enhanced by vitamin B2 (2), IL-1 (50), and IFN-γ (16). It has been suggested that severity of disease is related to propensity toward Th1 (resistant) versus Th2 (susceptible) (29), and macrophage (resistant) versus neutrophil (susceptible) immune responses (28, 38), although there is not complete agreement on this point within the literature (19). Th1 cells may participate in part by triggering TNF-α-mediated hypersensitivity to *P. aeruginosa* (8). Interestingly, susceptible mice have been shown to have a defect in TNF-α production (10, 26). Macrophages and neutrophils are important effector cells (30), with neutrophil accumulation mediated through CD11/CD18 cells (36) and cytokine-induced neutrophil chemoattractant (CINC)-2α (1). Transgenic cystic fibrosis mice exhibit reduced early clearance of *P. aeruginosa* from the respiratory tract (39).

Interference with research
Numerous publications have reported on the effects of *P. aeruginosa* on research. Most reports are from experimental and/or in vitro studies. Effects include early death follow-

ing exposure to radiation, cyclophosphamide treatment, CMV infection, or cold stress (31); increased severity of infection following airway trauma (52); induction of pulmonary fibrosis (23); stimulation of T-cell proliferation (6, 41); induction of apoptosis in the thymus (51), the liver (41), and possibly elsewhere (4); inhibition of wound healing (13); increased production of cytokines (40); inhibition of macrophage function by bacterial rhamnolipids (22); possible T-cell-dependent immune suppression mediated by the polysaccharide fraction of LPS (12); altered fluid transport across the lung epithelium (35); increased cardiac excitability and enhanced vulnerability to hypoxic insults (20); inhibition of protein synthesis in the liver and increases in levels of transaminase activity (41); and altered behavioral and clinical pathologic parameters following experimental infection of surgical wounds (3). In addition, rodents with streptozotocin-induced diabetes mellitus are more susceptible to *P. aeruginosa* infection (17). Natural infection of laboratory rodents could alter research studies involving the cardiopulmonary, dermal, enterohepatic, lymphoreticular, nervous, and respiratory systems.

Diagnosis and control
Diagnosis of *P. aeruginosa* infection is by culture and identification of characteristic colony morphology. Given the ubiquitous nature of *P. aeruginosa,* it is not practical to attempt to eliminate this organism from, or prevent its entry into, conventional animal facilities. To prevent buildup of the organism in the immediate environment of the facility, it is important to practice high standards of husbandry through such practices as frequent water bottle changes or flushing of automatic watering systems. Where the need exists to house immune-compromised animals under barrier conditions, autoclaving all cage, feed, and water stocks, and preventing contamination from the caretakers, should prevent entry of the organism. In addition, acidification or chlorination of water will keep infections in immune-compromised animals to a minimum. Animals showing clinical signs may be treated with antibiotics. However, at that point they are likely of limited value as research animals, and antibiotic treatment itself may alter host physiology (53) or paradoxically increase pathogen virulence (18).

Salmonella enterica

Agent
Salmonella enterica serotype Enteritidis and the roughly 1,500 serotypes of that species are gram-negative, non-endospore-forming bacteria that colonize the intestinal tracts of a wide variety of host animals. The primary importance of *Salmonella* serotypes is as zoonotic agents and as pathogens in immuno-compromised mice and rats.

Epidemiology
Salmonella serotype Typhimurium is the most common serotype infecting laboratory rodents, although the prevalence of asymptomatic carriers is unknown but likely low. Transmission is by ingestion of contaminated feed ingredients and water, and contact with contaminated bedding and animal facility personnel (25).

Clinical signs
Reports of natural outbreaks of disease are rare in the literature, likely because most infections are asymptomatic in normal hosts. When clinical effects are observed, reproduction is most prominently affected, while other signs are nonspecific (18). Diarrhea is an uncommon finding. Many host, pathogen, and environmental factors determine pathologic findings and severity of infection, including host age and genotype; makeup of intestinal flora; nutritional state; immune status; presence of concurrent infections; bacterial serotype; and environmental stressors such as food and water deprivation, temperature, iron deficiency, and experimental manipulations (25). Inbred mouse strains have a wide range of suscepti-

bility to *S. enterica*. Susceptible strains include DBA/1, BALB/c, C57BL/6, C3H/HeJ, and 129SV. Relatively resistant strains include C3H/HeN, A/J, and DBA/2. Susceptibility is determined by at least three distinct genetic loci (1).

Pathology
Following ingestion, *S. enterica* colonizes and invades the mucosa and Peyer's patches in the distal ileum (27). From those sites the organism reaches the mesenteric lymph nodes and gains access to the vascular system, to be distributed throughout the body. Lesion development depends on distribution of the pathogen. Organs most commonly colonized include the terminal small intestine and the large intestine, lymph nodes, liver, and spleen. Hallmarks of the infection include local hyperemia, focal necrosis, and pyogranulomatous inflammation, consistent with septicemic disease; and also in the intestine, crypt epithelial hyperplasia (29). Immunodeficient rodents are more severely affected (34). Numerous virulence factors have been identified, including LPS, enterotoxins, and fimbriae (35, 36, 38). Concerning the latter, there appears to be a synergistic effect of the four known fimbrial operons, *lpf, pef, fim,* and *agf,* on bacterial colonization and development of disease, and therefore on virulence (40).

A combination of innate and acquired immune mechanisms control infection with *S. enterica* (23). For example, in the preimmune phase of infection, neutrophils inactivate organisms implanting in the liver and spleen, control the subsequent proliferation of *S. enterica* in those organs, and prevent dissemination of the pathogen to other sites (5). IFN-γ (30) and TGF-β (8) appear also to be involved in the early phase of infection, while IFN-γ may also contribute to pathology in septic shock (14). Later, bacterial clearance is mediated by CD4$^+$ T cells with a subsequent humoral response and, to a lesser extent, CD8$^+$ cells (2, 15, 23, 24); and is regulated in part by the H-2 complex. TNF-α and IL-18 are also involved in immunity, although their phases of action are incompletely known (7, 20). IL-18 is likely involved in neutrophil accumulation (28).

Interference with research
Reported interference of *Salmonella* serotypes with research includes induced resistance or increased mortality due to copathogen infection, suppression of growth of transplantable tumors, reduced blood glucose and hepatic enzyme levels, reduced intestinal enzyme levels (25); progressive loss of CD4$^+$ T cells, accelerated T-cell apoptosis, loss of accessory molecules on macrophages (12); and increased rates of crypt cell proliferation resulting in substantial growth of the small intestine (26). Interestingly, infection with *S. enterica* serotype Typhimurium delayed the course of autoimmune disease in (NZB $\times$ NZW) F1 mice, likely through induction of polyreactive antibodies (21). In addition to the changes observed with infection, there is a large body of literature concerning the effects of *Salmonella* lipopolysaccharide and other cellular components, on mouse and/or rat systems under experimental, and often in vitro, conditions. These effects include mitogenic activity (37); stimulation of cytokine production (4); enhancement of microbial invasion (17); lung damage and decreased circulating leukocyte counts (31); recruitment of neutrophils to the lung, likely due to the chemoattractant properties of macrophage-inflammatory protein 2 (MIP-2) (13); induction of vasodilation of isolated rat skeletal muscle arterioles (10); decreased amino acid incorporation into proteins (16); altered guanine nucleotide regulatory (G) protein function (19); activation of the nuclear transcription factor κB and expression of E-selectin messenger RNA in hepatocytes, Kupffer cells, and endothelial cells (6); mortality in neonates and stimulation of adherent splenic cell thromboxane (TX)B2, IL-6, and nitrite production (3); altered development of the hypothalamic-pituitary-adrenal axis with long-term effects on stress responses (33); al-

tered glucose metabolism (11); increased expression of Mac-1 (CD11b/CD18) adhesion glycoproteins on neutrophils (42); increased calcitonin gene-related peptide (CGRP) and neuropeptide Y (NPY) levels in plasma (41); induction of reactive oxygen species which may affect enterocyte lipid peroxidation and viability (22); induction of immunosuppressive NK cells (32); and altered liver levels of 1,2-diacylglycerol and ceramide (39). It remains to be discerned which of these latter observations extend to the mouse or rat infected with *S. enterica*. Mice and/or rats infected with *S. enterica* serve as models of enteritis (27), typhoid fever, and other septicemic diseases (9). Clearly, natural infection of mice or rats with *S. enterica* has the potential to complicate a wide variety of studies involving several body systems, including the cardiovascular, endocrine, enterohepatic, hematopoietic, lymphoreticular, reproductive, and respiratory systems.

Diagnosis and control
Diagnosis of *S. enterica* infection is by culture on agar plates after enrichment in selenite broth. While antibiotic regimens effective against salmonellosis have been developed, their widespread use in the laboratory animal facility setting is neither practical, nor likely to effect complete eradication of the organism. Control includes strict adherence to good husbandry practices. Because *S. enterica* is zoonotic, persons working with infected or potentially infected animals should be instructed to exercise a high degree of personal hygiene.

Staphylococcus aureus

Agent
Staphylococcus aureus is a gram-positive, coagulase-positive coccus that commonly inhabits the skin, upper respiratory tract, and lower digestive tract of many animals, including laboratory rodents.

Epidemiology
S. aureus is most often a commensal organism. In fact, it can easily be recovered from the skin and mucus membranes of many animals, including rats and mice. Transmission is direct, and entry into the body is by breaks in normal barriers.

Clinical signs
Disease caused by *S. aureus* is uncommon. When it does occur, it frequently occurs following physiologic changes in the host (e.g., stress, immune suppression). A variety of clinical presentations have been reported in rats and mice. These include tail lesions, ulcerative dermatitis, and traumatic pododermatitis in rats; and facial abscesses, ulcerative dermatitis, preputial gland abscesses, and penile self-mutilation in mice (11, 20).

Pathology
The hallmark of *S. aureus* infection is suppurative inflammation, with abscess formation in virtually any organ. Most commonly, infection occurs in the skin and subcutaneous tissues, but may also be found in the upper airways, lungs, conjunctiva, and other tissues. Lesions are more severe in immune-deficient hosts. For example, the iNOS-deficient mouse is more susceptible to disease than immune-competent mice (17). In addition, the genetic background of various inbred strains of mice may influence outcome of infection. For example, IL-4 appears to be protective in 129SV mice, but detrimental in C57BL/6 mice (14). In wound infections, *S. aureus* may act synergistically with other pathogens such as *P. aeruginosa* (12). Immunity to *S. aureus* is primarily through complement-mediated killing by neutrophils. Cellular recognition of *S. aureus* is through toll-like receptors (24). Cell-mediated immunity may also be important, and may secondarily contribute to the pathogenesis of some lesions. Nitric oxide (18), INF-γ, TNF, and IL-6 (19) are induced during infection. Interestingly, female and castrated male CD-1 mice are more susceptible

to certain strains of *S. aureus,* suggesting a hormonal influence on resistance (27).

Interference with research
S. aureus produces several biologically active products, including hemolysins, leukocidins, nuclease, coagulase, lipase, hyaluronidase, exotoxins, collagen-binding proteins, protein A, and enterotoxins (25). Many of these may be degraded by phagocytic cells into other active products (9). The effects of these products and their metabolites are numerous. The following list is not exhaustive and includes cell lysis (13); increases in pulmonary microvascular permeability (16, 21); contractile dysfunction (3, 22); shock and multiple organ failure (7); epidermolysis (1); and induction of excess sleep, fever, cytokines indicative of a Th1 response, and IL-1 receptor antagonist (9, 23). Staphylococcal enterotoxins have been termed superantigens on the basis of their ability to stimulate polyclonal proliferative responses of murine and human T lymphocytes and in other ways alter immune responses (2, 6, 8, 10, 28). In addition, infection with *S. aureus* has been shown to alter behavior in open-field testing. Infected rats have alterations in plasma fibrinogen, serum glucose, total leukocyte counts, and wound histology scores (5, 15). Lastly, in vitro studies have shown that *S. aureus* induces high levels of IL-6 and IL-12 production (4) and apoptosis (26) in cultured osteoblasts. Clearly, natural infection of laboratory mice and rats could compromise a variety of studies involving multiple body systems, most prominently the dermal, lymphoreticular, and respiratory systems; and alter numerous physiologic parameters.

Diagnosis and control
Diagnosis of clinical staphylococcosis is by culture and colony identification. Colonization of conventionally housed rodents is unavoidable. Regardless, caretakers must be fully aware of the role played by good personal hygiene and adherence to standard operating procedures in preventing overwhelming exposure. Individual cases of staphylococcal abscess can usually be successfully treated by draining and application of antibiotic ointment. Hairless strains of mice are prone to *S. aureus* abscess formation secondary to biting. Aggressive animals should be separated from cagemates to decrease the occurrence of abscesses. Natural infection of immunodeficient rodents can be prevented but at great expense by barrier facility housing. However, this may be necessary to prevent infection and to ensure accomplishment of specific research objectives.

Streptococcus pneumoniae

Agent
Streptococcus pneumoniae is a gram-positive diplococcus. More than 80 strains, grouped by capsular type, have been reported.

Epidemiology
The current prevalence of *S. pneumoniae* in animal colonies is unknown, but is likely high. Transmission is primarily by aerosol from infected humans. The organism is considered a commensal under most conditions, although host strain susceptibility differences have been reported (9). Typically, a carrier state is established in the nasal passages and middle ears.

Clinical signs
Clinical signs are uncommon, although natural outbreaks of disease have been reported (6). When present, clinical signs are nonspecific and may include dyspnea, weight loss, hunched posture, and snuffling (6).

Pathology
Infection begins in a bronchopulmonary segment and spreads centrifugally (6). The infection spreads from the lung to the pleura, pericardium, and by septicemic spread, to the rest of the body. The affected lung is first edematous, then becomes consolidated and eventually cleared of cellular debris (15). There may be suppurative or fibrinous lesions throughout the respiratory tract and adjacent structures. These most commonly include

suppurative rhinitis and otitis media, but may include similar changes in and around the deeper tissues of the respiratory tract. In this regard, pus formation is a common sequela to streptococcal infection, particularly at mucocutaneous junctions or serosal surfaces. Septicemia may result in suppurative lesion establishment in virtually any organ, with death a common sequela. Mice deficient for the toll-like receptor 2 are highly susceptible to *S. pneumoniae* meningitis because of reduced bacterial clearing and enhanced inflammation (4). Athymic mice are not more susceptible to disease (14). Virulence is related to several bacterial components, among them pneumolysin, a multifunctional toxin with distinct cytolytic and complement-activating activities (3, 13).

Host immunity is primarily humoral (2, 11), with considerable help from the complement and mononuclear phagocytic systems, C-reactive protein (7), TNF-α (8), and pulmonary surfactant (10). IL-10 production is induced following *S. pneumoniae* infection and attenuates the proinflammatory cytokine response within the lungs, hampers effective clearance of the infection, and shortens survival (12). Mouse strains differing in their tendency to favor Th1 versus Th2 cellular responses do not differ in their clinical response to *S. pneumoniae* infection (5).

Interference with research
Rats and mice experimentally infected with *S. pneumoniae* serve as models of several human disease conditions. Natural or experimental infections of laboratory rats and mice with *S. pneumoniae* have been shown to alter hepatic metabolism, serum biochemical levels, blood pH and electrolytes, thyroid function, and respiratory parameters (6), and to induce production of nuclear factor-κB in lung lavage cells (1); and they could be expected to interfere with a variety of studies depending on bacterial distribution following septicemic spread. Organ systems likely to be affected include the cardiovascular, enterohepatic, lymphoreticular, and respiratory systems.

Diagnosis and control
Diagnosis of *S. pneumoniae* infection is by culture. While individual or small numbers of clinical cases may be treated with antibiotics, widespread usage of antibiotics will limit animal losses but are unlikely to eradicate the pathogen. Prevention of disease involves strict adherence to sound husbandry standard operating procedures (SOPs). The cost of eliminating the organism from colonies must be evaluated in light of the intended use of the animals. Personnel working with potentially infected laboratory animals should be informed that *S. pneumoniae* is zoonotic, and therefore, strict adherence to personal hygiene is warranted.

FUNGI

Pneumocystis carinii

Agent
Pneumocystis carinii was recently reclassified as a fungus (39). Using a variety of parameters, recent studies have demonstrated the existence of multiple strains, differing in host specificity (4, 24, 27, 35, 36, 41).

Epidemiology
P. carinii is a common inhabitant of the respiratory tracts of laboratory mice and rats. It is a pathogen only under conditions of induced or inherent immune deficiency. Transmission is by inhalation of infective cysts (38). Placental transmission does not occur (17). Host strain and gender may affect susceptibility to infection (20).

Clinical signs
Clinical signs are absent in immunecompetent animals. Infection has been detected and clinical signs induced following several weeks of corticosteroid administration (40). Clinical signs in immunosuppressed or immunodeficient mice and rats include wasting, rough hair coat, dyspnea, cyanosis, and death (26).

Pathology
P. carinii establishes in the lungs. In general, no lesions are observed. However, pathologic changes occur in the lungs of mice and rats lacking an adequate immune system. In these animals, gross changes include enlarged, dark, and rubbery lungs. Microscopic changes include alveolar septal thickening and alveolar filling with foamy, eosinophilic material consisting of organisms, dead host cells, serum protein, and pulmonary surfactant (11, 12, 13). Pneumonia may be exacerbated by the presence of coinfecting pneumotropic pathogens (33). The attachment of *P. carinii* to lung cells may play a role in the pathophysiology of *P. carinii* pneumonia (1) and may be enhanced by surfactant-associated protein-A (SP-A) (43). Immunity is age related (14); is by both humoral and cell-mediated mechanisms, with $CD4^+$ cells, macrophages, and neutrophils having major direct or indirect roles in killing organisms (3, 5, 16, 19, 22, 28, 34, 44); and involves a network of inflammatory events (6). Glycoprotein A is the immunodominant antigen of *P. carinii* (15).

Interference with research
Under conditions of asymptomatic infection, it is likely that *P. carinii* has minimal if any impact on host physiology. Experimentally, *P. carinii* has been demonstrated to alter alveolar capillary membrane permeability (45) and uptake of tracheally administered compounds (25); to elevate levels of arachidonic acid metabolites (8), SP-A (29), TNF (18), IL-1 (10), IL-6 (9), and other cytokines (44); induce nitrite production by pulmonary macrophages (37); and inhibit lung surfactant protein B expression (7). It must be kept in mind that most of these studies were conducted in immune-compromised animals. It is not known to what extent similar physiologic alterations might occur in naturally infected, asymptomatic animals. In addition, in vitro studies have shown *P. carinii* glycoprotein A inhibits surfactant phospholipid secretion by rat alveolar type II cells (23). Mice and rats have been used as models of opportunistic human *P. carinii* pneumonia (2, 21, 30, 31). Infected mice and rats are likely to develop severe pneumocystosis following immune suppression and will be rendered unsuitable for most experimental purposes, especially those involving the lymphoreticular and respiratory systems.

Diagnosis and control
Historically, diagnosis of pneumocystosis has been accomplished by special staining of pulmonary tissue sections or exudates, or by serologic methods (42). More recently, PCR has been used to detect *P. carinii* DNA in lungs and other tissues (32). There is no effective antimicrobial therapy for eradicating *P. carinii* from rodent colonies. Control is generally not practiced, since *P. carinii* is nearly ubiquitous and does not cause disease in immune-competent animals. Exclusion of the organism from immune-deficient animals would require cesarean rederivation and barrier maintenance.

PARASITES

Acariasis (mite infestation)

Agents
While many species of mites infest wild rodents (1), only three species of nonburrowing mites are commonly found on laboratory mice and rats. *Myobia musculi* and *Myocoptes musculinus* infest mice, and *Radfordia ensifera* infests rats. Mice are much more commonly infested than are rats.

Epidemiology
Despite marked improvements in laboratory animal facilities and husbandry practices, mite infestation remains problematic. Life cycles of all three mites are direct, with all stages (egg, nymph, and adult) present on the host. Consequently, hairless mice are not susceptible. Life cycles require roughly 3 weeks for completion. Transmission is by direct contact. Once a facility is infested, eradication of the parasites is achievable but labor-intensive.

Clinical signs
Clinical signs vary in severity depending on host factors and mite species. Among mice, C57BL/6 and related strains are most susceptible to severe disease because of severe type 1 hypersensitivity reactions (6). *M. musculi* is considered the more pathogenic of the three common species because it alone feeds on skin secretions and interstitial fluid (but not on blood), while *M. musculinus* and *R. ensifera* feed more superficially. Infestation may be asymptomatic, or may cause wasting; scruffiness; pruritus; patchy alopecia, which may be extensive; accumulation of fine bran-like material, mostly over affected areas; self-trauma to the point of excoriation or amputation; and secondary pyoderma (2, 4). Lesions are most common on the dorsum, primarily on the back of the neck and interscapular region.

Pathology
Pathologic changes include hyperkeratosis, erythema, mast cell infiltration, ulcerative dermatitis, splenic lymphoid and lymph node hyperplasia, and eventual secondary amyloidosis (3, 4).

Interference with research
Mite infestation has reportedly caused secondarily amyloidosis; altered behavior (6); selective increases in serum IgG1, IgE, and IgA, and depletion of IgM and IgG3; lymphocytopenia; granulocytosis; increased production of IL-4; and decreased IL-2 (3, 4, 5). These immunologic changes are consistent with a Th-2 type response, with marked systemic consequences (3). Natural infestation of laboratory rodents could interfere with a variety of study types, most notably those involving the dermal and lymphoreticular systems, but also those studies in which behavioral or nutritional parameters are measured.

Diagnosis and control
Diagnosis of mite infestation is accomplished by examination of the pelage for mites. Of course this is more successful in animals with darkly colored coats. Alternatively, diagnosis may be achieved by placing a recently euthanized animal on a sheet of black paper and placing it in the refrigerator for a few minutes. As the carcass cools, the mites will abandon the carcass and can be observed on the dark paper. Treatment of an existing infestation is by topical treatment with ivermectin (8), combined with rigorous cleansing of the animal room, the caging, and all items coming in contact with caging; and restriction of entry into the facility. Treatment of transgenic or inbred mice with ivermectin should be attempted cautiously, since toxicity has been reported in some strains of mice (7). Animals should always be certified mite-free prior to entry into the facility.

Encephalitozoon cuniculi

Agent
Encephalitozoon cuniculi is a microsporidian protozoan parasite infecting a wide range of hosts, including laboratory mice and rats. At least three strains have been identified on the basis of host specificity and other criteria (5).

Epidemiology
Prevalence remains high in many rabbitries, and rabbits may serve as a source of infection for mice and rats (8). In contrast, prevalence is low in modern rodent facilities. The primary significance of *E. cuniculi* in laboratory rodents is as a contaminant of transplantable tumors (8). In addition to infected tumors, transmission is by exposure to infectious urine. Following ingestion, sporoplasm from infectious spores gains entrance to host intestinal epithelium, where multiplication occurs. Continued multiplication results in eventual host cell rupture, with dissemination to other organs, including brain, kidneys, liver, and lungs (8).

Clinical signs
Infection is usually asymptomatic in immunocompetent rodents.

Pathology
Mouse strains differ in susceptibility to infection, with C57BL/6, DBA/1, and 129J being

highly susceptible; C57BL/10, DBA/2, and AKR exhibiting intermediate susceptibility; and BALB/c, A/J, and SJL being relatively resistant (8). In contrast to immunocompetent mice, athymic (nu/nu) and other immune-deficient mice experience high mortality with infection (4, 7). Lesions are most commonly found in the kidneys and brain. In the kidneys, lesions consist of intracellular parasites in the renal tubular epithelium and inflammatory changes, with eventual focal destruction of tubules and replacement by fibrous connective tissue, resulting in pitting of the renal surface (8). In the brain, lesions consist of meningoencephalitis. In rats, but not in mice, there is also multifocal granulomatous inflammation (8). Immunity is primarily cellular, with both $CD4^+$ and $CD8^+$ T cells serving essential roles in controlling infection (2). In addition, macrophage microbicidal activity is important and may involve nitrite (NO_2) (3, 7).

Interference with research
Infection with *E. cuniculi* may cause very subtle changes in host physiology. These may include transient increases in NK cell activity, hepatosplenomegaly with ascites, altered brain and kidney cytoarchitecture, altered host responses to transplanted tumors, reduced cellular and humoral responses to a variety of immunogens (8), and induction of cytokine production (1). *E. cuniculi* infection of mice is used as a model of human microsporidiosis (9). Natural infection of laboratory mice and rats would compromise studies involving the enterohepatic, lymphoreticular, nervous, and urinary systems.

Diagnosis and control
Historically, diagnosis of encephalitozoonosis has been accomplished by demonstrating spores in stained urine samples or tissue sections, by finding typical histologic lesions, and by using serologic methods (6, 8). There is no effective antimicrobial treatment that will successfully eradicate *E. cuniculi* from an animal facility. Although *E. cuniculi* may be transmitted transplacentally, cesarean rederivation, with serologic testing of offspring, is effective in eradicating the pathogen. Rodents should not be housed near rabbits, unless the rabbits are known to be free of *E. cuniculi*.

Giardia muris

Agent
Giardia muris is a flagellated intestinal protozoan. The genus *Giardia* is the only genus known to include parasites possessing a median body. This is a morphologic feature that assists in identification of the parasite, and appears as a "claw hammer" under light microscopy. Two median bodies may be present in *G. muris*. The median body appears to function as a repository of cytoskeletal elements.

Epidemiology
Infections are occasionally detected in laboratory rodent colonies. Strains of *G. muris*-infected mice and rats may be host specific (7). The life cycle is direct. Infectious, environmentally resistant cysts are passed in the feces. Excystation occurs following ingestion. The minimum infectious dose for a mouse is approximately 10 cysts (18). Shortly after excystment, trophozoites divide longitudinally and colonize the mucosal surface of the proximal small intestine, adhering to columnar cells near the bases of intestinal villi, and moving within the mucus layer on the mucosa (10).

Clinical signs
Most infections are asymptomatic. When apparent, clinical signs are nonspecific and include weight loss, stunted growth, rough hair coat, and enlarged abdomen. In athymic or otherwise immunocompromised hosts, clinical signs may be more severe, and may include diarrhea and death, and cyst shedding may be prolonged (2, 13).

Pathology
Following ingestion and excystation, infection establishes in the small intestine, principally in the midjejunum. Pathologic changes include villous blunting; increased numbers of intraepithelial lymphocytes, goblet cells, and mast

cells; and alterations in intestinal disaccharidase content (21). Strain differences in susceptibility have been observed. Resistant mouse strains include DBA/2, B10.A, C57BL/6, and SJL/2. In contrast, relatively more susceptible strains include BALB/c, C3H/He, A/J, and Crl:ICR (10, 20, 21). The bases for these differences are unknown, although both MHC and non-MHC genes appear to influence the outcome of primary *G. muris* infections (19). In addition, male mice shed cysts in their feces longer than female mice do and trophozoites are present in their intestines for a longer period than in female mice (3). Immune responses to *G. muris* include both cellular and humoral mechanisms, in addition to innate components such as mast cells, macrophages, and rarely, eosinophils (6, 11, 12, 16, 21). IgA plays a central role in clearance of *G. muris* (8). Cytokines produced by stimulated immune cells removed from mice at different stages of experimental infection are indicative of a Th2-type response (5). However, this is not essential for protection (16). Mechanisms responsible for elimination of a primary infection may not be identical with those required to resist a secondary infection (5, 17).

Interference with research
Reported effects of *G. muris* include alterations in intestinal mucosal immune responses (9) and disaccharidase levels (4). The latter may be mediated, at least in part, by T lymphocytes (14). Additionally, there may be transient reduction in immunoresponsiveness to sheep erythrocytes (1), increased severity of concurrent infections in athymic (*nu/nu*) mice (2), increased permeability of the small intestinal epithelial barrier due to changes in tight junctions (15), and in chronic cases, hypogammaglobulinemia (16) and jejunal brush-border microvillus alterations (14). Natural infection of laboratory mice and rats with *G. muris* could interfere with studies involving the enterohepatic and lymphoreticular systems.

Diagnosis and control
Diagnosis of giardiasis is accomplished by light microscopic examination of intestinal content or fecal wet mounts, and following fecal flotation. Control is usually not attempted because of the generally nonpathogenic nature of the infection. For studies where *Giardia*-free mice are needed, eradication can be accomplished by cesarean rederivation and barrier maintenance. Metronidazole may be useful for controlling clinical infections but will not eradicate the pathogen (1).

Oxyurids (pinworms)

Agents
Pinworms commonly infecting laboratory rodents include the rat pinworm *Syphacia muris* and in mice, *Syphacia obvelata* and *Aspiculuris tetraptera*. Both *S. obvelata* and *S. muris* are capable of infecting humans.

Epidemiology
Prevalence of infection with rodent pinworms remains high (10, 12, 13), even in well-managed animal colonies. Prevalence is generally greater than 50% for rat pinworms, and less than 50% for mouse pinworms. Life cycles are direct, with adult worms inhabiting the cecum and colon. Eggs are deposited in the perianal region of the host (*Syphacia* spp.) or are excreted with the feces (*A. tetraptera*). The eggs are very light and will aerosolize, resulting in widespread environmental contamination. Embryonated eggs are infective to another rodent and can survive for extended periods at room temperature.

Clinical signs
Pinworm burden in an infected rodent population is a function of age, sex, and host immune status (4). In enzootically infected colonies, weanling animals develop the greatest parasite loads, males are more heavily parasitized than females, and pinworm numbers diminish with increasing age of the host. Laboratory-adapted strains of mice appear to be more resistant to infection when compared with wild mice (4). Athymic (*nu/nu*) mice are reportedly more susceptible to infection (6). While infections are usually subclinical, rectal prolapse, intussusception, fecal impaction,

poor weight gain, and rough hair coat have been reported in heavily infected rodents, although generally without adequate exclusion of other pathogens (10).

Pathology
Light parasite burdens are without pathologic lesions. In contrast, very heavy parasite loads may lead to catarrhal enteritis, liver granulomas, and perianal irritation. Immunity to oxyuriasis is mostly humoral, as for many other helminthiases. In this regard, *Syphacia*-specific antibodies have been demonstrated in pinworm-infected mice (15).

Interference with research
There are few reports documenting the effects of pinworms on research. For this reason, many believe that pinworm infections are of no consequence to research efforts. However, this may not always be the case. In one study, for example, pinworm infection resulted in significantly higher antibody production to sheep erythrocytes (15). Others report impaired intestinal electrolyte transport (7), accelerated development of the hepatic monooxygenase system (9), decreased weight gain (16), reduced occurrence of adjuvant-induced arthritis (11), and modification of induction of neonatal autoimmune disease and pathogenic Th2 memory responses (1). In humans, *Enterobius vermicularis* has been associated with lower intelligence quotients than for uninfected peers (2). It is not known whether rodent pinworms affect learning ability of their hosts. Interestingly, McNair and Timmons (8) reported that mice infected with *A. tetraptera* and *S. obvelata* exhibited less exploratory behavior than did uninfected controls. This finding has not been supported by the work of others using rats infected with *S. muris* (17). So, while many consider pinworm infection irrelevant in laboratory rodents, specific research goals may justify the eradication of pinworms from an animal colony. Specifically, studies involving the dermal, enterohepatic, lymphoreticular, and musculoskeletal systems may be adversely affected.

Diagnosis and control
Diagnosis of oxyuriasis is by examination of clear cellophane tape, touched to the perianal area and then placed on a microscope slide (*Syphacia* spp.) or by examination of coverslips following fecal flotation (*A. tetraptera*). The preferred method of eradication involves feeding fenbendazole-medicated feed (5). Other anthelmintic treatments may be equally successful, although more labor intensive (14). Those intending to use treated rats in behavioral studies should consider foregoing fenbendazole treatment, and opt for another effective anthelmintic. Fenbendazole has been shown to alter behavior in offspring of dams treated for pinworms (3). Eradication efforts are facilitated by strict adherence to sanitation protocols.

Spironucleus muris

Agent
Spironucleus muris (formerly *Hexamita muris*) is a second flagellated protozoan. Host-specific strains of *S. muris* have been identified (8).

Epidemiology
The prevalence of *S. muris* is unknown, but in the author's experience, appears to be high. The biology of *S. muris* appears to be much like that of *G. muris*; however, because of the inability to culture *S. muris*, considerably less is known about this organism. Infectious cysts are passed in the feces. The minimum infective dose for a mouse is one cyst (9). Following ingestion, excystation occurs and trophozoites colonize the crypts of Lieberkuhn in the small intestine. Inbred mouse strains, differing in major histocompatibility type, differ in the magnitude and course of infection, with 129/J mice shedding significantly fewer cysts than BALB/c, ByJ, C3H/HeJ, and DBA/1J mice (1).

Clinical signs
Infections with *S. muris* are asymptomatic in immunocompetent adult mice and rats. However, weanling and immunodeficient mice may develop clinical disease. Several investi-

TABLE 2-1. Body systems known or likely to be affected by the pathogen indicated

Pathogen	Cardio-vascular	Dermal	Endocrine	Entero-hepatic	Hema-topoietic	Lympho-reticular	Musculo-skeletal	Nervous	Reproductive	Respiratory	Urinary
Adenoviruses	X		X	X	X	X		X			X
Cytomegalovirus	X		X	X	X					X	
Ectromelia virus		X		X	X	X					X
H-1 virus							X	X	X		
Kilham rat virus	X			X	X	X		X	X		X
Lactate dehydrogenase-elevating virus				X	X	X		X			
Lymphocytic choriomeningitis virus	X			X	X	X		X			X
Minute virus of mice				X	X	X		X		X	
Mouse hepatitis virus			X	X	X	X		X			
Mouse mammary tumor virus						X					
Mouse parvovirus-1				X	X	X					
Mouse rotavirus				X				X			
Mouse thymic virus				X	X	X					
Pneumonia virus of mice					X					X	
Rat rotavirus-like agent				X							
Reovirus-3	X	X		X	X	X					
Sendai virus		X				X			X	X	
Sialodacryoadenitis virus		X		X		X			X	X	
Theiler's murine encephalomyelitis virus				X			X	X			
Cilia-associated respiratory bacillus						X				X	
Citrobacter rodentium				X		X			X		

PATHOGENS OF RATS AND MICE

Clostridium piliforme
Corynebacterium kutscheri
Corynebacterium spp. in athymic mice
Helicobacter spp.
Klebsiella pneumotropica
Mycoplasma pulmonis
Pasteurella pneumotropica
Pseudomonas aeruginosa
Salmonella enterica
Staphylococcus aureus
Streptococcus pneumoniae
Pneumocystis carinii
Acariasis
Encephalitozoon cuniculi
Giardia muris
Oxyurids
Spironucleus muris

gators have reported that young mice may develop diarrhea, dehydration, weight loss, rough hair coat, lethargy, abdominal distension, hunched posture, and may occasionally die (6, 10), although in none of the reported cases were other potential causes for clinical signs adequately excluded.

Pathology

In athymic (*nu/nu*) and lethally irradiated mice, *S. muris* causes severe chronic enteritis and weight loss (5). In severe infections the intestine is reddened and filled with fluid and gas. The crypts are hyperplastic and may be distended with trophozoites, microvilli and villi may be shortened, and enterocyte turnover is increased; inflammation is minimal (6, 10).

Interference with research

A limited number of reports have implicated *S. muris* as a confounding factor in biomedical research. *S. muris* has been shown to increase the severity of copathogen infection (2), increase mortality following cadmium-treatment (4), and alter macrophage function and lymphocyte responsiveness to sheep erythrocytes, mitogens, and tetanus toxoid (3, 6, 7).

Diagnosis and control

Diagnosis of *S. muris* infection is by histologic examination of intestinal sections stained with periodic acid-Schiff, or silver stains; or by light microscopic examination of intestinal content or fecal wet mounts. Phase-contrast microscopy is useful when examining wet mounts, because it allows one to distinguish the cysts of *S. muris* from yeasts. There is no antiprotozoal therapy that completely eliminates *S. muris*. Additionally, it is difficult to find or obtain mice or rats free of *S. muris*. Because the organism is generally considered nonpathogenic, eradication is rarely considered necessary, but can be accomplished with cesarean rederivation and barrier maintenance. When it is necessary to obtain *S. muris*-free animals, potential vendors should be asked to specifically test for the organism prior to shipping.

REFERENCES
INTRODUCTION
1. **Baker, D. G.** 1998. Natural pathogens of laboratory mice, rats, and rabbits and their effects on research. *Clin. Microbiol. Rev.* **11**:231–266.

VIRUSES
Adenoviruses
1. **Blailock, Z. R., E. R. Rabin, and J. L. Melnick.** 1967. Adenovirus endocarditis in mice. *Science* **157**:69–70.
2. **Cauthen, A. N., C. C. Brown, and K. R. Spindler.** 1999. *In vitro* and *in vivo* characterization of a mouse adenovirus type 1 early region 3 null mutant. *J. Virol.* **73**:8640–8646.
3. **Charles, P. C., X. Chen, M. S. Horwitz, and C. F. Brosnan.** 1999a. Differential chemokine induction by the mouse adenovirus type-1 in the central nervous system of susceptible and resistant strains of mice. *J. Neurovirol.* **5**:55–64.
4. **Charles, P. C., J. D. Guida, C. F. Brosnan, and M. S. Horwitz.** 1998. Mouse adenovirus type-1 replication is restricted to vascular endothelium in the CNS of susceptible strains of mice. *Virology* **245**:216–228.
5. **Charles, P. C., K. S. Weber, B. Cipriani, and C. F. Brosnan.** 1999b. Cytokine, chemokine and chemokine receptor mRNA expression in different strains of normal mice: implications for establishment of a Th1/Th2 bias. *J. Neuroimmunol.* **100**:64–73.
6. **Einarsson, O., G. P. Geba, Z. Zhu, M. Landry, and J. A. Elias.** 1996. Interleukin-11: stimulation *in vivo* and *in vitro* by respiratory viruses and induction of airways hyperresponsiveness. *J. Clin. Invest.* **97**:915–924.
7. **Ginder, D. R.** 1964. Increased susceptibility of mice infected with mouse adenoviruses to *Escherichia coli*-induced pyelonephritis. *J. Exp. Med.* **120**:1117–1128.
8. **Guida, J. D., G. Fejer, L. A. Pirofski, C. F. Brosnan, and M. S. Horwitz.** 1995. Mouse adenovirus type 1 causes a fatal hemorrhagic encephalomyelitis in adult C57BL/6 but not BALB/c mice. *J. Virol.* **69**:7674–7681.
9. **Hamelin, C., and G. Lussier.** 1988. Genotypic differences between the mouse adenovirus strains FL and K87. *Experientia* **44**:65–66.
10. **Hartley, J. W., and W. P. Rowe.** 1960. A new mouse virus apparently related to the adenovirus group. *Virology* **11**:645–647.
11. **Hashimoto, K., T. Sugiyama, M. Yoshikawa, and S. Sasaki.** 1970. Intestinal resistance in the experimental enteric infection of mice with a mouse adenovirus. I. Growth of the virus and appearance of a neutralizing substance in the intestinal tract. *Jpn. J. Microbiol.* **14**:381–395.

12. Heck, F. C., Jr., W. C. Sheldon, and C. A. Gleiser. 1972. Pathogenesis of experimentally produced mouse adenovirus infection in mice. *Am. J. Vet. Res.* **33**:841–846.
13. Kajon, A. E., C. C. Brown, and K. R. Spindler. 1998. Distribution of mouse adenovirus type 1 in intraperitoneally and intranasally infected adult outbred mice. *J. Virol.* **72**:1219–1223.
14. Kring, S. C., C. S. King, and K. R. Spindler. 1995. Susceptibility and signs associated with mouse adenovirus type 1 infection of adult outbred Swiss mice. *J. Virol.* **69**:8084–8088.
15. Kring, S. C., and K. R. Spindler. 1996. Lack of effect of mouse adenovirus type 1 infection on cell surface expression of major histocompatibility complex class I antigens. *J. Virol.* **70**:5495–5502.
16. Margolis, G., L. Kilham, and E. M. Hoenig. 1974. Experimental adenovirus infection of the mouse adrenal gland. I. Light microscopic observations. *Am. J. Pathol.* **75**:363–372.
17. Markine-Goriaynoff, D., J. T. van der Logt, C. Truyens, T. D. Nguyen, F. W. Heessen, G. Bigaignon, Y. Carlier, and J. P. Coutelier. 2000. IFN-γ-independent IgG2a production in mice infected with viruses and parasites. *Int. Immunol.* **12**:223–230.
18. National Research Council. 1991. *Infectious Diseases of Mice and Rats: a Report of the Institute of Laboratory Animal Resources Committee on Infectious Diseases of Mice and Rats.* National Academy Press, Washington, D.C.
19. Smith, K., C. C. Brown, and K. R. Spindler. 1998. The role of mouse adenovirus type 1 early region 1A in acute and persistent infections in mice. *J. Virol.* **72**:5699–5706.
20. Spindler, K. R., L. Fang, M. L. Moore, G. N. Hirsch, C. C. Brown, and A. Kajon. 2001 SJL/J mice are highly susceptible to infection by mouse adenovirus type 1. *J. Virol.* **75**:12039–12046.
21. Takeuchi, A., and K. Hashimoto. 1976. Electron microscopy study of experimental enteric adenovirus infection in mice. *Infect. Immun.* **13**:569–580.
22. Umehara, K., M. Hirakawa, and K. Hashimoto. 1984. Fluctuation of antiviral resistance in the intestinal tracts of nude mice infected with a mouse adenovirus. *Microbiol. Immunol.* **28**:679–690.
23. Van der Veen, J., and A. Mes. 1973. Experimental infection with mouse adenovirus in adult mice. *Arch. Gesamte Virusforsch.* **42**:235–241.

Cytomegalovirus

1. Berencsi, K., V. Endresz, D. Klurfeld, L. Kari, D. Kritchevsky, and E. Gonczol. 1998. Early atherosclerotic plaques in the aorta following cytomegalovirus infection of mice. *Cell. Adhes. Commun.* **5**:39–47.
2. Bolger, G., N. Lapeyre, M. Rheaume, P. Kibler, C. Bousquet, M. Garneau, and M. Cordingley. 1999. Acute murine cytomegalovirus infection: a model for determining antiviral activity against CMV induced hepatitis. *Antivir. Res.* **44**:155–165.
3. Booth, T. W., A. A. Scalzo, C. Carrello, P. A. Lyons, H. E. Farrell, G. R. Singleton, and G. R. Shellam. 1993. Molecular and biological characterization of new strains of murine cytomegalovirus isolated from wild mice. *Arch. Virol.* **132**:209–220.
4. Bruggeman, C. A., H. Meijer, P. H. J. Dormans, W. M. H. Debie, G. E. L. M. Grauls, and C. P. A. van Boven. 1982. Isolation of a cytomegalovirus-like agent from wild rats. *Arch. Virol.* **73**:231–241.
5. Cassell, H. S., P. Price, S. D. Olver, and G. C. Yeoh. 1998. The association between murine cytomegalovirus induced hepatitis and the accumulation of oval cells. *Int. J. Exp. Pathol.* **79**:433–441.
6. Cavanaugh, V. J., L. G. Guidotti, and F. V. Chisari. 1998. Inhibition of hepatitis B virus replication during adenovirus and cytomegalovirus infections in transgenic mice. *J. Virol.* **72**:2630–2637.
7. Collins, T., C. Pomeroy, and M. C. Jordan. 1993. Detection of latent cytomegalovirus DNA in diverse organs of mice. *J. Infect. Dis.* **168**:725–729.
8. Cretney, E., M. A. Degli-Esposti, E. H. Densley, H. E. Farrell, N. J. Davis-Poynter, and M. J. Smyth. 1999. m144, a murine cytomegalovirus (MCMV)-encoded major histocompatibility complex class I homologue, confers tumor resistance to natural killer cell-mediated rejection. *J. Exp. Med.* **190**:435–444.
9. Dangler, C. A., S. F. Baker, M. Kariuki Njenga, and S. H. Chia. 1995. Murine cytomegalovirus-associated arteritis. *Vet. Pathol.* **32**:127–133.
10. Duan, Y., and S. S. Atherton. 1996. Immunosuppression induces transcription of murine cytomegalovirus glycoprotein H in the eye and at non-ocular sites. *Arch. Virol.* **141**:411–423.
11. Fairweather, D., C. M. Lawson, A. J. Chapman, C. M. Brown, T. W. Booth, J. M. Papadimitriou, and G. R. Shellam. 1998. Wild isolates of murine cytomegalovirus induce myocarditis and antibodies that cross-react with virus and cardiac myosin. *Immunology* **94**:263–270.

12. Fleck, M., E. R. Kern, T. Zhou, B. Lang, and J. D. Mountz. 1998. Murine cytomegalovirus induces a Sjogren's syndrome-like disease in C57Bl/6-lpr/lpr mice. *Arthritis Rheum.* **41:**2175–2184.
13. Furrarah, A. M., and C. Sweet. 1994. Studies of the pathogenesis of wild-type virus and six temperature-sensitive mutants of mouse cytomegalovirus. *J. Med. Virol.* **43:**317–330.
14. Goetz, L., and C. Pomeroy. 1996. Impact of prophylactic ganciclovir on bronchoalveolar lavage lymphocyte numbers and phenotypes in murine cytomegalovirus-induced reactivation of *Toxoplasma* pneumonia. *J. Lab. Clin. Med.* **128:**384–391.
15. Griffiths, M. M., C. B. Smith, L. S. Wei, and S. C. Ting-Yu. 1991. Effects of rat cytomegalovirus infection on immune functions in rats with collagen induced arthritis. *J. Rheumatol.* **18:**497–504.
16. Hamano, S., H. Yoshida, H. Takimoto, K. Sonoda, K. Osada, X. He, Y. Minamishima, G. Kimura, and K. Nomoto. 1998. Role of macrophages in acute murine cytomegalovirus infection. *Microbiol. Immunol.* **42:**607–616.
17. Hangai, M., Y. Kaneda, H. Tanihara, and Y. Honda. 1996. In vivo gene transfer into the retina mediated by a novel liposome system. *Investig. Ophthalmol. Vis. Sci.* **37:**2678–2685.
18. Huber, B. T., P. N. Hsu, and N. Sutkowski. 1996. Virus-encoded superantigens. *Microbiol. Rev.* **60:**473–482.
19. Inkinen, K., A. Soots, L. Krogerus, C. Bruggeman, J. Ahonen, and I. Lautenschlager. 2002. Cytomegalovirus increases collagen synthesis in chronic rejection in the rat. *Nephrol. Dial. Transplant.* **17:**772–779.
20. Karupiah, G., T. E. Sacks, D. M. Klinman, T. N. Fredrickson, J. W. Hartley, J. H. Chen, and H. C. Morse, III. 1998. Murine cytomegalovirus infection-induced polyclonal B cell activation is independent of $CD4^+$ T cells and CD40. *Virology* **240:**12–26.
21. Kloover, J. S., A. P. Soots, L. A. Krogerus, H. O. Kauppinen, R. J. Loginov, K. L. Holma, C. A. Bruggeman, P. J. Ahonen, and I. T. Lautenschlager. 2000. Rat cytomegalovirus infection in kidney allograft recipients is associated with increased expression of intracellular adhesion molecule-1, vascular adhesion molecule-1, and their ligans leukocyte function antigen-1 and very late antigen-4 in the graft. *Transplantation* **27:**1641–2647.
22. Kloover, J. S., A. E. van den Bogaard, J. G. van Dam, G. E. Grauls, C. Vink, and C. A. Bruggeman. 2002. Persistent rat cytomegalovirus (RCMV) infection of the salivary glands contribute to the anti-RCMV humoral immune response. *Virus Res.* **85:**163–172.
23. Koskinen, P., K. Lemstrom, H. Bruning, M. Daemen, C. Bruggeman, and P. Hayry. 1995. Cytomegalovirus infection induces vascular wall inflammation and doubles arteriosclerotic changes in rat cardiac allografts. *Transplant. Proc.* **27:**574–575.
24. Kosugi, I., H. Kawasaki, Y. Arai, and Y. Tsutsui. 2002. Innate immune responses to cytomegalovirus infection in the developing mouse brain and their evasion by virus-infected neurons. *Am. J. Pathol.* **161:**919–928.
25. Lee, S. H., S. Girard, D. Macina, M. Busa, A. Zafer, A. Belouchi, P. Gros, and S. M. Vidal. 2001. Susceptibility to mouse cytomegalovirus is associated with deletion of an activating natural killer cell receptor of the C-type lectin superfamily. *Nat. Genet.* **28:**42–45.
26. Mitchell, B. M., A. Leung, and J. G. Stevens. 1996. Murine cytomegalovirus DNA in peripheral blood of latently infected mice is detectable only in monocytes and polymorphonuclear leukocytes. *Virology* **223:**198–207.
27. Mori, T., K. Ando, K. Tanaka, Y. Ikeda, and Y. Koga. 1997. Fas-mediated apoptosis of the hematopoietic progenitor cells in mice infected with murine cytomegalovirus. *Blood* **89:**3565–3573.
28. **National Research Council.** 1991. *Infectious Diseases of Mice and Rats: a Report of the Institute of Laboratory Animal Resources Committee on Infectious Diseases of Mice and Rats.* National Academy Press, Washington, D.C.
29. Ninomiya, T., H. Takimoto, G. Matsuzaki, S. Hamano, H. Yoshido, Y. Yoshikai, G. Kimura, and K. Nomoto. 2000. $V\gamma 1^+$ $\gamma\delta$ T cells play protective roles at an early phase of murine cytomegalovirus infection through production of interferon-γ. *Immunology* **99:**187–194.
30. O'Donoghue, H. L., C. M. Lawson, and W. D. Reed. 1990. Autoantibodies to cardiac myosin in mouse cytomegalovirus myocarditis. *Immunology* **71:**20–28.
31. Olver, S. D., and P. Price. 1998. Contrasting phenotypes of liver-infiltrating leucocytes isolated from MCMV-infected BALB/c and C57Bl/6 mice. *Int. J. Exp. Pathol.* **79:**33–46.
32. Osborn, J. E. 1982. Cytomegalovirus and other herpesviruses, p. 267–292. *In* H. L. Foster, H. D. Small, and J. G. Fox (ed.), *The Mouse in Biomedical Research,* vol. II. *Diseases.* Academic Press, New York, N.Y.
33. Palmon, A., S. Tel-or, E. Shai, B. Rager-Zisman, and Y. Burstein. 2000. Development of a highly sensitive quantitative competitive

34. Peacock, C. D., and P. Price. 1999. The role of IL-12 in the control of MCMV is fundamentally different in mice with a retroviral immunodeficiency syndrome (MAIDS). *Immunol. Cell. Biol.* **77**:131–138.
35. Pollock, J. L., and H. W. Virgin, IV. 1995. Latency, without persistence, of murine cytomegalovirus in the spleen and kidney. *J. Virol.* **69**:1762–1768.
36. Price, P., S. D. Olver, M. Silich, T. Z. Nador, S. Yerkovich, and S. G. Wilson. 1996. Adrenalitis and the adrenocortical response of resistant and susceptible mice to acute murine cytomegalovirus infection. *Eur. J. Clin. Invest.* **26**:811–819.
37. Redpath, S., A. Angulo, N. R. Gascoigne, and P. Ghazal. 1999. Murine cytomegalovirus infection down-regulates MHC class II expression on macrophages by induction of IL-10. *J. Immunol.* **162**:6701–6707.
38. Ruzek, M. C., A. H. Miller, S. M. Opal, B. D. Pearce, and C. A. Biron. 1997. Characterization of early cytokine responses and an interleukin (IL)-6-dependent pathway of endogenous glucocorticoid induction during murine cytomegalovirus infection. *J. Exp. Med.* **185**:1185–1192.
39. Shanley, J. D., R. S. Thrall, and S. J. Forman. 1997. Murine cytomegalovirus replication in the lungs of athymic BALB/c nude mice. *J. Infect. Dis.* **175**:309–315.
40. Shinmura, Y., I. Kosugi, M. Keneta, and Y. Tsutsui. 1999. Migration of virus-infected neuronal cells in cerebral slice cultures of developing mouse brains after *in vitro* infection with murine cytomegalovirus. *Acta Neuropathol.* **98**:590–596.
41. Stals, F. S., G. Steinhoff, S. S. Wagenaar, J. P. van Breda Vriesman, A. Haverich, P. Dormans, F. Moeller, and C. A. Bruggeman. 1996. Cytomegalovirus induces interstitial lung disease in allogeneic bone marrow transplant recipient rats independent of acute graft-versus-host response. *Lab. Invest.* **74**:343–352.
42. Tay, C. H., and R. M. Welsh. 1997. Distinct organ-dependent mechanisms for the control of murine cytomegalovirus infection by natural killer cells. *J. Virol.* **71**:267–275.
43. Tsutsui, Y., A. Kashiwai, N. Kawamura, S. Aiba-Masago, and I. Kosugi. 1995. Prolonged infection of mouse brain neurons with murine cytomegalovirus after pre- and perinatal infection. *Arch. Virol.* **140**:1725–1736.
44. Wang, L. L., D. T. Chu, A. O. Dokun, and W. M. Yokoyama. 2000. Inducible expression of the gp49B inhibitory receptor on NK cells. *J. Immunol.* **164**:5215–5220.
45. Ziegler, H., W. Muranyi, H. G. Burgert, E. Kremmer, and U. H. Koszinowski. 2000. The luminal part of the murine cytomegalovirus glycoprotein gp40 catalyzes the retention of MHC class I molecules. *EMBO J.* **19**:870–881.

Ectromelia virus
1. Born, T. L., L. A. Morrison, D. J. Esteban, T. VandenBos, L. G Thebeau, N. Chen, M. K. Spriggs, J. E. Sims, and R. M. Buller. 2000. A poxvirus protein that binds to and inactivates IL-18, and inhibits NK cell response. *J. Immunol.* **164**:3246–3254.
2. Brownstein, D. G., and L. Gras. 1997. Differential pathogenesis of lethal mousepox in congenic DBA/2 mice implicates natural killer cell receptor NKR-P1 in necrotizing hepatitis and the fifth component of complement in recruitment of circulating leukocytes to spleen. *Am. J. Pathol.* **150**:1407–1420.
3. Chen, N., R. M. Buller, E. M. Wall, and C. Upton. 2000. Analysis of host response modifier ORF's of ectromelia virus, the causative agent of mousepox. *Virus Res.* **66**:155–173.
4. Delano, M. L., and D. G. Brownstein. 1995. Innate resistance to lethal mousepox is genetically linked to the NK gene complex on chromosome 6 and correlates with early restriction of virus replication by cells with an NK phenotype. *J. Virol.* **69**:5875–5877.
5. Dick, E. J., Jr., C. L. Kittell, H. Meyer, P. L. Farrar, S. L. Ropp, J. J. Esposito, R. M. L. Buller, H. Neubauer, Y. H. Kang, and A. E. McKee. 1996. Mousepox outbreak in a laboratory mouse colony. *Lab. Anim. Sci.* **46**:602–611.
6. Fenner, F. 1981. Mousepox (Infectious ectromelia): past, present, and future. *Lab. Anim. Sci.* **31**:553–559.
7. Karupiah, G., R. M. Buller, N. Van Rooijen, C. J. Duarte, and J. Chen. 1996. Different roles for CD4$^+$ and CD8$^+$ T lymphocytes and macrophage subsets in the control of a generalized virus infection. *J. Virol.* **70**:8301–8309.
8. Karupiah, G., J. H. Chen, C. F. Nathan, S. Mahalingam, and J. D. MacMickling. 1998. Identification of nitric oxide synthase 2 as an innate resistance locus against ectromelia virus infection. *J. Virol.* **72**:7703–7706.
9. Gierynska, M., F. N. Toka, I. S. Cespedes, A. Schollenberger, E. Malicka, A. Popis, and M. G. Niemialtowski. 2000. Homing studies on distribution of ectromelia (mousepox) virus-specific T cells adoptively transferred into syngeneic H-2d mice: paradigm of lymphocyte migration. *Viral Immunol.* **13**:107–123.

10. **Lipman, N. S., S. Perkins, H. Nguyen, M. Pfeffer, and H. Meyer.** 2000. Mousepox resulting from use of ectromelia virus-contaminated, imported mouse serum. *Comp. Med.* **50:**426–435.
11. **Mossman, K., C. Upton, R. M. Buller, and G. McFadden.** 1995. Species specificity of ectromelia virus and vaccinia virus interferon-γ binding proteins. *Virology* **208:**762–769
12. **Mullbacher, A., P. Waring, R. Tha Hla, T. Tran, S. Chin, T. Stehle, C. Museteanu, and M. M. Simon.** 1999. Granzymes are the essential downstream effector molecules for the control of primary virus infections by cytolytic leukocytes. *Proc. Natl. Acad. Sci. USA* **96:**13950–13955.
13. **National Research Council.** 1991. *Infectious Diseases of Mice and Rats: a Report of the Institute of Laboratory Animal Resources Committee on Infectious Diseases of Mice and Rats.* National Academy Press, Washington, D.C.
14. **Neubauer, H., M. Pfeffer, and H. Meyer.** 1997. Specific detection of mousepox virus by polymerase chain reaction. *Lab. Anim.* **31:**201–205.
15. **Niemialtowski, M. G., I. Spohr de Faundez, M. Gierynska, E. Malicka, F. N. Toka, A. Schollenberger, and A. Popis.** 1994. The inflammatory and immune response to mousepox (infectious ectromelia) virus. *Acta Virol.* **38:**299–307.
16. **Senkevich, T. G., E. V. Koonin, and R. M. Buller.** 1994. A poxvirus protein with a RING zinc finger motif is of crucial importance for virulence. *Virology* **198:**118–128.
17. **Smith, V. P., and N. A. Alcami.** 2000. Expression of secreted cytokine and chemokine inhibitors by ectromelia virus. *J. Virol.* **74:**8460–8471.
18. **Smith, V. P., N. A. Bryant, and A. Alcami.** 2000. Ectromelia, vaccinia and cowpox viruses encode secreted interleukin-18-binding proteins. *J. Gen. Virol.* **81:**1223–1230.
19. **Toka, F. N., M. G. Niemialtowski, I. Spohr de Faundez, and M. Gierynska.** 1996. Cytotoxic T lymphocyte control during ectromelia (mousepox) virus infection: interaction between MHC-restricted cells analyzed by non-radioactive fluorometry. *Acta Virol.* **40:**239–244.

H-1 virus

1. **Besselsen, D. G., C. L. Besch-Williford, D. J. Pintel, C. L. Franklin, R. R. Hook, Jr., and L. K. Riley.** 1995. Detection of H-1 parvovirus and Kilham rat virus by PCR. *J. Clin. Microbiol.* **33:**1699–1703.
2. **Faisst, S., D. Guittard, A. Benner, J. Y. Cesbron, J. R. Schlehofer, J. Rommelaere, and T. Dupressoir.** 1998. Dose-dependent regression of HeLa cell-derived tumours in SCID mice after parvovirus H-1 infection. *Int. J. Cancer* **75:**584–589.
3. **Gripenberg-Lerche, C., and P. Toivanen.** 1993. *Yersinia* associated arthritis in SHR rats: effect of the microbial status of the host. *Ann. Rheum. Dis.* **52:**223–228.
4. **Jacoby, R. O., L. Ball-Goodrich, D. G. Besselsen, M. D. McKisic, L. K. Riley, and A. L. Smith.** 1996. Rodent parvovirus infections. *Lab. Anim. Sci.* **46:**370–380.
5. **Kraft, V., and B. Meyer.** 1990. Seromonitoring in small laboratory animal colonies. A five year survey: 1984–1988. *Z. Verstierkd.* **33:**29–35.
6. **National Research Council.** 1991. *Infectious Diseases of Mice and Rats: a Report of the Institute of Laboratory Animal Resources Committee on Infectious Diseases of Mice and Rats.* National Academy Press, Washington, D.C.
7. **Ohshima, T., M. Iwama, Y. Ueno, F. Sugiyama, T. Nakajima, A. Fukamizu, and K. Yagami.** 1998. Induction of apoptosis *in vitro* and *in vivo* by H-1 parvovirus infection. *J. Gen. Virol.* **79:**3067–3071.
8. **Ran, Z., B. Rayet, J. Rommelaere, and S. Faisst.** 1999. Parvovirus H-1-induced cell death: influence of intracellular NAD consumption on the regulation of necrosis and apoptosis. *Virus Res.* **65:**161–174.
9. **Ruffolo, P. R., G. Margolis, and L. Kilham.** 1966. The induction of hepatitis by prior partial hepatectomy in resistant adult rats injected with H-1 virus. Light and electron microscopy and virologic studies. *Am. J. Pathol.* **49:**795–824.
10. **Schuster, G. S., G. B. Caughman, and N. L. O'Dell.** 1991. Altered lipid metabolism in parvovirus-infected cells. *Microbios* **66:**143–155.
11. **Van Pachterbeke, C., M. Tuynder, A. Brandenburger, G. Leclercq, M. Borras, and J. Rommelaere.** 1997. Varying sensitivity of human mammary carcinoma cells to the toxic effect of parvovirus H-1. *Eur. J. Cancer* **33:**1648–1653.
12. **Zenner, L., and J. P. Regnault.** 2000. Ten-year long monitoring of laboratory mouse and rat colonies in French facilities: a retrospective study. *Lab. Anim.* **34:**76–83.

Kilham rat virus

1. **Chung, Y. H., H. S. Jun, Y. Kang, K. Hirasawa, B. R. Lee, N. Van Rooijen, and J. W. Yoon.** 1997. Role of macrophages and macrophage-derived cytokines in the pathogenesis of Kilham rat virus-induced autoimmune diabetes in diabetes-resistant BioBreeding rats. *J. Immunol.* **159:**466–471.

2. Chung, Y. H., H. S. Jun, M. Son, M. Bao, H. Y. Bae, Y. Kang, and J. W. Yoon. 2000. Cellular and molecular mechanism for Kilham rat virus-induced autoimmune diabetes in DR-BB rats. *J. Immunol.* **165:**2866–2876.
3. Coleman, G. L., R. O. Jacoby, P. N. Bhatt, A. L. Smith, and A. M. Jonas. 1983. Naturally occurring lethal parvovirus infection in juvenile and young adult rats. *Vet. Pathol.* **20:**44–45.
4. Gabaldon, M., C. Capdevila, and A. Zuniga. 1992. Effect of spontaneous pathology and thrombin on leukocyte adhesion to rat aortic endothelium. *Atherosclerosis* **93:**217–228.
5. Gaertner, D. J., R. O. Jacoby, E. A. Johnson, F. X. Paturzo, and A. L. Smith. 1995. Persistent rat virus infection in juvenile athymic rats and its modulation by antiserum. *Lab. Anim. Sci.* **45:**249–253.
6. Gripenberg-Lerche, C., and P. Toivanen. 1993. *Yersinia* associated arthritis in SHR rats: effect of the microbial status of the host. *Ann. Rheum. Dis.* **52:**223–228.
7. Jacoby, R. O., L. Ball-Goodrich, D. G. Besselsen, M. D. McKisic, L. K. Riley, and A. L. Smith. 1996. Rodent parvovirus infections. *Lab. Anim. Sci.* **46:**370–380.
8. National Research Council. 1991. *Infectious Diseases of Mice and Rats: a Report of the Institute of Laboratory Animal Resources Committee on Infectious Diseases of Mice and Rats.* National Academy Press, Washington, D.C.
9. Nicklas, W., V. Kraft, and B. Meyer. 1993. Contamination of transplantable tumors, cell lines, and monoclonal antibodies with rodent viruses. *Lab. Anim. Sci.* **43:**296–300.
10. Schuster, G. S., G. B. Caughman, and N. L. O'Dell. 1991. Altered lipid metabolism in parvovirus-infected cells. *Microbios* **66:**143–155.

Lactate dehydrogenase-elevating virus
1. Anderson, G. W., G. A. Palmer, R. R. Rowland, C. Even, and P. G. Plagemann. 1995. Lactate dehydrogenase-elevating virus entry into the central nervous system and replication in anterior horn neurons. *J. Gen. Virol.* **76:**581–592.
2. Anderson, G. W., R. R. Rowland, G. A. Palmer, C. Even, and P. G. Plagemann. 1995. Lactate dehydrogenase–elevating virus replication persists in liver, spleen, lymph node, and testis tissues and results in accumulation of viral RNA in germinal centers, concomitant with polyclonal activation of B cells. *J. Virol.* **69:**5177–5188.
3. Chen, Z., K. Li, and P. G. Plagemann. 2000. Neuropathogenicity and sensitivity to antibody neutralization of lactate dehydrogenase-elevating virus are determined by polylactosaminoglycan chains on the primary envelope glycoprotein. *Virology* **266:**88–98.
4. Chen, Z., R. R. Rowland, G. W. Anderson, G. A. Palmer, and P. G. Plagemann. 1997. Coexistence in lactate dehydrogenase-elevating virus pools of variants that differ in neuropathogenicity and ability to establish a persistent infection. *J. Virol.* **71:**2913–2920.
5. Coutelier, J. P., J. Van Broeck, and S. F. Wolf. 1995. Interleukin-12 gene expression after viral infection in the mouse. *J. Virol.* **69:**1955–1958.
6. Even, C., R. R. Rowland, and P. G. Plagemann. 1995. Cytotoxic T cells are elicited during acute infection of mice with lactate dehydrogenase-elevating virus but disappear during the chronic phase of infection. *J. Virol.* **69:**5666–5676.
7. Even, C., R. R. Rowland, and P. G. Plagemann. 1995. Mouse hepatitis virus infection of mice causes long-term depletion of lactate dehydrogenase-elevating virus-permissive macrophages and T lymphocyte alterations. *Virus Res.* **39:**355–364
8. Faaberg, K. S., G. A. Palmer, C. Even, G. W. Anderson, and P. G. Plagemann. 1995. Differential glycosylation of the ectodomain of the primary envelope glycoprotein of two strains of lactate dehydrogenase-elevating virus that differ in neuropathogenicity. *Virus Res.* **39:**331–340.
9. Gomez, K. A., J. Coutelier, P. A. Mathieu, L. Lustig, and L. A. Retegui. 2000. Autoantibodies to cryptic epitopes elicited by infection with lactate dehyrogenase-elevating virus. *Scand. J. Immunol.* **51:**447–453.
10. Gomez, K. A., J. P. Coutelier, and L. A. Retegui. 1997. Changes in the specificity of antibodies in mice infected with lactate dehydrogenase-elevating virus. *Scand. J. Immunol.* **46:**168–174.
11. Goto, K., A. Takakura, M. Yoshimura, Y. Ohnishi, and T. Itoh. 1998. Detection and typing of lactate dehydrogenase-elevating virus RNA from transplantable tumors, mouse liver tissues, and cell lines, using polymerase chain reaction. *Lab. Anim. Sci.* **48:**99–102.
12. Hayashi, T., S. Hashimoto, and A. Kawashima. 1994. Effect of infection by lactic dehydrogenase virus on expression of intercellular adhesion molecule-1 on vascular endothelial cells of pancreatic islets in streptozotocin-induced insulitis of CD-1 mice. *Int. J. Exp. Pathol.* **75:**211–217.
13. Hayashi, T., H. Iwata, T. Hasegawa, M. Ozaki, H. Yamamoto, and T. Onodera.

1991. Decrease in neutrophil migration induced by endotoxin and suppression of interleukin-1 production by macrophages in lactic dehydrogenase virus-infected mice. *J. Comp. Pathol.* **104:** 161–170.

14. **Hayashi, T., Y. Koike, T. Hasegawa, M. Tsurudome, M. Ozaki, H. Yamamoto, and T. Onodera.** 1991. Inhibition of contact sensitivity by interferon in mice infected with lactic dehydrogenase virus. *J. Comp. Pathol.* **104:**357–366.

15. **Hayashi, T., T. Onodera, and H. Yamamoto.** 1992. Detection of the binding of IgG2a and IgG2b on the surface of macrophages from mice chronically infected with lactic dehydrogenase virus. *J. Comp. Pathol.* **107:**35–40.

16. **Hayashi, T., M. Ozaki, Y. Ami, T. Onodera, and H. Yamamoto.** 1992. Increased superoxide anion release by peritoneal macrophages in mice with a chronic infection of lactic dehydrogenase virus. *J. Comp. Pathol.* **106:**93–98.

17. **Kameyama, Y., and T. Hayashi.** 1994. Suppression of development of glomerulonephritis in NZB×NZWF1 mice by persistent infection with lactic dehydrogenase virus: relations between intercellular adhesion molecule-1 expression on endothelial cells and leucocyte accumulation in glomeruli. *Int. J. Exp. Pathol.* **75:** 295–304.

18. **Lawson, C. M.** 2000. Evidence for mimicry by viral antigens in animal models of autoimmune disease including myocarditis. *Cell. Mol. Life Sci.* **57:**552–560.

19. **Li, K., T. Schuler, Z. Chen, G. E. Glass, J. E. Childs, and P. G. Plagemann.** 2000. Isolation of lactate dehydrogenase-elevating viruses from wild house mice and their biological and molecular characterization. *Virus Res.* **67:**153–162.

20. **Lipman, N. S., K. Henderson, and W. Shek.** 2000. False negative results using RT-PCR for detection of lactate dehydrogenase-elevating virus in a tumor cell line. *Comp. Med.* **50:**255–256.

21. **Markine-Goriaynoff, D., J. T. van der Logt, C. Truyens, T. D. Nguyen, F. W. Heessen, G. Bigaignon, Y. Carlier, and J. P. Coutelier.** 2000. IFN-γ-independent IgG2a production in mice infected with viruses and parasites. *Int. Immunol.* **12:**223–230.

22. **Meite, M., S. Leonard, M. E. Idrissi, S. Izui, P. L. Masson, and J. P. Coutelier.** 2000. Exacerbation of autoantibody-mediated hemolytic anemia by viral infection. *J. Virol.* **74:**6045–6049.

23. **Monteyne, P., P. G. Coulie, and J. P. Coutelier.** 2000. Analysis of the Fv1 alleles involved in the susceptibility of mice to lactate dehydrogenase-elevating virus-induced polioencephalomyelitis. *J. Neurovirol.* **6:**89–93.

24. **Monteyne, P., M. Meite, and J.P. Coutelier.** 1997. Involvement of CD4$^+$ cells in the protection of C58 mouse against polioencephalomyelitis induced by lactate dehydrogenase-elevating virus. *J. Neurovirol.* **3:**380–384.

25. **Mori, I., T. Hayashi, S. Kitazima, and H. Yamamoto.** 1992. Binding of asparaginase to mouse monocytes. *Int. J. Exp. Pathol.* **73:**585–592.

26. **National Research Council.** 1991. *Infectious Diseases of Mice and Rats: a Report of the Institute of Laboratory Animal Resources Committee on Infectious Diseases of Mice and Rats.* National Academy Press, Washington, D.C.

27. **Nicklas, W., V. Kraft, and B. Meyer.** 1993. Contamination of transplantable tumors, cell lines, and monoclonal antibodies with rodent viruses. *Lab. Anim. Sci.* **43:**296–300.

28. **Ohnishi, Y., M. Yoshimura, and Y. Ueyama.** 1995. Lactic dehydrogenase virus (LDHV) contamination in human tumor xenografts and its elimination. *J. Natl. Cancer Inst.* **87:** 538–539.

29. **Schlenker, E. H., Q. A. Jones, R. R. Rowland, M. Steffen-Bien, and W. A. Cafruny.** 2001. Age-dependent poliomyelitis in mice is associated with respiratory failure and viral replication in the central nervous system and lung. *J. Neurovirol.* **7:**265–271.

30. **van den Broek, M. F., R. Sporri, C. Even, P. G. Plagemann, E. Hanseler, H. Hengartner, and R. M. Zinkernagel.** 1997. Lactate dehydrogenase-elevating virus (LDV): lifelong coexistence of virus and LDV-specific immunity. *J. Immunol.* **159:**1585–1588.

31. **Zitterkopf, N. L., T. R. Haven, M. Huela, D. S. Bradley, and W. A. Cafruny.** 2002. Transplacental lactate dehydrogenase-elevating virus (LDV) transmission: immune inhibition of umbilical cord infection, and correlation of fetal virus susceptibility with development of F4/80 antigen expression. *Placenta* **23:**438–446.

Lymphocytic choriomeningitis virus

1. **Bartholdy, C., J. P. Christensen, D. Wodarz, and A. R. Thomsen.** 2000. Persistent virus infection despite chronic cytotoxic T-lymphocyte activation in gamma interferon-deficient mice infected with lymphocytic choriomeningitis virus. *J. Virol.* **74:**10304–10311.

2. **Barton, L. L., and N. J. Hyndman.** 2000. Lymphocytic choriomeningitis virus: reemerging central nervous system pathogen. *Pediatrics* **105:** E35.

3. **Binder, D., J. Fehr, H. Hengartner, and R. M. Zinkernagel.** 1997. Virus-induced tran-

sient bone marrow aplasia: major role of interferon-α/β during acute infection with the noncytopathic lymphocytic choriomeningitis virus. *J. Exp. Med.* **185**:517–530.
4. Borrow, P., C. F. Evans, and M. B. Oldstone. 1995. Virus-induced immunosuppression: immune system-mediated destruction of virus-infected dendritic cells results in generalized immune suppression. *J. Virol.* **69**:1059–1070.
5. Christensen, J. P., J. Johansen, O. Marker, and A. R. Thomsen. 1995. Circulating intercellular adhesion molecule-1 (ICAM-1) as an early and sensitive marker for virus-induced T cell activation. *Clin. Exp. Immunol.* **102**:268–273.
6. Ciurea, A., P. Klenerman, L. Hunziker, E. Horvath, B. Odermatt, A. F. Ochsenbein, H. Hengartner, and R. M. Zinkernagel. 1999. Persistence of lymphocytic choriomeningitis virus at very low levels in immune mice. *Proc. Natl. Acad. Sci. USA* **96**:11964–11969.
7. Colle, J. H., M. F. Saron, and P. Truffa-Bachi. 1993. Altered cytokine genes expression by conA-activated spleen cells from mice infected by lymphocytic choriomeningitis virus. *Immunol. Lett.* **35**:247–253.
8. de la Torre, J. C., M. Mallory, M. Brot, L. Gold, G. Koob, M. B. Oldstone, and E. Masliah. 1996. Viral persistence in neurons alters synaptic plasticity and cognitive functions without destruction of brain cells. *Virology* **220**:508–515.
9. Dykewicz, C. A., V. M. Dato, S. P. Fisher-Hoch, M. V. Howarth, G. I. Perez-Oronoz, S. M. Ostroff, H. Gary, Jr., L. B. Schonberger, and J. B. McCormick. 1992. Lymphocytic choriomeningitis outbreak associated with nude mice in a research institute. *JAMA* **267**:1349–1353.
10. El Azami El Idrissi, M., G. Mazza, P. Monteyne, C. J. Elson, M. J. Day, C. J. Pfau, and J. P. Coutelier. 1998. Lymphocytic choriomeningitis virus-induced alterations of T helper-mediated responses in mice developing autoimmune hemolytic anemia during the course of infection. *Proc. Soc. Exp. Biol. Med.* **218**:349–356.
11. Gold, L. H., M. D. Brot, I. Polis, R. Schroeder, A. Tishon, J. C. de la Torre, M. B. Oldstone, and G. F. Koob. 1994. Behavioral effects of persistent lymphocytic choriomeningitis virus infection in mice. *Behav. Neural Biol.* **62**:100–109.
12. Gossmann, J., J. Lohler, O. Utermohlen, and F. Lehmann-Grube. 1995. Murine hepatitis caused by lymphocytic choriomeningitis virus. II. Cells involved in pathogenesis. *Lab. Invest.* **72**:559–570.
13. Guidotti, L. G., P. Borrow, M. V. Hobbs, B. Matzke, I. Gresser, M. B. Oldstone, and F. V. Chisari. 1996. Viral cross talk: intracellular inactivation of the hepatitis B virus during an unrelated viral infection of the liver. *Proc. Natl. Acad. Sci. USA* **93**:4589–4594.
14. Kagi, D., and H. Hengartner. 1996. Different roles for cytotoxic T cells in the control of infections with cytopathic versus noncytopathic viruses. *Curr. Opin. Immunol.* **8**:472–477.
15. Kagi, D., P. Seiler, J. Pavlovic, B. Ledermann, K. Burki, R. M. Zinkernagel, and H. Hengartner. 1995. The roles of perforin- and Fas-dependent cytotoxicity in protection against cytopathic and noncytopathic viruses. *Eur. J. Immunol.* **25**:3256–3262.
16. Mazza, G., M. E. el Idrissi, J. P. Coutelier, A. Corato, C. J. Elson, C. J. Pfau, and M. J. Day. 1997. Infection of C3HeB/FeJ mice with the docile strain of lymphocytic choriomeningitis virus induces autoantibodies specific for erythrocyte Band 3. *Immunology* **91**:239–245.
17. Morita, C., K. Tsuchiya, H. Ueno, Y. Muramatsu, A. Kojimahara, H. Suzuki, N. Miyashita, K. Moriwaki, M. L. Jin, X. L. Wu, and F. S. Wang. 1996. Seroepidemiological survey of lymphocytic choriomeningitis virus in wild house mice in China with particular reference to their subspecies. *Microbiol. Immunol.* **40**:313–315.
18. Moskophidis, D., M. Battegay, M. van den Broek, E. Laine, U. Hoffmann-Rohrer, and R. M. Zinkernagel. 1995. Role of virus and host variables in virus persistence or immunopathological disease caused by a non-cytolytic virus. *J. Gen. Virol.* **76**:381–391.
19. National Research Council. 1991. *Infectious Diseases of Mice and Rats: a Report of the Institute of Laboratory Animal Resources Committee on Infectious Diseases of Mice and Rats.* National Academy Press, Washington, D.C.
20. Nicklas, W., V. Kraft, and B. Meyer. 1993. Contamination of transplantable tumors, cell lines, and monoclonal antibodies with rodent viruses. *Lab. Anim. Sci.* **43**:296–300.
21. Orange, J. S., and C. A. Biron. 1996. An absolute and restricted requirement for IL-12 in natural killer cell IFN-γ production and antiviral defense. Studies of natural killer and T cell responses in contrasting viral infections. *J. Immunol.* **156**:1138–1142.
22. Ou, R., S. Zhou, L. Huang, and D. Moskophidis. 2001. Critical role for α/β and γ interferons in persistence of lymphocytic choriomeningitis virus by clonal exhaustion of cytotoxic T cells. *J. Virol.* **75**:8407–8423.

23. Peacock, C. D., M. Y. Lin, J. R. Ortaldo, and R. M. Welsh. 2000. The virus-specific and allospecific cytotoxic T-lymphocyte response to lymphocytic choriomeningitis virus is modified in a subpopulation of CD8[+] T cells coexpressing the inhibitory major histocompatibility complex class I receptor Ly49G2. *J. Virol.* **74:**7032–7038.
24. Percy, D. H., and S. W. Barthold. 2001. *Pathology of Laboratory Rodents and Rabbits,* 2nd ed. Iowa State University Press, Ames.
25. Rai, S. K., D. S. Cheung, M. S. Wu, T. F. Warner, and M. S. Salvato. 1996. Murine infection with lymphocytic choriomeningitis virus following gastric inoculation. *J. Virol.* **70:**7213–7218.
26. Slifka, M. K., and R. Ahmed. 1996. Long-term antibody production is sustained by antibody-secreting cells in the bone marrow following acute viral infection. *Ann. N. Y. Acad. Sci.* **797:**166–176.
27. Spence, P. M., V. Sriram, L. Van Kaer, J. A. Hobbs, and R. R. Brutkiewicz. 2001. Generation of cellular immunity to lymphocytic choriomeningitis virus is independent of CD1d1 expression. *Immunology* **104:**168–174.
28. Sydora, B. C., B. D. Jamieson, R. Ahmed, and M. Kronenberg. 1996. Intestinal intraepithelial lymphocytes respond to systemic lymphocytic choriomeningitis virus infection. *Cell. Immunol.* **167:**161–169.
29. Varga, S. M., and R. M. Welsh. 2000. High frequency of virus-specific interleukin-2-producing CD4[+] T cells and Th1 dominance during lymphocytic choriomeningitis virus infection. *J. Virol.* **74:**4429–4432.

Minute virus of mice
1. Besselsen, D. G., D. J. Pintel, G. A. Purdy, C. L. Besch-Williford, C. L. Franklin, R. R. Hook, Jr., and L. K. Riley. 1996. Molecular characterization of newly recognized rodent parvoviruses. *J. Gen. Virol.* **77:**899–911.
2. Besselsen, D. G., A. M. Wagner, and J. K. Loganbill. 2000. Effect of mouse strain and age on detection of Mouse Parvovirus 1 by use of serologic testing and polymerase chain reaction analysis. *Comp. Med.* **50:**498–502.
3. Brownstein, D. G., A. L. Smith, R. O. Jacoby, E. A. Johnson, G. Hansen, and P. Tattersall. 1991. Pathogenesis of infection with a virulent allotropic variant of minute virus of mice and regulation by host genotype. *Lab. Invest.* **65:**357–364.
4. Colomar, M. C., B. Hirt, and P. Beard. 1998. Two segments in the genome of the immunosuppressive minute virus of mice determine the host-cell specificity, control viral DNA replication and affect viral RNA metabolism. *J. Gen. Virol.* **79:**581–586.
5. Hansen, G. M., F. X. Paturzo, and A. L. Smith. 1999. Humoral immunity and protection of mice challenged with homotypic or heterotypic parvovirus. *Lab. Anim. Sci.* **49:**380–384.
6. Jacoby, R. O., E. A. Johnson, L. Ball-Goodrich, A. L. Smith, and M. D. McKisic. 1995. Characterization of mouse parvovirus infection by in situ hybridization. *J. Virol.* **69:**3915–3919.
7. Kapil, S. 1995. Minute virus of mice (MVM) nucleic acid production in susceptible and resistant strains of mice and F1 hybrids. *Comp. Immunol. Microbiol. Infect. Dis.* **18:**245–252.
8. National Research Council. 1991. *Infectious Diseases of Mice and Rats: a Report of the Institute of Laboratory Animal Resources Committee on Infectious Diseases of Mice and Rats.* National Academy Press, Washington, D.C.
9. Nicklas, W., V. Kraft, and B. Meyer. 1993. Contamination of transplantable tumors, cell lines, and monoclonal antibodies with rodent viruses. *Lab. Anim. Sci.* **43:**296–300.
10. Ramirez, J. C., A. Fairen, and J. M. Almendral. 1996. Parvovirus minute virus of mice strain I multiplication and pathogenesis in the newborn mouse brain are restricted to proliferative areas and to migratory cerebellar young neurons. *J. Virol.* **70:**8109–8116.
11. Redig, A. J., and D. G. Besselsen. 2001. Detection of rodent parvoviruses by use of fluorogenic nuclease polymerase chain reaction assays. *Comp. Med.* **51:**326–331.
12. Segovia, J. C., J. A. Bueren, and J. M. Almendral. 1995. Myeloid depression follows infection of susceptible newborn mice with the parvovirus minute virus of mice (strain I). *J. Virol.* **69:**3229–3232.
13. Segovia, J. C., J. M. Gallego, J. A. Bueren, and J. M. Almendral. 1999. Severe leukopenia and dysregulated erythropoiesis in SCID mice persistently infected with the parvovirus minute virus of mice. *J. Virol.* **73:**1774–1784.
14. Zenner, L., and J. P. Regnault. 2000. Ten-year long monitoring of laboratory mouse and rat colonies in French facilities: a retrospective study. *Lab. Anim.* **34:**76–83.

Mouse hepatitis virus
1. Barthold, S. W., D. S. Beck, and A. L. Smith. 1993. Enterotropic coronavirus (mouse hepatitis virus) in mice: influence of host age and strain on infection and disease. *Lab. Anim. Sci.* **43:**276–284.
2. Barthold, S. W., and A. L. Smith. 1992. Viremic dissemination of mouse hepatitis virus-

JHM following intranasal inoculation of mice. *Arch. Virol.* **122**:35–44.
3. **Belyavskyi, M., E. Belyavskaya, G. A. Levy, and J. L. Leibowitz.** 1998. Coronavirus MHV-3-induced apoptosis in macrophages. *Virology* **250**:41–49.
4. **Belyavskyi, M., G. A. Levy, and J. L. Leibowitz.** 1998. The pattern of induction of apoptosis during infection with MHV-3 correlates with strain variation in resistance and susceptibility to lethal hepatitis. *Adv. Exp. Med. Biol.* **440**:619–625.
5. **Besselsen, D. G., A. M. Wagner, and J. K. Loganbill.** 2002. Detection of rodent coronaviruses by sue of fluorogenic reverse transcriptase-polymerase chain reaction analysis. *Comp. Med.* **52**:111–116.
6. **Braunwald, J., H. Nonnenmacher, C. A. Pereira, and A. Kirn.** 1991. Increased susceptibility to mouse hepatitis virus type 3 (MHV3) infection induced by a hypercholesterolaemic diet with increased adsorption of MHV3 to primary hepatocyte cultures. *Res. Virol.* **142**:5–15.
7. **Casebolt, D. B., B. Qian, and C. B. Stephensen.** 1997. Detection of enterotropic mouse hepatitis virus fecal excretion by polymerase chain reaction. *Lab. Anim. Sci.* **47**:6–10.
8. **Chen, B. P., and T. E. Lane.** 2002. Lack of nitric oxide synthase type 2 (NOS2) results in reduced neuronal apoptosis and mortality following mouse hepatitis virus infection of the central nervous system. *J. Neurovirol.* **8**:58–63.
9. **Cray, C., M. O. Mateo, and N. H. Altman.** 1993. In vitro and long-term in vivo immune dysfunction after infection of BALB/c mice with mouse hepatitis virus strain A59. *Lab. Anim. Sci.* **43**:169–174.
10. **de Souza, M. S., A. L. Smith, and K. Bottomly.** 1991. Infection of BALB/cByJ mice with the JHM strain of mouse hepatitis virus alters in vitro splenic T cell proliferation and cytokine production. *Lab. Anim. Sci.* **41**:99–105.
11. **Ding, J. W., Q. Ning, M. F. Liu, A. Lai, K. Peltekian, L. Fung, C. Holloway, H. Yeger, M. J. Phillips, and G. A. Levy.** 1998. Expression of the fg12 and its protein product (prothrombinasse) in tissues during murine hepatitis virus strain-3 (MHV-3) infection. *Adv. Exp. Med. Biol.* **440**:609–618.
12. **Dufour, J. H., M. Dziejman, M. T. Liu, J. H. Leung, T. E. Lane, and A. D. Luster.** 2002. IFN-γ-inducible protein 10 (IP-10; CXCL10)-deficient mice reveal a role for IP-10 in effector T cell generation and trafficking. *J. Immunol.* **168**:3195–3204.
13. **Even, C., R. R. Rowland, and P. G. Plagemann.** 1995. Mouse hepatitis virus infection of mice causes long-term depletion of lactate dehydrogenase-elevating virus-permissive macrophages and T lymphocyte alterations. *Virus Res.* **39**:355–364.
14. **Fallon, M. T., W. H. Benjamin, Jr., T. R. Schoeb, and D. E. Briles.** 1991. Mouse hepatitis virus strain UAB infection enhances resistance to *Salmonella typhimurium* in mice by inducing suppression of bacterial growth. *Infect. Immun.* **59**:852–856.
15. **Gagne, S., L. Thibodeau, and L. Lamontagne.** 1998. Clonal deletion of some V beta$^+$ T cells in peripheral lymphocytes from C57BL/6 mice infected with MHV3. *Adv. Exp. Med. Biol.* **440**:485–489.
16. **Godfraind, C., K. V. Holmes, and J. P. Coutelier.** 1995. Thymus involution induced by mouse hepatitis virus A59 in BALB/c mice. *J. Virol.* **69**:6541–6547.
17. **Godfraind, C., S. G. Langreth, C. B. Cardellichio, R. Knobler, J. P. Coutelier, M. Dubois-Dalcq, and K. V. Holmes.** 1995. Tissue and cellular distribution of an adhesion molecule in the carcinoembryonic antigen family that serves as a receptor for mouse hepatitis virus. *Lab. Invest.* **73**:615–627.
18. **Glass, W. G., B. P. Chen, M. T. Liu, and T. E. Lane.** 2002. Mouse hepatitis virus infection of the central nervous system: chemokine-mediated regulation of host defense and disease. *Virol. Immunol.* **15**:261–272.
19. **Homberger, F. R.** 1997. Enterotropic mouse hepatitis virus. *Lab. Anim. Sci.* **31**:97–115.
20. **Homberger, F. R., and S. W. Barthold.** 1992. Passively acquired challenge immunity to enterotropic coronavirus in mice. *Arch. Virol.* **126**:35–43.
21. **Homberger, F. R., S. W. Barthold, and A. L. Smith.** 1992. Duration and strain-specificity of immunity to enterotropic mouse hepatitis virus. *Lab. Anim. Sci.* **42**:347–351.
22. **Homberger, F. R., and P. E. Thomann.** 1994. Transmission of murine viruses and mycoplasma in laboratory mouse colonies with respect to housing conditions. *Lab. Anim.* **28**:113–120.
23. **Hooks, J. J., C. Percopo, Y. Wang, and B. Detrick.** 1993. Retina and retinal pigment epithelial cell autoantibodies are produced during murine coronavirus retinopathy. *J. Immunol.* **151**:3381–3389.
24. **Huang, D. S., S. N. Emancipator, D. R. Fletcher, M. E. Lamm, and M. B. Mazanec.** 1996. Hepatic pathology resulting from mouse hepatitis virus S infection in severe combined immunodeficiency mice. *Lab. Anim. Sci.* **46**:167–173.

25. Jolicoeur, P., and L. Lamontagne. 1995. Impairment of bone marrow pre-B and B cells in MHV3 chronically-infected mice. *Adv. Exp. Med. Biol.* **380**:193–195.
26. Komurasaki, Y., C. N. Nagineni, Y. Wang, and J. J. Hooks. 1996. Virus RNA persists within the retina in coronavirus-induced retinopathy. *Virology* **222**:446–450.
27. Kyuwa, S. 1997. Replication of murine coronaviruses in mouse embryonic stem cell lines. *Exp. Anim.* **46**:311–313.
28. Kyuwa, S., K. Machii, A. Okumura, and Y. Toyoda. 1996. Characterization of T cells expanded *in vivo* during primary mouse hepatitis virus infection in mice. *J. Vet. Med. Sci.* **58**:431–437.
29. Kyuwa, S., K. Machii, and S. Shibata. 1996. Role of CD4$^+$ and CD8$^+$ T cells in mouse hepatitis virus infection in mice. *Exp. Anim.* **45**:81–83.
30. Lamontagne, L., S. Lusignan, and C. Page. 2001. Recovery from mouse hepatitis virus infection depends on recruitment of CD8$^+$ cells rather than activation of intrahepatic CD4$^+\alpha\beta^-$TCR^{inter} or NK$^-$T cells. *Clin. Immunol.* **101**:345–356.
31. Lardans, V., C. Godfraind, J. T. van der Logt, W. A. Heessen, M. D. Gonzalez, and J. P. Coutelier. 1996. Polyclonal B lymphocyte activation induced by mouse hepatitis virus A59 infection. *J. Gen. Virol.* **77**:1005–1009.
32. Lavi, E., Q. Wang, S. R. Weiss, and N. K. Gonatas. 1996. Syncytia formation induced by coronavirus infection is associated with fragmentation and rearrangement of the Golgi apparatus. *Virology* **221**:325–334.
33. Lee, S. K., H. Y. Youn, A. Hasegawa, H. Nakayama, and N. Goto. 1994. Apoptotic changes in the thymus of mice infected with mouse hepatitis virus, MHV-2. *J. Vet. Med. Sci.* **56**:879–882.
34. Liang, S.-C., W.-C. Lian, F.-J. Leu, P.-J. Lee, A.-J. Chao, C.-C. Hong, and W.-F. Chen. 1995. Epizootic of low-virulence hepatotropic murine hepatitis virus in a nude mice breeding colony in Taiwan. *Lab. Anim. Sci.* **45**:519–522.
35. Macy, J. D., G. A. Cameron, S. L. Ellis, E. A. Hill, and S. R. Compton. 2002. Assessment of static isolator cages with automatic watering when used with conventional husbandry techniques as a factor in the transmission of mouse hepatitis virus. *Contemp. Top. Lab. Anim. Sci.* **41**:30–35.
36. Matthews, A. E., S. R. Weiss, M. J. Shlomchik, L. G. Hannum, J. L. Gombold, and Y. Paterson. 2001. Antibody is required for clearance of infectious murine hepatitis virus A59 from the central nervous system, but not from the liver. *J. Immunol.* **167**:5254–5263.
37. Morrell, J. M. 1999. Techniques of embryo transfer and facility decontamination used to improve the health and welfare of transgenic mice. *Lab. Anim.* **33**:201–206.
38. National Research Council. 1991. *Infectious Diseases of Mice and Rats: a Report of the Institute of Laboratory Animal Resources Committee on Infectious Diseases of Mice and Rats.* National Academy Press, Washington, D.C.
39. Nicklas, W., V. Kraft, and B. Meyer. 1993. Contamination of transplantable tumors, cell lines, and monoclonal antibodies with rodent viruses. *Lab. Anim. Sci.* **43**:296–300.
40. Nicklas, W., and J. Weiss. 2000. Survey of embryonic stem cells for murine infective agents. *Comp. Med.* **50**:410–411.
41. Ohtsuka, N., and F. Taguchi. 1997. Mouse susceptibility to mouse hepatitis virus infection is linked to viral receptor genotype. *J. Virol.* **71**:8860–8863.
42. Orcutt, R. P., R. S. Phelan, and J. G. Geistfeld. 2001. Exclusion of mouse hepatitis virus from a filtered, plastic rodent shipping container during an in transit field challenge. *Contemp. Top. Lab. Anim. Sci.* **40**:32–35.
43. Perlman, S., N. Sun, and E. M. Barnett. 1995. Spread of MHV-JHM from nasal cavity to white matter of spinal cord. Transneuronal movement and involvement of astrocytes. *Adv. Exp. Med. Biol.* **380**:73–78.
44. Pewe, L., J. Haring, and S. Perlman. 2002. CD4 T-cell-mediated demyelination is increased in the absence of gamma interferon with mouse hepatitis virus. *J. Virol.* **76**:7329–7333.
45. Pewe, L., S. Xue, and S. Perlman. 1997. Cytotoxic T-cell-resistant variants arise at early times after infection in C57BL/6 but not in SCID mice infected with a neurotropic coronavirus. *J. Virol.* **71**:7640–7647.
46. Phillips, J. J., M. Chua, G. Rall, and S. Weiss. 2002. Murine coronavirus spike glycoprotein mediates degree of viral spread, inflammation, and virus-induced immunopathology in the central nervous system. *Virology* **301**:109.
47. Rehg, J. E., M. A. Blackman, and L. A. Toth. 2001. Persistent transmission of mouse hepatitis virus by transgenic mice. *Comp. Med.* **51**:369–374.
48. Schijns, V. E., C. M. Wierda, M. van Hoeij, and M. C. Horzinek. 1996. Exacerbated viral hepatitis in IFN-gamma receptor-deficient mice is not suppressed by IL-12. *J. Immunol.* **157**:815–821.

49. **Schwob, J. E., S. Saha, S. L. Youngtob, and B. Jubelt.** 2001. Intranasal inoculation with the olfactory bulb line variant of mouse hepatitis virus causes extensive destruction of the olfactory bulb and accelerated turnover of neurons in the olfactory epithelium of mice. *Chem. Senses* **26**:937–952.
50. **Steffan, A. M., C. A. Pereira, A. Bingen, M. Valle, J. P. Martin, F. Koehren, C. Royer, J. L. Gendrault, and A. Kirn.** 1995. Mouse hepatitis virus type 3 infection provokes a decrease in the number of sinusoidal endothelial cell fenestrae both *in vivo* and *in vitro*. *Hepatology* **22**:395–401.
51. **Suzuki, H., W. Kiatipattanasakul, S. Kajikawa, S. Tsutsui, H. Nakayama, N. Goto, and K. Doi.** 1997. Age-related changes in susceptibility of mice to low-virulent mouse hepatitis virus (MHV-2-CC) infection. *Exp. Anim.* **46**:211–218.
52. **Suzuki, H., K. Yorozu, T. Watanabe, M. Nakura, and J. Adachi.** 1996. Rederivation of mice by means of *in vitro* fertilization and embryo transfer. *Exp. Anim.* **45**:33–38.
53. **Taguchi, F., A. Yamada, and K. Fujiwara.** 1979. Asymptomatic infection of mouse hepatitis virus in the rat. *Arch. Virol.* **59**:275–279.
54. **Tahara, S., C. Bergmann, G. Nelson, R. Anthony, T. Dietlin, S. Kyuwa, and S. Stohlman.** 1993. Effects of mouse hepatitis virus infection on host cell metabolism. *Adv. Exp. Med. Biol.* **342**:111–116.
55. **Takakura, A., Y. Ohnishi, T. Itoh, M. Yoshimura, K. Urano, and Y. Ueyama.** 2000. Decontamination of human xenotransplantable tumor with mouse hepatitis virus by implantation in nude rat: a case report. *Exp. Anim.* **49**:39–41.
56. **Torrecilhas, A. C., E. Faquim-Mauro, A. V. Da Silva, and I. A. Abrahamsohn.** 1999. Interference of natural mouse hepatitis virus infection with cytokine production and susceptibility to *Trypanosoma cruzi*. *Immunology* **96**:381–388.
57. **Uetsuka, K., H. Nakayama, and N. Goto.** 1996. Hepatitogenicity of three plaque purified variants of hepatotropic mouse hepatitis virus, MHV-2 in athymic nude mice. *Exp. Anim.* **45**:183–187.
58. **Vacha, J., V. Znojil, M. Pospisil, J. Hola, and I. Pipalova.** 1994. Microcytic anemia and changes in ferrokinetics as late after-effects of glucan administration in murine hepatitis virus-infected C57BL/10ScSnPh mice. *Int. J. Immunopharmacol.* **16**:51–60.
59. **Vassao, R. C., M. T. de Franco, D. Hartz, M. Modolell, A. E. Sippel, and C. A. Pereira.** 2000. Down-regulation of Bgpl (a) viral receptor by interferon-γ is related to the antiviral state and resistance to mouse hepatitis virus 3 infection. *Virology* **274**:278–283.
60. **Verinaud, L., I. J. Camargo, J. Vassallo, J. K. Sakurada, and H. A. Rangel.** 1999. Lymphoid organ alterations enhanced by sublethal doses of coronaviruses in experimentally induced *Trypanosoma cruzi* infection in mice. *Lab. Anim. Sci.* **49**:35–41.
61. **Wang, Y., M. Burnier, B. Detrick, and J. J. Hooks.** 1996. Genetic predisposition to coronavirus-induced retinal disease. *Investig. Ophthalmol. Vis. Sci.* **37**:250–254.
62. **Wang, R. F., W. L. Campbell, W. W. Cao, R. M. Colvert, M. A. Holland, and C. E. Cerniglia.** 1999. Diagnosis of mouse hepatitis virus contamination in mouse populations by using nude mice and RT-PCR. *Mol. Cell. Probes* **13**:29–33.
63. **Wijburg, O. L., M. H. Heemskerk, C. J. Boog, and N. Van Rooijen.** 1997. Role of spleen macrophages in innate and acquired immune responses against mouse hepatitis virus strain A59. *Immunology* **92**:252–258.
64. **Wijburg, O. L., M. H. Heemskerk, A. Sanders, C. J. Boog, and N. Van Rooijen.** 1996. Role of virus-specific $CD4^+$ cytotoxic T cells in recovery from mouse hepatitis virus infection. *Immunology* **87**:34–41.
65. **Wilberz, S., H. J. Partke, F. Dagnaes-Hansen, and L. Herberg.** 1991. Persistent MHV (mouse hepatitis virus) infection reduces the incidence of diabetes mellitus in non-obese diabetic mice. *Diabetologia* **34**:2–5.
66. **Yamada, Y. K., and M. Yabe.** 2000. Sequence analysis of major structural proteins of newly isolated mouse hepatitis virus. *Exp. Anim.* **49**:61–66.
67. **Yamada, Y. K., M. Yabe, K. Takimoto, K. Nakayama, and M. Saitoh.** 1998. Application of nested polymerase chain reaction to detection of mouse hepatitis virus in fecal specimens during a natural outbreak in an immunodeficient mouse colony. *Exp. Anim.* **47**:261–264.
68. **Zenner, L., and J. P. Regnault.** 2000. Ten-year long monitoring of laboratory mouse and rat colonies in French facilities: a retrospective study. *Lab. Anim.* **34**:76–83.
69. **Zhou, J., S. A. Stohlman, R. Atkinson, D. R. Hinton, and N. W. Marten.** 2002. Matrix metalloproteinase expression correlates with virulence following neurotropic mouse hepatitis virus infection. *J. Virol.* **76**:7374–7384.

Mouse mammary tumor virus
1. **Acha-Orbea, H., D. Finke, A. Attinger, S. Schmid, N. Wehrli, S. Vacheron, I. Xena-

rios, L. Scarpellino, K. M. Toellner, I. C. MacLennan, and S. A. Luther. 1999. Interplays between mouse mammary tumor virus and the cellular and humoral immune response. *Immunol. Rev.* **168**:287–303.
2. Bentvelzen, P., and J. Briinkhof. 1980. Ubiquity of natural antibodies to the mammary tumour virus in mice. *Arch. Gesamte Wulstforsch.* **50**:193–203.
3. Bolander, F. F., Jr. 1994. The effect of mouse mammary tumor virus receptor activation on mammary epithelial cell sensitivity toward prolactin. *Biochem. Biophys. Res. Commun.* **205**:524–528.
4. Bolander, F. F., Jr., and M. E. Blackstone. 1990. Thyroid hormone requirement for retinoic acid induction of mouse mammary tumor virus expression. *J. Virol.* **64**:5192–5193.
5. Champagne, E., L. Scarpellino, P. Lane, and H. Acha-Orbea. 1996. CD28/CTLA4-B7 interaction is dispensable for T cell stimulation by mouse mammary tumor virus superantigen but not for B cell differentiation and virus dissemination. *Eur. J. Immunol.* **26**:1595–1602.
6. Erny, K. M., J. Peli, J. F. Lambert, V. Muller, and H. Diggelmann. 1996. Involvement of the Tpl-2/cot oncogene in MMTV tumorigenesis. *Oncogene* **13**:2015–2020.
7. Fernandes, G., B. Chandrasekar, D. A. Troyer, J. T. Venkatraman, and R. A. Good. 1995. Dietary lipids and calorie restriction affect mammary tumor incidence and gene expression in mouse mammary tumor virus/v-Ha-ras transgenic mice. *Proc. Natl. Acad. Sci. USA* **92**:6494–6498.
8. Gill, R., H. Wang, H. Bluethmann, A. Iglesias, and W. Z. Wei. 1994. Activation of natural killer cells by mouse mammary tumor virus C4 in BALB/c and T-cell receptor V beta 2-transgenic mice. *Cancer Res.* **54**:1529–1535.
9. Karapetian, O., A. N. Shakhov, J. P. Kraehenbuhl, and H. Acha-Orbea. 1994. Retroviral infection of neonatal Peyer's patch lymphocytes: the mouse mammary tumor virus model. *J. Exp. Med.* **180**:1511-1516.
10. Le Bon, A., B. Lucas, F. Vasseur, C. Penit, and M. Papiernik. 1996. *In vivo* T cell response to viral superantigen. Selective migration rather than proliferation. *J. Immunol.* **156**:4602–4608.
11. Matsuzawa, A., H. Nakano, T. Yoshimoto, and K. Sayama. 1995. Biology of mouse mammary tumor virus (MMTV). *Cancer Lett.* **90**:3–11.
12. Miconnet, I., T. Roger, M. Seman, and M. Bruley-Rosset. 1995. Critical role of endogenous Mtv in acute lethal graft-versus-host disease. *Eur. J. Immunol.* **25**:364–368.
13. Mukhopadhyay, R., D. Medina, and J. S. Butel. 1995. Expression of the mouse mammary tumor virus long terminal repeat open reading frame promotes tumorigenic potential of hyperplastic mouse mammary epithelial cells. *Virology* **211**:74–93.
14. Muller, W. J., C. L. Arteaga, S. K. Muthuswamy, P. M. Siegel, M. A. Webster, R. D. Cardiff, K. S. Meise, F. Li, S. A. Halter, and R. J. Coffey. 1996. Synergistic interaction of the Neu proto-oncogene product and transforming growth factor alpha in the mammary epithelium of transgenic mice. *Mol. Cell. Biol.* **16**:5726–5736.
15. Nabarra, B., C. Desaymard, A. C. Wache, and M. Papiernik. 1996. Mouse mammary tumor virus production by thymic epithelial cells *in vivo*. *Eur. J. Immunol.* **26**:2724–2730.
16. National Research Council. 1991. *Infectious Diseases of Mice and Rats: a Report of the Institute of Laboratory Animal Resources Committee on Infectious Diseases of Mice and Rats*. National Academy Press, Washington, D.C.
17. Shakhov, A. N., H. Wang, H. Acha-Orbea, R. J. Pauley, and W. Z. Wei. 1993. A new infectious mammary tumor virus in the milk of mice implanted with C4 hyperplastic alveolar nodules. *Eur. J. Immunol.* **23**:2765–2769.
18. Vacheron, S., S. A. Luther, and H. Acha-Orbea. 2002. Preferential infection of immature dendritic cells and B cells by mouse mammary tumor virus. *J. Immunol.* **168**:3470–3476.
19. Van Nie, R., and J. Hilgers. 1976. Genetic analysis of mammary tumor induction and expression of mammary tumor virus antigen in hormone-treated ovariectomized GR mice. *J. Natl. Cancer Inst.* **56**:27–32.
20. Wajjwalku, W., M. Takahashi, O. Miyaishi, J. Lu, K. Sakata, T. Yokoi, S. Saga, M. Imai, M. Matsuyama, and M. Hoshino. 1991. Tissue distribution of mouse mammary tumor virus (MMTV) antigens and new endogenous MMTV loci in Japanese laboratory mouse strains. *Jpn. J. Cancer Res.* **82**:1413–1420.
21. Wrona, T., and J. P. Dudley. 1996. Major histocompatibility complex class II I-E-independent transmission of C3H mouse mammary tumor virus. *J. Virol.* **70**:1246–1249.
22. Xu, L., T. J. Wrona, and J. P. Dudley. 1996. Exogenous mouse mammary tumor virus (MMTV) infection induces endogenous MMTV sag expression. *Virology* **215**:113–123.
23. Yamazaki, K., E. A. Boyse, J. Bard, M. Curran, D. Kim, S. R. Ross, and G. K. Beauchamp. 2002. Presence of mouse mammary tumor virus specifically alters the body odor of mice. *Proc. Natl. Acad. Sci. USA* **99**:5612–5615.

24. Yoshimoto, T., H. Nagase, H. Nakano, A. Matsuzawa, and H. Nariuchi. 1996. Deletion of CD4+ T cells by mouse mammary tumor virus (FM) superantigen with broad specificity of T cell receptor beta-chain variable region. *Virology* **223**:387–391.

Mouse parvovirus-1
1. Besselsen, D. G., D. J. Pintel, G. A. Purdy, C. L. Besch-Williford, C. L. Franklin, R. R. Hook, Jr., and L. K. Riley. 1996. Molecular characterization of newly recognized rodent parvoviruses. *J. Gen. Virol.* **77**:899–911.
2. Besselsen, D. G., A. M. Wagner, and J. K. Loganbill. 2000. Effect of mouse strain and age on detection of Mouse Parvovirus 1 by use of serologic testing and polymerase chain reaction analysis. *Comp. Med.* **50**:498–502.
3. Hansen, G. M., F. X. Paturzo, and A. L. Smith. 1999. Humoral immunity and protection of mice challenged with homotypic or heterotypic parvovirus. *Lab. Anim. Sci.* **49**:380–384.
4. Jacoby, R. O., L. Ball-Goodrich, D. G. Besselsen, M. D. McKisic, L. K. Riley, and A. L. Smith. 1996. Rodent parvovirus infections. *Lab. Anim. Sci.* **46**:370–380.
5. Jacoby, R. O., E. A. Johnson, L. Ball-Goodrich, A. L. Smith, and M. D. McKisic. 1995. Characterization of mouse parvovirus infection by in situ hybridization. *J. Virol.* **69**:3915–3919.
6. McKisic, M. D., D. W. Lancki, G. Otto, P. Padrid, S. Snook, D. C. Cronin, II, P. D. Lohmar, T. Wong, and F. W. Fitch. 1993. Identification and propagation of a putative immunosuppressive orphan parvovirus in cloned T cells. *J. Immunol.* **150**:419–428.
7. McKisic, M. D., J. D. Macy, Jr., M. L. Delano, R. O. Jacoby, F. X. Paturzo, and A. L. Smith. 1998. Mouse parvovirus infection potentiates allogeneic skin graft rejection and induces syngeneic graft rejection. *Transplantation* **65**:1436–1446.
8. Riley, L. K., R. Knowles, G. Purdy, N. Salmone, D. Pintel, R. R. Hook, Jr., C. L. Franklin, and C. L. Besch-Williford. 1996. Expression of recombinant parvovirus NS1 protein by a baculovirus and application to serologic testing of rodents. *J. Clin. Microbiol.* **34**:440–444.
9. Shek, W. R., F. X. Paturzo, E. A. Johnson, G. M. Hansen, and A. L. Smith. 1998. Characterization of mouse parvovirus infection among BALB/c mice from an enzootically infected colony. *Lab. Anim. Sci.* **48**:294–297.
10. Smith, A. L., R. O. Jacoby, E. A. Johnson, F. X. Paturzo, and P. N. Bhatt. 1993. In vivo studies with an "orphan" parvovirus of mice. *Lab. Anim. Sci.* **43**:175–182.
11. Ueno, Y., M. Iwama, T. Ohshima, F. Sugiyama, A. Takakura, T. Itoh, and K. Yagami. 1998. Prevalence of "orphan" parvovirus infections in mice and rats. *Exp. Anim.* **47**:207–210.

Mouse rotavirus
1. Angel, J., B. Tang, N. Feng, H. B. Greenberg, and D. Bass. 1997. Studies of the role for NSP4 in the pathogenesis of homologous murine rotavirus diarrhea. *J. Infect. Dis.* **177**:455–458.
2. Beisner, B., D. Kool, A. Marich, and I. H. Holmes. 1998. Characterization of G serotype dependent non-antibody inhibitors of rotavirus in normal mouse serum. *Arch. Virol.* **143**:1277–1294.
3. Blutt, S. E., K. L. Warfield, D. E. Lewis, and M. E. Conner. 2002. Early response to rotavirus infection involves massive B cell activation. *J. Immunol.* **168**:5716–5721.
4. Burns, J. W., A. A. Krishnaney, P. T. Vo, R. V. Rouse, L. J. Anderson, and H. B. Greenberg. 1995. Analyses of homologous rotavirus infection in the mouse model. *Virology* **207**:143–153.
5. Chen, C. C., M. Baylor, and D. M. Bass. 1993. Murine intestinal mucins inhibit rotavirus infection. *Gastroenterology* **105**:84–92.
6. Collins, J., W. G. Starkey, T. S. Walls, G. J. Clarke, K. K. Worton, A. J. Spencer, S. J. Haddon, M. P. Osborne, D. C. A. Candy, and J. Stephen. 1988. Intestinal enzyme profiles in normal and rotavirus-infected mice. *J. Pediatr. Gastroenterol. Nutr.* **7**:264–272.
7. Eiden, J., H. M. Lederman, S. Vonderfecht, and R. Yolken. 1986. T-cell-deficient mice display normal recovery from experimental rotavirus infection. *J. Virol.* **57**:706–708.
8. Franco, M. A., N. Feng, and H. B. Greenberg. 1996. Molecular determinants of immunity and pathogenicity of rotavirus infection in the mouse model. *J. Infect. Dis.* **174**:S47–S50.
9. Franco, M. A., and H. B. Greenberg. 1999. Immunity to rotavirus infection in mice. *J. Infect. Dis.* **179**:S466–S469.
10. Guimaraes, M. A., C. M. Nozawa, A. C. Guimaraes, and S. Ramos. 1997. Rotavirus and reovirus interaction with mouse peritoneal resident phagocytic cells. *Braz. J. Med. Biol. Res.* **30**:1187–1190.
11. Horie, Y., O. Nakagomi, Y. Koshimura, T. Nakagomi, Y. Suzuki, T. Oka, S. Sasaki, Y. Matsuda, and S. Watanabe. 1999. Diarrhea induction by rotavirus NSP4 in the homologous mouse model system. *Virology* **262**:398–407.
12. Ijaz, M. K., M. I. Sabara, T. Alkarmi, P. J. Frenchick, K. F. Ready, M. Longson, F. K.

Dar, and L. A. Babiuk. 1993. Characterization of two rotaviruses differing in their *in vitro* and *in vivo* virulence. *J. Vet. Med. Sci.* **55:**963–971.

13. Ijaz, M. K., M. I. Sabara, P. J. Frenchick, and L. A Babiuk. 1987. Assessment of intestinal damage in rotavirus infected neonatal mice by a D-xylose absorption test. *J. Virol. Methods* **18:**153–157.

14. Katyal, R., S. V. Rana, K. Vaiphei, S. Ohja, K. Singh, and V. Singh. 1999. Effect of rotavirus infection on small gut pathophysiology in a mouse model. *J. Gastroenterol. Hepatol.* **14:**779–784.

15. Little, L. M., and J. A. Shadduck. 1982. Pathogenesis of rotavirus infection in mice. *Infect. Immun.* **38:**755–763.

16. Lundgren, O., A. T. Peregrin, K. Persson, S. Kordasti, I. Uhnoo, and L. Svenson. 2000. Role of the enteric nervous system in the fluid and electrolyte secretion of rotavirus diarrhea. *Science* **287:**491–495.

17. McNeal, M. M., R. L. Broome, and R. L. Ward. 1994. Active immunity against rotavirus infection in mice is correlated with viral replication and titers of serum rotavirus IgA following vaccination. *Virology* **204:**642–650.

18. McNeal, M. M., M. N. Rae, and R. L. Ward. 1997. Evidence that resolution of rotavirus infection in mice is due to both CD4 and CD8 cell-dependent activities. *J. Virol.* **71:**8735–8742.

19. McNeal, M. M., J. L. Van Cott, A. H. Choi, M. Basu, J. A. Flint, S. C. Stone, J. D. Clements, and R. L. Ward. 2002. CD4 T cells are the only lymphocytes needed to protect mice against rotavirus shedding after intranasal immunization with a chimeric VP6 protein and the adjuvant LT(R192G). *J. Virol.* **76:**560–568.

20. McNeal, M. M., and R. L. Ward. 1995. Long-term production of rotavirus antibody and protection against reinfection following a single infection of neonatal mice with murine rotavirus. *Virology* **211:**474–480.

21. Morrey, J. D., R. W. Sidwell, R. L. Noble, B. B. Barnett, and A. W. Mahoney. 1984. Effects of folic acid malnutrition on rotaviral infection in mice. *Proc. Soc. Exp. Biol. Med.* **176:**77–83.

22. Morris, A. P., J. K. Scott, J. M. Ball, C. Q. Zeng, W. K. O'Neal, and M. K. Estes. 1999. NSP4 elicits age-dependent diarrhea and Ca^{++} mediated I^- influx into intestinal crypts of CF mice. *Am. J. Physiol.* **277:**G431–G444.

23. National Research Council. 1991. *Infectious Diseases of Mice and Rats: a Report of the Institute of Laboratory Animal Resources Committee on Infectious Diseases of Mice and Rats*. National Academy Press, Washington, D.C.

24. Newsome, P. M., and K. A. Coney. 1985. Synergistic rotavirus and *Escherichia coli* diarrheal infection of mice. *Infect. Immun.* **47:**573–574.

25. Noble, R. L., R. W. Sidwell, A. W. Mahoney, B. B. Barnett, and R. S. Splendlove. 1983. Influence of malnutrition and alterations in dietary protein on murine rotaviral disease. *Proc. Soc. Exp. Biol. Med.* **173:**417–426.

26. Percy, D. H., and S. W. Barthold. 2001. *Pathology of Laboratory Rodents and Rabbits*, 2nd ed. Iowa State University Press, Ames.

27. Riepenhoff-Talty, M., T. Dharakul, E. Kowalski, S. Michalak, and P. L. Ogra. 1987. Persistent rotavirus infection in mice with severe combined immunodeficiency. *J. Virol.* **61:**3345–3348.

28. Sagher, F. A., J. A. Dodge, D. H. Simpson, and P. Evans. 1991. Kinetics of viral replication in experimental rotavirus infection: effects of high dietary fat. *J. Pediatr. Gastroenterol. Nutr.* **13:**83–89.

29. Shaw, R. D., S. J. Hempson, and E. R. Mackow. 1995. Rotavirus diarrhea is caused by nonreplicating viral particles. *J. Virol.* **69:**5946–5950.

30. Sodhi, C. P., R. Katyal, S. V. Rana, S. Attri, and V. Singh. 1996. Study of oxidative-stress in rotavirus infected infant mice. *Indian J. Med. Res.* **104:**245–249.

31. Tatti, K., J. Gentsch, W. Shieh, T. Ferebee-Harris, M. Lynch, J. Bresee, B. Jiang, S. Zaki, and R. Glass. 2002. Molecular and immunological methods to detect rotavirus in formalin-fixed tissue. *J. Virol. Methods* **105:**305.

32. Williams, M. B., J. R. Rose, L. S. Rott, M. A. Franco, H. B. Greenberg, and E. C. Butcher. 1998. The memory B cell subset responsible for the secretory IgA response and protective humoral immunity to rotavirus expresses the intestinal homing receptor, $\alpha_4\beta_7$. *J. Immunol.* **161:**4227–4235.

33. Willoughby, R. E. 1993. Rotaviruses preferentially bind O-linked sialylglycoconjugates and sialomucins. *Glycobiology* **3:**437–445.

Mouse thymic virus

1. Athanassious, R., and G. Lussier. 1992. Mouse thymic virus infection: ultrastructural and immunocytochemical studies of infected thymus cells. *J. Exp. Anim. Sci.* **35:**63–70.

2. Cohen, P. L., S. S. Cross, and D. E. Mosier. 1975. Immunolgic effects of neonatal infection with mouse thymic virus. *J. Immunol.* **115:**706–710.

3. Cross, S. S., H. C. Morse, III, and R. Asofsky. 1976. Neonatal infection with mouse thymic

virus. Differential effects on T cells mediating the graft-versus-host reaction. *J. Immunol.* **117**:635–638.
4. Morse, S. S. 1987. Mouse thymic necrosis virus: A novel murine lymphotropic agent. *Lab. Anim. Sci.* **37**:717–725.
5. National Research Council. 1991. *Infectious Diseases of Mice and Rats: a Report of the Institute of Laboratory Animal Resources Committee on Infectious Diseases of Mice and Rats.* National Academy Press, Washington, D.C.
6. St-Pierre, Y., E. F. Potworowski, and G. F. Lussier. 1987. Transmission of mouse thymic virus. *J. Gen. Virol.* **68**:1173–1176.
7. Wood, B. A., W. Dutz, and S. S. Cross. 1981. Neonatal infection with mouse thymic virus: Spleen and lymph node necrosis. *J. Gen. Virol.* **57**:139–147.

Pneumonia virus of mice
1. Boot, R., H. van Herck, and J. van der Logt. 1996. Mutual viral and bacterial infections after housing rats of various breeders within an experimental unit. *Lab. Anim.* **30**:42–45.
2. Carthew, P., and S. Sparrow. 1980. A comparison in germ-free mice of the pathogenesis of Sendai virus and mouse pneumonia virus infection. *J. Pathol.* **130**:153–158.
3. Carthew, P., and S. Sparrow. 1980. Persistence of pneumonia virus of mice and Sendai virus in germ-free (*nu/nu*) mice. *Br. J. Exp. Pathol.* **61**:172–175.
4. Domachowske, J. B., C. A. Bonville, K. D. Dyer, A. J. Easton, and H. F. Rosenberg. 2000. Pulmonary eosinophilia and production of MIP-1-a are prominent responses to infection with pneumonia virus of mice. *Cell. Immunol.* **200**:98–104.
5. Domachowske, J. B., C. A. Bonville, A. J. Easton, and H. F. Rosenberg. 2002. Differential expression of proinflammatory cytokine genes *in vivo* in response to pathogenic and nonpathogenic pneumovirus infections. *J. Infect. Dis.* **186**:8–14.
6. Lussier, G. 1988. Potential detrimental effects of rodent viral infections on long-term experiments. *Vet. Res. Commun.* **12**:199–217.
7. Miyata, H., M. Kishikawa, H. Kondo, C. Kai, Y. Watanabe, K. Ohsawa, and H. Sato. 1995. New isolates of pneumonia virus of mice (PVM) from Japanese rat colonies and their characterization. *Exp. Anim.* **44**:95-104.
8. National Research Council. 1991. *Infectious Diseases of Mice and Rats: a Report of the Institute of Laboratory Animal Resources Committee on Infectious Diseases of Mice and Rats.* National Academy Press, Washington, D.C.
9. Randhawa, J. S., P. Chambers, C. R. Pringle, and A. J. Easton. 1995. Nucleotide sequences of the genes encoding the putative attachment glycoprotein (G) of mouse and tissue culture-passaged strains of pneumonia virus of mice. *Virology* **207**:240–245.
10. Richter, C. B., J. E. Thigpen, C. S. Richter, and J. M. Mackenzie, Jr. 1988. Fatal pneumonia with terminal emaciation in nude mice caused by pneumonia virus of mice. *Lab. Anim. Sci.* **38**:255–261.
11. Rosenberg, H. F. and J. B. Domachowske. 2001. Eosinophils, eosinophil ribonucleases, and their role in host defense against respiratory virus pathogens. *J. Leukoc. Biol.* **70**:691–198.
12. Schuurman, H.-J., E. B. Bell, K. Gärtner, H. J. Hedrich, A. K. Hansen, B. C. Kruijt, P. de Vrey, R. Leyten, S. J. Maeder, R. Moutier, U. Mohnle, J. Vankerkom, R. Boot, R. Broekhuizen, J. Dormans, H. van Herck, P. G. C. Hermans, J. Hoekman, J. van der Logt, M. van Wiik, J. G. Vos, and L. F. M. van Zutphen. 1992. Comparative evaluation of the immune status of congenitally athymic and euthymic rat strains bred and maintained at different institutes: 1. Euthymic rats. *J. Exp. Anim. Sci.* **35**:16–32.
13. Zenner, L., and J. P. Regnault. 2000. Ten-year long monitoring of laboratory mouse and rat colonies in French facilities: a retrospective study. *Lab. Anim.* **34**:76–83.

Rat rotavirus-like agent
1. National Research Council. 1991. *Infectious Diseases of Mice and Rats: a Report of the Institute of Laboratory Animal Resources Committee on Infectious Diseases of Mice and Rats.* National Academy Press, Washington, D.C.
2. Salim, A. F., A. D. Phillips, and M. Farthing. 1990. Pathogenesis of gut virus infection. *Baillieres Clin. Gastroenterol.* **4**:593–607.
3. Salim, A. F., A. D. Phillips, J. A. Walker-Smith, and M. J. Farthing. 1995. Sequential changes in small intestinal structure and function during rotavirus infection in neonatal rats. *Gut* **36**:231–238.
4. Vonderfecht, S. L., A. C. Huber, J. J. Eiden, L. C. Mader, and R. H. Yolken. 1984. Infectious diarrhea of infant rats produced by a rotavirus-like agent. *J. Virol.* **52**:94–98.
5. Vonderfecht, S. L., and J. K. Schemmer. 1993. Purification of the IDIR strain of group B rotavirus and identification of viral structural proteins. *Virology* **194**:277–283.
6. Yolken, R. H., C. Ojeh, I. A. Khatri, U. Sajjan, and J. F. Forstner. 1994. Intestinal mucins inhibit rotavirus replication in an oligosaccharide-dependent manner. *J. Infect. Dis.* **169**:1002–1006.

Reovirus-3

1. al-Sheboul, S., D. Crosley, and T. A. Steele. 1996. Inhibition of reovirus-stimulated murine natural killer cell cytotoxicity by cyclosporine. *Life Sci.* **59:**1675–1682.
2. Barkon, M. L., B. L. Haller, and H. W. Virgin, IV. 1996. Circulating immunoglobulin G can play a critical role in clearance of intestinal reovirus infection. *J. Virol.* **70:**1109–1116.
3. Barthold, S. W., A. L. Smith, and P. N. Bhatt. 1993. Infectivity, disease patterns, and serologic profiles of reovirus serotypes 1, 2, and 3 in infant and weanling mice. *Lab. Anim. Sci.* **43:**425–430.
4. Bennette, J. G. 1960. Isolation of a non-pathogenic tumour-destroying virus from mouse ascites. *Nature* **187:**72–73.
5. Cook, I. 1963. Reovirus type 3 infection in laboratory mice. *Aust. J. Exp. Biol. Med. Sci.* **41:**651–660.
6. Cuff, C. F., C. K. Cebra, E. Lavi, E. H. Molowitz, D. H. Rubin, and J. J. Cebra. 1991. Protection of neonatal mice from fatal reovirus infection by immune serum and gut derived lymphocytes. *Adv. Exp. Med. Biol.* **310:**307–315.
7. Derrien, M. and B. N. Fields. 1999. Reovirus type 3 clone 9 increases interleukin-1α level in the brain of neonatal, but not adult, mice. *Virology* **257:**35–44.
8. Fan, J. Y., C. S. Boyce, and C. S. Cuff. 1998. T-Helper 1 and T-Helper 2 cytokine responses in gut-associated lymphoid tissue following enteric reovirus infection. *Cell. Immunol.* **188:**55–63.
9. Farone, A. L., C. W. Frevert, M. B. Farone, M. J. Morin, B. N. Fields, J. D. Paulauskis, and L. Kobzik. 1996. Serotype-dependent induction of pulmonary neutrophilia and inflammatory cytokine gene expression by reovirus. *J. Virol.* **70:**7079–7084.
10. Farone, A. L., P. C. O'Brien, and D. C. Cox. 1993. Tumor necrosis factor-alpha induction by reovirus serotype 3. *J. Leukoc. Biol.* **53:**133–137.
11. Hicks, J., S. H. Zhu, and J. Barrish. 2001. Neonatal syncytial giant cell hepatitis with paramyxoviral-like inclusions. *Ultrastruct. Pathol.* **25:**65–71.
12. Klein, J. O., G. M. Green, T. G. Tilles, E. H. Kass, and M. Finland. 1969. Effect of intranasal reovirus infection in antibacterial activity of mouse lung. *J. Infect. Dis.* **119:**43–50.
13. Kollmorgen, G. M., D. C. Cox, J. J. Killion, J. L. Cantrell, and W. A. Sansing. 1976. Immunotherapy of EL4 lymphoma with reovirus. *Cancer Immunol. Immunother.* **1:**239–244.
14. Major, A. S. and C. F. Cuff. 1997. Enhanced mucosal and systemic immune response to intestinal reovirus infection in β2-microglobulin-deficient mice. *J. Virol.* **71:**5782–5789.
15. Meek, R. B., III, B. M. McGrew, C. F. Cuff, A. S. Berrebi, G. A. Spirou, and S. J. Wetmore. 1999. Immunologic and histologic observations in reovirus-induced otitis media in the mouse. *Ann. Otol. Rhinol. Laryngol.* **108:**31–38.
16. Morin, M. J., A. Warner, and B. N. Fields. 1996. Reovirus infection in rat lungs as a model to study the pathogenesis of viral pneumonia. *J. Virol.* **70:**541–548.
17. National Research Council. 1991. *Infectious Diseases of Mice and Rats: a Report of the Institute of Laboratory Animal Resources Committee on Infectious Diseases of Mice and Rats.* National Academy Press, Washington, D.C.
18. Nelson, J. B., and G. S. Tarnowski. 1960. An oncolytic virus recovered from Swiss mice during passage of an ascites tumour. *Nature* **188:**866–867.
19. Nicklas, W., V. Kraft, and B. Meyer. 1993. Contamination of transplantable tumors, cell lines, and monoclonal antibodies with rodent viruses. *Lab. Anim. Sci.* **43:**296–300.
20. Oberhaus, S. M., R. L. Smith, G. H. Clayton, T. S. Dermody, and K. L. Tyler. 1997. Reovirus infection and tissue injury in the mouse central nervous system are associated with apoptosis. *J. Virol.* **71:**2100–2106.
21. Parashar, K., M. J. Tarlow, and M. A. McCrae. 1992. Experimental reovirus type 3-induced murine biliary tract disease. *J. Pediatr. Surg.* **27:**843–847.
22. Sansing, W. A., J. J. Killion, and G. M. Kollmorgen. 1977. Evaluation of time and dose in treating mammary adenocarcinoma with immunostimulants. *Cancer Immunol. Immunother.* **2:**63–68.
23. Sharpe, A. H., and B. N. Fields. 1985. Pathogenesis of viral infections. Basic concepts derived from the reovirus model. *N. Engl. J. Med.* **312:**486–497.
24. Sherry, B., C. J. Baty, and M. A. Blum. 1996. Reovirus-induced acute myocarditis in mice correlates with viral RNA synthesis rather than generation of infectious virus in cardiac myocytes. *J. Virol.* **70:**6709–6715.
25. Stanley, N. F. 1974. The reovirus murine models. *Prog. Med. Virol.* **18:**257–272.
26. Steele, T. A., and D. C. Cox. 1995. Reovirus type 3 chemoimmunotherapy of murine lymphoma is abrogated by cyclosporine. *Cancer Biother.* **10:**307–315.
27. Theiss, J. C., G. D. Stoner, and A. K. Kniazeff. 1978. Effect of reovirus infection on pul-

monary tumor response to urethane in strain A mice. *J. Natl. Cancer Inst.* **61**:131–134.
28. **Tyler, K. L., M. A. Mann, B. N. Fields, and H. W. Virgin, IV.** 1993. Protective antireovirus monoclonal antibodies and their effects on viral pathogenesis. *J. Virol.* **67**:3446–3453.
29. **Virgin, H. W., IV, M. A. Mann, and K. L. Tyler.** 1994. Protective antibodies inhibit reovirus internalization and uncoating by intracellular proteases. *J. Virol.* **68**:6719–6729.
30. **Virgin, H. W., IV, and K. L. Tyler.** 1991. Role of immune cells in protection against and control of reovirus infection in neonatal mice. *J. Virol.* **65**:5157–5164.

Sendai virus
1. **Akaike, T., S. Fujii, A. Kato, J. Yoshitake, Y. Miyamoto, T. Sawa, S. Okamoto, M. Suga, M. Asakawa, Y. Nagai, and H. Maeda.** 2000. Viral mutation accelerated by nitric oxide production during infection *in vivo*. *FASEB J.* **14**:1447–1454.
2. **Bitzer, M., F. Prinz, M. Bauer, M. Spiegel, W. J. Neubert, M. Gregor, K. Schulze-Osthoff, and U. Lauer.** 1999. Sendai virus infection induces apoptosis through activation of caspase-8 (FLICE) and caspase-3 (CPP32). *J. Virol.* **73**:702–708.
3. **Brownstein, D. G., and E. C. Weir.** 1987. Immunostimulation in mice infected with Sendai virus. *Am. J. Vet. Res.* **12**:1692–1696.
4. **Cormier, Y., E. Israel-Assayag, M. Fournier, and G. M. Tremblay.** 1993. Modulation of experimental hypersensitivity pneumonitis by Sendai virus. *J. Lab. Clin. Med.* **121**:683–688.
5. **Costas, M. A., D. Mella, M. Criscuolo, A. Diaz, S. Finkielman, V. E. Nahmod, and E. Arzt.** 1993. Superinduction of mitogen-stimulated interferon-gamma production and other lymphokines by Sendai virus. *J. Interferon Res.* **13**:407–412.
6. **Finberg, R., H. Cantor, B. Benacerraf, and S. Burakoff.** 1980. The origins of alloreactivity: Differentiation of prekiller cells to virus infection results in alloreactive cytolytic T lymphocytes. *J. Immunol.* **124**:1858–1860.
7. **Fukushima, T., K. Sekizawa, M. Yamaya, S. Okinaga, M. Satoh, and H. Sasaki.** 1995. Viral respiratory infection increases alveolar macrophage cytoplasmic motility in rats: role of NO. *Am. J. Physiol.* **268**:L399–L406.
8. **Garlinghouse, L. E., and G. L. Van Hoosier.** 1978. Studies on adjuvant-induced arthritis, tumor transplantability and serologic response to bovine serum albumin in Sendai virus infected rats. *Am. J. Vet. Res.* **39**:297–300.
9. **Hasan, M. K., A. Kato, M. Muranaka, R. Yamaguchi, Y. Sakai, I. Hatano, M. Tashiro, and Y. Nagai.** 2000. Versatility of the accessory C proteins of Sendai virus: contribution to virus assembly as an additional role. *J. Virol.* **74**:5619–5628.
10. **Homberger, F. R., and P. E. Thomann.** 1994. Transmission of murine viruses and mycoplasma in laboratory mouse colonies with respect to housing conditions. *Lab. Anim.* **28**:113–120.
11. **Hua, J., M. J. Liao, and A. Rashidbaigi.** 1996. Cytokines induced by Sendai virus in human peripheral blood leukocytes. *J. Leukoc. Biol.* **60**:125–128.
12. **Huang, C., K. Kiyotani, Y. Fujii, N. Fukuhara, A. Kato, Y. Nagai, T. Yoshida, and T. Sakaguchi.** 2000. Involvement of the zinc-binding capacity of Sendai virus V protein in viral pathogenesis. *J. Virol.* **74**:7834–7841.
13. **Itoh, T., H. Iwai, and K. Ueda.** 1991. Comparative lung pathology of inbred strain of mice resistant and susceptible to Sendai virus infection. *J. Vet. Med. Sci.* **53**:275–279.
14. **Iwai, H., A. Morioka, Y. Shoya, Y. Obta, M. Goto, R. Kirisawa, H. Okada, and T. Yoshino.** 1998. Protective effect of passive immunization against TNF-alpha in mice infected with Sendai virus. *Exp. Anim.* **47**:49–54.
15. **Jacoby, R. O., P. N. Bhatt, S. W. Barthold, and D. G. Brownstein.** 1994. Sendai viral pneumonia in aged BALB/c mice. *Exp. Gerontol.* **29**:89–100.
16. **Jecker, P., A. McWilliam, A. Marsh, P. G. Holt, W. J. Mann, R. Pabst, and J. Westermann.** 2001. Acute laryngotracheitis in the rat induced by Sendai virus: the influx of six different types of immunocompetent cells into the laryngeal mucosa differs strongly between the subglottic and the glottic compartment. *Laryngoscope* **111**:1645–1651.
17. **Kay, M. M. B.** 1978. Long term subclinical effects of parainfluenza (Sendai) infection on immune cells of aging mice. *Proc. Soc. Exp. Biol. Med.* **158**:326–331.
18. **Kenyon, A. J.** 1983. Delayed wound healing in mice associated with viral alteration of macrophages. *Am. J. Vet. Res.* **44**:652–656.
19. **Knott, P. G., P. J. Henry, A. S. McWilliams, P. J. Rigby, L. B. Fernandes, and R. G. Goldie.** 1996. Influence of parainfluenza-1 respiratory tract viral infection on endothelin receptor-effector systems in mouse and rat tracheal smooth muscle. *Br. J. Pharmacol.* **119**:291–298.
20. **Komatsu, T., Takeuchi, K., Tokoo, J., Y. Tanaka, and B. Gotoh.** 2000. Sendai virus blocks alpha interferon signaling to signal transducers and activators of transcription. *J. Virol.* **74**:2477–2480.

21. **Lavilla-Apelo, C., H. Kida, and H. Kanagawa.** 1992. The effect of experimental infection of mouse preimplantation embryos with paramyxovirus Sendai. *J. Vet. Med. Sci.* **54:**335–340.
22. **Liang, S. C., T. R. Schoeb, J. K. Davis, J. W. Simecka, G. H. Cassell, and J. R. Lindsey.** 1995. Comparative severity of respiratory lesions of sialodacryoadenitis virus and Sendai virus infections in LEW and F344 rats. *Vet. Pathol.* **32:**661–667.
23. **Liang, S. C., J. W. Simecka, J. R. Lindsey, G. H. Cassell, and J. K. Davis.** 1999. Antibody responses after Sendai virus infection and their role in upper and lower respiratory tract disease in rats. *Lab. Anim. Sci.* **49:**385–394.
24. **Makino, S., S. Seko, H. Nakao, and K. Mikazuki.** 1972. An epizootic of Sendai virus infection in a rat colony. *Exp. Anim.* **22:**275–280.
25. **Matsuya, Y., T. Kusano, S. Endo, N. Takahashi, and I. Yamane.** 1978. Reduced tumorigenicity by addition *in vitro* of Sendai virus. *Eur. J. Cancer* **14:**837–850.
26. **Mo, X. Y., M. Sangster, S. Sarawar, C. Coleclough, and P. C. Doherty.** 1995. Differential antigen burden modulates the gamma interferon but not the immunoglobulin response in mice that vary in susceptibility to Sendai virus pneumonia. *J. Virol.* **69:**5592–5598.
27. **Mo, X. Y., S. R. Sarawar, and P. C. Doherty.** 1995. Induction of cytokines in mice with parainfluenza pneumonia. *J. Virol.* **69:**1288–1291.
28. **Mo, X. Y., R. A. Tripp, M. Y. Sangster, and P. C. Doherty.** 1997. The cytotoxic T-lymphocytes response to Sendai virus is unimpaired in the absence of gamma interferon. *J. Virol.* **71:**1906–1910.
29. **National Research Council.** 1991. *Infectious Diseases of Mice and Rats: a Report of the Institute of Laboratory Animal Resources Committee on Infectious Diseases of Mice and Rats.* National Academy Press, Washington, D.C.
30. **Peck, R. M., G. J. Eaton, E. B. Peck, and S. Litwin.** 1983. Influence of Sendai virus on carcinogenesis in strain A mice. *Lab. Anim. Sci.* **33:**154–156.
31. **Percy, D. H., D. C. Auger, and B. A. Croy.** 1994. Signs and lesions of experimental Sendai virus infection in two genetically distinct strains of SCID/beige mice. *Vet. Pathol.* **31:**67–73.
32. **Roberts, N. J.** 1982. Different effects of influenza virus, respiratory syncytial virus, and Sendai virus on human lymphocytes and macrophages. *Infect. Immun.* **35:**1142–1146.
33. **Sakaguchi, T., K. Kiyotani, M. Sakaki, Y. Fujii, and T. Yoshida.** 1994. A field isolate of Sendai virus: its high virulence to mice and genetic divergence form prototype strains. *Arch. Virol.* **135:**159–164.
34. **Sakai, Y., K. Kiyotani, M. Fukumura, M. Asakawa, A. Kato, T. Shioda, T. Yoshida, A. Tanaka, M. Hasegawa, and Y. Nagai.** 1999. Accommodation of foreign genes into the Sendai virus genome: sizes of inserted genes and viral replication. *FEBS Lett.* **456:**221–226.
35. **Sakai, K., T. Kohri, M. Tashiro, Y. Kishino, and H. Kido.** 1994. Sendai virus infection changes the subcellular localization of tryptase Clara in rat bronchiolar epithelial cells. *Eur. Respir. J.* **7:**686–692.
36. **Skiadopoulos, M. H., S. R. Surman, J. M. Riggs, W. R. Elkins, M. St. Claire, M. Nishio, D. Garcin, D. Kolakofsky, P. L. Collins, and B. R. Murphy.** 2002. Sendai virus, a murine parainfluenza virus type 1, replicates to a level similar to human PIV1 in the upper and lower respiratory tract of African green monkeys and chimpanzees. *Virology* **297:**153–160.
37. **Sorden, S. D., and W. L. Castleman.** 1995. Virus-induced increases in bronchiolar mast cells in Brown Norway rats are associated with both local mast cell proliferation and increases in blood mast cell precursors. *Lab. Invest.* **73:**197–204.
38. **Sorkness, R. L., W. L. Castleman, A. Kumar, M. R. Kaplan, and R. F. Lamanske, Jr.** 1999. Prevention of chronic postbronchiolitis airway sequelae with IFN-gamma treatment in rats. *Am. J. Respir. Crit. Care Med.* **160:**705–710.
39. **Sorkness, R., R. F. Lemanske, Jr., and W. L. Castleman.** 1991. Persistent airway hyperresponsiveness after neonatal viral bronchiolitis in rats. *J. Appl. Physiol.* **70:**375–383.
40. **Sorkness, R. L., H. Mehta, M. R. Kaplan, M. Miyasaka, S. L. Hefle, and R. F. Lemanske, Jr.** 2000. Effect of ICAM-1 blockade on lung inflammation and physiology during acute viral bronchiolitis in rats. *Pediatr. Res.* **47:**819–824.
41. **Streilein, J. W., J. A. Shadduck, and S. P. Pakes.** 1981. Effects of splenectomy and Sendai virus infection on rejection of male skin isografts by pathogen free C57BL/6 female mice. *Transplantation* **32:**34–37.
42. **Tanabayashi, K., and R. W. Compans.** 1996. Functional interaction of paramyxovirus glycoproteins: identification of a domain in Sendai virus HN which promotes cell fusion. *J. Virol.* **70:**6112–6118.
43. **Topham, D. J., and P. C. Doherty.** 1998. Longitudinal analysis of the acute Sendai virus-specific CD4+ T cell response and memory. *J. Immunol.* **161:**4530–4535.
44. **Uhl, E. W., L. L. Moldawar, W. W. Busse, T. J. Jack, and W. L. Castleman.** 1998. In-

creased tumor necrosis factor-alpha (TNF-α) gene expression in parainfluenza type 1 (Sendai) virus-induced bronchiolar fibrosis. *Am. J. Pathol.* **152:**513–522.
45. Usherwood, E. J., R. J. Hogan, G. Crowther, S. L. Surman, T. L. Hogg, J. D. Altman, and D. L. Woodland. 1999. Functionally heterogeneous CD8+ T-cell memory is induced in Sendai virus infection of mice. *J. Virol.* **73:**7278–7286.
46. Winter, J. B., A. S. Gouw, M. Groen, C. Wildevuur, and J. Prop. 1994. Respiratory viral infections aggravate airway damage caused by chronic rejection in rat lung allografts. *Transplantation* **57:**418–422.
47. Yamawaki, I., P. Geppetti, C. Bertrand, B. Chan, P. Massion, G. Piedimonte, and J. A. Nadel. 1995. Viral infection potentiates the increase in airway blood flow produced by substance P. *J. Appl. Physiol.* **79:**398–404.
48. Yoshihara, S., B. Chan, I. Yamawaki, P. Geppetti, F. L. Ricciardolo, P. P. Massion, and J. A. Nadel. 1995. Plasma extravasation in the rat trachea induced by cold air is mediated by tachykinin release from sensory nerves. *Am. J. Respir. Crit. Care Med.* **151:**1011–1017.

Sialodacryoadenitis virus
1. Barthold, S. W., M. S. de Souza, and A. L. Smith. 1990. Susceptibility of laboratory mice to intranasal and contact infection with coronaviruses of other species. *Lab. Anim. Sci.* **40:**481–485.
2. Bihun, C. G., and D. H. Percy. 1995. Morphologic changes in the nasal cavity associated with sialodacryoadenitis virus infection in the Wistar rat. *Vet. Pathol.* **32:**1–10.
3. Boschert, K. R., T. R. Schoeb, D. B. Chandler, and D. L. Dillehay. 1988. Inhibition of phagocytosis and interleukin-1 production in pulmonary macrophages from rats with sialodacryoadenitis virus infection. *J. Leukoc. Biol.* **44:**87–92.
4. Hajjar, A. M., R. F. DiGiacomo, J. K. Carpenter, S. A. Bingel, and T. C. Moazed. 1991. Chronic sialodacryoadenitis virus (SDAV) infection in athymic rats. *Lab. Anim. Sci.* **41:**22–25.
5. Jacoby, R. O., P. N. Bhatt, and A. M. Jonas. 1979. Viral diseases, p. 271–306. *In* H. J. Baker, J. R. Lindsey, and S. H. Weisbroth (ed.), *The Laboratory Rat*, vol. I: *Biology and Diseases*. Academic Press, New York, N.Y.
6. Kojima, A., and A. Okaniwa. 1991. Antigenic heterogeneity of sialodacryoadenitis virus isolates. *J. Vet. Med. Sci.* **53:**1059–1063.
7. La Regina, M., L. Woods, P. Klender, D. J. Gaertner, and F. X. Paturzo. 1992. Transmission of sialodacryoadenitis virus (SDAV) from infected rats to rats and mice through handling, close contact, and soiled bedding. *Lab. Anim. Sci.* **42:**344–346.
8. Liang, S. C., T. R. Schoeb, J. K. Davis, J. W. Simecka, G. H. Cassell, and J. R. Lindsey. 1995. Comparative severity of respiratory lesions of sialodacryoadenitis virus and Sendai virus infections in LEW and F344 rats. *Vet. Pathol.* **32:**661–667.
9. **National Research Council.** 1991. *Infectious Diseases of Mice and Rats: a Report of the Institute of Laboratory Animal Resources Committee on Infectious Diseases of Mice and Rats*. National Academy Press, Washington, D.C.
10. Nichols, P. W., T. R. Schoeb, J. K. Davis, M. K. Davidson, and J. R. Lindsey. 1992. Pulmonary clearance of *Mycoplasma pulmonis* in rats with respiratory viral infections or of susceptible genotype. *Lab. Anim. Sci.* **42:**454–457.
11. Nunoya, T., M. Itabashi, S. Kudow, M. Hayashi, and M. Tajima. 1977. An epizootic outbreak of sialodacryoadenitis in rats. *Jpn. J. Vet. Sci.* **39:**445–450.
12. Percy, D. H., M. A. Hayes, T. E. Kocal, and Z. W. Wojcinski. 1988. Depletion of salivary gland epidermal growth factor by sialodacryoadenitis virus infection in the Wistar rat. *Vet. Pathol.* **25:**183–192.
13. Percy, D. H., K. L. Williams, and B. A. Croy. 1991. Experimental sialodacryoadenitis virus infection in severe combined immunodeficient mice. *Can. J. Vet. Res.* **55:**89–90.
14. Schoeb, T. R., M. M. Juliana, P. W. Nichols, J. K. Davis, and J. R. Lindsey. 1993. Effects of viral and mycoplasmal infections, ammonia exposure, vitamin A deficiency, host age, and organism strain on adherence of *Mycoplasma pulmonis* in cultured rat tracheas. *Lab. Anim. Sci.* **43:**417–424.
15. Schunk, M. K., D. H. Percy, and S. Rosendal. 1995. Effect of time of exposure to rat coronavirus and *Mycoplasma pulmonis* on respiratory tract lesions in the Wistar rat. *Can. J. Vet. Res.* **59:**60–66.
16. Utsumi, K., T. Maeda, H. Tatsumi, and K. Fijiwara. 1978. Some clinical and epizootiological observations of infectious sialoadenitis in rats. *Exp. Anim.* **27:**283–287.
17. Utsumi, K., K. Maeda, Y. Yokota, S. Fukagawa, and K. Fujiwara. 1991. Reproductive disorders in female rats infected with sialodacryoadenitis virus. *Jikken Dobutsu* **40:**361–365.
18. Wickham, L. A., Z. Huang, R. W. Lambert, and D. A. Sullivan. 1997. Effect of sialodacryoadenitis virus exposure on acinar epithelial

cells from the rat lacrimal gland. *Ocul. Immunol. Inflamm.* **5:**181–195.
19. **Wickham, L. A., Z. Huang, R. W. Lambert, and D. A. Sullivan.** 1994. Sialodacryoadenitis virus infection of rat lacrimal gland acinar cells. *Adv. Exp. Med. Biol.* **350:**193–196.
20. **Yoo, D., Y. Pei, N. Christie, and M. Cooper.** 2000. Primary structure of the sialodacryoadenitis virus genome: sequence of the structural-protein region and its application for differential diagnosis. *Clin. Diagn. Lab. Immunol.* **7:**568–573.

Theiler's murine encephalomyelitis virus

1. **Abzug, M. J.** 1993. Identification of trophoblastic giant cells as the initial principal target of early gestational murine enterovirus infection. *Placenta* **14:**137–148.
2. **Azoulay-Cayla, A., S. Dethlefs, B. Perarnau, E. L. Larsson-Sciard, F. A. Lemonnier, M. Brahic, and J. F. Bureau.** 2000. H-2D$^{b-/-}$ mice are susceptible to persistent infection by Theiler's virus. *J. Virol.* **74:**5470–5476.
3. **Bureau, J. F., K. M. Drescher, L. R. Pease, T. Vikoren, M. Delcroix, L. Zoecklein, M. Brahic, and M. Rodriquez.** 1998. Chromosome 14 contains determinants that regulate susceptibility to Theiler's virus-induced demyelination in the mouse. *Genetics* **148:**1941–1949.
4. **Gomez, R. M., J. E. Rinehart, R. Wollmann, and R. P. Roos.** 1996. Theiler's murine encephalomyelitis virus-induced cardiac and skeletal muscle disease. *J. Virol.* **70:**8926–8933.
5. **Ha-Lee, Y. M., K. Dillon, B. Kosaras, R. Sidman, P. Revell, R. Fujinamik, and M. Chow.** 1995. Mode of spread to and within the central nervous system after oral infection of neonatal mice with the DA strain of Theiler's murine encephalomyelitis virus. *J. Virol.* **69:**7354–7361.
6. **Inoue, A., C. S. Koh, H. Yahikozawa, N. Yanagisawa, H. Yagita, Y. Ishihara, and B. S. Kim.** 1996. The level of tumor necrosis factor-alpha producing cells in the spinal cord correlates with the degree of Theiler's murine encephalomyelitis virus-induced demyelinating disease. *Int. Immunol.* **8:**1001–1008.
7. **Kang, B. S., M. A. Lyman, and B. S. Kim.** 2002. The majority of infiltrating CD8$^+$ T cells in the central nervous system of susceptible SJL/J mice infected with Theiler's virus are virus specific and fully functional. *J. Virol.* **76:**6577–6585.
8. **Krinke, G. J., and A. Zurbriggen.** 1997. Spontaneous demyelinating myelopathy in aging laboratory mice. *Exp. Toxicol. Pathol.* **49:**501–503.
9. **Larsson-Sciard, E. L., S. Dethlefs, and M. Brahic.** 1997. *In vivo* administration of interleukin-2 protects susceptible mice from Theiler's virus persistence. *J. Virol.* **71:**797–799.
10. **Lipton, H. L., B. S. Kim, H. Yahikozawa, and C. F. Nadler.** 2001. Serological evidence that *Mus musculus* is the natural host of Theiler's murine encephalomyelitis virus. *Virus Res.* **76:**79–86.
11. **Martinat, C., N. Jarousse, M. C. Prevost, and M. Brahic.** 1999. The GDVII strain of Theiler's virus spreads via axonal transport. *J. Virol.* **73:**6093–6098.
12. **McGavern, D. B., P. D. Murray, C. Rivera-Quinones, J. D. Schmelzer, P. A. Low, and M. Rodriguez.** 2000. Axonal loss results in spinal cord atrophy, electrophysiological abnormalities and neurological deficits following demyelination in a chronic inflammatory model of multiple sclerosis. *Brain* **123:**519–531.
13. **Molina-Holgado, E., A. Arevalo-Martin, A. Castrillo, L. Bosca, J. M. Vela, and C. Guaza.** 2002. Interleukin-4 and interleukin-10 modulate nuclear factor κB activity and nitric oxide synthase-2 expression in Theiler's murine encephalomyelitis virus-infected brain astrocytes. *J. Neurochem.* **81:**1242–1252.
14. **Molina-Holgado, E., A. Arevalo-Martin, S. Ortiz, J. M. Vela, and C. Guaza.** 2002. Theiler's virus infection induces the expression of cyclooxygenase-2 in murine astrocytes: inhibition by the anti-inflammatory cytokines interleukin-4 and interleukin-10. *Neurosci. Lett.* **324:**237–241.
15. **National Research Council.** 1991. *Infectious Diseases of Mice and Rats: a Report of the Institute of Laboratory Animal Resources Committee on Infectious Diseases of Mice and Rats.* National Academy Press, Washington, D.C.
16. **Nicholson, S. M., J. D. Peterson, S. D. Miller K. Wang, M. C. Dal Canto, and R. W. Melvold.** 1994. BALB/c substrain differences in susceptibility to Theiler's murine encephalomyelitis virus-induced demyelinating disease. *J. Neuroimmunol.* **52:**19–24.
17. **Ohara, Y., T. Himeda, K. Asakura, and M. Sawada.** 2002. Distinct cell death mechanisms by Theiler's murine encephalomyelitis virus (TMEV) infection in microglia and macrophage. *Neurosci. Lett.* **327:**41–44.
18. **Olsberg, C., A. Pelka, S. Miller, C. Waltenbaugh, T. M. Creighton, M. C. Dal Canto, H. Lipton, and R. Melvold.** 1993. Induction of Theiler's murine encephalomyelitis virus (TMEV)-induced demyelinating disease in genetically resistant mice. *Reg. Immunol.* **5:**1–10.
19. **Percy, D. H., and S. W. Barthold.** 2001. *Pathology of Laboratory Rodents and Rabbits,* 2nd ed. Iowa State University Press, Ames.

20. Ranschoff, R. M., T. Wei, K. D. Pavelko, J. C. Lee, P. D. Murray, and M. Rodriguez. 2002. Chemokine expression in the central nervous system of mice with a viral disease resembling multiple sclerosis: roles of CD4$^+$ and CD8$^+$ T cells and viral persistence. *J. Virol.* **76:**2217–2224.

21. Rossi, C. P., M. Delcroix, I. Huitinga, A. McAllister, N. van Rooijen, E. Claassen, and M. Brahic. 1997. Role of macrophages during Theiler's virus infection. *J. Virol.* **71:**3336–3340.

22. Rubio, N., and C. Torres. 1991. IL-1, IL-2 and IFN-γ production by Theiler's virus-induced encephalomyelitic SJL/J mice. *Immunology* **74:**284–289.

23. Theil, D. J., I. Tsunoda, J. E. Libbey, T. J. Derfuss, and R. S. Fujinami. 2000. Alterations in cytokine but not chemokine mRNA expression during three distinct Theiler's virus infections. *J. Neuroimmunol.* **104:**22–30.

24. Tompkins, S. M., K. G. Fuller, and S. D. Miller. 2002. Theiler's virus-mediated autoimmunity: local presentation of CNS antigens and epitope spreading. *Ann. N. Y. Acad. Sci.* **958:**26–38.

25. Trottier, M., B. P. Schlitt, and H. L. Lipton. 2002. Enhanced detection of Theiler's virus RNA copy equivalents in the mouse central nervous system by real-time RT-PCR. *J. Virol. Methods* **103:**89–99.

26. Tsunoda, I., and R. S. Fujinami. 1996. Two models for multiple sclerosis: experimental allergic encephalomyelitis and Theiler's murine encephalomyelitis virus. *J. Neuropathol. Exp. Neurol.* **55:**673–686.

27. Tsunoda, I., C. I. Kurtz, and R. S. Fujinami. 1997. Apoptosis in acute and chronic central nervous system disease induced by Theiler's murine encephalomyelitis virus. *Virology* **228:**388–393.

28. Zheng, L., M. A. Calenoff, and M. C. Dal Canto. 2001. Astrocytes, not microglia, are the main cells responsible for viral persistence in Theiler's murine encephalomyelitis virus infection leading to demyelination. *J. Neuroimmunol.* **118:**256–267.

BACTERIA

Cilia-associated respiratory bacillus

1. Brogden, K. A., R. C. Cutlip, and H. D. Lehmkuhl. 1993. Cilia-associated respiratory bacillus in wild rats in central Iowa. *J. Wildl. Dis.* **29:**123–126.

2. Cundiff, D. D., and C. Besch-Williford. 1992. Respiratory disease in a colony of rats. *Lab. Anim.* **21:**16–19.

3. Cundiff, D. D., C. L. Besch-Williford, R. R. Hook, Jr., C. L. Franklin, and L. K. Riley. 1994. Characterization of cilia-associated respiratory bacillus isolates from rats and rabbits. *Lab. Anim. Sci.* **44:**305–312.

4. Franklin, C. L., J. D. Pletz, L. K. Riley, B. A. Livingston, R. R. Hook, Jr., and C. L. Besch-Williford. 1999. Detection of cilia-associated respiratory (CAR) bacillus in nasal-swab specimens from infected rats by use of polymerase chain reaction. *Lab. Anim. Sci.* **49:**114–117.

5. Griffith, J. W., W. J. White, P. J. Danneman, and C. M. Lang. 1988. Cilia-associated respiratory (CAR) bacillus infection in obese mice. *Vet. Pathol.* **25:**72–76.

6. Hook, R. R., Jr., C. L. Franklin, L. K. Riley, B. A. Livingston, and C. L. Besch-Williford. 1998. Antigenic analysis of cilia-associated respiratory (CAR) bacillus isolates by use of monoclonal antibodies. *Lab. Anim. Sci.* **48:**234–239.

7. Kawano, A., M. Nenoi, S. Matsushita, T. Matsumoto, and K. Mita. 2000. Sequence of 16S rRNA gene of rat-origin cilia-associated respiratory (CAR) bacillus SMR strain. *J. Vet. Med. Sci.* **62:**797–800.

8. Kendall, L. V., L. K. Riley, R. R. Hook, Jr., C. L. Besch-Williford, and C. L. Franklin. 2000. Antibody and cytokine responses to the cilium-associated respiratory bacillus in BALB/c and C57BL/6 mice. *Infect. Immun.* **68:**4961–4967.

9. Kendall, L. V., L. K. Riley, R. R. Hook, Jr., C. L. Besch-Williford, and C. L. Franklin. 2002. Characterization of lymphocyte subsets in the bronchiolar lymph nodes of BALB/c mice infected with cilia-associated respiratory bacillus. *Comp. Med.* **52:**322–327.

10. Kendall, L. V., L. K. Riley, R. R. Hook, Jr., C. L. Besch-Williford, and C. L. Franklin. 2001. Differential interleukin-10 and gamma interferon mRNA expression in lungs of cilium-associated respiratory bacillus-infected mice. *Infect. Immun.* **69:**3697–3702.

11. Matsushita, S., and H. Joshima. 1989. Pathology of rats intranasally inoculated with the cilia-associated respiratory bacillus. *Lab. Anim.* **23:**89–95.

12. Matsushita, S., J. Joshima, T. Matsumoto, and K. Fukutsu. 1989. Transmission experiments of cilia-associated respiratory bacillus in mice, rabbits, and guinea pigs. *Lab. Anim.* **23:**96–102.

13. Matsushita, S., and E. Suzuki. 1995. Prevention and treatment of cilia-associated respiratory bacillus in mice by use of antibiotics. *Lab. Anim. Sci.* **45:**503–507.

14. **Medina, L. V., J. D. Fortman, R. M. Bunte, and B. T. Bennett.** 1994. Respiratory disease in a rat colony: identification of CAR bacillus without other respiratory pathogens by standard diagnostic screening methods. *Lab. Anim. Sci.* **44:** 521–525.
15. **National Research Council.** 1991. *Infectious Diseases of Mice and Rats: a Report of the Institute of Laboratory Animal Resources Committee on Infectious Diseases of Mice and Rats.* National Academy Press, Washington, D.C.
16. **Schoeb, T. R., M. K. Davidson, and J. K. Davis.** 1997. Pathogenicity of cilia-associated respiratory (CAR) bacillus isolates for F344, LEW, and SD rats. *Vet. Pathol.* **34:**263–270.
17. **Schoeb, T. R., K. Dybvig, K. F. Keisling, M. K. Davidson, and J. K. Davis.** 1997. Detection of *Mycoplasma pulmonis* in cilia-associated respiratory bacillus isolates and in respiratory tracts of rats by nested PCR. *J. Clin. Microbiol.* **35:**1667–1670.
18. **Shoji-Darkye, Y., T. Itoh, and N. Kagiyama.** 1991. Pathogenesis of CAR bacillus in rabbits, guinea pigs, Syrian hamsters, and mice. *Lab. Anim. Sci.* **41:**567–571.

Citrobacter rodentium
1. **Barthold, S. W., G. L. Coleman, R. O. Jacoby, E. M. Livstone, and A. M. Jonas.** 1978. Transmissible murine colonic hyperplasia. *Vet. Pathol.* **15:**223–236.
2. **Barthold, S. W., and A. M. Jonas.** 1977. Morphogenesis of early 1,2-dimethylhydrazine-induced lesions and latent period reduction of colon carcinogenesis in mice by a variant of *Citrobacter freundii*. *Cancer Res.* **37:**4352–4360.
3. **Barthold, S. W., G. W. Osbaldiston, and A. M. Jonas.** 1977. Dietary, bacterial and host genetic interactions in the pathogenesis of transmissible murine colonic hyperplasia. *Lab. Anim. Sci.* **27:**938–945.
4. **Brennan, P. C., T. E. Fritz, R. J. Flynn, and C. M. Poole.** 1965. *Citrobacter freundii* associated with diarrhea in laboratory mice. *Lab. Anim. Care* **15:**266–275.
5. **Deng, W., Y. Li, B. A. Vallance, and B. B. Finlay.** 2001. Locus of enterocyte effacement from *Citrobacter rodentium*: sequence analysis and evidence for horizontal transfer among attaching and effacing pathogens. *Infect. Immun.* **69:**6323–6335.
6. **Frankel, G., A. D. Phillips, M. Novakova, H. Field, D. C. Candy, D. B. Schauer, G. Douce, and G. Dougan.** 1996. Intimin from enteropathogenic *Escherichia coli* restores murine virulence to a *Citrobacter rodentium* eaeA mutant: induction of an immunoglobulin A response to intimin and EspB. *Infect. Immun.* **64:**5315–5325.
7. **Ghaem-Maghami, M., C. P. Simmons, S. Daniell, M. Pizza, D. Lewis, G. Frankel, and G. Dougan.** 2001. Intimin-specific immune responses prevent bacterial colonization by the attaching-effacing pathogen *Citrobacter rodentium*. *Infect. Immun.* **69:**5597–5605.
8. **Higgins, L. M., G. Frankel, G. Douce, G. Dougan, and T. T. MacDonald.** 1999. *Citrobacter rodentium* infection in mice elicits a mucosal Th1 cytokine response and lesions similar to those in murine inflammatory bowel disease. *Infect. Immun.* **67:**3031–3039.
9. **Hubbard, A. L., D. J. Harrison, C. Moyes, and S. McOrist.** 1998. Direct detection of eae-positive bacteria in human and veterinary colorectal specimens by PCR. *J. Clin. Microbiol.* **36:** 2326–2330.
10. **Luperchio, S. A., J. V. Newman, C. A. Dangler, M. D. Schrenzel, D. J. Brenner, A. G. Steigerwalt, and D. B. Schauer.** 2000. *Citrobacter rodentium*, the causative agent of transmissible murine colonic hyperplasia, exhibits clonality: synonymy of *C. rodentium* and mouse-pathogenic *Escherichia coli*. *J. Clin. Microbiol.* **38:** 4343–4350.
11. **Luperchio, S. A., and D. B. Schauer.** 2001. Molecular pathogenesis of *Citrobacter rodentium* and transmissible murine colonic hyperplasia. *Microb. Infect.* **3:**333–340.
12. **Maggio-Price, L., K. L. Nicholson, K. M. Kline, T. Birkebak, I. Suzuki, D. L. Wilson, D. Schauer, and P. J. Fink.** 1998. Diminished reproduction, failure to thrive, and altered immunologic function in a colony of T-cell receptor transgenic mice: possible role of *Citrobacter rodentium*. *Lab. Anim. Sci.* **48:**145–155.
13. **Malstrom, C., and S. James.** 1998. Inhibition of murine splenic and mucosal lymphocyte function by enteric bacterial products. *Infect. Immun.* **66:**3120–3127.
14. **National Research Council.** 1991. *Infectious Diseases of Mice and Rats: a Report of the Institute of Laboratory Animal Resources Committee on Infectious Diseases of Mice and Rats.* National Academy Press, Washington, D.C.
15. **Newman, J. V., T. Kosaka, B. J. Sheppard, J. G. Fox, and D. B. Schauer.** 2001. Bacterial infection promotes colon tumorigenesis in $Apc^{Min/+}$ mice. *J. Infect. Dis.* **184:**227–230.
16. **Schauer, D. B., and S. Falkow.** 1993. The eae gene of *Citrobacter freundii* biotype 4280 is necessary for colonization in transmissible murine colonic hyperplasia. *Infect. Immun.* **61:**4654–4661.
17. **Schauer, D. B., B. A. Zabel, I. F. Pedraza, C. M. O'Hara, A. G. Steigerwalt, and D. J. Brenner.** 1995. Genetic and biochemical char-

acterization of *Citrobacter rodentium* sp. nov. *J. Clin. Microbiol.* **33:**2064–2068.

18. **Simmons, C. P., N. S. Goncalves, M. Ghaem-Maghami, M. Bajab-Elliot, S. Clare, B. Neves, G. Frankel, G. Dougan, and T. T. MacDonald.** 2002. Impaired resistance and enhanced pathology during infection with a noninvasive, attaching-effacing enteric bacterial pathogen, *Citrobacter rodentium*, in mice lacking IL-12 or IFN-γ. *J. Immunol.* **168:**1804–1812.

19. **Vallance, B. A., W. Deng, L. A. Knodler, and B. B. Finley.** 2002. Mice lacking T and B lymphocytes develop transient colitis and crypt hyperplasia yet suffer impaired bacterial clearance during *Citrobacter rodentium* infection. *Infect. Immun.* **70:**2070–2081.

20. **Van Ogtrop, M. L., H. F. Guiot, H. Mattie, and R. van Furth.** 1991. Modulation of the intestinal flora of mice by parenteral treatment with broad-spectrum cephalosporins. *Antimicrob. Agents Chemother.* **35:**976–982.

Clostridium piliforme

1. **Boot, R., H. van Herck, and J. van der Logt.** 1996. Mutual viral and bacterial infections after housing rats of various breeders within an experimental unit. *Lab. Anim.* **30:**42–45.

2. **Duncan, A. J., R. J. Carman, G. J. Olsen, and K. H. Wilson.** 1993. Assignment of the agent of Tyzzer's disease to *Clostridium piliforme* comb. nov. on the basis of 16S rRNA sequence analysis. *Int. J. Syst. Bacteriol.* **43:**314–318.

3. **Franklin, C. L., S. L. Motzel, C. L. Besch-Williford, R. R. Hook, Jr., and L. K. Riley.** 1994. Tyzzer's infection: host specificity of *Clostridium piliforme* isolates. *Lab. Anim. Sci.* **44:**568–572.

4. **Fries, A. S.** 1978. Demonstration of antibodies to *Bacillus piliformis* in SPF colonies and experimental transplacental infection by *Bacillus piliformis* in mice. *Lab. Anim.* **12:**23–26.

5. **Fries, A. S.** 1980. Studies on Tyzzer's disease: comparison between *Bacillus piliformis* strains from mouse, rat and rabbit. *Lab. Anim.* **14:**61–63.

6. **Fries, A. S., and O. Ladefoged.** 1979. The influence of *Bacillus piliformis* (Tyzzer) infections on the reliability of pharmacokinetic experiments in mice. *Lab. Anim.* **13:**257–261.

7. **Goto, K., and T. Itoh.** 1996. Detection of *Clostridium piliforme* by enzymatic assay of amplified cDNA in microtitration plates. *Lab. Anim. Sci.* **46:**493–496.

8. **Hansen, A. K., H. V. Andersen, and O. Svendsen.** 1994. Studies on the diagnosis of Tyzzer's disease in laboratory rat colonies with antibodies against *Bacillus piliformis* (*Clostridium piliforme*). *Lab. Anim. Sci.* **44:**424–429.

9. **Livingston, R. S., C. L. Franklin, C. L. Besch-Williford, R. R. Hook, Jr., and L. K. Riley.** 1996. A novel presentation of *Clostridium piliforme* infection (Tyzzer's disease) in nude mice. *Lab. Anim. Sci.* **46:**21–25.

10. **Motzel, S. L., J. K. Meyer, and L. K. Riley.** 1991. Detection of serum antibodies to *Bacillus piliformis* in mice and rats using an enzyme-linked immunosorbent assay. *Lab. Anim.* **41:**26–30.

11. **National Research Council.** 1991. *Infectious Diseases of Mice and Rats: a Report of the Institute of Laboratory Animal Resources Committee on Infectious Diseases of Mice and Rats.* National Academy Press, Washington, D.C.

12. **Thunert, A., L. C. Jonas, S. Rehm, and E. Sickel.** 1985. Transmission and course of Tyzzer's disease in euthymic and thymus aplastic nude Han:RNU rats. *Z. Versterkd.* **27:**241–248.

13. **Van Andel, R. A., C. L. Franklin, C. L. Besch-Williford, R. R. Hook, Jr., and L. K. Riley.** 2000. Prolonged perturbations of tumour necrosis factor-α and interferon-γ in mice inoculated with *Clostridium piliforme. J. Med. Microbiol.* **49:**557–563.

14. **Van Andel, R. A., C. L. Franklin, C. L. Besch-Williford, R. R. Hook, Jr., and L. K. Riley.** 2000. Role of interleukin-6 in determining the course of murine Tyzzer's disease. *J. Med. Microbiol.* **49:**171–176.

15. **Van Andel, R. A., R. R. Hook, Jr., C. L. Franklin, C. L. Besch-Williford, N. van Rooijen, and L. K. Riley.** 1997. Effects of neutrophil, natural killer cell, and macrophage depletion on murine *Clostridium piliforme* infection. *Infect. Immun.* **65:**2725–2731.

16. **Van Andel, R. A., R. R. Hook, Jr., C. L. Franklin, C. L. Besch-Williford, and L. K. Riley.** 1998. Interleukin-12 has a role in mediating resistance of murine strains to Tyzzer's disease. *Infect. Immun.* **66:**4942–4946.

17. **Waggie, K. S., C. T. Hansen, J. R. Ganaway, and T. S. Spencer.** 1981. A study of mouse strain susceptibility to *Bacillus piliformis* (Tyzzer's disease): The association of B-cell function and resistance. *Lab. Anim. Sci.* **31:**139–142.

Corynebacterium kutscheri

1. **Amao, H., T. Akimoto, Y. Komukai, T. Sawada, M. Saito, and K. W. Takahashi.** 2002. Detection of *Corynebacterium kutscheri* from the oral cavity of rats. *Exp. Anim.* **51:**99–102.

2. **Amao, H., Y. Komukai, T. Akimoto, M. Sugiyama, K. W. Takahashi, T. Sawada, and M. Saito.** 1995. Natural and subclinical *Corynebacterium kutscheri* infection in rats. *Lab. Anim. Sci.* **45:**11–14.

3. **Amao, H., Y. Komukai, M. Sugiyama, T. R. Saito, K. W. Takahashi, and M. Saito.**

1993. Differences in susceptibility of mice among various strains to oral infection with *Corynebacterium kutscheri*. *Jikken Dobutsu* **42:**539–545.
4. **Amao, H., Y. Komukai, M. Sugiyama, K. W. Takahashi, T. Sawada, and M. Saito.** 1995. Natural habitats of *Corynebacterium kutscheri* in subclinically infected ICGN and DBA/2 strains of mice. *Lab. Anim. Sci.* **45:**6–10.
5. **Hirst, R. G., and R. Campbell.** 1977. Mechanisms of resistance to *Corynebacterium kutscheri* in mice. *Infect. Immun.* **17:**319–324.
6. **Juhr, N. C., and J. Horn.** 1975. Modellinfektion mit *Corynebacterium kutscheri* bei der maus. *Z. Versitierkd.* **17:**129–141.
7. **Kita, E., N. Kamikaidou, D. Ku, A. Nakano, N. Katsui, and S. Kashiba.** 1992. Nonspecific stimulation of host defense by *Corynebacterium kutscheri*. III. Enhanced cytokine induction by the active moiety of *C. kutscheri*. *Nat. Immun.* **11:**46–55.
8. **Komukai, Y., H. Amao, N. Goto, Y. Kusajima, T. Sawada, M. Saito, and K. W. Takahashi.** 1999. Sex differences in susceptibility of ICR mice to oral infection with *Corynebacterium kutscheri*. *Exp. Anim.* **48:**37–42.
9. **National Research Council.** 1991. *Infectious Diseases of Mice and Rats: a Report of the Institute of Laboratory Animal Resources Committee on Infectious Diseases of Mice and Rats.* National Academy Press, Washington, D.C.
10. **Weisbroth, S. H.** 1979. Bacterial and mycotic diseases, p. 193–241. *In* H. J. Baker, J .R. Lindsey, and S. H. Weisbroth (ed.), *The Laboratory Rat*, vol. I. Academic Press, New York, N.Y.
11. **Weisbroth, S. H., and S. Scher.** 1968. *Corynebacterium kutscheri* infection in the mouse. I. Report of an outbreak, bacteriology, and pathology of spontaneous infections. *Lab. Anim. Care* **18:**451–458.

Corynebacterium spp. in athymic mice
1. **Clifford, C. B., B. J. Walton, T. H. Reed, M. B. Coyle, W. J. White, and H. L. Amyx.** 1995. Hyperkeratosis in athymic nude mice caused by a coryneform bacterium: microbiology, transmission, clinical signs, and pathology. *Lab. Anim. Sci.* **45:**131–139.
2. **Duga, S., A. Gobbi, R. Asselta, L. Crippa, M. L. Tenchini, T. Simonic, and E. Scanziani.** 1998. Analysis of the 16S rRNA gene sequence of the coryneform bacterium associated with hyperkeratotic dermatitis of athymic nude mice and development of a PCR-based detection assay. *Mol. Cell. Probes* **12:**191–199.
3. **Field, K., G. Greenstein, M. Smith, S. Herrmann, and J. Gizzi.** 1995. Hyperkeratosis-associated coryneform in athymic nude mice. *Lab. Anim. Sci.* **45:**469.
4. **Gobbi, A., L. Crippa, and E. Scanziani.** 1999. *Corynebacterium bovis* infection in hirsute mice. *Lab. Anim. Sci.* **49:**209–211.
5. **Gobbi, A., L. Crippa, and E. Scanziani.** 1999. *Corynebacterium bovis* infection in waltzing mice. *Lab. Anim. Sci.* **49:**132–133.
6. **Richter, C. B., K. L. Klingenberger, D. Hughes, H. S. Friedman, and D. I. Schenkman.** 1990. D2 coryneforms as a cause of severe hyperkeratotic dermatitis in athymic nude mice. *Lab. Anim. Sci.* **40:**545.
7. **Scanziani, E., A. Gobbi, L. Crippa, A. M. Giusti, R. Giavazzi, E. Cavalletti, and M. Luini.** 1997. Outbreaks of hyperkeratotic dermatitis of athymic nude mice in northern Italy. *Lab. Anim.* **31:**206–211.
8. **Scanziani, E., A. Gobbi, L. Crippa, A. M. Giusti, E. Pesenti, E. Cavaletti, and M. Luini.** 1998. Hyperkeratosis-associated coryneform infection in severe combined immunodeficient mice. *Lab. Anim.* **32:**330–336.

Helicobacter spp.
1. **Breidert, M., S. Miehlke, A. Glasow, Z. Orban, M. Stolte, G. Ehninger, E. Bayerdörffer, O. Nettesheim, U. Halm, A. Haidan, and S. R. Bornstein.** 1999. Leptin and its receptor in normal human gastric mucosa and in *Helicobacter pylori*-associated gastritis. *Scand. J. Gastroenterol.* **34:**954–961.
2. **Burich, A., R. Hershberg, K. Waggie, W. Zeng, T. Brabb, G. Westrich, J. L. Viney, and L. Maggio-Price.** 2001. Helicobacter-induced inflammatory bowel disease in IL-10⁻ and T cell-deficient mice. *Am. J. Physiol.* **281:** G764–G778.
3. **Canella, K. A., B. A. Diwan, P. L. Gorelick, P. J. Donovan, M. A. Sipowicz, K. S. Kasprzak, C. M. Weghorst, E. G. Snyderwine, C. D. Davis, L. K. Keefer, S. A. Kyrtopoulos, S. S. Hecht, M.Wang, L. M. Anderson, and J. M. Rice.** 1996. Liver tumorigenesis by *Helicobacter hepaticus*: considerations of mechanism. *In Vivo* **10:**285–292.
4. **Chomarat, P., M. A. Sipowicz, B. A. Diwan, L. W. Fornwald, Y. C. Awasthi, M. R. Anver, J. M. Rice, L. M. Anderson, and C. P. Wild.** 1997. Distinct time courses of increase in cytochromes P450, 1A2, 2A5 and glutathione S-transferases during the progressive hepatitis associated with *Helicobacter hepaticus*. *Carcinogenesis* **18:**2179–2190.
5. **Dewhirst, F. E., J. G. Fox, E. N. Mendes, B. J. Paster, C. E. Gates, C. A. Kirkbride, and K. A. Eaton.** 2000. 'Flexispira rappini' strains represent at least 10 *Helicobacter* taxa. *Int. J. Syst. Evol. Microbiol.* **50:**1781–1787.

6. Diwan, B. A., J. M. Ward, D. Ramljak, and L. M. Anderson. 1997. Promotion by *Helicobacter hepaticus*-induced hepatitis of hepatic tumors initiated by N-nitrosodimethylamine in male A/JCr mice. *Toxicol. Pathol.* **25**:597–605.

7. Drazenovich, N. L., C. L. Franklin, R. S. Livingston, and D. G. Besselsen. 2002. Detection of rodent *Helicobacter* spp. by use of fluorogenic nuclease polymerase chain reaction assays. *Comp. Med.* **52**:347–353.

8. Erdman, S., J. G. Fox, C. A. Dangler, D. Feldman, and B. H. Horwitz. 2001. Typhlocolitis in NF-κB-deficient mice. *J. Immunol.* **166**:1443–1447.

9. Foltz, C. J., J. G. Fox, R. Cahill, J. C. Murphy, L. Yan, B. Shames, and D. B. Schauer. 1998. Spontaneous inflammatory bowel disease in multiple mutant mouse lines: association with colonization by *Helicobacter hepaticus*. *Helicobacter* **3**:69–78.

10. Fox, J. G., F. E. Dewhirst, J. G. Tully, B. J. Paster, L. Yan, N. S. Taylor, M. J. Collins, Jr., P. L. Gorelick, and J. M. Ward. 1994. *Helicobacter hepaticus* sp. nov., a microaerophilic bacterium isolated from livers and intestinal mucosal scrapings from mice. *J. Clin. Microbiol.* **32**:1238–1245.

11. Fox, J. G., and A. Lee. 1997. The role of *Helicobacter* species in newly recognized gastrointestinal tract diseases of animals. *Lab. Anim. Sci.* **47**:222–255.

12. Fox, J. G., X. Li, L. Yan, R. J. Cahill, R. Hurley, R. Lewis, and J. C. Murphy. 1996. Chronic proliferative hepatitis in A/JCr mice associated with persistent *Helicobacter hepaticus* infection: a model of helicobacter-induced carcinogenesis. *Infect. Immun.* **64**:1548–1558.

13. Fox, J. G., J. A. MacGregor, Z. Shen, X. Li, R. Lewis, and C. A. Dangler. 1998. Comparison of methods of identifying *Helicobacter hepaticus* in B6C3F1 mice used in a carcinogenesis bioassay. *J. Clin. Microbiol.* **36**:1382–1387.

14. Fox, J. G., L. L. Yan, F. E. Dewhirst, B. J. Paster, B. Shames, J. C. Murphy, A. Hayward, J. C. Belcher, and E. N. Mendes. 1995. *Helicobacter bilis* sp. nov., a novel *Helicobacter* species isolated from bile, livers, and intestines of aged, inbred mice. *J. Clin. Microbiol.* **33**:445–454.

15. Fox, J. G., L. Yan, B. Shames, J. Campbell, J. C. Murphy, and X. Li. 1996. Persistent hepatitis and enterocolitis in germfree mice infected with *Helicobacter hepaticus*. *Infect. Immun.* **64**:3673–3681.

16. Franklin, C. L., P. L. Gorelick, L. R. Riley, F. E. Dewhirst, R. S. Livingston, J. M. Ward, C. S. Beckwith, and J. G. Fox. 2001. *Helicobacter typhlonius* sp. Nov., a novel murine urease-negative *Helicobacter* species. *J. Clin. Microbiol.* **39**:3920–3926.

17. Goto, K., K. I. Ishihara, A. Kuzuoka, Y. Ohnishi, and T. Itoh. 2001. Contamination of transplantable human tumor-bearing lines by *Helicobacter hepaticus* and its elimination. *J. Clin. Microbiol.* **39**:3703–3704.

18. Goto, K., H. Ohashi, A. Takakura, and T. Itoh. 2000. Current status of *Helicobacter* contamination of laboratory mice, rats, gerbils, and house musk shrews in Japan. *Curr. Microbiol.* **41**:161–166.

19. Grehan, M., G. Tamotia, B. Robertson, and H. Mitchell. 2002. Detection of *Helicobacter* colonization of the murine lower bowel by genus-specific PCR-denaturing gradient gel electrophoresis. *Appl. Environ. Microbiol.* **68**:5164–5166.

20. Hailey, J. R., J. K. Haseman, J. R. Bucher, A. E. Radovsky, D. E. Malarkey, R. T. Miller, A. Nyska, and R. R. Maronpot. 1998. Impact of *Helicobacter hepaticus* infection in B6C3F1 mice from twelve National Toxicology Program two-year carcinogenesis studies. *Toxicol. Pathol.* **26**:602–611.

21. Haines, D. C., P. L. Gorelick, J. K. Battles, K. M. Pike, R. J. Anderson, J. G. Fox, N. S. Taylor, Z. Shen, F. E. Dewhirst, M. R. Anver, and J. M. Ward. 1998. Inflammatory large bowel disease in immunodeficient rats naturally and experimentally infected with *Helicobacter bilis*. *Vet. Pathol.* **35**:202–208.

22. Ihrig, M., M. D. Schrenzel, and J. G. Fox. 1999. Differential susceptibility to hepatic inflammation and proliferation in AXB recombinant inbred mice chronically infected with *Helicobacter hepaticus*. *Am. J. Pathol.* **155**:571–582.

23. Jiang, H. Q., N. Kushnir, M. C. Thurnheer, N. A. Boss, and J. J. Cebra. 2002. Monoassociation of SCID mice with *Helicobacter muridarum*, but not four other enterics, provokes IBD upon receipt of T cells. *Gastroenterology* **122**:1346–1354.

24. Karkas, J., A. McCullen, A. Smith, and A. R. Banknieder. 2000. *Helicobacter* and PCR testing: What do the results really mean? *Contemp. Top. Lab. Anim. Sci.* **39**:94.

25. Kullberg, M. C., A. G. Rothfuchs, D. Jankovic, P. Caspar, T. A. Wynn, P. L. Gorelick, A. W. Cheever, and A. Sher. 2001. *Helicobacter hepaticus*-induced colitis in interleukin-10-deficient mice: cytokine requirements for the induction and maintenance of intestinal inflammation. *Infect. Immun.* **69**:4232–4241.

26. Lee, A., M. W. Phillips, J. L. O'Rourke, B. J. Paster, F. E. Dewhirst, G. J. Fraser, J. G. Fox, L. I. Sly, P. J. Romaniuk, and

T. J. Trust. 1992. *Helicobacter muridarum* sp. nov., a microaerophilic helical bacterium with a novel ultrastructure isolated from the intestinal mucosa of rodents. *Int. J. Syst. Bacteriol.* **42:**27–36.

27. Li, X., J. G. Fox, M. T. Whary, L. Yan, B. Shames, and Z. Zhao. 1998. SCID/NCr mice naturally infected with *Helicobacter hepaticus* develop progressive hepatitis, proliferative typhlitis, and colitis. *Infect. Immun.* **66:**5477–5484.

28. Livingston, R. S., L. K. Riley, R. R. Hook, Jr., C. L. Besch-Williford, and C. L. Franklin. 1999. Cloning and expression of an immunogenic membrane-associated protein of *Helicobacter hepaticus* for use in an enzyme-linked immunosorbent assay. *Clin. Diagn. Lab. Immunol.* **6:**745–750.

29. Livingston, R. S., L. K. Riley, E. K. Steffan, C. L. Besch-Williford, R. R. Hook, Jr., and C. L. Franklin. 1997. Serodiagnosis of *Helicobacter hepaticus* infection in mice by an enzyme-linked immunosorbent assay. *J. Clin. Microbiol.* **35:**1236–1238.

30. Maggio-Price, L., D. Shows, K. Waggie, Z. Burich, W. Zeng, S. Excobar, P. Morrissey, and J. L. Viney. 2002. *Helicobacter bilis* infection accelerates and *H. hepaticus* infection delays the development of colitis in multiple drug resistance-deficient$^{mdr1a-/-}$ mice. *Am. J. Pathol.* **160:**739–751.

31. Mahler, M., H. G. Bedigian, B. L. Burgett, R. J. Bates, M. E. Hogan, and J. P. Sundberg. 1998. Comparison of four diagnostic methods for detection of *Helicobacter* species in laboratory mice. *Lab. Anim. Sci.* **48:**85–91.

32. Malarkey, D. E., T. V. Ton, J. R. Hailey, and T. R. Devereux. 1997. A PCR-RFLP method for the detection of *Helicobacter hepaticus* in frozen or fixed liver from B6C3F1 mice. *Toxicol. Pathol.* **25:**606–612.

33. Mendes, E. N., D. M. Queiroz, F. E. Dewhirst, B. J. Paster, S. B. Moura, and J. G. Fox. 1996. *Helicobacter trogontum* sp. nov., isolated from the rat intestine. *Int. J. Syst. Bacteriol.* **46:**916–921.

34. Mohammadi, M., J. Nedrud, R. Redline, N. Lycke, and S. J. Czinn. 1997. Murine CD4 T-cell response to *Helicobacter* infection: TH1 cells enhance gastritis and TH2 cells reduce bacterial load. *Gastroenterology* **113:**1848–1857.

35. Nyska, A., R. R. Maronpot, S. R. Eldridge, J. K. Haseman, and J. R. Hailey. 1997. Alteration in cell kinetics in control B6C3F1 mice infected with *Helicobacter hepaticus*. *Toxicol. Pathol.* **25:**591–596.

36. Robertson, B. R., J. L. O'Rourke, P. Vandamme, S. L. On, and A. Lee. 2001. *Helicobacter ganmani* sp. nov., a urease-negative anaerobe isolated from the intestines of laboratory mice. *Int. J. Syst. Evol. Microbiol.* **51:**1881–1889.

37. Schauer, D. B., N. Ghori, and S. Falkow. 1993. Isolation and characterization of "*Flexispira rappini*" from laboratory mice. *J. Clin. Microbiol.* **31:**2709–2714.

38. Shames, B., J. G. Fox, F. Dewhirst, L. Yan, Z. Shen, and N. S. Taylor. 1995. Identification of widespread *Helicobacter hepaticus* infection in feces in commercial mouse colonies by culture and PCR assay. *J. Clin. Microbiol.* **33:**2968–2972.

39. Shen, Z., J. G. Fox, F. E. Dewhirst, B. J. Paster, C. J. Foltz, L. Yan, B. Shames, and L. Perry. 1997. *Helicobacter rodentium* sp. nov., a urease-negative *Helicobacter* species isolated from laboratory mice. *Int. J. Syst. Bacteriol.* **47:**627–634.

40. Shomer, N. H., C. A. Dangler, R. P. Marini, and J. G. Fox. 1998. *Helicobacter bilis/Helicobacter rodentium* co-infection associated with diarrhea in a colony of SCID mice. *Lab. Anim. Sci.* **48:**455–459.

41. Shomer, N. H., C. A. Dangler, M. D. Schrenzel, and J. G. Fox. 1997. *Helicobacter bilis*-induced inflammatory bowel disease in SCID mice with defined flora. *Infect. Immun.* **65:**4858–4864.

42. Shomer, N. H., C. A. Dangler, M. D. Schrenzel, M. T. Whary, S. Xu, Y. Feng, B. J. Paster, F. E. Dewhirst, and J. G. Fox. 2001. Cholangiohepatitis and inflammatory bowel disease induced by a novel urease-negative *Helicobacter* species in A/J and Tac:ICR:HascidfRF mice. *Exp. Biol. Med.* **226:**420–428.

43. Singletary, K. B., C. A. Kloster, and D. G. Baker. Optimal age at fostering for derivation of *Helicobacter hepaticus*-free mice. *Comp. Med.*, in press.

44. Sutton, P., J. Wilson, R. Genta, D. Torrey, A. Savinainen, J. Pappo, and A. Lee. 1999. A genetic basis for atrophy: dominant non-responsiveness and *Helicobacter* induced gastritis in F(1) hybrid mice. *Gut* **45:**335–340.

45. Truett, G. E., J. A. Walker, and D. G. Baker. 2000. Eradication of *Helicobacter sp.* by neonatal transfer. *Comp. Med.* **50:**426–433.

46. Ward, J. M., M. R. Anver, D. C. Haines, J. M. Melhorn, P. Gorelick, L. Yan, and J. G. Fox. 1996. Inflammatory large bowel disease in immunodeficient mice naturally infected with *Helicobacter hepaticus*. *Lab. Anim. Sci.* **46:**15–20.

47. Ward, J. M., R. E. Benveniste, C. H. Fox, J. K. Battles, M. A. Gonda, and T. G. Tully. 1996. Autoimmunity in chronic active *Helicobacter hepatitis* of mice. Serum antibodies and expression

of heat shock protein 70 in liver. *Am. J. Pathol.* **148**:509–517.
48. Ward, J. M., J. G. Fox, M. R. Anver, D. C. Haines, C. V. George, M. J. Collins, Jr., P. L. Gorelick, K. Nagashima, M. A. Gonda, R. V. Gilden, J. G. Tully, R. J. Russell, R. E. Benveniste, B. J. Paster, F. E. Dewhirst, J. C. Donovan, L. M. Anderson, and J. M. Rice. 1994. Chronic active hepatitis and associated liver tumors in mice caused by a persistent bacterial infection with a novel *Helicobacter* species. *J. Natl. Cancer Inst.* **86**:1222–1227.
49. Weisbroth, S. H. 1999. The rodent Helicobacters: Present status of diagnostic detection and guidelines for institutional procurement standards. *Lab. Anim.* **28**:41–45.
50. Whary, M. T., J. H. Cline, A. E. King, C. A. Corcoran, S. Xu, and J. G. Fox. 2000. Containment of *Helicobacter hepaticus* by use of husbandry practices. *Comp. Med.* **50**:78–81.
51. Whary, M. T., J. Cline, A. King, Z. Ge, Z. Shen, B. Sheppard, and J. G. Fox. 2001. Long-term colonization levels of *Helicobacter hepaticus* in the cecum of hepatitis-prone A/JCr mice are significantly lower than those in hepatitis-resistant C57BL/6 mice. *Comp. Med.* **51**:413–417.
52. Whary, M. T., J. H. Cline, A. E. King, K. M. Hewes, D. Chojnacky, A. Salvarrey, and J. G. Fox. 2000. Monitoring sentinel mice for *Helicobacter hepaticus*, *H. rodentium*, and *H. bilis* infection by use of polymerase chain reaction analysis and serologic testing. *Comp. Med.* **50**:436–443.
53. Young, V. B., K. A. Knox, and D. B. Schauer. 2000. Cytolethal distending toxin sequence and activity in the enterohepatic pathogen *Helicobacter hepaticus*. *Infect. Immun.* **68**:184–191.

Klebsiella pneumoniae
1. Bolister, N. J., H. E. Johnson, and C. M. Wathes. 1992. The ability of airborne *Klebsiella pneumoniae* to colonize mouse lungs. *Epidemiol. Infect.* **109**:121–131.
2. Brijlal, S., A. V. Lakshmi, M. S. Bamji, and P. Suresh. 1996. Flavin metabolism during respiratory infection in mice. *Br. J. Nutr.* **76**:453–462.
3. Camprubi, S., S. Merino, V. J. Benedi, and J. M. Tomas. 1993. The role of the O-antigen lipopolysaccharide and capsule on an experimental *Klebsiella pneumoniae* infection of the rat urinary tract. *FEMS Microbiol. Lett.* **111**:9–13.
4. Chhibber, S., and J. Bajaj. 1995. Polysaccharide-iron-regulated cell surface protein conjugate vaccine: its role in protection against *Klebsiella pneumoniae*-induced lobar pneumonia. *Vaccine* **13**:179–184.
5. Dickneite, G., and J. Czech. 1994. Combination of antibiotic treatment with the thrombin inhibitor recombinant hirudin for the therapy of experimental *Klebsiella pneumoniae* sepsis. *Thromb. Haemostasis* **71**:768–772.
6. De Bont, N., M. G. Netea, P. N. Demacker, B. J. Kullberg, J. W. Van Der Meer, and A. F. Stalenhoef. 2000. Apolipoprotein E-deficient mice have an impaired immune response to *Klebsiella pneumoniae*. *Eur. J. Clin. Invest.* **30**:818–822.
7. Flamm, H. 1957. *Klebsiella*-Enzootic in einer Mauszucht. *Schweiz. Z. Pathol. Bakteriol.* **20**:23–27.
8. Greenberger, M. J., S. L. Kunkel, R. M. Strieter, N. W. Lukacs, J. Bramson, J. Gauldie, F. L. Graham, M. Hitt, J. M. Danforth, and T. J. Standiford. 1996. IL-12 gene therapy protects mice in lethal *Klebsiella pneumonia*. *J. Immunol.* **157**:3006–3012.
9. Haghgoo, S., T. Hasegawa, M. Nadai, L. Wang, T. Nabeshima, and N. Kato. 1995. Effect of a bacterial lipopolysaccharide on biliary excretion of a beta-lactam antibiotic, cefoperazone, in rats. *Antimicrob. Agents Chemother.* **39**:2258–2261.
10. Hansen, A. K. 1995. Antibiotic treatment of nude rats and its impact on the aerobic bacterial flora. *Lab. Anim.* **29**:37–44.
11. Hartwich, J., and M. T. Shouman. 1965. Untersuchungen uber gehauft auftretende *Klebsiella*-infectionen bei versuchsratten. *Z. Verstierkd.* **6**:141–146.
12. Hirakata, Y., N. Furuya, T. Matsumoto, K. Tateda, and K. Yamaguchi. 1996. Experimental endogenous septicaemia caused by *Klebsiella pneumoniae* and *Escherichia coli* in mice. *J. Med. Microbiol.* **44**:211–214.
13. Hochepied, T., W. Van Molle, F. G. Berger, H. Baumann, and C. Libert. 2000. Involvement of the acute phase protein a_1-acid glycoprotein in nonspecific resistance to a lethal gram-negative infection. *J. Biol. Chem.* **275**:14903–14909.
14. Iizawa, Y., T. Nishi, M. Kondo, and A. Imada. 1991. Examination of host defense factors responsible for experimental chronic respiratory tract infection caused by *Klebsiella pneumoniae* in mice. *Microbiol. Immunol.* **35**:615–622.
15. Jackson, N. N., H. G. Wall, C. A. Miller, and M. Rogul. 1980. Naturally acquired infections of *Klebsiella pneumoniae* in Wistar rats. *Lab. Anim.* **14**:357–361.
16. Kohashi, O., T. Ono, K. Ohki, T. Soejima, T. Moriya, A. Umeda, Y. Meno, K. Amako,

S. Funakosi, M. Masuda, and N. Fujii. 1992. Bactericidal activities of rat defensins and synthetic rabbit defensins on Staphylococci, *Klebsiella pneumoniae* (Chedid, 277, and 8N3), *Pseudomonas aeruginosa* (mucoid and nonmucoid strains), *Salmonella typhimurium* (Ra, Rc, Rd, and Re of LPS mutants) and *Escherichia coli*. *Microbiol. Immunol.* **36:**369–380.

17. Malaviya, R., T. Ikeda, E. Ross, and S. N. Abraham. 1996. Mast cell modulation of neutrophil influx and bacterial clearance at sites of infection through TNF-α. *Nature* **381:**77–80.

18. Malina, J., J. Hofmann, and J. Franek. 1991. Informative value of a mouse model of *Klebsiella pneumoniae* infection used as a host-resistance assay. *Folia Microbiol.* **36:**183–191.

19. Mancuso, P., T. J. Standiford, T. Marshall, and M. Peters-Golden. 1998. 5-Lipoxygenase reaction products modulate alveolar phagocytosis of *Klebsiella pneumoniae*. *Infect. Immun.* **66:**5140–5146.

20. National Research Council. 1991. *Infectious Diseases of Mice and Rats: a Report of the Institute of Laboratory Animal Resources Committee on Infectious Diseases of Mice and Rats.* National Academy Press, Washington, D.C.

21. Netea, M. G., W. L. Blok, B. J. Kullberg, M. Bemelmans, M. T. Vogels, W. A. Buurman, and J. W. van der Meer. 1995. Pharmacologic inhibitors of tumor necrosis factor production exert differential effects in lethal endotoxemia and in infection with live microorganisms in mice. *J. Infect. Dis.* **171:**393–399.

22. O'Brien, A. D., T. J. Standiford, K. A. Bucknell, S. E. Wilcoxen, and R. Paine, III. 1999. Role of alveolar epithelial cell intercellular adhesion molecule-1 in host defense against *Klebsiella pneumoniae*. *Am. J. Physiol.* **276:**L961–L970.

23. Rani, M., R. K. Gupta, and S. Chhibber. 1990. Protection against *Klebsiella pneumoniae* induced lobar pneumonia in rats with lipopolysaccharide and related antigens. *Can. J. Microbiol.* **36:**885–890.

24. Schneemilch, H. D. 1976. A naturally acquired infection of laboratory mice with *Klebsiella* capsule type 6. *Lab. Anim.* **10:**305–310.

25. Standiford, T. J., R. M. Strieter, M. J. Greenberger, and S. L. Kunkel. 1996. Expression and regulation of chemokines in acute bacterial pneumonia. *Biol. Signals* **5:**203–208.

26. Tsai, W. C., R. M. Strieter, J. M. Wilkowski, K. A. Bucknell, M. D. Burdick, S. A. Lira, and T. J. Standiford. 1998. Lung-specific transgenic expression of KC enhances resistance to *Klebsiella pneumoniae* in mice. *J. Immunol.* **161:**2435–2440.

27. van Enckevort, F. H., C. G. Sweep, P. N. Span, M. G. Netea, A. R. Hermus, and B. J. Kullberg. 2001. Reduced adrenal response and increased mortality after systemic *Klebsiella pneumoniae* infection in interleukin-6-deficient mice. *Eur. Cytokine Netw.* **12:**581–586.

28. Verleye, M., I. Heulard, J. R. Stephens, R. H. Levy, and J. M. Gillardin. 1995. Effects of citrulline malate on bacterial lipopolysaccharide induced endotoxemia in rats. *Arzneim.-Forsch.* **45:**712–715.

29. Vogels, M. T., I. J. Lindley, J. H. Curfs, W. M. Eling, and J. W. van der Meer. 1993. Effects of interleukin-8 on nonspecific resistance to infection in neutropenic and normal mice. *Antimicrob. Agents Chemother.* **37:**276–280.

30. Vogels, M. T., E. J. Mensink, K. Ye, O. C. Boerman, C. M. Verschueren, C. A. Dinarello, and J. W. van der Meer. 1994. Differential gene expression for IL-1 receptor antagonist, IL-1, and TNF receptors and IL-1 and TNF synthesis may explain IL-1-induced resistance to infection. *J. Immunol.* **153:**5772–5780.

31. Wang, E., N. Ouellet, M. Simard, I. Fillion, Y. Bergeron, D. Beauchamp, and M. G. Bergeron. 2001. Pulmonary and systemic host response to *Streptococcus pneumoniae* and *Klebsiella pneumoniae* bacteremia in normal and immunosuppressed mice. *Infect. Immun.* **69:**5294–5304.

32. Watanaba, H. 1992. Study on lymphocyte-response in early stage of respiratory infection—a view point from experimental *Klebsiella pneumoniae* pneumonia. *Kansen Shogaku Zasshi* **66:**696–708.

33. Yokochi, T., Y. Fujii, I. Nakashima, J. Asai, M. Kiuchi, K. Kojima, and N. Kato. 1993. A murine model of experimental autoimmune lens-induced uveitis using *Klebsiella* O3 lipopolysaccharide as a potent immunological adjuvant. *Int. J. Exp. Pathol.* **74:**573–582.

34. Yoshida, K., T. Matsumoto, K. Tateda, K. Uchida, S. Tsujimoto, Y. Iwakurai, and K. Yamaguchi. 2001. Protection against pulmonary infection with *Klebsiella pneumoniae* in mice by interferon-gamma through activation of phagocytic cells and stimulation of production of other cytokines. *J. Med. Microbiol.* **50:**959–964.

35. Yoshida, K., T. Matsumoto, K. Tateda, K. Uchida, S. Tsujimoto, and K. Yamaguchi. 2000. Role of bacterial capsule in local and systemic inflammatory responses of mice during pulmonary infection with *Klebsiella pneumoniae*. *J. Med. Microbiol.* **49:**1003–1010.

36. Yoshida, K., T. Matsumoto, K. Tateda, K. Uchida, S. Tsujimoto, and K. Yamaguchi. 2001. Induction of interleukin-10 and down-regulation of cytokine production by *Klebsiella*

pneumoniae capsule in mice with pulmonary infection. *J. Med. Microbiol.* **50:**456–461.

Mycoplasma pulmonis
1. **Baluk, P., J. J. Bowden, P. M. Lefevre, and D. M. McDonald.** 1997. Upregulation of substance P receptors in angiogenesis associated with chronic airway inflammation in rats. *Am. J. Physiol.* **273:**L565–L571.
2. **Bowden, J. J., P. Baluk, P. M. Lefevre, T. R. Schoeb, J. R. Lindsey, and D. M. McDonald.** 1996. Sensory denervation by neonatal capsaicin treatment exacerbates *Mycoplasma pulmonis* infection in rat airways. *Am. J. Physiol.* **270:**L393–L403.
3. **Brown, M. B., and D. A. Steiner.** 1996. Experimental genital mycoplasmosis: time of infection influences pregnancy outcome. *Infect. Immun.* **64:**2315–2321.
4. **Cartner, S. C., J. R. Lindsey, J. Gibbs-Erwin, G. H. Cassell, and J. W. Simecka.** 1998. Roles of innate and adaptive immunity in respiratory mycoplasmosis. *Infect. Immun.* **66:**3485–3491.
5. **Cartner, S. C., J. W. Simecka, D. E. Briles, G. H. Cassell, and J. R. Lindsey.** 1996. Resistance to mycoplasmal lung disease in mice is a complex genetic trait. *Infect. Immun.* **64:**5326–5331.
6. **Cartner, S. C., J. W. Simecka, J. R. Lindsey, G. H. Cassell, and J. K. Davis.** 1995. Chronic respiratory mycoplasmosis in C3H/HeN and C57BL/6N mice: lesion severity and antibody response. *Infect. Immun.* **63:**4138–4142.
7. **Cassell, G. H.** 1982. The pathogenic potential of mycoplasmas: *Mycoplasma pulmonis* as a model. *Rev. Infect. Dis.* **4:**S18–S34.
8. **Dahlqvist, K., E. Y. Umemoto, J. J. Brokaw, M. Dupuis, and D. M. McDonald.** 1999. Tissue macrophages associated with angiogenesis in chronic airway inflammation in rats. *Am. J. Respir. Cell. Mol. Biol.* **20:**237–247.
9. **Davidson, M. K., J. R. Lindsey, M. B. Brown, T. R. Schoeb, and G. H. Cassell.** 1981. Comparison of methods for detection of *Mycoplasma pulmonis* in experimentally and naturally infected rats. *J. Clin. Microbiol.* **14:**644–646.
10. **Davis, J. K., M. K. Davidson, Y. R. Schoeb, and J. R. Lindsey.** 1992. Decreased intrapulmonary killing of *Mycoplasma pulmonis* after short-term exposure to NO_2 is associated with damaged alveolar macrophages. *Am. Rev. Respir. Dis.* **145:**406–411.
11. **Faulkner, C. B., M. K. Davidson, J. K. Davis, T. R. Schoeb, J. W. Simecka, and J. R. Lindsey.** 1995. Acute *Mycoplasma pulmonis* infection associated with coagulopathy in C3H/HeN mice. *Lab. Anim. Sci.* **45:**368–372.
12. **Faulkner, C. B., J. W. Simecka, M. K. Davidson, J. K. Davis, T. R. Schoeb, J. R. Lindsey, and M. P. Everson.** 1995. Gene expression and production of tumor necrosis factor alpha, interleukin 1, interleukin 6, and gamma interferon in C3H/HeN and C57BL/6N mice in acute *Mycoplasma pulmonis* disease. *Infect. Immun.* **63:**4084–4090.
13. **Hickman-Davis, J. M., J. Gibbs-Erwin, J. R. Lindsey, and S. Matalon.** 1999. Surfactant protein A mediates mycoplasmacidal activity of alveolar macrophages by production of peroxynitrite. *Proc. Natl. Acad. Sci. USA* **96:**4953–4958.
14. **Hickman-Davis, J. M., S. M. Michalek, J. Gibbs-Erwin, and J. R. Lindsay.** 1997. Depletion of alveolar macrophages exacerbates respiratory mycoplasmosis in mycoplasma-resistant C57BL mice but not mycoplasma-susceptible C3H mice. *Infect. Immun.* **65:**2278–2282.
15. **Homberger, F. R., and P. E. Thomann.** 1994. Transmission of murine viruses and mycoplasma in laboratory mouse colonies with respect to housing conditions. *Lab. Anim.* **28:**113–120.
16. **Hsu, H. C., H. G. Zhang, G. G. Song, J. Xie, D. Liu, P. A. Yang, M. Fleck, W. Wintersberger, T. Zhou, C. K. Edwards, III, and J. D. Mountz.** 2001. Defective Fas ligand-mediated apoptosis predisposes to development of a chronic erosive arthritis subsequent to *Mycoplasma pulmonis* infection. *Arthritis Rheum.* **44:**2146–2159.
17. **Iglauer, F., W. Deutsch, K. Gartner, and G. O. Schwarz.** 1992. The influence of genotypes and social ranks in the clinical course of an experimental infection with *Mycoplasma pulmonis* (MRM) in inbred rats. *Zentbl. Vetmed. Reihe B* **39:**672–682.
18. **Jones, H. P., L. Tabor, X. Sun, M. D. Woolard, and J. W. Simecka.** 2002. Depletion of $CD8^+$ T cells exacerbates $CD4^+$ Th cell-associated inflammatory lesions during murine mycoplasma respiratory disease. *J. Immunol.* **168:**3493–3501.
19. **Lai, W. C., G. Linton, M. Bennett, and S. P. Pakes.** 1993. Genetic control of resistance to *Mycoplasma pulmonis* infection in mice. *Infect. Immun.* **61:**4615–4621.
20. **Lai, W. C., S. P. Pakes, K. Ren, Y. S. Lu, and M. Bennett.** 1997. Therapeutic effect of DNA immunization of genetically susceptible mice infected with virulent *Mycoplasma pulmonis*. *J. Immunol.* **158:**2513–2516.
21. **Lambert, L. C., H. Q. Trummell, A. Singh, G. H. Cassell, and R. J. Bridges.** 1998. *Mycoplasma pulmonis* inhibits electrogenic ion

transport across murine tracheal epithelial cell monolayers. *Infect. Immun.* **66:**272–279.
22. **McDonald, D. M.** 2001. Angiogenesis and remodeling of airway vasculature in chronic inflammation. *Am. J. Respir. Crit. Care Med.* **164:**S39–S45.
23. **McIntosh, J. C., J. W. Simecka, S. E. Ross, J. K. Davis, E. J. Miller, and G. H. Cassell.** 1992. Infection-induced airway fibrosis in two rat strains with differential susceptibility. *Infect. Immun.* **60:**2936–2942.
24. **Minion, F. C., and K. Jarvill-Taylor.** 1994. Membrane-associated hemolysin activities in mycoplasmas. *FEMS Microbiol. Lett.* **116:**101–106.
25. **Modric, S., A. I. Webb, and M. Davidson.** 1999. Effect of respiratory tract disease on pharmacokinetics of tilmicosin in rats. *Lab. Anim. Sci.* **49:**248–253.
26. **Murphy, T. J., G. Thurston, T. Ezaki, and D. M. McDonald.** 1999. Endothelial cell heterogeneity in venules of mouse airways induced by polarized inflammatory stimulus. *Am. J. Pathol.* **155:**93–103.
27. **Naot, Y., S. Merchav, E. Ben-David, and H. Ginsburg.** 1979. Mitogenic activity of *Mycoplasma pulmonis*. I. Stimulation of rat B and T lymphocytes. *Immunology* **36:**399–406.
28. **National Research Council.** 1991. *Infectious Diseases of Mice and Rats: a Report of the Institute of Laboratory Animal Resources Committee on Infectious Diseases of Mice and Rats.* National Academy Press, Washington, D.C.
29. **Nohr, D., A. Buob, K. Gartner, and E. Weihe.** 1996. Changes in pulmonary calcitonin gene-related peptide and protein gene product 9.5 innervation in rats infected with *Mycoplasma pulmonis*. *Cell Tissue Res.* **283:**215–219.
30. **Percy, D. H., and S. W. Barthold.** 2001. *Pathology of Laboratory Rodents and Rabbits,* 2nd ed. Iowa State University Press, Ames.
31. **Reyes, L., D. A. Steiner, J. Hutchinson, B. Crenshaw, and M. B. Brown.** 2000. *Mycoplasma pulmonis* genital disease: effect of rat strain on pregnancy outcome. *Comp. Med.* **50:**622–627.
32. **Romero-Rojas, A., C. Ponce-Hernandez, A. Ciprian, S. Estrada-Parra, and J. W. Hadden.** 2001. Immunomodulatory properties of *Mycoplasma pulmonis*. I. Characterization of the immunomodulatory activity. *Int. Immunopharmacol.* **1:**1679–1688.
33. **Romero-Rojas, A., C. Ponce-Hernandez, S. E. Mendoza, J. A. Reyes-Esparza, S. Estrada-Parra, and J. W. Hadden.** 2001. Immunomodulatory properties of *Mycoplasma pulmonis*. II. Studies on the mechanisms of immunomodulation. *Int. Immunopharmacol.* **1:**1689–1697.
34. **Romero-Rojas, A., J. A. Reyes-Esparza, S. Estrada-Parra, and J. W. Hadden.** 2001. Immunomodulatory properties of *Mycoplasma pulmonis*. III. Lymphocyte stimulation and cytokine production by *Mycoplasma pulmonis* products. *Int. Immunopharmacol.* **1:**1699–1707.
35. **Ross, S. E., J. W. Simecka, G. P. Gambill, J. K. Davis, and G. H. Cassell.** 1992. *Mycoplasma pulmonis* possesses a novel chemoattractant for B lymphocytes. *Infect. Immun.* **60:**669–674.
36. **Sandstedt, K., A. Berglof, R. Feinstein, G. Bolske, B. Evengard, and C. I. Smith.** 1997. Differential susceptibility to *Mycoplasma pulmonis* intranasal infection in X-linked immunodeficient (xid), severe combined immunodeficient (scid), and immunocompetent mice. *Clin. Exp. Immunol.* **108:**490–496.
37. **Schoeb, T. R., K. Dybvig, K. F. Keisling, M. K. Davidson, and J. K. Davis.** 1997. Detection of *Mycoplasma pulmonis* in cilia-associated respiratory bacillus isolates and in respiratory tracts of rats by nested PCR. *J. Clin. Microbiol.* **35:**1667–1670.
38. **Schoeb, T. R., M. M. Juliana, P. W. Nichols, J. K. Davis, and J. R. Lindsey.** 1993. Effects of viral and mycoplasmal infections, ammonia exposure, vitamin A deficiency, host age, and organism strain on adherence of *Mycoplasma pulmonis* in cultured rat tracheas. *Lab. Anim. Sci.* **43:**417–424.
39. **Schunk, M. K., D. H. Percy, and S. Rosendal.** 1995. Effect of time of exposure to rat coronavirus and *Mycoplasma pulmonis* on respiratory tract lesions in the Wistar rat. *Can. J. Vet. Res.* **59:**60–66.
40. **Simecka, J. W.** 1999. β-chemokines are produced in lungs of mice with mycoplasma respiratory disease. *Curr. Microbiol.* **39:**163–167.
41. **Steffen, M. J., and J. L. Ebersole.** 1992. Effects of aging on exocrine immune responses to *Mycoplasma pulmonis*. *Mech. Ageing Dev.* **66:**131–147.
42. **Steiner, D. A., E. W. Uhl, and M. B. Brown.** 1993. In utero transmission of *Mycoplasma pulmonis* in experimentally infected Sprague-Dawley rats. *Infect. Immun.* **61:**2985–2990.
43. **Tanaka, H., S. Abe, and H. Tamura.** 1998. Pathological changes by the imbalance of host T helper lymphocyte subsets in *Mycoplasma pulmonis* pneumonia of mice. *Kansen Shogaku Zasshi* **72:**342–346.
44. **Taylor-Robinson, D., and P. M. Furr.** 2000. Observations on the antibiotic treatment of experimentally induced mycoplasmal infections in mice. *J. Antimicrob. Chemother.* **45:**903–907.

45. **Timenetsky, J., and R. R. De Luca.** 1998. Detection of *Mycoplasma pulmonis* from rats and mice of São Paulo, Brazil. *Lab. Anim. Sci.* **48:** 210–213.

46. **Yamamoto, H., H. Sato, K. Yagami, J. Arikawa, M. Furuya, T. Kurosawa, K. Mannen, K. Matsubayashi, Y. Nishimune, T. Shibahara, T. Ueda, and T. Itoh.** 2001. Microbiological contamination in genetically modified animals and proposals for a microbiological test standard for national universities in Japan. *Exp. Anim.* **50:**397–407.

47. **Yancey, A. L., H. L. Watson, S. C. Cartner, and J. W. Simecka.** 2001. Gender is a major factor in determining the severity of mycoplasma respiratory disease in mice. *Infect. Immun.* **69:** 2865–2871.

48. **Yoshimura, M., S. Endo, K. Ishihara, T. Itoh, A. Takakura, Y. Ueyama, and Y. Ohnishi.** 1997. Quarantine for contaminated pathogens in transplantable human tumors or infections in tumor bearing mice. *Exp. Anim.* **46:** 161–164.

Pasteurella pneumotropica

1. **Artwohl, J. E., J. C. Flynn, R. M. Bunte, O. Angen, and K. C. Herold.** 2000. Outbreak of *Pasteurella pneumotropica* in a closed colony of STOCK-CD28tm1Mak mice. *Contemp. Top. Lab. Anim. Sci.* **39:**39–41.

2. **Boot, R., and M. Bisgaard.** 1995. Reclassification of 30 Pasteurellaceae strains isolated from rodents. *Lab. Anim.* **29:**314–319.

3. **Boot, R., H. van Herck, and J. van der Logt.** 1996. Mutual viral and bacterial infections after housing rats of various breeders within an experimental unit. *Lab. Anim.* **30:**42–45.

4. **Burek, J. D., G. C. Jersey, C. K. Whitehair, and G. R. Carter.** 1972. The pathology and pathogenesis of *Bordetella bronchiseptica* and *Pasteurella pneumotropica* infection in conventional and germfree rats. *Lab. Anim. Sci.* **22:**844–849.

5. **Carthew, P., and J. Gannon.** 1981. Secondary infection of rat lungs with *Pasteurella pneumotropica* after Kilham rat virus infection. *Lab. Anim.* **15:** 219–221.

6. **Chapes, S. K., D. A. Mosier, A. D. Wright, and M. L. Hart.** 2001. MHCII, Tlr4 and Nramp1 genes control host pulmonary resistance against the opportunistic bacterium *Pasteurella pneumotropica*. *J. Leukoc. Biol.* **69:**381–386.

7. **Czuprynski, C. J., and A. K. Sample.** 1990. Interactions of *Haemphilus–Actinobacillus–Pasteurella* bacteria with phagocytic cells. *Can. J. Vet. Res.* **54:**S36–S40.

8. **Dickie, P., P. Mount, D. Purcell, G. Miller, T. Fredrickson, L. J. Chang, and M. A. Martin.** 1996. Myopathy and spontaneous *Pasteurella pneumotropica*-induced abscess formation in an HIV-1 transgenic mouse model. *J. Acquir. Immune Defic. Syndr. Hum. Retrovirol.* **13:**101–116.

9. **Goelz, M. F., J. E. Thigpen, J. Mahler, W. P. Rogers, J. Locklear, B. J. Weigler, and D. B. Forsythe.** 1996. Efficacy of various therapeutic regimens in eliminating *Pasteurella pneumotropica* from the mouse. *Lab. Anim. Sci.* **46:** 280–285.

10. **Harkness, J. E., and J. E. Wagner.** 1975. Self-mutilation in mice associated with otitis media. *Lab. Anim. Sci.* **25:**315–318.

11. **Hong, C. C., and R. D. Ediger.** 1978. Chronic necrotizing mastitis in rats caused by *Pasteurella pneumotropica*. *Lab. Anim. Sci.* **28:**317–320.

12. **Kodjo, A., L. Villard, F. Veillet, F. Escande, E. Borges, F. Maurin, J. Bonnod, and Y. Richard.** 1999. Identification by 16S rDNA fragment amplification and determination of genetic diversity by random amplified polymorphic DNA analysis of *Pasteurella pneumotropica* isolated from laboratory rodents. *Lab. Anim. Sci.* **49:**49–53.

13. **Macy, J. D., Jr., E. C. Weir, S. R. Compton, M. J. Shlomchik, and D. G. Brownstein.** 2000. Dual infection with *Pneumocystis carinii* and *Pasteurella pneumotropica* in B cell-deficient mice: diagnosis and therapy. *Comp. Med.* **50:**49–55.

14. **McGinn, M. D., D. Bean-Knudsen, and R. W. Ermel.** 1992. Incidence of otitis media in CBA/J and CBA/CaJ mice. *Hear. Res.* **59:**1–6.

15. **Mikazuki, K., T. Hirasawa, H. Chiba, K. Takahashi, Y. Sakai, S. Ohhara, and H. Nenui.** 1994. Colonization pattern of *Pasteurella pneumotropica* in mice with latent pasteurellosis. *Jikken Dobutsu* **43:**375–379.

16. **Mikazuki, K., K. Takahashi, K. Nanba, and Y. Hayashi.** 1987. Selective media for *Pasteurella pneumotropica*. *Jikken Dobutsu* **36:**229–237.

17. **Nakai, N., C. Kawaguchi, K. Nawa, S. Kobayashi, Y. Katsuta, and M. Watanabe.** 2000. Detection and elimination of contaminating microorganisms in transplantable tumors and cell lines. *Exp. Anim.* **49:**309–313.

18. **National Research Council.** 1991. *Infectious Diseases of Mice and Rats: a Report of the Institute of Laboratory Animal Resources Committee on Infectious Diseases of Mice and Rats*. National Academy Press, Washington, D.C.

19. **Nozu, R., K. Goto, H. Ohashi, A. Takakura, and T. Itoh.** 1999. Evaluation of PCR as a means of identification of *Pasteurella pneumotropica*. *Exp. Anim.* **48:**51–54.

20. **Scharmann, W., and A. Heller.** 2001. Survival and transmissibility of *Pasteurella pneumotropica*. *Lab. Anim.* **35:**163–166.

21. Suzuki, H., K. Yorozu, T. Watanabe, M. Nakura, and J. Adachi. 1996. Rederivation of mice by means of *in vitro* fertilization and embryo transfer. *Exp. Anim.* **45:**33–38.
22. Ueno, Y., R. Shimizu, R. Nozu, S. Takahashi, M. Yamamoto, F. Sugiyama, A. Takakura, T. Itoh, and K. Yagami. 2002. Elimination of *Pasteurella pneumotropica* from a contaminated mouse colony by oral administration of Enrofloxacin. *Exp. Anim.* **51:**401–405.
23. Wang, R. F., W. Campbell, W. W. Cao, C. Summage, R. S. Steele, and C. E. Cerniglia. 1996. Detection of *Pasteurella pneumotropica* in laboratory mice and rats by polymerase chain reaction. *Lab. Anim. Sci.* **46:**81–85.

Pseudomonas aeruginosa
1. Amano, H., K. Oishi, F. Sonoda, M. Senba, A. Wada, H. Nakagawa, and T. Nagatake. 2000. Role of cytokine-induced neutrophil chemoattractant-2 (CINC-2) a in a rat model of chronic bronchopulmonary infections with *Pseudomonas aeruginosa*. *Cytokine* **12:**1662–1668.
2. Araki, S., M. Suzuki, M. Fujimoto, and M. Kimura. 1995. Enhancement of resistance to bacterial infection in mice by vitamin B2. *J. Vet. Med. Sci.* **57:**599–602.
3. Bradfield, J. F., T. R. Schachtman, R. M. McLaughlin, and E. K. Steffen. 1992. Behavioral and physiologic effects of inapparent wound infection in rats. *Lab. Anim. Sci.* **42:**572–578.
4. Buommino, E., F. Morelli, S. Metafora, F. Rossano, B. Perfetto, A. Baroni, and M. A. Tufano. 1999. Porin from *Pseudomonas aeruginosa* induces apoptosis in an epithelial cell line derived from rat seminal vesicles. *Infect. Immun.* **67:**4794–4800.
5. Dietrich, H. M., D. Khaschabi, and B. Albini. 1996. Isolation of *Enterococcus durans* and *Pseudomonas aeruginosa* in a SCID mouse colony. *Lab. Anim.* **30:**102–107.
6. Dixon, D. M., and M. L. Misfeldt. 1994. Proliferation of immature T cells within the splenocytes of athymic mice by *Pseudomonas* exotoxin A. *Cell. Immunol.* **158:**71–82.
7. Dunkley, M. L., R. L. Clancy, and A. W. Cripps. 1994. A role for CD4$^+$ T cells from orally immunized rats in enhanced clearance of *Pseudomonas aeruginosa* from the lung. *Immunology* **83:**362–369.
8. Fruh, R., B. Blum, H. Mossmann, H. Domdey, and B. U. von Specht. 1995. TH1 cells trigger tumor necrosis factor alpha-mediated hypersensitivity to *Pseudomonas aeruginosa* after adoptive transfer into SCID mice. *Infect. Immun.* **63:**1107–1112.
9. Furuya, N., Y. Hirakata, K. Tomono, T. Matsumoto, K. Tateda, M. Kaku, and K. Yamaguchi. 1993. Mortality rates amongst mice with endogenous septicaemia caused by *Pseudomonas aeruginosa* isolates from various clinical sources. *J. Med. Microbiol.* **39:**141–146.
10. Gosselin, D., J. DeSanctis, M. Boule, E. Skamene, C. Matouk, and D. Radzioch. 1995. Role of tumor necrosis factor alpha in innate resistance to mouse pulmonary infection with *Pseudomonas aeruginosa*. *Infect. Immun.* **63:**3272–3278.
11. Gupta, S. K., S. A. Masinick, J. A. Hobden, R. S. Berk, and L. D. Hazlett. 1996. Bacterial proteases and adherence of *Pseudomonas aeruginosa* to mouse cornea. *Exp. Eye Res.* **62:**641–650.
12. Haslov, K., A. Fomsgaard, K. Takayama, J. S. Fomsgaard, P. Ibsen, M. B. Fauntleroy, P. W. Stashak, C. E. Taylor, and P. J. Baker. 1992. Immunosuppressive effects induced by the polysaccharide moiety of some bacterial lipopolysaccharides. *Immunobiology* **186:**378–393.
13. Heggers, J. P., S. Haydon, F. Ko, P. G. Hayward, S. Carp, and M. C. Robson. 1992. *Pseudomonas aeruginosa* exotoxin A: its role in retardation of wound healing: the 1992 Lindberg Award. *J. Burn Care Rehabil.* **13:**512–518.
14. Hirakata, Y., N. Furuya, K. Tateda, T. Matsumoto, and K. Yamaguchi. 1995. The influence of exo-enzyme S and proteases on endogenous *Pseudomonas aeruginosa* bacteraemia in mice. *J. Med. Microbiol.* **43:**258–261.
15. Johansen, H. K., F. Espersen, S. S. Pedersen, H. P. Hougen, J. Rygaard, and N. Hoiby. 1993. Chronic *Pseudomonas aeruginosa* lung infection in normal and athymic rats. *APMIS* **101:**207–225.
16. Johansen, H. K., H. P. Hougen, J. Rygaard, and N. Hoiby. 1996. Interferon-gamma (IFN-γ) treatment decreases the inflammatory response in chronic *Pseudomonas aeruginosa* pneumonia in rats. *Clin. Exp. Immunol.* **103:**212–218.
17. Kitahara, Y., T. Ishibashi, Y. Harada, M. Takamoto, and K. Tanaka. 1981. Reduced resistance to *Pseudomonas* septicemia in diabetic mice. *Clin. Exp. Immunol.* **43:**590–598.
18. Kobayashi, T., K. Tateda, T. Matsumoto, S. Miyazaki, A. Watanabe, T. Nukiwa, and K. Yamaguchi. 2001. Macrolide-treated *Pseudomonas aeruginosa* induces paradoxical host responses in the lungs of mice and a high mortality rate. *J. Antimicrob. Chemother.* **50:**59–66.
19. Kondratieva, T. K., N. V. Kobets, S. V. Khaidukov, V. V. Yeremeev, I. V. Lyadova, A. S. Apt, M. F. Tam, and M. M. Stevenson. 2000. Characterization of T cell clones derived from lymph nodes and lungs of *Pseudomonas aeruginosa*-susceptible and resistant mice following

immunization with heat-killed bacteria. *Clin. Exp. Immunol.* **121:**275–282.
20. **Kwiatkowska-Patzer, B., J. A. Patzer, and L. J. Heller.** 1993. *Pseudomonas aeruginosa* exotoxin A enhances automaticity and potentiates hypoxic depression of isolated rat hearts. *Proc. Soc. Exp. Biol. Med.* **202:**377–383.
21. **Mahenthiralingam, E., and D. P. Speert.** 1995. Nonopsonic phagocytosis of *Pseudomonas aeruginosa* by macrophages and polymorphonuclear leukocytes requires the presence of the bacterial flagellum. *Infect. Immun.* **63:**4519–4523.
22. **Marshall, J. C., M. B. Ribeiro, P. T. Chu, O. D. Rotstein, and P. A. Sheiner.** 1993. Portal endotoxemia stimulates the release of an immunosuppressive factor from alveolar and splenic macrophages. *J. Surg. Res.* **55:**14–20.
23. **McIntosh, J. C., J. W. Simecka, S. E. Ross, J. K. Davis, E. J. Miller, and G. H. Cassell.** 1992. Infection-induced airway fibrosis in two rat strains with differential susceptibility. *Infect. Immun.* **60:**2936–2942.
24. **Meyer, J. M., A. Neely, A. Stintzi, C. Georges, and I. A. Holder.** 1996. Pyoverdin is essential for virulence of *Pseudomonas aeruginosa*. *Infect. Immun.* **64:**518–523.
25. **Miyazaki, S., T. Matsumoto, K. Tateda, A. Ohno, and K. Yamaguchi.** 1995. Role of exotoxin A in inducing severe *Pseudomonas aeruginosa* infections in mice. *J. Med. Microbiol.* **43:**169–175.
26. **Morissette, C., C. Francoeur, C. Darmond-Zwaig, and F. Gervais.** 1996. Lung phagocyte bactericidal function in strains of mice resistant and susceptible to *Pseudomonas aeruginosa*. *Infect. Immun.* **64:**4984–4992.
27. **Morissette, C., E. Skamene, and F. Gervais.** 1995. Endobronchial inflammation following *Pseudomonas aeruginosa* infection in resistant and susceptible strains of mice. *Infect. Immun.* **63:**1718–1724.
28. **Moser, C., H. P. Hougen, Z. Song, J. Rygaard, A. Kharazmi, and N. Hoiby.** 1999. Early immune response in susceptible and resistant mice strains with chronic *Pseudomonas aeruginosa* lung infection determines the type of T-helper cell response. *APMIS* **107:**1093–1100.
29. **Moser, C., H. K. Johansen, Z. Song, H. P. Hougen, J. Rygaard, and N. Hoiby.** 1997. Chronic *Pseudomonas aeruginosa* lung infection is more severe in Th2 responding BALB/c mice compared to TH1 responding C3H/HeN mice. *APMIS* **105:**838–842.
30. **Nakano, Y., T. Kasahara, N. Mukaida, Y. C. Ko, M. Nakano, and K. Matsushima.** 1994. Protection against lethal bacterial infection in mice by monocyte-chemotactic and -activating factor. *Infect. Immun.* **62:**377–383.
31. **National Research Council.** 1991. *Infectious diseases of mice and rats: A report of the Institute of Laboratory Animal Resources Committee on Infectious Diseases of Mice and Rats.* National Academy Press, Washington, D.C.
32. **O'Callaghan, R. J., L. L. Engel, J. A. Hobden, M. C. Callegan, L. C. Green, and J. M. Hill.** 1996. *Pseudomonas* keratitis. The role of an uncharacterized exoprotein, protease IV, in corneal virulence. *Investig. Ophthalmol. Vis. Sci.* **37:**534–543.
33. **Percy, D. H., and S. W. Barthold.** 2001. *Pathology of Laboratory Rodents and Rabbits,* 2nd ed. Iowa State University Press, Ames.
34. **Pier, G. B., G. Meluleni, and J. B. Goldberg.** 1995. Clearance of *Pseudomonas aeruginosa* from the murine gastrointestinal tract is effectively mediated by O-antigen-specific circulating antibodies. *Infect. Immun.* **63:**2818–2825.
35. **Pittet, J. F., S. Hashimoto, M. Pian, M. C. McElroy, G. Nitenberg, and J. P. Wiener-Kronish.** 1996. Exotoxin A stimulates fluid reabsorption from distal airspaces of lung in anesthetized rats. *Am. J. Physiol.* **270:**L232–L241.
36. **Qin, L., W. M. Quinlan, N. A. Doyle, L. Graham, J. E. Sligh, F. Takei, A. L. Beaudet, and C. M. Doerschuk.** 1996. The roles of CD11/CD18 and ICAM-1 in acute *Pseudomonas aeruginosa*-induced pneumonia in mice. *J. Immunol.* **157:**5016–5021.
37. **Sakata, Y., T. Akaike, M. Suga, S. Ijiri, M. Ando, and H. Maeda.** 1996. Bradykinin generation triggered by *Pseudomonas* proteases facilitates invasion of the systemic circulation by *Pseudomonas aeruginosa*. *Microbiol. Immunol.* **40:**415–423.
38. **Sapru, K., P. K. Stotland, and M. M. Stevenson.** 1999. Quantitative and qualitative differences in bronchoalveolar inflammatory cells in *Pseudomonas aeruginosa*-resistant and -susceptible mice. *Clin. Exp. Immunol.* **115:**103–109.
39. **Schroeder, T. H., N. Reiniger, G. Meluleni, M. Grout, F. T. Coleman, and G. B. Pier.** 2001. Transgenic cystic fibrosis mice exhibit reduced early clearance of *P. aeruginosa* from the respiratory tract. *J. Immunol.* **166:**7410–7418.
40. **Schultz, M. J., A. W. Rijneveld, S. Florquin, P. Speelman, S. J. Van Deventer, and T. van der Poll.** 2001. Impairment of host defense by exotoxin A in *Pseudomonas aeruginosa* pneumonia in mice. *J. Med. Microbiol.* **50:**822–827.
41. **Schumann, J., S. Angermuller, R. Bang, M. Lohoff, and G. Tiegs.** 1998. Acute hepatotoxicity of *Pseudomonas aeruginosa* exotoxin A in mice

depends on T cells and TNF. *J. Immunol.* **161:** 5745–5754.

42. **Schumann, J., H. Bluethmann, and G. Tiegs.** 2000. Synergism of *Pseudomonas aeruginosa* exotoxin A with endotoxin, superantigen, or TNF results in TNFR1- and TNFR2-dependent liver toxicity in mice. *Immunol. Lett.* **74:**165–172.

43. **Shellito, J., S. Nelson, and R. U. Sorensen.** 1992. Effect of pyocyanine, a pigment of *Pseudomonas aeruginosa,* on production of reactive nitrogen intermediates by murine alveolar macrophages. *Infect. Immun.* **60:**3913–3915.

44. **Stevenson, M. M., T. K. Kondratieva, A. S. Apt, M. F. Tam, and E. Skamene.** 1995. *In vitro* and *in vivo* T cell responses in mice during bronchopulmonary infection with mucoid *Pseudomonas aeruginosa. Clin. Exp. Immunol.* **99:**98–105.

45. **Takase, H., H. Nitanai, K. Hoshino, and T. Otani.** 2000. Impact of siderophore production on *Pseudomonas aeruginosa* infections in immunosuppressed mice. *Infect. Immun.* **68:**1834–1839.

46. **Tam, M., G. J. Snipes, and M. M. Stevenson.** 1999. Characterization of chronic bronchopulmonary *Pseudomonas aeruginosa* infection in resistant and susceptible inbred mouse strains. *Am. J. Respir. Cell. Mol. Biol.* **20:**710–719.

47. **Tamura, Y., S. Suzuki, and T. Sawada.** 1992. Role of elastase as a virulence factor in experimental *Pseudomonas aeruginosa* infection in mice. *Microb. Pathog.* **12:**237–244.

48. **Tang, H. B., E. DiMango, R. Bryan, M. Gambello, B. H. Iglewski, J. B. Goldberg, and A. Prince.** 1996. Contribution of specific *Pseudomonas aeruginosa* virulence factors to pathogenesis of pneumonia in a neonatal mouse model of infection. *Infect. Immun.* **64:**37–43.

49. **Urano, T., K. Noguchi, G. Jiang, and K. Tsukumi.** 1995. Survey of *Pseudomonas aeruginosa* contamination in human beings and laboratory animals. *AADE Ed. J.* **44:**233–239.

50. **Vogels, M. T., W. M. Eling, A. Otten, and J. W. van der Meer.** 1995. Interleukin-1 (IL-1)-induced resistance to bacterial infection: role of the type I IL-1 receptor. *Antimicrob. Agents Chemother.* **39:**1744–1747.

51. **Wang, S. D., K. J. Huang, Y. S. Lin, and H. Y. Lei.** 1994. Sepsis-induced apoptosis of the thymocytes in mice. *J. Immunol.* **152:**5014–5021.

52. **Yamaguchi, T., and H. Yamada.** 1991. Role of mechanical injury on airway surface in the pathogenesis of *Pseudomonas aeruginosa. Am. Rev. Respir. Dis.* **144:**1147–1152.

53. **Yokochi, T., K. Narita, A. Morikawa, K. Takahashi, Y. Kato, T. Sugiyama, N. Koide, M. Kawai, M. Fukada, and T. Yoshida.** 2000. Morphological change in *Pseudomonas aeruginosa* following antibiotic treatment of experimental infection in mice and its relation to susceptibility to phagocytosis and to release of endotoxin. *Antimicrob. Agents Chemother.* **44:**205–206.

Salmonella enterica

1. **Caron, J., J. C. Loredo-Osti, L. Laroche, E. Skamene, K. Morgan, and D. Malo.** 2002. Identification of genetic loci controlling bacterial clearance in experimental *Salmonella enteritidis* infection: an unexpected role of *Nramp1* (S1c11a1) in the persistence of infection in mice. *Genes Immun.* **3:**196–204.

2. **Chen, Z. M., and M. K. Jenkins.** 1999. Clonal expansion of antigen-specific CD4 T cells following infection with *Salmonella typhimurium* is similar in susceptible (Ity^s) and resistant (Ity^r) BALB/c mice. *Infect. Immun.* **67:**2025–2029.

3. **Cochran, J. B., H. Chen, M. La Via, V. Cusumano, G. Teti, and J. A. Cook.** 1995. Age-related mortality and adherent splenic cell mediator production to endotoxin in the rat. *Shock* **4:**450–454.

4. **Cohen, L., B. David, and J. M. Cavaillon.** 1991. Interleukin-3 enhances cytokine production by LPS-stimulated macrophages. *Immunol. Lett.* **28:**121–126.

5. **Conlan, J. W.** 1997. Critical roles of neutrophils in host defense against experimental systemic infections of mice by *Listeria monocytogenes, Salmonella typhimurium,* and *Yersinia enterocolitica. Infect. Immun.* **65:**630–635.

6. **Essani, N. A., G. M. McGuire, A. M. Manning, and H. Jaeschke.** 1996. Endotoxin-induced activation of the nuclear transcription factor κB and expression of E-selectin messenger RNA in hepatocytes, Kupffer cells, and endothelial cells *in vivo. J. Immunol.* **156:**2956–2963.

7. **Everest, P., M. Roberts, and G. Dougan.** 1998. Susceptibility to *Salmonella typhimurium* infection and effectiveness of vaccination in mice deficient in the tumor necrosis factor a p55 receptor. *Infect. Immun.* **66:**3355–3364.

8. **Galdiero, M., A. Marcatili, G. Cipollaro de l'Ero, T. Nuzzo, C. Bentivoglio, M. Galdiero, and C. Romano Carratelli.** 1999. Effect of transforming growth factor β on experimental *Salmonella typhimurium* infection in mice. *Infect. Immun.* **67:**1432–1438.

9. **Genovese, F., G. Mancuso, M. Cuzzola, V. Cusumano, F. Nicoletti, B. Bendtzen, and G. Teti.** 1996. Improved survival and antagonistic effect of sodium fusidate on tumor necrosis factor alpha in a neonatal mouse model of endotoxin shock. *Antimicrob. Agents Chemother.* **40:** 1733–1735.

10. Glembot, T. M., L. D. Britt, and M. A. Hill. 1996. Endotoxin interacts with tumor necrosis factor-a to induce vasodilation of isolated rat skeletal muscle arterioles. *Shock* **5**:251–257.

11. Goto, M., W. P. Zeller, and R. C. Lichtenberg. 1994. Decreased gluconeogenesis and increased glucose disposal without hyperinsulinemia in 10-day-old rats with endotoxic shock. *Metabolism* **43**:1248–1254.

12. Gupta, S. 1998. Priming of T-cell responses in mice by porins of *Salmonella typhimurium*. *Scand. J. Immunol.* **48**:136–143.

13. Gupta, S., L. Feng, T. Yoshimura, J. Redick, S. M. Fu, and C. E. Rose, Jr. 1996. Intra-alveolar macrophage-inflammatory peptide 2 induces rapid neutrophil localization in the lung. *Am. J. Respir. Cell. Mol. Biol.* **15**:656–663.

14. Heinzel, F. P. 1990. The role of IFN-γ in the pathology of experimental endotoxemia. *J. Immunol.* **145**:2920–2924.

15. Hess, J., C. Ladel, D. Miko, and S. H. Kaufmann. 1996. *Salmonella typhimurium aroA$^-$* infection in gene-targeted immunodeficient mice: major role of CD4$^+$ TCR-$\alpha\beta$ cells and IFN-γ in bacterial clearance independent of intracellular location. *J. Immunol.* **156**:3321–3326.

16. Holecek, M., F. Skopec, L. Sprongl, and M. Pecka. 1995. Protein metabolism in specific tissues of endotoxin-treated rats: effect of nutritional status. *Physiol. Res.* **44**:399–406.

17. Islam, A. F., N. D. Moss, Y. Dai, M. S. Smith, A. M. Collins, and G. D. Jackson. 2000. Lipopolysaccharide-induced biliary factors enhance invasion of *Salmonella enteritidis* in a rat model. *Infect. Immun.* **68**:1–5.

18. Lentsch, R. H., B. K. Kirchner, L. W. Dixon, and J. E. Wagner. 1983. A report of an outbreak of *Salmonella oranienburg* in a hybrid mouse colony. *Vet. Microbiol.* **8**:105–109.

19. Makhlouf, M., S. H. Ashton, J. Hildebrandt, N. Mehta, T. W. Gettys, P. V. Halushka, and J. A. Cook. 1996. Alterations in macrophage G proteins are associated with endotoxin tolerance. *Biochim. Biophys. Acta* **1312**:163–168.

20. Mastroeni, P., S. Clare, S. Khan, J. A. Harrison, C. E. Hormaeche, H. Okamura, M. Kurimoto, and G. Dougan. 1999. Interleukin 18 contributes to host resistance and γ interferon production in mice infected with virulent *Salmonella typhimurium*. *Infect. Immun.* **67**:478–483.

21. Matsiota-Bernard, P., B. Hentati, S. Pie, N. Legakis, C. Nauciel, and S. Avrameas. 1996. Beneficial effect of *Salmonella typhimurium* infection and of immunoglobulins from *S. typhimurium*-infected mice on the autoimmune disease of (NZB x NZW) F1 mice. *Clin. Exp. Immunol.* **104**:228–235.

22. Mehta, A., S. Singh, and N. K. Ganguly. 1999. Effect of *Salmonella typhimurium* enterotoxin (S-LT) on lipid peroxidation and cell viability levels of isolated rat enterocytes. *Mol. Cell. Biochem.* **196**:175–181.

23. Mittrucker, H. W., and S. H. Kaufmann. 2000. Immune response to infection with *Salmonella typhimurium* in mice. *J. Leukoc. Biol.* **67**:457–463.

24. Mixter, P. F., V. Camerini, B. J. Stone, V. L. Miller, and M. Kronenberg. 1994. Mouse T lymphocytes that express a $\gamma\delta$ T-cell antigen receptor contribute to resistance to *Salmonella* infection *in vivo*. *Infect. Immun.* **62**:4618–4621.

25. National Research Council. 1991. *Infectious Diseases of Mice and Rats: a Report of the Institute of Laboratory Animal Resources Committee on Infectious Diseases of Mice and Rats*. National Academy Press, Washington, D.C.

26. Naughton, P. J., G. Grant, S. W. Ewen, R. J. Spencer, D. S. Brown, A. Pusztai, and S. Bardocz. 1995. *Salmonella typhimurium* and *Salmonella enteritidis* induce gut growth and increase the polyamine content of the rat small intestine *in vivo*. *FEMS Immunol. Med. Microbiol.* **12**:251–258.

27. Naughton, P. J., G. Grant, R. J. Spencer, S. Bardocz, and A. Pusztai. 1996. A rat model of infection by *Salmonella typhimurium* or *S. enteritidis*. *J. Appl. Bacteriol.* **81**:651–656.

28. Netea, M. G., G. Fantuzzi, B. J. Kullberg, R. J. Stuyt, E. J. Pulido, R. C. McIntyre, Jr., L. A. Joosten, J. W. Van der Meer, and C. A. Dinarello. 2000. Neutralization of IL-18 reduces neutrophil tissue accumulation and protects mice against lethal *Escherichia coli* and *Salmonella typhimurium* endotoxemia. *J. Immunol.* **164**:2644–2649.

29. Percy, D. H., and S. W. Barthold. 2001. *Pathology of Laboratory Rodents and Rabbits*, 2nd ed. Iowa State University Press, Ames.

30. Pie, S., P. Truffa-Bachi, M. Pla, and C. Nauciel. 1997. Th1 response in *Salmonella typhimurium*-infected mice with a high or low rate of bacterial clearance. *Infect. Immun.* **65**:4509–4514.

31. Rose, C. E., Jr., C. A. Juliano, D. E. Tracey, T. Yoshimura, and S. M. Fu. 1994. Role of interleukin-1 in endotoxin-induced lung injury in the rat. *Am. J. Respir. Cell. Mol. Biol.* **10**:214–221.

32. Schwacha, M. G., J. J. Meissler, Jr., and T. K. Eisenstein. 1998. *Salmonella typhimurium* infection in mice induces nitric oxide-mediated immunosuppression through a natural killer cell-mediated pathway. *Infect. Immun.* **66**:5862–5866.

33. **Shanks, N., S. Larocque, and M. J. Meaney.** 1995. Neonatal endotoxin exposure alters the development of the hypothalamic-pituitary-adrenal axis: early illness and later responsivity to stress. *J. Neurosci.* **15:**376–384.
34. **Sinha, K., P. Mastroeni, J. Harrison, R. D. de Hormaeche, and C. E. Hormaeche.** 1997. *Salmonella typhimurium aroA, htrA,* and *aroD htrA* mutants cause progressive infections in athymic (*nu/nu*) BALB/c mice. *Infect. Immun.* **65:**1566–1569.
35. **Stone, B. J., and V. L. Miller.** 1995. *Salmonella enteritidis* has a homologue of tolC that is required for virulence in BALB/c mice. *Mol. Microbiol.* **17:**701–712.
36. **Suzuki, S., K. Komase, H. Matsui, A. Abe, K. Kawahara, Y. Tamura, M. Kijima, H. Danbara, M. Nakamura, and S. Sato.** 1994. Virulence region of plasmid pNL2001 of *Salmonella enteritidis. Microbiology* **140:**1307–1318.
37. **Sveen, K., and N. Skaug.** 1992. Comparative mitogenicity and polyclonal B cell activation capacity of eight oral or nonoral bacterial lipopolysaccharides in cultures of spleen cells from athymic (nu/nu-BALB/c) and thymic (BALB/c) mice. *Oral Microbiol. Immunol.* **7:**71–77.
38. **Thorns, C. J., C. Turcotte, C. G. Gemmell, and M. J. Woodward.** 1996. Studies into the role of the SEF14 fimbrial antigen in the pathogenesis of *Salmonella enteritidis. Microb. Pathog.* **20:**235–246.
39. **Turinsky, J., B. P. Bayly, and D. M. O'Sullivan.** 1991. 1,2-Diacylglycerol and ceramide levels in rat liver and skeletal muscle *in vivo. Am. J. Physiol.* **261:**E620–E627.
40. **van der Velden, A. W., A. J. Bäumler, R. M. Tsolis, and F. Heffron.** 1998. Multiple fimbrial adhesins are required for full virulence of *Salmonella typhimurium* in mice. *Infect. Immun.* **66:**2803–2808.
41. **Wang, X., S. B. Jones, Z. Zhou, C. Han, and R. R. Fiscus.** 1992. Calcitonin gene-related peptide (CGRP) and neuropeptide Y (NPY) levels are elevated in plasma and decreased in vena cava during endotoxin shock in the rat. *Circ. Shock* **36:**21–30.
42. **Witthaut, R., A. Farhood, C. W. Smith, and H. Jaeschke.** 1994. Complement and tumor necrosis factor-alpha contribute to Mac-1 (CD11b/CD18) up-regulation and systemic neutrophil activation during endotoxemia *in vivo. J. Leukoc. Biol.* **55:**105–111.

Staphylococcus aureus
1. **Bailey, C. J., B. P. Lockhart, M. B. Redpath, and T. P. Smith.** 1995. The epidermolytic (exfoliative) toxins of *Staphylococcus aureus. Med. Microbiol. Immunol.* **184:**53–61.
2. **Benedettini, G., G. DeLibero, L. Mori, and M. Campa.** 1984. *Staphylococcus aureus* inhibits contact sensitivity to oxazolone by activating suppressor B cells in mice. *Int. Arch. Allergy Appl. Immunol.* **73:**269–273.
3. **Bhakdi, S., and J. Tranum-Jensen.** 1991. Alpha-toxin of *Staphylococcus aureus. Microbiol. Rev.* **55:**733–751.
4. **Bost, K. L., W. K. Ramp, N. C. Nicholson, J. L. Bento, I. Marriott, and M. C. Hudson.** 1999. *Staphylococcus aureus* infection of mouse or human osteoblasts induces high levels of interleukin-6 and interleukin-12 production. *J. Infect. Dis.* **180:**1912–1920.
5. **Bradfield, J. F., T. R. Schachtman, R. M. McLaughlin, and E. K. Steffen.** 1992. Behavioral and physiologic effects of inapparent wound infection in rats. *Lab. Anim. Sci.* **42:**572–578.
6. **Das, T., G. Sa, and P. K. Ray.** 1999. Mechanisms of protein A superantigen-induced signal transduction for proliferation of mouse B cell. *Immunol. Lett.* **70:**43–51.
7. **De Kimpe, S. J., M. Kengatharan, C. Thiemermann, and J. R. Vane.** 1995. The cell wall components peptidoglycan and lipoteichoic acid from *Staphylococcus aureus* act in synergy to cause shock and multiple organ failure. *Proc. Natl. Acad. Sci. USA* **92:**10359–10363.
8. **Fierabracci, A., L. Hammond, M. Lowdell, L. Chiovato, A. W. Goode, G. F. Bottazzo, and R. Mirakian.** 1999. The effect of staphylococcal enterotoxin B on thyrocyte HLA molecule expression. *J. Autoimmun.* **12:**305–314.
9. **Fincher, E. F., IV, L. Johannsen, L. Kapas, S. Takahashi, and J. M. Krueger.** 1996. Microglia digest *Staphylococcus aureus* into low molecular weight biologically active compounds. *Am. J. Physiol.* **271:**149–156.
10. **Gelfand, E. W., J. Saloga, and G. Lack.** 1995. Modification of immediate hypersensitivity responses by staphylococcal enterotoxin B. *J. Clin. Immunol.* **15:**37S–41S.
11. **Haraguchi, M., M. Hino, H. Tanaka, and M. Maru.** 1997. Naturally occurring dermatitis associated with *Staphylococcus aureus* in DS-Nh mice. *Exp. Anim.* **46:**225–229.
12. **Hendricks, K. J., T. A. Burd, J. O. Anglen, A. W. Simpson, G. D. Christensen, and B. J. Gainor.** 2001. Synergy between *Staphylococcus aureus* and *Pseudomonas aeruginosa* in a rat model of complex orthopaedic wounds. *J. Bone Joint Surg. Am. Vol.* **83:**855–861.
13. **Hildebrand, A., M. Pohl, and S. Bhakdi.** 1991. *Staphylococcus aureus* alpha-toxin. Dual

mechanism of binding to target cells. *J. Biol. Chem.* **266:**17195–17200.

14. Hultgren, O., M. Kopf, and A. Tarkowski. 1999. Outcome of *Staphylococcus aureus*-triggered sepsis and arthritis in IL-4-deficient mice depends on the genetic background of the host. *Eur. J. Immunol.* **29:**2400–2405.

15. Kilcullen, J. K., Q. P. Ly, T. H. Chang, S. M. Levenson, and J. J. Steinberg. 1998. Nonviable *Staphylococcus aureus* and its peptidoglycan stimulate macrophage recruitment, angiogenesis, fibroplasia, and collagen accumulation in wounded rats. *Wound Repair Regen.* **6:**149–156.

16. McElroy, M. C., H. R. Harty, G. E. Hosford, G. M. Boylan, J. F. Pittet, and T. J. Foster. 1999. Alpha-toxin damages the air-blood barrier of the lung in a rat model of *Staphylococcus aureus*-induced pneumonia. *Infect. Immun.* **67:**5541–5544.

17. McInnes, I. B., B. Leung, X. Q. Wei, G. C. Gemmell, and F. Y. Liew. 1998. Septic arthritis following *Staphylococcus aureus* infection in mice lacking inducible nitric oxide synthase. *J. Immunol.* **160:**308–315.

18. McKay, D. M., J. Lu, S. Jedrzkiewicz, W. Ho, and K. A. Sharkey. 1999. Nitric oxide participates in the recovery of normal jejunal epithelial ion transport following exposure to the superantigen *Staphylococcus aureus* enterotoxin B. *J. Immunol.* **163:**4519–4526.

19. Nakane, A., M. Okamoto, M. Asano, M. Kohanawa, and T. Minagawa. 1995. Endogenous gamma interferon, tumor necrosis factor, and interleukin-6 in *Staphylococcus aureus* infection in mice. *Infect. Immun.* **63:**1165–1172.

20. National Research Council. 1991. *Infectious Diseases of Mice and Rats: a Report of the Institute of Laboratory Animal Resources Committee on Infectious Diseases of Mice and Rats*. National Academy Press, Washington, D.C.

21. Seeger, W., R. G. Birkemeyer, L. Ermert, N. Suttorp, S. Bhakdi, and H. R. Duncker. 1990. Staphylococcal alpha-toxin-induced vascular leakage in isolated perfused rabbit lungs. *Lab. Invest.* **63:**341–349.

22. Sibelius, U., U. Grandel, M. Buerke, D. Mueller, L. Kiss, H. J. Kraemer, R. Braun-Dullaeus, W. Haberbosch, W. Seeger, and F. Grimminger. 2000. Staphylococcal a toxin provokes coronary vasoconstriction and loss in myocardial contractility in perfused rat hearts: role of thromboxane generation. *Circulation* **101:**78–85.

23. Sinha, P., A. K. Ghosh, T. Das, G. Sa, and P. K. Ray. 1999. Protein A of *Staphylococcus aureus* evokes Th1 type response in mice. *Immunol. Lett.* **67:**157–165.

24. Takeuchi, O., K. Hoshino, and S. Akira. 2000. Cutting edge: TLR2-deficient and MyD88-deficient mice are highly susceptible to *Staphylococcus aureus* infection. *J. Immunol.* **165:**5392–5396.

25. Tao, M., H. Yamashita, K. Watanabe, and T. Nagatake. 1999. Possible virulence factors of *Staphylococcus aureus* in a mouse septic model. *FEMS Immunol. Med. Microbiol.* **23:**135–146.

26. Tucker, K. A., S. S. Reilly, C. S. Leslie, and M. C. Hudson. 2000. Intracellular *Staphylococcus aureus* induces apoptosis in mouse osteoblasts. *FEMS Microbiol. Lett.* **186:**151–156.

27. Yanke, S. J., M. E. Olson, H. D. Davies, and D. A. Hart. 2000. A CD-2 mouse model of infection with *Staphylococcus aureus*: influence of gender on infection with MRSA and MSSA isolates. *Can. J. Microbiol.* **46:**920–926.

28. Yoon, K. S., R. H. Fitzgerald, Jr., S. Sud, Z. Song, and P. H. Wooley. 1999. Experimental acute hematogenous osteomyelitis in mice. II. Influence of *Staphylococcus aureus* infection on T-cell immunity. *J. Orthop. Res.* **17:**382–391.

Streptococcus pneumoniae

1. Amory-Rivier, C. F., J. Mohler, J. P. Bedos, E. Azoulay-Dupuis, D. Henin, M. Muffat-Joly, C. Carbon, and P. Moine. 2000. Nuclear factor-κB activation in mouse lung lavage cells in response to *Streptococcus pneumoniae* pulmonary infection. *Crit. Care Med.* **28:**3249–3256.

2. Arva, E., U. Dahlgren, R. Lock, and B. Andersson. 1996. Antibody response in bronchoalveolar lavage and serum of rats after aerosol immunization of the airways with a well-adhering and a poorly adhering strain of *Streptococcus pneumoniae*. *Int. Arch. Allergy Immunol.* **109:**35–43.

3. Benton, K. A., J. C. Paton, and D. E. Briles. 1997. Differences in virulence for mice among *Streptococcus pneumoniae* strains of capsular types 2, 3, 4, 5, and 6 are not attributable to differences in pneumolysin production. *Infect. Immun.* **65:**1237–1244.

4. Echchannaoui, H., K. Frei, C. Schnell, S. L. Leib, W. Zimmerli, and R. Landmann. 2002. Toll-like receptor 2-deficient mice are highly susceptible to *Streptococcus pneumoniae* meningitis because of reduced bacterial clearing and enhanced inflammation. *J. Infect. Dis.* **186:**798–806.

5. Gabr, U., Y. S. Won, S. Boonlayangoor, K. Thompson, F. M. Baroody, and R. M. Na-

clerio. 2001. C57BL/6 and BALB/c mice have similar neutrophil response to acute *Streptococcus pneumoniae* sinus infections. *Arch. Otolaryngol. Head Neck Surg.* **127:**985–990.

6. **National Research Council.** 1991. *Infectious Diseases of Mice and Rats: a Report of the Institute of Laboratory Animal Resources Committee on Infectious Diseases of Mice and Rats.* National Academy Press, Washington, D.C.

7. **Szalai, A. J., D. E. Briles, and J. E. Volanakis.** 1996. Role of complement in C-reactive-protein-mediated protection of mice from *Streptococcus pneumoniae. Infect. Immun.* **64:**4850–4853.

8. **Takashima, K., K. Tateda, T. Matsumoto, Y. Iizawa, M. Nakao, and K. Yamaguchi.** 1997. Role of tumor necrosis factor alpha in pathogenesis of pneumococcal pneumonia in mice. *Infect. Immun.* **65:**257–260.

9. **Takashima, K., K. Tateda, T. Matsumoto, T. Ito, Y. Iizawa, M. Nakao, and M. Yamaguchi.** 1996. Establishment of a model of penicillin-resistant *Streptococcus pneumoniae* pneumonia in healthy CBA/J mice. *J. Med. Microbiol.* **45:**319–322.

10. **Tino, M. J., and J. R. Wright.** 1996. Surfactant protein A stimulates phagocytosis of specific pulmonary pathogens by alveolar macrophages. *Am. J. Physiol.* **270:**L677–L688.

11. **Van den Dobbelsteen, G. P., K. Brunekreef, H. Kroes, N. van Rooijen, and E. P. van Rees.** 1993. Enhanced triggering of mucosal immune responses by reducing splenic phagocytic functions. *Eur. J. Immunol.* **23:**1488–1493.

12. **Van der Poll, T., A. Marchant, C. V. Keogh, M. Goldman, and S. F. Lowry.** 1996. Interleukin-10 impairs host defense in murine pneumococcal pneumonia. *J. Infect. Dis.* **174:**994–1000.

13. **Watson, D. A., D. M. Musher, and J. Verhoef.** 1995. Pneumococcal virulence factors and host immune responses to them. *Eur. J. Clin. Microbiol. Infect. Dis.* **14:**479–490.

14. **Winkelstein, J. A., and A. J. Swift.** 1975. Host defense against the pneumococcus in T-lymphocyte deficient, nude mice. *Infect. Immun.* **12:**1222–1223.

15. **Wood, W. B., Jr.** 1941. Studies on the mechanisms of recovery in pneumococcal pneumonia. I. The action of type specific antibody upon the pulmonary lesion of experimental pneumonia. *J. Exp. Med.* **73:**201–222.

FUNGI

Pneumocystis carinii

1. **Aliouat, E. M., E. Dei-Cas, A. Ouaissi, F. Palluault, B. Soulez, and D. Camus.** 1993. *In vitro* attachment of *Pneumocystis carinii* from mouse and rat origin. *Biol. Cell.* **77:**209–217.

2. **Armstrong, M. Y., A. L. Smith, and F. F. Richards.** 1991. *Pneumocystis carinii* pneumonia in the rat model. *J. Protozool.* **38:**136S–138S.

3. **Bartlett, M. S., W. C. Angus, M. M. Shaw, P. J. Durant, C. H. Lee, J. M. Pascale, and J. W. Smith.** 1998. Antibody to *Pneumocystis carinii* protects rats and mice from developing pneumonia. *Clin. Diagn. Lab. Immunol.* **5:**74–77.

4. **Bauer, N. L., J. R. Paulsrud, M. S. Bartlett, J. W. Smith, and C. E. Wilde, III.** 1993. *Pneumocystis carinii* organisms obtained from rats, ferrets, and mice are antigenically different. *Infect. Immun.* **61:**1315–1319.

5. **Beck, J. M., R. L. Newbury, B. E. Palmer, M. L. Warnock, P. K. Byrd, and H. B. Kaltreider.** 1996. Role of CD8+ lymphocytes in host defense against *Pneumocystis carinii* in mice. *J. Lab. Clin. Med.* **128:**477–487.

6. **Beck, J. M., A. M. Prestion, and M. R. Gyetko.** 1999. Urokinase-type plasminogen activator in inflammatory cell recruitment and host defense against *Pneumocystis carinii* in mice. *Infect. Immun.* **67:**879–884.

7. **Beers, M. F., E. N. Atochina, A. M. Preston, and J. M. Beck.** 1999. Inhibition of lung surfactant protein B expression during *Pneumocystis carinii* pneumonia in mice. *J. Lab. Clin. Med.* **133:**423–433.

8. **Castro, M., T. I. Morgenthaler, O. A. Hoffman, J. E. Standing, M. S. Rohrbach, and A. H. Limper.** 1993. *Pneumocystis carinii* induces the release of arachidonic acid and its metabolites from alveolar macrophages. *Am. J. Respir. Cell. Mol. Biol.* **9:**73–81.

9. **Chen, W., E. A. Havell, F. Gigliotti, and A. G. Harmsen.** 1993. Interleukin-6 production in a murine model of *Pneumocystis carinii* pneumonia: relation to resistance and inflammatory response. *Infect. Immun.* **61:**97–102.

10. **Chen, W., E. A. Havell, L. L. Moldawer, K. W. McIntyre, R. A. Chizzonite, and A. G. Harmsen.** 1992. Interleukin 1: an important mediator of host resistance against *Pneumocystis carinii. J. Exp. Med.* **176:**713–718.

11. **Chen, W., J. W. Mills, and A. G. Harmsen.** 1992. Development and resolution of *Pneumocystis carinii* pneumonia in severe combined immunodeficient mice: a morphological study of host inflammatory responses. *Int. J. Exp. Pathol.* **73:**709–720.

12. **Deerberg, F., G. Pohlmeyer, M. Wullenweber, and H. J. Hedrich.** 1993. History and pathology of an enzootic *Pneumocystis carinii* pneumonia in athymic Han:RNU and Han:NZNU rats. *J. Exp. Anim. Sci.* **36:**1–11.

13. **el-Nassery, S. M., A. E. Rahmy, W. M. el Gebaly, and H. A. Sadaka.** 1994. *Pneumocystis carinii*: recognition of the infection in albino rats using different stains. *J. Egypt. Soc. Parasitol.* **24:** 285–294.
14. **Garvy, B. A., and M. H. Qureshi.** 2000. Delayed inflammatory response to *Pneumocystis carinii* infection in neonatal mice is due to an inadequate lung environment. *J. Immunol.* **165:**6480–6486.
15. **Gigliotti, F., and T. McCool.** 1996. Glycoprotein A is the immunodominant antigen of *Pneumocystis carinii* in mice following immunization. *Parasitol. Res.* **82:**90–91.
16. **Hanano, R., K. Reifenberg, and S. H. Kaufmann.** 1996. T- and B-lymphocyte-independent formation of alveolar macrophage-derived multinucleated giant cells in murine *Pneumocystis carinii* pneumonia. *Infect. Immun.* **64:**2821–2823.
17. **Ito, M., T. Tsugane, K. Kobayashi, K. Kuramochi, K. Hioki, T. Furuta, and T. Nomura.** 1991. Study on placental transmission of *Pneumocystis carinii* in mice using immunodeficient SCID mice as a new animal model. *J. Protozool.* **38:**218S–219S.
18. **Kolls, J. K., J. M. Beck, S. Nelson, W. R. Summer, and J. Shellito.** 1993. Alveolar macrophage release of tumor necrosis factor during murine *Pneumocystis carinii* pneumonia. *Am. J. Respir. Cell. Mol. Biol.* **8:**370–376.
19. **Kolls, J. K., S. Habetz, M. K. Shean, C. Vazquez, J. A. Brown, D. Lei, P. Schwarzenberger, P. Ye, S. Nelson, W. R. Summer, and J. E. Shellito.** 1999. IFNγ and CD8+ T cells restore host defenses against *Pneumocystis carinii* in mice depleted of CD4+ T cells. *J. Immunol.* **162:**2890–2894.
20. **Kovacevic, S., and M. Knezevic.** 1995. Pulmonary pathohistological changes in mice in experimental infection with *Pneumocystis carinii*. *Vojnosanit. Pregl.* **52:**3–8.
21. **Kunz, S., U. Junker, J. Blaser, B. Joos, B. Meyer, O. Zak, and T. O'Reilly.** 1995. The SCID mouse as an experimental model for the evaluation of anti-*Pneumocystis carinii* therapy. *J. Antimicrob. Chemother.* **36:**137–155.
22. **Laursen, A. L., N. Obel, J. Rungby, and P. L. Andersen.** 1993. Phagocytosis and stimulation of the respiratory burst in neutrophils by *Pneumocystis carinii*. *J. Infect. Dis.* **168:**1466–1471.
23. **Lipschik, G. Y., J. F. Treml, S. D. Moore, and M. F. Beers.** 1997. *Pneumocystis carinii* glycoprotein A inhibits surfactant phospholipid secretion by rat alveolar type II cells. *J. Infect. Dis.* **177:**182–187.
24. **Mazars, E., K. Guyot, I. Durand, E. Dei-Cas, S. Boucher, S. B. Abderrazak, A. L. Banuls, M. Tibayrenc, and D. Camus.** 1997. Isoenzyme diversity in *Pneumocystis carinii* from rats, mice, and rabbits. *J. Infect. Dis.* **175:**655–660.
25. **Mordelet-Dambrine, M., C. Danel, R. Farinotti, G. Urzua, L. Barritault, and G. J. Huchon.** 1992. Influence of *Pneumocystis carinii* pneumonia on serum and tissue concentrations of pentamidine administered to rats by tracheal injections. *Am. Rev. Respir. Dis.* **146:**735–739.
26. **National Research Council.** 1991. *Infectious Diseases of Mice and Rats: a Report of the Institute of Laboratory Animal Resources Committee on Infectious Diseases of Mice and Rats.* National Academy Press, Washington, D.C.
27. **Nielsen, M. H., O. P. Settnes, E. M. Aliouat, J. C. Cailliez, and E. Dei-Cas.** 1998. Different ultrastructural morphology of *Pneumocystis carinii* derived from mice, rats, and rabbits. *APMIS* **106:**771–779.
28. **Paine, P., III, A. M. Preston, S. Wilcoxen, H. Jin, B. B. Siu, S. B. Morris, J. A. Reed, G. Ross, J. A. Whitsett, and J. M. Beck.** 2000. Granulocyte-macrophage colony-stimulating factor in the innate immune response to *Pneumocystis carinii* pneumonia in mice. *J. Immunol.* **164:**2602–2609.
29. **Phelps, D. S., T. M. Umstead, R. M. Rose, and J. A. Fishman.** 1996. Surfactant protein-A levels increase during *Pneumocystis carinii* pneumonia in the rat. *Eur. Respir. J.* **9:**565–570.
30. **Pohlmeyer, G., and F. Deerberg.** 1993. Nude rats as a model of natural *Pneumocystis carinii* pneumonia: sequential morphological study of lung lesions. *J. Comp. Pathol.* **109:**217–230.
31. **Powles, M. A., D. C. McFadden, L. A. Pittarelli, and D. M. Schmatz.** 1992. Mouse model for *Pneumocystis carinii* pneumonia that uses natural transmission to initiate infection. *Infect. Immun.* **60:**1397–1400.
32. **Rabodonirina, M., R. Wilmotte, E. Dannaoui, F. Persat, G. Bayle, and M. Mojon.** 1997. Detection of *Pneumocystis carinii* DNA by PCR amplification n various rat organs in experimental pneumocystosis. *J. Med. Microbiol.* **46:** 665–668.
33. **Roths, J. B., A. L. Smith, and C. L. Sidman.** 1993. Lethal exacerbation of *Pneumocystis carinii* pneumonia in severe combined immunodeficiency mice after infection by pneumonia virus of mice. *J. Exp. Med.* **177:**1193–1198.
34. **Rudmann, D. G., A. M. Preston, M. W. Moore, and J. M. Beck.** 1998. Susceptibility to *Pneumocystis carinii* in mice is dependent on simultaneous deletion of IFNγ and type 1 and 2 TNF receptor genes. *J. Immunol.* **161:**360–366.

35. Schaffzin, J. K., and J. R. Stringer. 2000. The major glycoprotein expression sites of two special forms of rat *Pneumocystis carinii* differ in structure. *J. Infect. Dis.* **181:**1729–1739.
36. Shah, J. S., W. Pieciak, J. Liu, A. Buharin, and D. J. Lane. 1996. Diversity of host species and strains of *Pneumocystis carinii* is based on rRNA sequences. *Clin. Diagn. Lab. Immunol.* **3:**119–127.
37. Simonpoli, A. M., P. Rajogopalan-Levasseur, M. Brun-Pascaud, G. Bertrand, M. A. Pocidalo, and P. M. Girard. 1996. Influence of *Pneumocystis carinii* on nitrite production by rat alveolar macrophages. *J. Eukaryot. Microbiol.* **43:**400–403.
38. Soulez, B., F. Palluault, J. Y. Cesbron, E. Dei-Cas, A. Capron, and D. Camus. 1991. Introduction of *Pneumocystis carinii* in a colony of SCID mice. *J. Protozool.* **38:**123S–125S.
39. Stringer, J. R. 1993. The identity of *Pneumocystis carinii*: not a single protozoan, but a diverse group of exotic fungi. *Infect. Agents Dis.* **2:**109–117.
40. Sukura, A., T. Soveri, and L. A. Lindberg. 1991. Superiority of methylprednisolone over dexamethasone for induction of *Pneumocystis carinii* infection in rats. *J. Clin. Microbiol.* **29:**2331–2332.
41. Weinberg, G. A., and P. J. Durant. 1994. Genetic diversity of *Pneumocystis carinii* derived from infected rats, mice, ferrets, and cell cultures. *J. Eukaryot. Microbiol.* **41:**223–228.
42. Weisbroth, S. H., J. Geistfeld, S. P. Weisbroth, B. Williams, S. H. Feldman, M. J. Linke, S. Orr, and M. T. Cushion. 1999. Latent *Pneumocystis carinii* infection in commercial rat colonies: comparisons of inductive immunosuppressants plus histopathology, PCR, and serology as detection methods. *J. Clin. Microbiol.* **37:**1441–1446.
43. Williams, M. D., J. R. Wright, K. L. March, and W. J. Martin, II. 1996. Human surfactant protein A enhances attachment of *Pneumocystis carinii* to rat alveolar macrophages. *Am. J. Respir. Cell. Mol. Biol.* **14:**232–238.
44. Wright, T. W., C. J. Johnston, A. G. Harmsen, and J. N. Finkelstein. 1997. Analysis of cytokine mRNA profiles in the lungs of *Pneumocystis carinii*-infected mice. *Am. J. Respir. Cell. Mol. Biol.* **17:**491-500.
45. Yoneda, K., and P. D. Walzer. 1981. Mechanism of pulmonary alveolar injury in experimental *Pneumocystis carinii* pneumonia in the rat. *Br. J. Exp. Pathol.* **62:**339–346.

PARASITES

Acariasis (mite infestation)
1. Chung, S. L., S. J. Hwang, S. B. Kwon, D. W. Kim, J. B. Jun, and B. K. Cho. 1998. Outbreak of rat mite dermatitis in medical students. *Int. J. Dermatol.* **37:**591–594.
2. Iijima, O. T., H. Takeda, Y. Komatsu, T. Matsumiya, and H. Takahashi. 2000. Atopic dermatitis in NC/Jic mice associated with *Myobia musculi* infestation. *Comp. Med.* **50:**225–228.
3. Jungmann, P., A. Freitas, A. Bandeira, A. Nobrega, A. Coutinho, M. A. Marcos, and P. Minoprio. 1996a. Murine acariasis. II. Immunological dysfunction and evidence for chronic activation of Th-2 lymphocytes. *Scand. J. Immunol.* **43:**604–612.
4. Jungmann, P., J. L. Guenet, P. A. Cazenave, A. Coutinho, and M. Huerre. 1996b. Murine acariasis: I. Pathological and clinical evidence suggesting cutaneous allergy and wasting syndrome in BALB/c mouse. *Res. Immunol.* **147:**27–38.
5. Morita, E., S. Kaneko, T. Hiragun, T. Shindo, H. Shindo, T. Tanaka, T. Furukawa, A. Nobukiyo, and S. Yamamoto. 1999. Fur mites induce dermatitis associated with IgE hyperproduction in an inbred strain of mice, NC/Kuj. *J. Dermatol.* **19:**37–43.
6. National Research Council. 1991. *Infectious Diseases of Mice and Rats: a Report of the Institute of Laboratory Animal Resources Committee on Infectious Diseases of Mice and Rats.* National Academy Press, Washington, D.C.
7. Skopets, S., R. P. Wilson, J. W. Griffith, and C. M. Lang. 1996. Ivermectin toxicity in young mice. *Lab. Anim. Sci.* **46:**111–112.
8. Vachon, P., and L. Aubry. 1996. The use of ivermectin for the treatment of mites, *Myobia musculi* and *Myocoptes musculinus* in a colony of transgenic mice. *Can. Vet. J.* **37:**231–232.

Encephalitozoon cuniculi
1. Braunfuchsova, P., J. Kopecky, O. Ditrich, and B. Koudela. 1999. Cytokine response to infection with the microsporidian, *Encephalitozoon cuniculi*. *Folia Parasitol.* **46:**91–95.
2. Braunfuchsova, P., J. Salat, and J. Kopecky. 2002. Comparison of the significance of $CD4^+$ and $CD8^+$ T lymphocytes in the protection of mice against *Encephalitozoon cuniculi* infection. *J. Parasitol.* **88:**797–799.
3. Didier, E. S. 1995. Reactive nitrogen intermediates implicated in the inhibition of *Encephalitozoon cuniculi* (phylum microspora) replication in murine peritoneal macrophages. *Parasite Immunol.* **17:**405–412.

4. Didier, E. S., P. S. Varner, P. J. Didier, A. M. Aldras, N. J. Millichamp, M. Murphey-Corb, R. Bohm, and J. A. Shadduck. 1994. Experimental microsporidiosis in immunocompetent and immunodeficient mice and monkeys. *Folia Parasitol.* **41:**1–11.
5. Didier, E. S., C. R. Vossbrinck, M. D. Baker, L. B. Rogers, D. C. Bertucci, and J. A. Shadduck. 1995. Identification and characterization of three *Encephalitozoon cuniculi* strains. *Parasitology* **111:**411–421.
6. Enriquez, F. J., O. Ditrich, J. D. Palting, and K. Smith. 1997. Simple diagnosis of *Encephalitozoon* sp. microsporidial infections by using a pan-specific antiexospore monoclonal antibody. *J. Clin. Microbiol.* **35:**724–729.
7. Moretto, M., L. Casciotti, B. Durell, and I. A. Khan. 2000. Lack of CD4$^+$ T cells does not affect induction of CD8$^+$ T-cell immunity against *Encephalitozoon cuniculi* infection. *Infect. Immun.* **68:**6223–6232.
8. National Research Council. 1991. *Infectious Diseases of Mice and Rats: a Report of the Institute of Laboratory Animal Resources Committee on Infectious Diseases of Mice and Rats.* National Academy Press, Washington, D.C.
9. Snowden, K. F., E. S. Didier, J. M. Orenstein, and J. A. Shadduck. 1998. Animal models of human microsporidial infections. *Lab. Anim. Sci.* **48:**589–592.

Giardia muris

1. Belosevic, M., G. M. Faubert, and J. D. MacLean. 1985. Suppression of primary antibody response to sheep erythrocytes in susceptible and resistant mice infected with *Giardia muris*. *Infect. Immun.* **47:**21–25.
2. Boorman, G. A., P. H. C. Lina, C. Zurcher, and H. T. M. Nieuwerkerk. 1973. *Hexamita* and *Giardia* as a cause of mortality in congenitally thymus-less (nude) mice. *Clin. Exp. Immunol.* **15:**623–627.
3. Daniels, C. W., and M. Belosevic. 1995. Comparison of the course of infection with *Giardia muris* in male and female mice. *Int. J. Parasitol.* **25:**131–135.
4. Daniels, C. W., and M. Belosevic. 1995. Disaccharidase activity in male and female C57BL/6 mice infected with *Giardia muris*. *Parasitol. Res.* **81:**143–147.
5. Djamiatun, K., and G. M. Faubert. 1998. Exogenous cytokines released by spleen and Peyer's patch cells removed from mice infected with *Giardia muris*. *Parasite Immunol.* **20:**27–36.
6. Heyworth, M. F. 1992. Relative susceptibility of *Giardia muris* trophozoites to killing by mouse antibodies of different isotypes. *J. Parasitol.* **78:**73–76.
7. Kunstýr, I., U. Schoeneberg, and K. T. Friedhoff. 1992. Host specificity of *Giardia muris* isolates from mouse and golden hamster. *Parasitol. Res.* **78:**621–622.
8. Langford, T. D., M. P. Housley, M. Boes, J. Chen, M. F. Kagnoff, F. D. Gillin, and L. Eckmann. 2002. Central importance of immunoglobulin A in host defense against *Giardia* spp. *Infect. Immun.* **70:**11–18.
9. Ljungstrom, I., J. Holmgren, A.-M. Svennerholm, and A. Ferrante. 1985. Changes in intestinal fluid and mucosal immune responses to cholera toxin in *Giardia muris* infection and binding of cholera toxin to *Giardia muris* trophozoites. *Infect. Immun.* **50:**243–249.
10. National Research Council. 1991. *Infectious Diseases of Mice and Rats: a Report of the Institute of Laboratory Animal Resources Committee on Infectious Diseases of Mice and Rats.* National Academy Press, Washington, D.C.
11. Petro, T. M., R. R. Watson, D. E. Feely, and H. Darban. 1992. Suppression of resistance to *Giardia muris* and cytokine production in a murine model of acquired immune deficiency syndrome. *Reg. Immunol.* **4:**409–414.
12. Roberts-Thomson, I. C., and R. F. Anders. 1984. Cellular and humoral immunity in giardiasis, p. 185-200. *In* S. L. Erlandsen and E. A. Meyer (ed.), *Giardia and Giardiasis*. Plenum Press, New York, N.Y.
13. Romia, S. A., A. A. Abu-Zakham, H. M. al-Naggar, R. A. Atia, and A. F. Abu-Shady. 1990. The course of *Giardia muris* infection in immunocompetent and immunocompromised mice. *J. Egypt. Soc. Parasitol.* **20:**721–728.
14. Scott, K. G., M. R. Logan, G. M. Klammer, D. A. Teoh, and A. G. Buret. 2000. Jejunal brush border microvillous alterations in *Giardia muris*-infected mice: role of T lymphocytes and interleukin-6. *Infect. Immun.* **68:**3412–3418.
15. Scott, K. G., J. B. Middings, D. R. Kirk, S. P. Lees-Miller, and A. G. Buret. 2002. Intestinal infection with *Giardia* spp. reduces epithelial barrier function in a myosin light chain kinase-dependent fashion. *Gastroenterology* **123:**1179–1190.
16. Singer, S. M., and T. E. Nash. 2000. T-cell-dependent control of acute *Giardia lamblia* infections in mice. *Infect. Immun.* **68:**170–175.
17. Skea, D. L., and B. J. Underdown. 1991. Acquired resistance to *Giardia muris* in X-linked immunodeficient mice. *Infect. Immun.* **59:**1733–1738.

18. **Stachan, R., and I. Kunstýř.** 1983. Minimal infectious doses and prepatent periods in *Giardia muris, Spironucleus muris,* and *Tritrichomonas muris. Zentbl. Bakteriol. Mikrobiol. Hyg. A* **256:**249–256.
19. **Venkatesan, P., R. G. Finch, and D. Wakelin.** 1993. MHC haplotype influences primary *Giardia muris* infections in H-2 congenic strains of mice. *Int. J. Parasitol.* **23:**661–664.
20. **Venkatesan, P., R. G. Finch, and D. Wakelin.** 1996. Comparison of antibody and cytokine responses to primary *Giardia muris* infection in H-2 congenic strains of mice. *Infect. Immun.* **64:**4525–4533.
21. **Venkatesan, P., R. G. Finch, and D. Wakelin.** 1997. A comparison of mucosal inflammatory responses to *Giardia muris* in resistant B10 and susceptible BALB/c mice. *Parasite Immunol.* **19:**137–143.

Oxyurids (pinworms)
1. **Agersborg, S. S., K. M. Garza, and K. S. K. Tung.** 2001. Intestinal parasitism terminates self tolerance and enhances neonatal induction of autoimmune disease and memory. *Eur. J. Immunol.* **31:**851–859.
2. **Bahader, S. M., G. S. Ali, A. H. Shaalan, H. M. Khalil, and N. M. Khalil.** 1995. Effects of *Enterobius vermicularis* infection on intelligence quotient (I.Q.) and anthropometric measurements of Egyptian rural children. *J. Egypt. Soc. Parasitol.* **25:**183–194.
3. **Barron, S., B. J. Baseheart, T. M. Segar, T. Deveraux, and J. A. Willford.** 2000. The behavioral teratogenic potential of fenbendazole: a medication for pinworm infestation. *Neurotoxicol. Teratol.* **22:**871–877.
4. **Derothe, J. M., C. Loubes, A. Orth, F. Ranaud, and C. Moulia.** 1997. Comparison between patterns of pinworm infection (*Aspiculuris tetraptera*) in wild and laboratory strains of mice, *Mus musculus. Int. J. Parasitol.* **27:**645–651.
5. **Huerkamp, M. J., K. A. Benjamin, L. A. Zitzow, J. K. Pullium, J. A. Lloyd, W. D. Thompson, S. K. Webb, and N. D. Lehner.** 2000. Fenbendazole treatment without environmental decontamination eradicates *Syphacia muris* from rats in a large, complex research institution. *Contemp. Top. Lab. Anim. Sci.* **39:**9–12.
6. **Jacobson, R. H., and N. D. Reed.** 1974. The thymus dependency of resistance to pinworm infection in mice. *J. Parasitol.* **60:**976–979.
7. **Lubcke, R., F. A. Hutcheson, and G. O. Barbezat.** 1992. Impaired intestinal electrolyte transport in rats infested with the common parasite *Syphacia muris. Dig. Dis. Sci.* **37:**60–64.
8. **McNair, D. M., and E. H. Timmons.** 1977. Effects of *Aspiculuris tetraptera* and *Syphacia obvelata* on exploratory behavior of an inbred mouse strain. *Lab. Anim. Sci.* **27:**38–42.
9. **Mohn, G., and E. M. Philipp.** 1981. Effects of *Syphacia muris* and the anthelmintic fenbendazole on the microsomal monooxygenase system in mouse liver. *Lab. Anim.* **15:**89–95.
10. **National Research Council.** 1991. *Infectious Diseases of Mice and Rats: a Report of the Institute of Laboratory Animal Resources Committee on Infectious Diseases of Mice and Rats.* National Academy Press, Washington, D.C.
11. **Pearson, D. J., and G. Taylor.** 1975. The influence of the nematode *Syphacia obvelata* on adjuvant arthritis in rats. *Immunology* **29:**391–396.
12. **Pinto, R. M., L. Goncalves, D. Noronha, and D. C. Gomes.** 2001. Worm burdens in outbred and inbred laboratory rats with morphometric data on *Syphacia muris* (Yamaguti, 1935) Yamaguti, 1941 (Nematoda, Oxyuroidea). *Mem. Inst. Oswaldo Cruz* **96:**133–136.
13. **Pinto, R. M., J. J. Vicente, D. Noronha, L. Goncalves, and D. C. Gomes.** 1994. Helminth parasites of conventionally maintained laboratory mice. *Mem. Inst. Oswaldo Cruz.* **89:**33–40.
14. **Pritchett, K. R., and N. A. Johnston.** 2002. A review of treatments for the eradication of pinworm infections from laboratory rodent colonies. *Contemp. Top. Lab. Anim. Sci.* **41:**36–46.
15. **Sato, Y., H. K. Ooi, N. Nonaka, Y. Oku, and M. Kamiya.** 1995. Antibody production in *Syphacia obvelata* infected mice. *J. Parasitol.* **81:**559–562.
16. **Wagner, M.** 1988. The effect of infection with the pinworm (*Syphacia muris*) on rat growth. *Lab. Anim. Sci.* **38:**476–478.
17. **Webster, J. P.** 1994. The effect of *Toxoplasma gondii* and other parasites on activity levels in wild and hybrid *Rattus norvegicus. Parasitology* **109:**583–589.

Spironucleus muris
1. **Baker, D. G., S. Malineni, and H. W. Tayor.** 1998. Experimental infection of inbred mouse strains with *Spironucleus muris. Vet. Parasitol.* **77:**305–310.
2. **Boorman, G. A., P. H. C. Lina, C. Zurcher, and H. T. M. Nieuwerkerk.** 1973. *Hexamita* and *Giardia* as a cause of mortality in congenitally thymus-less (nude) mice. *Clin. Exp. Immunol.* **15:**623–627.
3. **Brett, S. J.** 1983. Immunodepression in *Giardia muris* and *Spironucleus muris* infections in mice. *Parasitology* **87:**507–515.

4. **Exon, J. H., N. M. Patton, and L. D. Koller.** 1975. Hexamitiasis in cadmium-exposed mice. *Arch. Environ. Health* **31**:463–464.
5. **Kunstýř, I., B. Meyer, and E. Ammerpohl.** 1977. Spironucleosis in nude mice: An animal model for immuno-parasitologic studies, p. 17–27. *In* Proceedings of the Second International Workshop on Nude Mice. Gustav Fischer Verlag, Stuttgart.
6. **National Research Council.** 1991. *Infectious Diseases of Mice and Rats: a Report of the Institute of Laboratory Animal Resources Committee on Infectious Diseases of Mice and Rats.* National Academy Press, Washington, D.C.
7. **Ruitenberg, E. J., and B. C. Kruyt.** 1975. Effect of intestinal flagellates on immune response in mice. *Parasitology* **71**:30.
8. **Schagemann, G., W. Bohnet, I. Kunstýř, and T. Friedhoff.** 1990. Host specificity of cloned *Spironucleus muris* in laboratory rodents. *Lab. Anim.* **24**:234–239.
9. **Stachan, R., and I. Kunstýř.** 1983. Minimal infectious doses and prepatent periods in *Giardia muris, Spironucleus muris,* and *Tritrichomonas muris. Zentbl. Bakteriol. Mikrobiol. Hyg. A* **256**:249–256.
10. **Whitehouse, A., M. P. France, S. E. Pope, J. E. Lloyd, and R. C. Ratcliffe.** 1993. *Spironucleus muris* in laboratory mice. *Aust. Vet. J.* **70**: 193.

PATHOGENS OF GERBILS

3

INTRODUCTION

The Mongolian gerbil (jird, desert rat, antelope rat, sand rat), *Meriones unguiculatus,* is the most commonly used laboratory subject of more than 100 species of rodents called "gerbil" (2). The Mongolian gerbil is used as an animal model in a variety of research areas, including studies of infectious diseases, auditory science, epilepsy, vascular science, microsomal enzyme activity, and others.

Few natural pathogens have been described for the Mongolian gerbil. Those most commonly found in laboratory colonies are discussed in this chapter. No viral pathogens are presented; however, gerbils are not resistant to infection with all viruses. In fact, the Mongolian gerbil has been experimentally infected with a variety of human and other animal viruses, including La Crosse virus (9), Borna disease virus (7), Venezuelan (11) and Western (3) equine encephalitis virus, Rift Valley fever virus (1), encephalomyocarditis virus (6), Hantavirus (12), and Reovirus 3 (13). Cell cultures established from gerbil tissues are susceptible to several DNA and RNA animal viruses (8). In addition, oxyurids (pinworms) are the only type of parasite discussed. Historically, the gerbil has been known to harbor the dwarf tapeworm, *Rodentolepis* (= *Hymenolepis*) *nana* (5), is susceptible to infection with *Hymenolepis diminuta* (4), and in one report was infected with *Demodex merioni* (10). However, these parasitisms are considered rare enough to justify their exclusion from this text. As discussed in the general introduction, modern husbandry practices have contributed to the decrease in the number of all pathogens of laboratory rodents, but especially of parasites.

BACTERIA

Clostridium piliforme

Agent
The biology of *Clostridium piliforme,* the causative agent of Tyzzer's disease, is more thoroughly discussed in chapters 2 and 4. *C. piliforme* is a gram-negative, filamentous, motile, endospore-forming, obligate intracellular bacterium.

Epidemiology
The Mongolian gerbil is highly susceptible to Tyzzer's disease. For this reason, the gerbil is an excellent sentinel for *C. piliforme* infection. Prevalence of infection remains high in many gerbil colonies. The extent to which strains isolated from gerbils are cross-infective to other rodent species is currently unknown. Protein and antigenic heterogeneity have been

demonstrated among isolates of *C. piliforme* (9), and Franklin and coworkers (3) have suggested that both cross-infective isolates and more host-specific isolates exist. This is supported by the report of Motzel and Riley (7), in which young gerbils showed no evidence of infection following exposure to bedding contaminated with two rat isolates of *C. piliforme*. Serologically, rabbit-origin *C. piliforme* has been shown to be cross-reactive with gerbil isolates (12), while others have demonstrated a lack of cross-reactivity between rat and gerbil isolates when purified *C. piliforme* flagella, rather than whole organisms, constitute the antigen preparation (1). Transmission is by ingestion of infectious endospores transferred from cage to cage by fomites, caretakers, or other vectors; or in contaminated food or bedding following inadequate sterilization of those materials.

Clinical signs

Infections in adult gerbils are often subclinical. In contrast, young gerbils, or highly stressed adults, may experience sudden death with few premonitory signs. When present, clinical signs may include watery diarrhea, rough hair coat, listlessness, and anorexia (2). Disease severity peaks within a week of infection (11).

Pathology

It is likely that pathologic changes in gerbils infected with *C. piliforme* involve the same three main phases as demonstrated in other animal species (13). These include the establishment of infection in the ileum and cecum, the ascension of the pathogen to the liver via the portal circulation, and hematogenous spread to other tissues, including the myocardium (8, 11). Gross changes usually, although not always (6), involve the liver (2) and consist of an enlarged and friable, yellow liver with multiple whitish spots throughout. A proteinaceous exudate may be found in the abdominal cavity (5). Histologic lesions include multifocal, necrotizing ileotyphlocolitis, hepatitis (6, 13), myocarditis (11), and occasionally, encephalitis (10). Lesions resolve following acute onset of disease (11).

Interference with research

Specific reports of *C. piliforme* altering research findings are not available. On the basis of clinical and pathologic effects noted in both natural and experimental infections of gerbils and other mammals, natural infections of gerbils are likely to severely alter the findings of studies involving the enterohepatic and cardiovascular systems, and less commonly, the central nervous system.

Diagnosis and control

Historically, diagnosis of *C. piliforme* infection was by serologic testing such as indirect fluorescent antibody assay, or by staining of tissue sections with Gram, periodic acid-Schiff (PAS), or silver stains. With either approach, diagnosis was difficult. Successful identification of infected animals was more likely when *C. piliforme*-free weanlings were used as sentinel animals for a suspect colony. Histologically, filamentous, intracellular organisms may be found at the periphery of lesions. More recently, PCR assay has become the diagnostic method of choice (4). Prevention includes testing of new animals prior to introduction into the colony. Control includes stress reduction and strict adherence to sanitation protocols. In addition, the author has found that positioning contaminated cages in front of an isolator set on negative pressure, thereby drawing air over the contaminated cages, with HEPA filtration in the exhaust port, considerably reduces the incidence of clinical disease in a known *C. piliforme*-positive colony, presumably by reducing the numbers of bacteria circulating within the room. Treatment is often difficult because of the acuteness of the disease and the intracellular nature of the pathogen (5). Tetracyclines may be useful for suppressing pathogen numbers. For a complete discussion of specific therapeutic control measures against *C. piliforme*, see Harkness and Wagner (5).

Staphylococcus aureus

Agent

The biology of *Staphylococcus aureus* is discussed more completely under pathogens of rats and mice. The interested reader is referred to chapters 2 and 6 for more information. In brief, *S. aureus* is a gram-positive, coagulase-positive coccus.

Epidemiology
S. aureus commonly inhabits the skin, upper respiratory tract, and lower digestive tract of many animals, including gerbils, in which it occasionally causes disease. The bacterium is ubiquitous. Transmission is primarily direct through physical contact. However, fomites may also vector the pathogen. While this means of spread is more relevant for immune-deficient mice, it may also on occasion play a role in exposure of gerbils to high numbers of bacteria.

Clinical signs
The most common clinical presentation of *S. aureus* infection in gerbils is "sore nose," or staphylococcal nasal dermatitis. Entry into the body is through breaks in normal barriers. These may result from a variety of causes. For example, nasal dermatitis may occur following behavioral changes, such as increased and excessive burrowing activity (3) and physiologic changes in the host, such as stress and immune suppression. Stress appears to be a common and particularly important facilitator of clinical disease in gerbils, likely due to stress-associated increases in porphyrin secretion from the harderian glands located behind the eyes. Porphyrin secretions are irritating, and may facilitate establishment of dermatitis (3). Porphyrin accumulations may also build up on the medial aspects of the forepaws during facial grooming, resulting in forepaw lesions. Other signs may include periocular alopecia and protrusion of the nictitating membrane (1).

Pathology
Histopathologic changes associated with staphylococcal dermatitis include acanthosis, hyperkeratosis, and inflammation. Staphylococcal lesions may also occur at other sites on the skin, secondary to bite wounds and other sources of trauma. Such conditions are much less common in gerbils than in many other rodents, likely due to the more sociable nature of gerbils. In addition to dermatitis, gerbils may potentially develop internal staphylococcal abscesses following surgical contamination.

Interference with research
The reader is referred to chapter 2 for a complete discussion of the potential physiologic effects of internal infection. To the author's knowledge, no reports exist on these conditions in gerbils, but it is not unreasonable to assume that gerbils would be similarly affected. While clinical infection of gerbils could compromise a variety of studies, depending on site of infection, clinical disease generally indicates a high level of stress within the colony. Physiologic changes associated with stress may greatly interfere with research findings in gerbils (2, 4, 5, 6) and other animals (7).

Diagnosis and control
Diagnosis of *S. aureus* infection is easily accomplished by culture and Gram staining. Colonization of conventionally housed gerbils is unavoidable. Prevention of clinical disease primarily depends on stress reduction. Local treatment with antibiotics and/or disinfectants is generally not necessary if the source of stress is identified and eliminated. For example, the author has found that single housing gerbils used to having one or more cage mates is sufficient stress to induce sore nose. Returning single-housed gerbils to a group or companion housing arrangement usually results in elimination of the dermatitis.

PARASITES

Oxyurids (pinworms)

Agent
The most common pinworm infecting laboratory gerbils is *Dentostomella translucida*. In addition, young gerbils may also become infected with *Syphacia muris* and *Syphacia obvelata,* although adult animals tend to rid themselves of infections with *Syphacia* spp. (2).

TABLE 3-1. Body systems known or likely to be affected by pathogen indicated

Pathogen	Cardio-vascular	Dermal	Endocrine	Entero-hepatic	Hema-topoietic	Lympho-reticular	Musculo-skeletal	Nervous	Reproductive	Respiratory	Urinary
Clostridium piliforme	X			X				X			
Staphylococcus aureus		X									
Oxyurids (pinworms)				X		X					

Epidemiology

The life cycles of pinworms infecting gerbils are direct and similar, with minor differences between them. *D. translucida* occurs in the anterior third of the small intestine, eggs are passed in the feces approximately 24 days postinfection (8), and become infective to the next host in as little as 5 days under experimental conditions (7). *S. muris* and *S. obvelata* inhabit the large intestine. Eggs are cemented to the perianal region, where they embryonate and drop off into the bedding, to await ingestion by another host. Pinworm eggs easily aerosolize, resulting in widespread environmental contamination. In general, embryonated pinworm eggs are thought to survive for extended periods at room temperature, although studies defining maximum survival times of *D. translucida* and *Syphacia* spp., under different conditions, have not been conducted.

Clinical signs

In most cases, pinworm infections result in no clinical signs, even in heavy infections.

Pathology

Infection with *D. translucida* may cause local accumulation of eosinophils and plasma cells, resulting in some thickening of the lamina propria in the villus tips (7).

Interference with research

While in other rodents, infection with *Syphacia* spp. has been shown to affect immune responses (1, 5, 6) and impair intestinal electrolyte transport (4), no similar findings have been demonstrated in gerbils infected with any pinworm species. However, studies supporting a definitive statement that there are no physiologic effects associated with oxyuriasis in gerbils have not been conducted. Specific research goals, especially those involving the enterohepatic or the lymphoreticular systems, may justify eradication of pinworms from the colony.

Diagnosis and control

Diagnosis is by examination of fecal flotations (*D. translucida*) or perianal tape preparations (*Syphacia* spp.). In most cases, pinworms may be eradicated using Fenbendazole-medicated chow (3). Careful attention to fomite or vector spread is necessary to prevent the spread or reintroduction of infection.

REFERENCES

INTRODUCTION

1. **Anderson, G. W., Jr., T. W. Slone, Jr., and C. J. Peters.** 1988. The gerbil *Meriones unguiculatus*, a model for Rift Valley fever viral encephalitis. *Arch. Virol.* **102:**187–196.
2. **Clark, J. D.** 1984. Biology and Diseases of Other Rodents, p. 183–206. *In* J. G. Fox, B. J. Cohen, and F. M. Loew (ed.), *Laboratory Animal Medicine.* Academic Press, Inc., New York, N.Y.
3. **Hayles, L. B.** 1972. Susceptibility of the Mongolian gerbil (*Meriones unguiculatus*) to Western equine encephalitis. *Can. J. Microbiol.* **18:**941–944.
4. **Johnson, S. S., and G. A. Conder.** 1996. Infectivity of *Hymenolepis diminuta* for the jird, *Meriones unguiculatus*, and utility of this model for anthelmintic studies. *J. Parasitol.* **82:**492–495.
5. **Lussier, G., and F. M. Loew.** 1970. Case report. Natural *Hymenolepis nana* infection in Mongolain gerbils (*Meriones unguiculatus*). *Can. Vet. J.* **11:**105–107.
6. **Matsuzaki, H., K. Doi, C. Doi, T. Onodera, and T. Mitsuoka.** 1989. Susceptibility of four species of small rodents to encephalomyocarditis (EMC) virus infection. *Jikken Dobutsu* **38:**357–361.
7. **Nakamura, Y., T. Nakaya, K. Hagiwara, N. Momiyama, Y. Kagawa, H. Taniyama, C. Ishihara, T. Sata, T. Kurata, and K. Ikuta.** 1999. High susceptibility of Mongolian gerbil (*Meriones unguiculatus*) to Borna disease virus. *Vaccine* **17:**480–489.
8. **Nawa, M.** 1983. A continuous cell line, GK, derived from the kidney tissue of Mongolian gerbil (*Meriones unguiculatus*) and its virological application. *Jpn. J. Med. Sci. Biol.* **36:**215–218.
9. **Osorio, J. E., and T. M. Yuill.** 1996. La Crosse viremias in Mongolian gerbils (*Meriones unguiculatus*). *Am. J. Trop. Med. Hyg.* **55:**567–569.
10. **Schwarzbrott, S. S., J. E. Wagner, and C. S. Frisk.** 1974. Demodecosis in the Mongolian gerbil (*Meriones unguiculatus*): a case report. *Lab. Anim. Sci.* **24:**666–668.
11. **Vaughan, J. A., M. Trpis, and M. J. Turrell.** 1999. *Brugia malayi* microfilariae (Nematoda: Filaridae) enhance the infectivity of Venezuelan equine encephalitis virus to *Aedes* mosquitoes (Diptera: Culicidae). *J. Med. Entomol.* **36:**758–763.
12. **Xu, X., S. L. Ruo, J. B. McCormick, and S. P. Fisher-Hoch.** 1992. Immunity to Hantavirus challenge in *Meriones unguiculatus* induced by vaccinia-vectored viral proteins. *Am. J. Trop. Med. Hyg.* **47:**397–404.
13. **Yukawa, M., T. Takeuchi, K. Mochizuki, Y. Inaba, H. Kamata, and T. Onodera.** 1993. Infection of reovirus type 3 in Mongolian gerbils (*Meriones unguiculatus*)-lesions in pancreas and brain. *J. Basic Microbiol.* **33:**147–152.

BACTERIA

Clostridium piliforme

1. **Boivin, G. P., R. R. Hook, Jr., and L. K. Riley.** 1994. Development of a monoclonal antibody-based competitive inhibition enzyme-linked immunosorbent assay for detection of *Bacillus piliformis* isolate-specific antibodies in laboratory animals. *Lab. Anim. Sci.* **44:**153–158.
2. **Clark, J. D.** 1984. Biology and diseases of other rodents, p. 183–206. *In* J. G. Fox, B. J. Cohen, and F. M. Loew (ed.), *Laboratory Animal Medicine.* Academic Press, Inc., New York, N.Y.
3. **Franklin, C. L., S. L. Motzel, C. L. Besch-Williford, R. R. Hook, Jr., and L. K. Riley.** 1994. Tyzzer's infection: host specificity of *Clostridium piliforme* isolates. *Lab. Anim. Sci.* **44:**568–572.
4. **Goto, K., and T. Itoh.** 1996. Detection of *Clostridium piliforme* by enzymatic assay of amplified cDNA in microtitration plates. *Lab. Anim. Sci.* **46:**493–496.
5. **Harkness, J. E., and J. E. Wagner.** 1995. *The Biology and Medicine of Rabbits and Rodents,* 4th ed. Williams & Wilkins, Media, Pa.
6. **Motzel, S. L., and S. V. Gibson.** 1990. Tyzzer disease in hamsters and gerbils from a pet store supplier. *J. Am. Vet. Med. Assoc.* **197:**1176–1178.
7. **Motzel, S. L., and L. K. Riley.** 1992. Subclinical infection and transmission of Tyzzer's disease in rats. *Lab. Anim. Sci.* **42:**439–443.
8. **National Research Council.** 1991. *Infectious Diseases of Mice and Rats: a Report of the Institute of Laboratory Animal Resources Committee on Infectious Diseases of Mice and Rats.* National Academy Press, Washington, D.C.
9. **Riley, L. K., C. Besch-Williford, and K. S. Waggie.** 1990. Protein and antigenic heterogeneity among isolates of *Bacillus piliformis. Infect. Immun.* **58:**1010–1016.

10. **Veazey, R. S., II, D. B. Paulsen, and D. O. Schaeffer.** 1992. Encephalitis in gerbils due to naturally occurring infection with *Bacillus piliformis* (Tyzzer's disease). *Lab. Anim. Sci.* **42:**516–518.
11. **Waggie, K. S., J. R. Ganaway, J. E. Wagner, and T. S. Spencer.** 1984. Experimentally induced Tyzzer's disease in Mongolian gerbils (*Meriones unguiculatus*). *Lab. Anim. Sci.* **34:**53–57.
12. **Waggie, K. S., T. S. Spencer, and J. R. Ganaway.** 1987. An enzyme-linked immunosorbent assay for detection of anti-*Bacillus piliformis* serum antibodies in rabbits. *Lab. Anim. Sci.* **37:**176–179.
13. **Yokomori, K., N. Okada, Y. Murai, N. Goto, and K. Fujiwara.** 1989. Enterohepatitis in Mongolian gerbils (*Meriones unguiculatus*) inoculated perorally with Tyzzer's organism (*Bacillus piliformis*). *Lab. Anim. Sci.* **39:**16–20.

Staphylococcus aureus
1. **Bresnahan, J. F., G. D. Smith, R. H. Lentsch, W. G. Barnes, and J. E. Wagner.** 1983. Nasal dermatitis in the Mongolian gerbil. *Lab. Anim. Sci.* **33:**258–263.
2. **Fenske, M.** 1986. Adrenal function in the Mongolian gerbil (*Meriones unguiculatus*): influence of confinement stress upon glucocorticosteroid, progesterone, dehydroepiandrosterone, testosterone, and androstenedione plasma levels, adrenal content and in-vitro secretion. *Exp. Clin. Endocrinol.* **87:**15–25.
3. **Harkness, J. E., and J. E. Wagner.** 1995. *The Biology and Medicine of Rabbits and Rodents*, 4th ed. Williams & Wilkins, Media, Pa.
4. **Heinzeller, T., B. N. Joshi, F. Nurnberger, and R. J. Reiter.** 1988. Effects of aggressive encounters on pineal melatonin formation in male gerbils (*Meriones unguiculatus*, Cricetidae). *J. Comp. Physiol.* **164:**91–94.
5. **Hull, E. M., E. Chapin, and C. Kastaniotis.** 1974. Effects of crowding and intermittent isolation on gerbils (*Meriones unguiculatus*). *Physiol. Behav.* **13:**723–727.
6. **Nagata, E., Y. Fukuuchi, K. Tanaka, S. Gomi, S. Takashima, B. Mihara, T. Shirai, S. Nogawa, and H. Nozaki.** 1993. Immobilization stress induces alterations of second-messenger systems in the gerbil brain. *Neurosci. Res.* **17:**31–38.
7. **Strange, K. S., L. R. Kerr, H. N. Andrews, J. T. Emerman, and J. Weinberg.** 2000. Psychosocial stressors and mammary tumor growth: an animal model. *Neurotoxicol. Teratol.* **22:**89–102.

PARASITES
Oxyurids (Pinworms)
1. **Agersborg, S. S., K. M. Garza, and K. S. K. Tung.** 2001. Intestinal parasitism terminates self tolerance and enhances neonatal induction of autoimmune disease and memory. *Eur. J. Immunol.* **31:**851–859.
2. **Clark, J. D.** 1984. Biology and diseases of other rodents, p. 183–206. *In* J. G. Fox, B. J. Cohen, and F. M. Loew (ed.), *Laboratory Animal Medicine*. Academic Press, Inc., New York, N.Y.
3. **Coghlan, L. G., D. R. Lee, B. Psencik, and D. Weiss.** 1993. Practical and effective eradication of pinworms (*Syphacia muris*) in rats by use of fenbendazole. *Lab. Anim. Sci.* **43:**481–487.
4. **Lubcke, R., F. A. Hutcheson, and G. O. Barbezat.** 1992. Impaired intestinal electrolyte transport in rats infested with the common parasite *Syphacia muris*. *Dig. Dis. Sci.* **37:**60–64.
5. **Pearson, D. J., and G. Taylor.** 1975. The influence of the nematode *Syphacia obvelata* on adjuvant arthritis in rats. *Immunolgy* **29:**391–396.
6. **Sato, Y., H. K. Ooi, N. Nonaka, Y. Oku, and M. Kamiya.** 1995. Antibody production in *Syphacia obvelata* infected mice. *J. Parasitol.* **81:**559–562.
7. **Smith, G. D., and T. G. Snider III.** 1988. Experimental infection and treatment of *Dentostomella translucida* in the Mongolian gerbil. *Lab. Animal. Sci.* **38:**339–340.
8. **Wightman, S. R., P. A. Pilitt, and J. E. Wagner.** 1978. *Dentostomella translucida* in the Mongolian gerbil (*Meriones unguiculatus*). *Lab. Anim. Sci.* **28:**290–296.

PATHOGENS OF HAMSTERS

4

INTRODUCTION

Hamsters are used in several areas of biomedical research, including infectious diseases, endocrinology, nutrition, reproduction, behavior, ophthalmology, olfaction, and others. At least eight species of hamster have served as research subjects. These include the Golden or Syrian hamster (*Mesocricetus auratus*), the Striped or Chinese hamster (*Cricetulus griseus*), the European hamster (*Cricetus cricetus*), the Dzungarian hamster (*Phodopus sungorus*), the South African hamster (*Mystromys albicaudatus*), the Turkish hamster (*Mesocricetus brandti*), the Rumanian hamster (*Mesocricetus newtoni*), and the Armenian hamster (*Cricetulus migratorius*) (1, 2, 3, 4). The Syrian hamster is the most widely used hamster in biomedical research, although Chinese hamster cells are also widely used for in vitro research. Therefore, more is known of the pathogens of the Syrian hamster than of the pathogens of other hamster species. Unless otherwise stated, all information presented will apply to the Syrian hamster. Important distinctions occur between the Syrian hamster and other hamster species. Those distinctions will be included where known. The interested reader is referred to the excellent text edited by Van Hoosier and McPherson (5) covering in detail the biology, diseases, care, and use of all major species of laboratory hamsters.

Compared with mice and rats, hamsters are relatively minor laboratory animal species. Therefore, as for most other minor species, little is known of the effects of natural pathogens of hamsters on research. Some information comes from pathogenicity and immunologic studies involving experimentally induced infections. These are, by design, somewhat limited in their scope of investigation. Greater dependence on information from experimental infections may not present the entire range of effects a pathogen may have during natural infection. The reader is therefore advised to consider the pathogenesis of the infection when deciding what influences the agent may have on one's research. A second source of information concerning potential effects of hamster pathogens on their hosts comes from reports of these agents infecting mice and/or rats. While the pathogenicity is probably very similar if not identical in most cases, caution should be exercised when extrapolating findings from these studies to the hamster.

VIRUSES

Lymphocytic choriomeningitis virus

Agent

Lymphocytic choriomeningitis virus (LCMV) is a noncytopathic single-stranded RNA (ssRNA) virus of the family *Arenaviridae*, genus *Arenavirus*. Multiple strains exist (12). Several animal species are susceptible to infection with LCMV.

Epidemiology

Within hamster colonies, prevalence of infection with LCMV has historically been low and is likely declining further (7, 14). Human outbreaks have been associated with hamsters purchased as pets (6, 13), suggesting that some commercial vendors of laboratory hamsters are potential sources of infection for laboratory workers. In addition, laboratory personnel may be at risk when working with hamsters receiving untested, contaminated, transplanted tumors (5, 8) or cell lines (18). Human infection generally results in "flu-like" symptoms, although viral meningitis or encephalomyelitis may also occur (19). LCMV does not appear to be highly contagious within hamster colonies. Transmission is primarily through contact with infectious urine or saliva (16) and so would be limited to cagemates or possibly other hamsters in the same room, so long as proper sanitary practices are followed by animal caretakers moving between rooms. Transmission may also be congenital with enzootic infection (10).

Clinical signs

Most infections in hamsters are subclinical, but severity of disease is influenced by host and viral strains, level of host immune competence, age of host at infection, as well as dose and route of inoculation (1, 3, 4). The patterns of disease presented for mouse infections are similarly observed in experimentally infected hamsters, and the interested reader is referred to that discussion. Some experimentally inoculated or congenitally infected hamsters clear the infection quickly, with immune response indicated by widespread lymphoid hyperplasia and/or perivascular infiltration, but with no lasting evidence of infection, while others develop progressive wasting disease characterized clinically by lethargy, weight loss, and diarrhea.

Pathology

Following infection and development of clinical disease, one observes a range of histologic changes, variably including chronic glomerulonephritis, ileitis, vasculitis, and lymphoid hyperplasia and/or infiltration; and with persistent viremia and virus shedding (1, 3, 9, 10). Viral distribution is nearly pantropic, and is especially localized in organs of the reticuloendothelial system (1). Therefore, mild inflammatory lesions may be found, in some cases, in nearly any organ (1).

For hamsters that respond to infection, immunity to LCMV infection is primarily cell mediated by $CD8^+$ T cells, although anti-LCMV antibodies also form and account for the antigen–antibody complexes sometimes found in arterioles and the renal glomerular basement membrane (2, 11, 15). Numbers of LCMV-specific memory T cells may be greatly reduced by concurrent or subsequent infection with other viruses. Likewise, LCMV infection may decrease numbers of memory T cells specific for other viruses (15), suggesting that LCMV infection could dramatically alter results of immunologic studies. Other components of immunity are presumed to be as described for mouse infections, although these have yet to be demonstrated in hamsters.

Interference with research

While specific reports are lacking, natural infection of hamsters with LCMV may confound a wide range of research studies, certainly including those of the cardiovascular, enterohepatic, lymphoreticular, and urinary systems. On the basis of results of murine infections, it is likely that LCMV could also interfere with studies involving the hematopoietic and nervous systems of hamsters, although this remains to be demonstrated. Lastly, natural infection of laboratory hamsters represents a serious risk to human health.

Diagnosis and control
Routine diagnosis of LCMV infection has traditionally involved serologic methods (17), although PCR assays are certainly feasible and are likely more sensitive. There is no effective treatment for LCMV infection in the hamster. Elimination of LCMV infection requires depopulation of the hamster colony, emphasizing the importance of preimportation testing, especially of hamster-derived tumors and cell lines.

Pneumonia virus of mice

Agent
Pneumonia virus of mice (PVM), an ssRNA virus, is one of the two member of the genus *Pneumovirus*, of the family *Paramyxoviridae*. The genus also includes respiratory syncytial virus (RSV), to which hamsters are also experimentally susceptible (6). These viruses differ from Morbilliviruses and Paramyxoviruses, other members of the family, in lacking neuraminidase, and in having a smaller nucleocapsid (8).

Epidemiology
Prevalence of PVM in hamster colonies appears to be low (1, 3). Transmission is by aerosol and contact exposure (2). The virus is thought to be unstable outside of the host (4), and therefore to be of low contagiousness.

Clinical signs
Clinical signs have not been reported in naturally seropositive hamsters.

Pathology
Like clinical signs, gross and histopathologic pulmonary changes have only been reported following experimental infection, and have consisted principally of interstitial pneumonia (5).

Interference with research
No effects of PVM on research have been reported. The reader is referred to the section on PVM infections in mice and rats for a general discussion of the physiologic effects of PVM in those species. It is possible that similar effects occur in hamsters. Therefore, natural infection of laboratory hamsters could affect studies involving the respiratory system.

Diagnosis and control
Diagnosis of PVM infection is by serology. The indirect fluorescent antibody test has been found particularly sensitive (3). Alternatively, PVM may be isolated following inoculation of BHK-21 cells, or others (4). Lastly, diagnosis should be possible by reverse transcription PCR, as described for bovine RSV infection (7). There is no effective treatment for PVM infection. Therefore, exclusion of the pathogen from the animal facility is very important. Exclusion efforts should begin with mouse importations, since laboratory mice represent a significant source of infection.

Sendai virus

Agent
Sendai virus (SV) is an ssRNA virus, and is a member of the family *Paramyxoviridae*, genus *Paramyxovirus* and species *parainfluenza 1*.

Epidemiology
Mice, rats, and hamsters are the only known reservoir hosts of SV. The virus is extremely contagious, and transmission is by contact and aerosol infection of the respiratory tract. Fortunately, there is no carrier state. Virus isolation from naturally infected hamsters is extremely rare. Seroprevalence of the exposure has been documented historically in a number of serologic surveys (9), although seroprevalence rates in hamsters have declined (8).

Clinical signs
Clinical signs have been observed in naturally and enzootically infected neonatal hamsters, and consisted chiefly of sudden death (12). Mortality in young hamsters may be related to increased susceptibility of neonatal respiratory epithelium to infection and cytopathic effects (13).

Pathology
Gross and histopathologic findings are similar to those described in susceptible mouse strains, and consist of focal interstitial pneumonia (12). Nonfatal cases may develop rhinitis, tracheitis, focal pulmonary consolidation, bronchitis, bronchioalveolitis, edema, and epithelial desquamation with basement membrane destruction and inflammation (2, 7, 10). Most lesions resolve within 12 days of infection (10). Likewise, SV can be recovered from the lungs of experimentally infected hamsters for only a few days (10). Others have reported hydrocephalus secondary to necrosis and fusion of ependymal cells lining the aqueduct of Sylvius in newborn hamsters experimentally infected with SV (3). Humoral immunity is detectable within 6 to 7 days of infection (10, 11), and is thought to control infection while promoting inflammatory lesions (2, 7). Cellular immunity is likely also involved, since cytotoxic T cells can be demonstrated against SV glycoproteins (1).

Interference with research
Sendai virus alters host physiology in many ways. Besides profoundly altering hamster pulmonary cytoarchitecture, SV may alter renal potassium flux (4) and accelerate apoptosis (6). The interested reader is referred to the discussion of SV in chapter 2, for a description of additional biological features of SV, which may impact research using hamsters. It is likely that even clinically unapparent, enzootic infection of hamsters would confound research involving the immune and/or respiratory systems.

Diagnosis and control
Diagnosis of SV infection is by serologic methods. Inactivated (5) and temperature-sensitive mutant vaccines (14) have been developed and advocated for the protection of newborn hamsters. However, it is doubtful that such efforts are practical, considering there is no carrier state. Purposeful exposure of all susceptible animals at risk and cessation of breeding within the colony should result in eventual elimination of the pathogen. Prevention of introduction of SV into the animal colony depends on strict adherence to preimportation serologic surveillance of hamsters, mice, and rats.

BACTERIA
Clostridium piliforme

Agent
Clostridium piliforme, formerly *Bacillus piliformis*, is the causative agent of Tyzzer's disease. *C. piliforme* is a gram-negative, filamentous, endospore-forming, obligate intracellular bacterium. Multiple strains of *C. piliforme* exist, and can be grouped antigenically (1), by protein profile (11), and by host specificity, with both cross-infective isolates and host-specific isolates known (4). While not generally considered zoonotic, at least one infection has been reported in a human with concurrent human immunodeficiency virus type 1 (HIV-1) infection (13).

Epidemiology
Prevalence rates in and among laboratory hamster colonies are generally unknown because reports are scant (9). Transmission is through fecal-oral spread, ultimately by ingestion of infectious spores, which may remain viable for many months. Therefore, inadequate sterilization of feed or bedding may facilitate entry of the pathogen into an animal facility. Transplacental transmission has been reported in mice (5) and guinea pigs (3), but not in hamsters.

Clinical signs

Among mice, susceptibility and disease severity are strain dependent and are worsened by stress. These aspects have not been investigated in the hamster. Clinical signs are generally restricted to sudden death, or may include watery, yellow diarrhea.

Pathology

Following infection, colonization occurs in the cecum, with subsequent hematogenous and lymphatic dissemination to various sites, most notably the liver and myocardium. Pathologic findings are as described in Tyzzer's disease of rats and mice, although gross liver lesions may be absent in hamsters (10). Immunity is primarily humoral, with innate resistance contributed by neutrophils and natural killer cells.

Interference with research

Few studies have reported physiologic effects of *C. piliforme* infection of hamsters, other than increased mortality. In mice, *C. piliforme* infection alters the pharmacokinetics of warfarin and trimethoprim (6) and the activity of hepatic transaminases, and increases serum interleukin 6 (IL-6) and IL-12 levels (14, 15); while in rats, susceptibility to experimentally induced arthritis may be altered (8). If investigated, similar effects may be found to occur in hamsters. Natural infection of laboratory hamsters would likely alter the findings of studies involving the cardiovascular and enterohepatic systems, and possibly the lymphoreticular system. Lastly, pharmacologic studies may also be affected. However, because some isolates of *C. piliforme* produce cytotoxins (12), the effects on research may be broader than is currently appreciated, and may extend to studies involving several other organ systems.

Diagnosis and control

Infections with *C. piliforme* may be diagnosed by tissue staining, egg inoculation, serology, and PCR assay (2, 7). *C. piliforme* has not been cultured on artificial media. Various antibiotic treatment regimens have been described, but these are inadequate for eradicating the pathogen from a colony. Therefore, strict attention to sanitation and stress reduction, coupled with testing and elimination of infected animals is required.

Lawsonia intracellularis

Agent

For many years the cause of proliferative ileitis (regional enteritis, terminal ileitis, atypical transmissible ileal hyperplasia, and other identifiers) in hamsters was unknown. Both infectious and noninfectious causes were reportedly associated with the condition (1, 2). For a long time it was thought that *Campylobacter* sp. and/or *Escherichia coli* were responsible. These agents were recovered from diseased hamsters in some studies, but not in others, and so eventually became viewed as secondary agents. Also, while these agents did often cause enteritis in experimental infections, the proliferative or hyperplastic component was frequently absent. Later, the causative agent was discovered and referred to simply as "intracellular *Campylobacter*-like organism." More recently, the agent was definitively identified as *Lawsonia intracellularis*. *L. intracellularis* is a small, gram-negative, curved, obligate intracellular bacterium. It causes disease in several other animal species, including swine, horses, monkeys, rabbits, ratites, and deer (4). Human infections have not been reported. The 16S ribosomal DNA from isolates obtained from several host species has been sequenced and found to be nearly indistinguishable between host species (1). Also, hamsters have been infected with isolates from swine and horses (1). These studies collectively suggest that isolates recovered from a range of host species are very closely related, if not identical. The organism can be grown in cell culture but not on artificial media, making taxonomic characterization difficult.

Epidemiology

Infection with *L. intracellularis* remains an important cause of morbidity and mortality in laboratory hamsters, although the prevalence is decreasing. Transmission is primarily fecal-oral, although complete transmission studies have not been reported. Transplacental infection is not thought to occur but has also not been thoroughly studied (1).

Clinical signs
Clinical signs are variable and nonspecific, and are most often seen in less than fully immunocompetent hamsters, including weanlings and pregnant dams (1). When present, clinical signs may include watery diarrhea, anorexia, runting, emaciation, dehydration, lethargy, and rough hair coat (6).

Pathology
Infection is characterized by segmental mucosal hypertrophy due to crypt and villous cell hyperplasia and proliferation; villous elongation and fusion; and varying degrees of necrosis, hemorrhage, abscessation, and granuloma formation. Serosal nodules and fibrinous peritoneal adhesions may also be present (6). Intracellular bacteria can be observed in tissues stained with periodic acid Schiff (PAS) or silver. Inflammation is not always present and may be caused or worsened by other, secondary pathogens (1). Lesions are found primarily in the ileum but may also extend into the stomach of hamsters (2). The mechanisms by which *L. intracellularis* localizes in specific regions of the gastrointestinal tract, enters host cells, and stimulates enterocyte hyperplasia are unknown.

Interference with research
Little information is available concerning the effects of *L. intracellularis* on host physiology. In a report of *L. intracellularis* in swine, the authors speculated that infection may result in disruption of normal processes of cell growth, differentiation, or apoptosis in the intestinal epithelium (5). Therefore, natural infection of laboratory hamsters with *L. intracellularis* would likely confound studies involving the enterohepatic system, and may affect those studies wherein nutritional indices, such as growth rate, are assessed.

Diagnosis and control
Diagnosis has traditionally been hampered by the need for special staining of appropriately selected intestine. Others have demonstrated antibody responses that may be useful for diagnosis (7). More recently, fecal PCR has been used, and will likely be the diagnostic test of choice in the future (3). There is no satisfactory antibiotic regimen for eradicating the infection. Antibiotic treatment may control clinical disease but will accomplish no more (1). High sanitary standards, reduced stress, and cage filter covers may reduce outbreak severity. Also, spontaneous clearing of the pathogen sometimes occurs after several weeks in individual animals. However, reliance on this for clearance of an entire colony is unreasonable. Eradication may be achieved by rederivation of infected animals. Animals should be certified free of infection prior to importation into the facility.

Staphylococcus aureus

Agent
Staphylococcus aureus is a gram-positive, coagulase-positive coccus that may live as an opportunistic pathogen in and on laboratory hamsters.

Epidemiology
As with many other species of mammals, silent infection with *S. aureus* is extremely common, if not ubiquitous.

Clinical signs
Most infections with *S. aureus* are asymptomatic. When staphylococcal disease occurs in the hamster, it usually consists of abscess formation in the skin, or less commonly, in deeper organs. Infection occurs following breaks in the skin, such as occurs with surgery, bite wounds, and cage trauma, and may remain localized or disseminate. Although the

hamster is more susceptible to wound infection than the rat (1), the incidence of clinical staphylococcal infections has historically been low (2).

Pathology

In hamsters, staphylococcal abscesses are most often found on and around the head. This is most likely due to fighting and cage trauma in this region. In hamsters, as in other laboratory animals, resistance to *S. aureus* is primarily through neutrophil release of microbicidal peptides belonging to the defensin family (4). Macrophages, specific antibodies, and cell-mediated immunity also contribute to pathogen elimination. Animal species differ in the kinetics of alveolar macrophage killing of *S. aureus*, with hamster alveolar macrophages requiring opsonization, and killing at a slower rate than human or rabbit macrophages (5). In an experimental hamster model, mucin was found to exacerbate staphylococcal pneumonia, possibly through interference with the mobility of resident phagocytic cells (7).

Interference with research

S. aureus produces a wide range of biologically active products, including enterotoxins which biologically can act as superantigens. The pathophysiology of staphylococcal dermatitis, as well as the known effects of *S. aureus* toxins and other products, is described in the section on *S. aureus* in chapter 2. Because of the wide range of effects elicited by staphylococcal products, systemic or localized clinical staphylococcal infection could compromise a wide variety of research efforts involving hamsters. For example, *S. aureus* has been shown to enhance early lesions of experimental *Leishmania braziliensis* infection (6) and, in combination with lynestrenol, a synthetic progesterone-like substance, alter the kinetics of experimental tumor growth (8).

Diagnosis and treatment

Staphylococcal infection is easily diagnosed using bacterial culture. Colonization of conventionally housed hamsters is unavoidable. Treatment with topical antibiotics usually eliminates clinical disease, but not the presence of the organism (3). Therefore, efforts should be directed at minimizing stress and skin trauma. To minimize pathogen spread, special attention should be directed toward ensuring that animal care personnel maintain a high degree of personal hygiene.

PARASITES

Demodex spp.

Agent

Hamsters may be infested with a variety of ectoparasites. Most common are infestations with *Demodex* mites (13). In addition to the Syrian hamster, *Demodex* spp. have been described in the less commonly used hamsters, including *Demodex sinocricetuli* in *Cricetulus barabensis* (4) and *Demodex cricetuli* in *C. migratorius* (7).

Epidemiology

In the Syrian hamster, two species are commonly found, often as a mixed infestation. *Demodex criceti* is a relatively nonpathogenic mite found in the epidermal "pits," whereas *Demodex aurati* is a pathogenic mite found in the sebaceous glands and hair follicles (13). Infestation is transmitted by contact, and occurs from dam to young shortly after birth (13). Male hamsters are often more heavily infested than females (11).

Clinical signs

Clinical signs are uncommon and are most often seen in aged or experimentally stressed hamsters (5, 12). Research on *Demodex folliculorum* infestations of human renal transplant patients suggests that in that host–parasite relationship increased susceptibility may not be entirely due to immunosuppression (1), while in generalized canine demodicosis, immunosuppression appears to play a major role in susceptibility to disease (8). When present,

TABLE 4-1. Body systems known or likely to be affected by pathogen indicated

Pathogen	Cardio-vascular	Dermal	Endocrine	Entero-hepatic	Hema-topoietic	Lympho-reticular	Musculo-skeletal	Nervous	Reproductive	Respiratory	Urinary
Lymphocytic choriomeningitis virus	X							X			X
Pneumonia virus of mice										X	
Sendai virus										X	X
Clostridium piliforme	X			X	X	X		X			
Lawsonia intracellularis				X							
Staphylococcus aureus		X				X					
Demodex spp.		X				X					X
Oxyurids (pinworms)				X							

clinical signs of *D. aurati* infestation may include scruffiness, patchy alopecia, drying and scaling of the skin, and scabbing (13). Infestation with *Demodex* spp. is only moderately pruritic.

Pathology

Histopathologic evidence of infestation is often not observed in immune-competent hosts. Lesions in clinical cases are usually limited to dermal changes associated with pruritus and alopecia (6). In addition, Murphy and coworkers (9) have suggested that infestation of hamsters with *D. aurati* may contribute to development of the nephrotic syndrome and renal amyloidosis. Lastly, Wolf and coworkers (14) have suggested that *Demodex* spp. may serve as vectors of other pathogens, including dermatophytes.

Interference with research

Little information is available specifically describing the effects of demodectic mange on hamster physiology. Nutting and Rauch (10) reported that experimental biotin deficiency resulted in a decrease in mite numbers, suggesting to this author that heavy infestation may alter findings of some nutritional studies. In addition, reports from other host-parasite models indicate an association between mite infestation and diabetes (3) and alterations in T-lymphocyte populations (2). Therefore, it is reasonable to assume that heavy infestation of laboratory hamsters with *Demodex* spp. could compromise research involving the dermal, lymphoreticular, and renal systems, as well as studies on host longevity and those in which nutritional parameters are measured. It is likely that mild infestations would have no effect, although the relationship between infestation and renal amyloidosis requires further study.

Diagnosis and control

Diagnosis of demodicosis is by examination of the hairs around areas of alopecia (13). Mites can also be visualized in skin scrapings dissolved in 10% KOH. Control is achieved by use of acaricidal preparations and attention to cage cleanliness (6). Because *D. criceti* and *D. aurati* are generally host specific, all infestations are transmitted from other hamsters, rather than other rodent species. Therefore, control efforts should be focused on preventing spread from infested colonies to susceptible animals.

Oxyurids (pinworms)

Agents

The most common pinworm infecting laboratory hamsters is thought to be *Syphacia obvelata*, the mouse pinworm (3), although en face examinations, necessary for accurate speciation of the worms, are rarely done. It is possible that many "*S. obvelata*" infections are actually *Syphacia mesocriceti*, since the two parasites are quite similar and the Syrian hamster is the natural host for *S. mesocriceti* (2). Through cohabitation, hamsters may also be infected with *Syphacia muris*, the rat pinworm (4).

Epidemiology

Relatively little is known of the life cycles of oxyurid parasites in hamsters. They are assumed to be similar to the life cycles of *S. obvelata* and *S. muris* in their natural hosts, and the reader is referred to chapter 2 for additional information.

Clinical signs

In most cases of hamster oxyuriasis, pinworm infections result in few clinical signs, even in heavy infections. Infections in other rodents are sometimes accompanied by clinical signs (6).

Pathology

Following infection, colonization occurs in the cecum and, to a lesser extent, the colon. In gerbils, infection in these sites causes local accumulation of eosinophils and plasma cells, resulting in some thickening of the lamina propria (5). It is likely that similar lesions occur in the hamster, although this has yet to be studied.

Interference with research

There is a growing body of literature concerning the effects of pinworms on their hosts (see chapter 2). No similar information is available for pinworm infections of hamsters. However, definitive studies concerning potential effects of pinworm infection on hamster research have not been reported. Given the effects of pinworms on other host species, it seems unwarranted to assert that there are no effects whatsoever on hamsters. In this author's view, specific research goals, especially those involving the enterohepatic and lymphoreticular systems, may justify the eradication of pinworms from a hamster colony.

Diagnosis and control

Diagnosis of pinworm infection is by examination of perianal tape preparations. Pinworms in most rodent species are best treated using fenbendazole-medicated rodent chow (1), although other treatment regimens have also proven successful (7). Careful attention to fomite or vector transmission is necessary to prevent reinfection, or infection from contaminated mouse colonies. Because other rodents are often the source of infection for hamsters, efforts to prevent introduction of oxyurids into the hamster colony should also be directed at controlling infection in those species.

REFERENCES

INTRODUCTION

1. **Cantrell, C. A., and D. Padovan.** 1987. Biology, care, and use in research, p. 369–387. *In* G. L. Van Hoosier and C. W. McPherson (ed.), *Laboratory Hamsters*. Academic Press, Inc., New York, N.Y.
2. **Chang, A., A. Diani, and M. Connell.** 1987. Biology and care, p. 305–319. *In* G. L. Van Hoosier, Jr., and C. W. McPherson (ed.), *Laboratory Hamsters*. Academic Press, Inc., New York, N.Y.
3. **Clark, J. D.** 1987. Historical perspectives and taxonomy, p. 3–7. *In* G. L. Van Hoosier, Jr., and C. W. McPherson (ed.), *Laboratory Hamsters*. Academic Press, Inc., New York, N.Y.
4. **Mohr, U., and H. Ernst.** 1987. Biology, care, and use in research, p. 351–366. *In* G. L. Van Hoosier, Jr., and C. W. McPherson (ed.), *Labo-*

ratory Hamsters. Academic Press, Inc., New York, N.Y.
5. Van Hoosier, G. L., Jr., and C. W. McPherson (ed.). 1987. *Laboratory Hamsters.* Academic Press, Inc., New York, N.Y.

VIRUSES
Lymphocytic choriomeningitis virus
1. Genovesi, E. V., A. J. Johnson, and C. J. Peters. 1988. Susceptibility and resistance of inbred strains of Syrian golden hamsters (*Mesocricetus auratus*) to wasting disease caused by lymphocytic choriomeningitis virus: pathogenesis of lethal and non-lethal infections. *J. Gen. Virol.* **69:**2209–2220.
2. Genovesi, E. V., A. J. Johnson, and C. J. Peters. 1989. Delayed type-hypersensitivity response of inbred strains of Syrian golden hamsters (*Mesocricetus auratus*) to lethal or non-lethal lymphocytic choriomeningitis virus (LCMV) infections. *Microb. Pathog.* **7:**347–360.
3. Genovesi, E. V., and C. J. Peters. 1987. Susceptibility of inbred Syrian golden hamsters (*Mesocricetus auratus*) to lethal disease by lymphocytic choriomeningitis virus. *Proc. Soc. Exp. Biol. Med.* **185:**250–261.
4. Genovesi, E. V., and C. J. Peters. 1987. Immunosuppression-induced susceptibility of inbred hamsters (*Mesocricetus auratus*) to lethal-disease by lymphocytic choriomeningitis virus infection. *Arch. Virol.* **97:**61–76.
5. Hinman, A. R., D. W. Fraser, R. G. Douglas, G. S. Bowen, L. Kraus, W. G. Winkler, and W. W. Rhodes. 1975. Outbreak of lymphocytic choriomeningitis virus infections in medical center personnel. *Am. J. Epidemiol.* **101:**103–110.
6. Hirsch, M. S., R. C. Moellering, Jr., H. G. Pope, and D. C. Poskanzer. 1974. Lymphocytic-choriomeningitis-virus infection traced to a pet hamster. *N. Engl. J. Med.* **291:**610–612.
7. Kraft, V., and B. Meyer. 1990. Seromonitoring in small laboratory animal colonies. A five year survey: 1984–1988. *Z. Verstierkd.* **33:**29–35.
8. Lewis, A. M., Jr., W. P. Rowe, H. C. Turner, and R. J. Huebner. 1965. Lymphocytic-choriomeningitis virus in hamster tumor: spread to hamsters and humans. *Science* **150:**363–364.
9. Parker, J. C., J. R. Ganaway, and C. S. Gillett. 1987. Viral diseases, p. 95–110. *In* G. L. Van Hoosier, Jr., and C. W. McPherson (ed.), *Laboratory Hamsters.* Academic Press, Inc., New York, N.Y.
10. Parker, J. C., H. J. Igel, R. K. Reynolds, A. M. Lewis, Jr., and W. P. Rowe. 1976. Lymphocytic choriomeningitis virus infection in fetal, newborn, and young adult Syrian hamsters (*Mesocricetus auratus*). *Infect. Immun.* **13:**967–981.
11. Percy, D. H., and S. W. Barthold. 2001. *Pathology of Laboratory Rodents and Rabbits*, 2nd ed. Iowa State University Press, Ames.
12. Reiserova, L., M. Kaluzova, S. Kaluz, A. C. Willis, J. Zavada, E. Zavodska, Z. Zavadova, F. Ciampor, J. Pastorek, and S. Pastorekova. 1999. Identification of MaTu-MX agent as a new strain of lymphocytic choriomeningitis virus (LCMV) and serological indication of horizontal spread of LCMV in human populations. *Virology* **257:**73–83.
13. Rousseau, M. C., M. F. Saron, P. Brouqui, and A. Bourgeade. 1997. Lymphocytic choriomeningitis virus in southern France: four case reports and a review of the literature. *Eur. J. Epidemiol.* **13:**817–823.
14. Sato, H., and H. Miyata. 1986. Detection of lymphocytic choriomeningitis virus antibody in colonies of laboratory animals in Japan. *Jikken Dobutsu* **35:**189–192.
15. Selin, L. K., K. Vergillis, R. M. Welsh, and S. R. Nahill. 1996. Reduction of otherwise remarkably stable virus-specific cytotoxic T lymphocyte memory by heterologous viral infections. *J. Exp. Med.* **183:**2489–2499.
16. Skinner, H. H., E. H. Knight, and L. S. Buckley. 1976. The hamster as a secondary reservoir host of lymphocytic choriomeningitis virus. *J. Hyg.* **76:**299–306.
17. Thacker, W. L., V. J. Lewis, J. H. Shaddock, and W. G. Winkler. 1982. Infection of Syrian hamsters with lymphocytic choriomeningitis virus: comparison of detection methods. *Am. J. Vet. Res.* **43:**1500–1502.
18. van der Zeijst, B. A., B. E. Noyes, M. E. Mirault, B. Parker, A. D. Osterhaus, E. A. Swyryd, N. Bleumink, M. C. Horzinek, and G. R. Stark. 1983. Persistent infection of some standard cell lines by lymphocytic choriomeningitis virus: transmission of infection by an intracellular agent. *J. Virol.* **48:**249–261.
19. Vanzee, B. E., R. G. Douglas, R. F. Betts, A. W. Bauman, D. W. Fraser, and A. R. Hinman. 1975. Lymphocytic choriomeningitis in university hospital personnel. Clinical features. *Am. J. Med.* **58:**803–809.

Pneumonia virus of mice
1. Kraft, V., and B. Meyer. 1990. Seromonitoring in small laboratory animal colonies. A five year survey: 1984–1988. *Z. Verstierkd.* **33:**29–35.
2. Miyata, H., M. Kishikawa, H. Kondo, C. Kai, Y. Watanabe, K. Ohsawa, and H. Sato. 1995. New isolates of pneumonia virus of mice (PVM) from Japanese rat colonies and their characterization. *Exp. Anim.* **44:**95–104.

3. Miyata, H., Y. Watanabe, H. Kondo, K. Yagami, and H. Sato. 1993. Serological evidence of pneumonia virus of mouse (PVM) infection in laboratory rats. *Jikken Dobutsu* **42:**371–376.
4. Parker, J. C., J. R. Ganaway, and C. S. Gillett. 1987. Viral diseases, p. 95–110. *In* G. L. Van Hoosier, Jr., and C. W. McPherson (ed.), *Laboratory Hamsters*. Academic Press, Inc., New York, N.Y.
5. Pearson, H. E., and M. D. Eaton. 1940. A virus pneumonia of Syrian hamsters. *Proc. Soc. Exp. Biol. Med.* **45:**677–679.
6. Skovikova, L. P., L. Y. Taros, and A. P. Volgarev. 1983. Respiratory syncytial virus infection in Syrian hamsters. I. Development of humoral immunity. *Acta Virol.* **27:**490–495.
7. Valarcher, J. F., H. Bourhy, J. Gelfi, and F. Schelcher. 1999. Evaluation of a nested reverse transcription-PCR assay based on the nucleoprotein gene for diagnosis of spontaneous and experimental bovine respiratory syncytial virus infection. *J. Clin. Microbiol.* **37:**1858–1862.
8. Zee, Y. C. 1999. Paramyxoviridae. *In* D. C. Hirsh and Y. C. Zee (ed.), *Veterinary Microbiology*. Blackwell Science, Inc., Malden, Mass.

Sendai virus
1. Al-Ahdal, M. N., I. Nakamura, and T. D. Flanagan. 1985. Cytotoxic T-lymphocyte reactivity with individual Sendai virus glycoproteins. *J. Virol.* **54:**53–57.
2. Blandford, G., and D. Charlton. 1977. Studies of pulmonary and renal immunopathology after nonlethal primary sendai viral infection in normal and cyclophosphamide-treated hamsters. *Am. Rev. Respir. Dis.* **115:**305–314.
3. Friedman, H. M., D. H. Gilden, F. S. Lief, D. Santoli, and H. Koprowski. 1975. Hydrocephalus produced by the 6/94 virus; A parainfluenza type 1 isolate from multiple sclerosis brain tissue. *Arch. Neurol.* **32:**408–413.
4. Fuchs, P., and E. Giberman. 1973. Enhancement of potassium influx, in baby hamster kidney cells and chicken erythrocytes, during adsorption of parainfluenza 1 (Sendai) virus. *FEBS Lett.* **31:**127–130.
5. Fukumi, H., and Y. Takeuchi. 1975. Vaccination against parainfluenza 1 virus (*typus muris*) infection in order to eradicate this virus in colonies of laboratory animals. *Dev. Biol. Stand.* **28:**477–481.
6. Garcin, D., G. Taylor, K. Tanebayashi, R. Compans, and D. Kolakofsky. 1998. The short Sendai virus leader region controls induction of programmed cell death. *Virology* **243:**340–353.
7. Kimsey, P. B., M. E. Goad, Z. B. Zhao, G. Brackee, and J. G. Fox. 1989. Methyl prednisolone acetate modulation of infection and subsequent pulmonary pathology in hamsters exposed to parainfluenza-1 virus (Sendai). *Am. Rev. Respir. Dis.* **140:**1704–1711.
8. Kraft, V., and B. Meyer. 1990. Seromonitoring in small laboratory animal colonies. A five year survey: 1984–1988. *Z. Verstierkd.* **33:**29–35.
9. Parker, J. C., M. D. Whiteman, and C. B. Richter. 1978. Susceptibility of inbred and outbred mouse strains to Sendai virus and prevalence of infection in laboratory rodents. *Infect. Immun.* **19:**123–130.
10. Percy, D. H., and D. J. Palmer. 1997. Pathogenesis of Sendai virus infection in the Syrian hamster. *Lab. Anim. Sci.* **47:**132–137.
11. Profeta, M. L. 1975. Anti-neuraminidase antibody response in hamsters experimentally infected with Sendai virus. *Ann. Sclavo.* **17:**884–892.
12. Profeta, M. L., F. S. Lief, and S. A. Plotkin. 1969. Enzootic sendai infection in laboratory hamsters. *Am. J. Epidemiol.* **89:**316–324.
13. Schiff, L. J. 1976. Replication of murine paramyxoviruses in hamster tracheal organ culture and comparison with standard tissue culture methods. *J. Clin. Microbiol.* **4:**248–252.
14. Tagaya, M., I. Mori, T. Miyadai, Y. Kimura, H. Ito, and K. Nakakuki. 1995. Efficacy of a temperature-sensitive Sendai virus vaccine in hamsters. *Lab. Anim. Sci.* **45:**233–238.

BACTERIA
Clostridium piliforme
1. Boivin, G. P., R. R. Hook, Jr., and L. K. Riley. 1993. Antigenic diversity in flagellar epitopes among *Bacillus piliformis* isolates. *J. Med. Microbiol.* **38:**177–182.
2. Boivin, G. P., R. R. Hook, Jr., and L. K. Riley. 1994. Development of a monoclonal antibody-based competitive inhibition enzyme-linked immunosorbent assay for detection of *Bacillus piliformis* isolate-specific antibodies in laboratory animals. *Lab. Anim. Sci.* **44:**153–158.
3. Boot, R., and H. C. Walvoort. 1984. Vertical transmission of *Bacillus piliformis* infection (Tyzzer's disease) in a guinea pig: case report. *Lab. Anim.* **18:**195–199.
4. Franklin, C. L., S. L. Motzel, C. L. Besch-Williford, R. R. Hook, Jr., and L. K. Riley. 1994. Tyzzer's infection: host specificity of *Clostridium piliforme* isolates. *Lab. Anim. Sci.* **44:**568–572.
5. Fries, A. S. 1978. Demonstration of antibodies to *Bacillus piliformis* in SPF colonies and experimental transplacental infection by *Bacillus piliformis* in mice. *Lab. Anim.* **12:**23–26.

6. **Fries, A. S., and O. Ladefoged.** 1979. The influence of *Bacillus piliformis* (Tyzzer) infections on the reliability of pharmacokinetic experiments in mice. *Lab. Anim.* **13:**257–261.
7. **Goto, K., and T. Itoh.** 1996. Detection of *Clostridium piliforme* by enzymatic assay of amplified cDNA segment in microtitration plates. *Lab. Anim. Sci.* **46:**493–496.
8. **Gripenberg-Lerche, C., and P. Toivanen.** 1994. Variability in the induction of experimental arthritis: *Yersinia* associated arthritis in Lewis rats. *Scand. J. Rheumatol.* **23:**124–127.
9. **Kraft, V., and B. Meyer.** 1990. Seromonitoring in small laboratory animal colonies. A five year survey: 1984–1988. *Z. Verstierkd.* **33:**29–35.
10. **Motzel, S. L., and S. V. Gibson.** 1990. Tyzzer disease in hamsters and gerbils from a pet store supplier. *J. Am. Vet. Med. Assoc.* **197:**1176–1178.
11. **Riley, L. K., C. Besch-Williford, and K. S. Waggie.** 1990. Protein and antigenic heterogeneity among isolates of *Bacillus piliformis*. *Infect. Immun.* **58:**1010–1016.
12. **Riley, L. K., C. J. Caffrey, V. S. Musille, and J. K. Meyer.** 1992. Cytotoxicity of *Bacillus piliformis*. *J. Med. Microbiol.* **37:**77–80.
13. **Smith, K. J., H. G. Skelton, E. J. Hilyard, T. Hadfield, R. S. Moeller, S. Tuur, C. Decker, K. F. Wagner, and P. Angritt.** 1996. *Bacillus piliformis* infection (Tyzzer's disease) in a patient infected with HIV-1: confirmation with 16S ribosomal RNA sequence analysis. *J. Am. Dermatol.* **34:**343–348.
14. **Van Andel, R. A., C. L. Franklin, C. L. Besch-Williford, R. R. Hook, Jr., and L. K. Riley.** 2000. Role of interleukin-6 in determining the course of murine Tyzzer's disease. *J. Med. Microbiol.* **49:**171–176.
15. **Van Andel, R. A., R. R. Hook, Jr., C. L. Franklin, C. L. Besch-Williford, and L. K. Riley.** 1998. Interleukin-12 has a role in mediating resistance of murine strains to Tyzzer's disease. *Infect. Immun.* **66:**4942–4946.

Lawsonia intracellularis
1. **Cooper, D. M., and C. J. Gebhart.** 1998. Comparative aspects of proliferative enteritis. *J. Am. Vet. Med. Assoc.* **212:**1446–1451.
2. **Frisk, C. S.** 1987. Bacterial and mycotic diseases, p. 112–133. *In* G. L. Van Hoosier, Jr. and C. W. McPherson (ed.), *Laboratory Hamsters*. Academic Press, Inc., New York, N.Y.
3. **Jordan, D. M., J. P. Knittel, M. B. Roof, K. Schwartz, D. Larson, and L. J. Hoffman.** 1999. Detection of *Lawsonia intracellularis* in swine using polymerase chain reaction methodology. *J. Vet. Diagn. Invest.* **11:**45–49.
4. **Klein, E. C., C. J. Gebhart, and G. E. Duhamel.** 1999. Fatal outbreaks of proliferative enteritis caused by *Lawsonia intracellularis* in young colony-raised rhesus macaques. *J. Med. Primatol.* **28:**11–18.
5. **McOrist, S., L. Roberts, S. Jasni, A. C. Rowland, G. H. Lawson, C. J. Gebhart, and B. Bosworth.** 1996. Developed and resolving lesions in porcine proliferative enteropathy: possible pathogenetic mechanisms. *J. Comp. Pathol.* **115:**35–45.
6. **Percy, D. H., and S. W. Barthold.** 2001. *Pathology of Laboratory Rodents and Rabbits*, 2nd ed. Iowa State University Press, Ames.
7. **Stills, H. F.** 1991. Isolation of an intracellular bacterium from hamsters (*Mesocricetus auratus*) with proliferative ileitis and reproduction of the disease with a pure culture. *Infect. Immun.* **59:**3227–3236.

Staphylococcus aureus
1. **Donnelly, T. M., and D. M. Stark.** 1985. Susceptibility of laboratory rats, hamsters, and mice to wound infection with *Staphylococcus aureus*. *Am. J. Vet. Res.* **46:**2634–2638.
2. **Hearst, B. R.** 1967. Low incidence of staphylococcal dermatitides in animals with high incidence of *Staphylococcus aureus*. 3. Preliminary study of laboratory animals. *Vet. Med. Small Anim. Clin.* **62:** 666–667.
3. **Ikeda, M., J. Arata, and N. Kashiwa.** 1984. Antibiotic effects on bacterial counts in skin lesions of experimental staphylococcal skin infections in the hamster. *J. Dermatol.* **11:**67–72.
4. **Mak, P., K. Wojcik, I. B. Thogersen, and A. Dubin.** 1996. Isolation, antimicrobial activities, and primary structures of hamster neutrophil defensins. *Infect. Immun.* **64:**4444–4449.
5. **Nguyen, B. Y., P. K. Peterson, H. A. Verbrugh, P. G. Quie, and J. R. Hoidal.** 1982. Differences in phagocytosis and killing by alveolar macrophages from humans, rabbits, rats, and hamsters. *Infect. Immun.* **36:**504–509.
6. **Potter, M. E., W. L. Chapman, Jr., W. L. Hanson, and J. L. Blue.** 1983. *Leishmania braziliensis*: effects of bacteria (*Staphylococcus aureus* and *Pasteurella multocida*) on the developing cutaneous leishmaniasis lesion in the golden hamster. *Exp. Parasitol.* **56:**107–118.
7. **Verghese, A., A. Catanese, and R. D. Arbeit.** 1988. *Staphylococcus aureus* pneumonia in hamsters with elastase-induced emphysema- the virulence enhancing activity of mucin. *Proc. Soc. Exp. Biol. Med.* **188:**1–6.
8. **Wybran, J., and L. Thiry.** 1978. Delay of tumor growth in hamsters treated with lynestrenol and effect of *Staphylococcus aureus* Cowan A. *J. Natl. Cancer Inst.* **61:**173–176.

PARASITES
Demodex spp.
1. **Aydingoz, I. E., T. Mansur, and B. Dervent.** 1997. *Demodex folliculorum* in renal transplant patients. *Dermatology* **195:**232–234.

2. **Caswell, J. L., J. A. Yager, W. M. Parker, and P. F. Moore.** 1997. A prospective study of the immunophenotype and temporal changes in the histologic lesions of canine demodicosis. *Vet. Pathol.* **34:**279–287.
3. **Clifford, C. W., and G. W. Fulk.** 1990. Association of diabetes, lash loss, and *Staphylococcus aureus* with infestation of eyelids by *Demodex folliculorum* (Acari: Demodicidae). *J. Med. Entomol.* **27:**467–470.
4. **Desch, C. E., Jr., and R. J. Hurley.** 1997. *Demodex sinocricetuli*: new species of hair follicle mite (Acari: Demodicidae) from the Chinese form of the striped hamster, *Cricetulus barabensis* (Rodentia: Muridae). *J. Med. Entomol.* **34:**317–320.
5. **Estes, P. C., C. B. Richter, and J. A. Franklin.** 1971. Demodectic mange in the golden hamster. *Lab. Anim. Sci.* **21:**825–828.
6. **Hasegawa, T.** 1995. A case report of the management of demodicosis in the golden hamster. *J. Vet. Med. Sci.* **57:**337–338.
7. **Hurley, R. J., and C. E. Desch, Jr.** 1994. *Demodex cricetuli*: new species of hair follicle mite (Acari: Demodicidae) from the Armenian hamster, *Cricetulus migratorius* (Rodentia: Cricetidae). *J. Med. Entomol.* **31:**529–533.
8. **Mozos, E., J. Perez, M. J. Day, R. Lucena, and P. J. Ginel.** 1999. Leishmaniosis and generalized demodicosis in three dogs: a clinicopathological and immunohistochemical study. *J. Comp. Pathol.* **120:**257–268.
9. **Murphy, J. C., J. G. Fox, and S. M. Niemi.** 1984. Nephrotic syndrome associated with renal amyloidosis in a colony of Syrian hamsters. *J. Am. Vet. Med. Assoc.* **185:**1359–1362.
10. **Nutting, W. B., and H. Rauch.** 1961. The effect of biotin deficiency in *Mesocricetus auratus* on parasites of the genus *Demodex*. *J. Parasitol.* **47:**319–322.
11. **Nutting, W. B., and H. Rauch.** 1963. Distribution of *Demodex aurati* in the host (*Mesocricetus auratus*) skin complex. *J. Parasitol.* **49:**323–329.
12. **Owen, D., and C. Young.** 1973. The occurrence of *Demodex aurati* and *Demodex criceti* in the Syrian hamster (*Mesocricetus auratus*) in the United Kingdom. *Vet. Rec.* **92:**282–284.
13. **Wagner, J. E.** 1987. Parasitic diseases, p. 135–156. *In* G. L. Van Hoosier, Jr., and C. W. McPherson (ed.), *Laboratory Hamsters*. Academic Press, Inc., New York, N.Y.
14. **Wolf, R., J. Ophir, J. Avigad, J. Lengy, and A. Krakowski.** 1988. The hair follicle mites (*Demodex* spp.). Could they be vectors of pathogenic microorganisms? *Acta Derm. Venereol.* **68:**535–537.

Oxyurids (Pinworms)

1. **Coghlan, L. G., D. R. Lee, B. Psencik, and D. Weiss.** 1993. Practical and effective eradication of pinworms (*Syphacia muris*) in rats by use of fenbendazole. *Lab. Anim. Sci.* **43:**481–487.
2. **Dick, T. A., J. C. Quentin, and R. S. Freeman.** 1973. Redescription of *Syphacia mesocriceti* (Nematoda: Oxyuroidea) parasite of the golden hamster. *J. Parasitol.* **59:**256–259.
3. **Hasslinger, M. A., and T. Wiethe.** 1987. Oxyurid infestation of small laboratory animals and its control with ivermectin. *Tieraerztl. Prax.* **15:**93–97.
4. **Ross, C. R., J. E. Wagner, S. R. Wightman, and S. E. Dill.** 1980. Experimental transmission of *Syphacia muris* among rats, mice, hamsters, and gerbils. *Lab. Anim. Sci.* **30:**35–37.
5. **Smith, G. D., and T. G. Snider III.** 1988. Experimental infection and treatment of *Dentostomella translucida* in the Mongolian gerbil. *Lab. Anim. Sci.* **38:**339–340.
6. **Tafts, L. F.** 1976. Pinworm infections in laboratory rodents: a review. *Lab. Anim.* **10:**1–13.
7. **Unay, E. S., and B. J. Davis.** 1980. Treatment of *Syphacia obvelata* in the Syrian hamster (*Mesocricetus auratus*) with piperazine citrate. *Am. J. Vet. Res.* **41:**2899–2900.

PATHOGENS OF GUINEA PIGS

5

INTRODUCTION

The guinea pig (*Cavia porcellus*) has for many years been an important laboratory animal species. Biomedical uses of guinea pigs have included studies of gnotobiology, nutrition, toxicology, complement biology, pulmonary physiology, opportunistic AIDS infections, and auditory research. Guinea pigs are susceptible to a wide range of pathogens. Despite tremendous improvements in laboratory animal husbandry, a significant number of guinea pigs used in research continue to harbor natural pathogens capable of altering research findings.

VIRUSES

Cytomegalovirus

Agent
A more complete discussion of the biology of the cytomegaloviruses (CMVs) is presented in chapter 2. CMVs are DNA viruses of the family *Herpesviridae,* subfamily Betaherpesvirinae.

Epidemiology
Guinea pig cytomegalovirus (GPCMV) has not been transmitted to other host species. Prevalence of infection in laboratory guinea pigs is unknown. At one time prevalence was assumed to be high (6). It is unlikely that is still the case. Transmission is transplacental (10, 11, 18), and by contact.

Clinical signs
Clinical signs are usually not observed in natural infections. One report described clinical disease in two guinea pigs, one of which died, presumably of natural GPCMV infection (26), although other causes of death were not entirely ruled out. In another report, GPCMV was considered responsible for fetal death and sow mortality in a breeding colony (21).

Pathology
Following infection, virus colonizes the ductal epithelium of salivary glands, as well as other tissues. While gross necropsy findings are generally absent, typical histologic findings include eosinophilic intranuclear inclusion bodies in ductal epithelium of the salivary glands and renal tubules. Less commonly, intracytoplasmic inclusion bodies may also be found (8, 27). Infected salivary gland cells are enlarged. Microscopic lesions, including inclusion bodies, have also been described in many other organs during generalized disease, including liver, spleen, lungs, and lymph nodes (21, 26). There is a considerable volume

of literature on central nervous system effects of GPCMV following experimental infection, which serves as a model for human infection (2, 7, 25). Lesions induced by artificial inoculation are similar to those resulting from natural infection, with the addition of mononuclear infiltration at the site of inoculation (27). Fetal host death is likely due to cytolysis of GPCMV-infected fetal cells by maternal cytolytic cells (14, 15).

Immunity to GPCMV is predominantly cell mediated (14), with humoral immunity playing a lesser role (3, 19). The temporal appearance of anti-GPCMV antibodies may be altered by pregnancy (4, 13, 16). Along these lines, considerable alteration of host immune-response capability occurs depending on time of infection. For example, acutely infected neonatal guinea pigs develop growth retardation, thymic hypoplasia, and splenomegaly. Depletion of T lymphocytes occurred in the thymuses and suppression of proliferative responses to mitogens occurred in splenic lymphocytes (29). In another report, granulocyte number and function were reduced in guinea pigs infected as weanlings (28).

Interference with research
There is a considerable body of literature on the in vitro effects of human CMV on various cellular functions. It is likely that similar mechanisms may be active in the guinea pig, although to date most have not been tested. For example, in vitro effects of human CMV include: inhibition of lysozyme release and intracellular acid phosphatase release in human monocytes (17); altered expression of major histocompatibility complex (MHC) class I antigen, interleukin 6 (IL-6) mRNA, transforming growth factor-β (TGF-β) (1, 20), and IL-2 receptor-α mRNA (9); modulation of angiogenesis due to down-regulation of thrombospondin-1 expression (5); attraction of human neutrophils by an alpha chemokine (22); and inhibition of hematopoietic cell line growth (24). In vivo, human CMV impairs fetal lung maturity, possibly because of reduced surfactant release and/or production (23). Natural infection of guinea pigs with CMV could confound research involving several organ systems, most notably the enterohepatic, hematopoietic, lymphoreticular, nervous, reproductive, respiratory, and urinary systems. In addition, studies in which growth rates are measured would likely also be affected.

Diagnosis and control
Diagnosis of CMV infection is by histopathologic examination, or by in situ hybridization (12). There is no effective treatment for CMV infection. CMVs may persist for long periods in the host, making elimination of the pathogen difficult. Screening animals prior to entry into the facility constitutes the most appropriate preventive measure.

Lymphocytic choriomeningitis virus

Agent
Lymphocytic choriomeningitis virus (LCMV) is a noncytopathic single-stranded RNA (ssRNA) virus in the family *Arenaviridae*. At least two strains exist. These differ in pathogenic potential for guinea pigs (1, 3, 4).

Epidemiology
Natural infection of guinea pigs with LCMV appears to be uncommon (2, 5). The primary importance of LCMV is as a zoonosis and as a contaminant of transplantable tumors and cultured cell lines. The biology of the virus is fully described in chapter 2, and the interested reader is referred there for details. It should be recognized, however, that comparatively little is known of the biology of the virus in guinea pigs, and there may be significant differences between infections in various hosts. Transmission is likely by exposure of mucous membranes and broken skin to infectious urine, saliva, and milk, through implantation of infected tumors, and possibly by ingestion. It is uncertain whether transovarian and transuterine transmission occurs in guinea pigs.

Clinical signs
Clinical signs of LCMV infection in guinea pigs are uncommon. Signs associated with

meningitis and hind-limb paralysis have been reported (6).

Pathology
Gross lesions may include pneumonia, pulmonary edema, pleural exudate, fatty liver, and splenomegaly (6). The microscopic hallmark of infection is lymphocytic infiltration of the meninges, liver, adrenals, kidneys, and lungs (6). Neutrophilic destruction of the splenic red pulp, focal bone marrow necrosis, lymphopenia, and death occur following infection with the more virulent WE strain (3, 4). Immunity to LCMV is primarily cellular, although virus-specific antibody is also induced (7).

Interference with research
Little information is available on the effects of LCMV on research in guinea pigs. Caution is warranted in extrapolating the findings of experimental infections in mice and other host species to guinea pigs. It is likely that natural infection of guinea pigs would compromise research involving the enterohepatic, hematopoietic, lymphoreticular, musculoskeletal, nervous, respiratory, and urinary systems, and would certainly serve as a source of human infection.

Diagnosis and control
Diagnosis historically was by mouse inoculation with suspect samples, but this has been replaced with serologic assays. It is expected that PCR assays and in situ hybridization will also be used. Control is best achieved by purchasing only LCMV-free animals of all susceptible species from reputable dealers.

BACTERIA

Bordetella bronchiseptica

Agent
Bordetella bronchiseptica is a gram-negative, beta-hemolytic, nonspore-forming rod commonly found inhabiting the respiratory tracts of a variety of domestic animals, including dogs, cats, rabbits, swine, horses, primates, and others. Multiple isolates and/or strains exist. These may be differentiated by pulsed-field gel electrophoresis following macrorestriction digestion with *Xba*I (2), antimicrobial drug susceptibility, nitrate reduction (1), immunoblotting using monoclonal antibodies against fimbrial antigens (4), and ribotyping with restriction enzyme *Pvu*II (16). These approaches may (4, 16), or may not (1, 2), be useful for predicting host specificity.

Epidemiology
Definitive studies examining host species cross-infectivity patterns of *B. bronchiseptica* have yet to be reported. Transmission is by direct contact, respiratory aerosol (18), and contaminated fomites, and it occurs early in life. Prevalence rates have historically been high (12), although more recent surveys are lacking.

Clinical signs
Within infected colonies, asymptomatic carriers are common, constituting up to 20% of resident guinea pigs. Many guinea pigs eventually clear the infection spontaneously. Conversion to clinical disease, most commonly seen in young guinea pigs, is precipitated by stresses such as dietary changes, vitamin C deficiency, rapid temperature change, heat, or overcrowding. The incubation period for the acute disease is 5 to 7 days, followed by sudden onset and signs lasting 2 to 3 days accompanied by high mortality rates. Clinical signs therefore occur relatively late in the course of infection and are often associated with pneumonia, and may include anorexia, depression, rough hair coat, weight loss, nasal and/or ocular discharges, dyspnea, and death. Abortions and stillbirths are also occasionally seen.

Pathology
Gross lesions include mucopurulent or catarrhal exudates in the upper respiratory tract and tympanic bullae (3, 19), anteroventral pulmonary consolidation, and pleuritis (15). Histologically the condition is characterized by suppurative bronchopneumonia and loss of normal pulmonary cytoarchitecture, with

variable amounts of fibrinous exudation in the terminal airway (15). Filamentous hemagglutinin (5), fimbriae (11), and possibly other factors, share roles in tracheal colonization. Immunity is primarily humoral, and is directed at least in part toward fimbriae (11).

Interference with research
B. bronchiseptica may alter host physiology in several ways. B. bronchiseptica produces toxins, such as the dermonecrotizing toxin (DNT) located in the intracellular space (13), which causes actin stress fiber formation through activation of Rho (14). Other toxins may affect peripheral blood vessels (6). Additional physiologic effects include: hyperresponsiveness to histamine, with increased vascular permeability and recruitment of nociceptive nerve-parasympathetic reflexes (8); modulation of host immune responses; induction of apoptosis; and inhibition of NF-κB activation (7, 21). Clinical or subclinical bordetellosis could compromise the usefulness of guinea pigs in a variety of research endeavors because of general depression of health and by direct effects on the cardiovascular, lymphoreticular, nervous, reproductive, respiratory, and urinary systems.

Diagnosis and control
Diagnosis is suggested by clinical signs and confirmed by bacterial culture, preferably using MacConkey's agar. Cultures can be taken from the respiratory tract or middle ear. In addition, enzyme-linked immunosorbent assay (ELISA) has also been used (20), and more recently, PCR has been used, targeting an upstream sequence of the flagellin gene (9). Radiography may be helpful in diagnosing otitis media (19). Clinically affected guinea pigs should be treated immediately, or preferably, culled. Treatment is often unrewarding, although sulfonamides and fluoroquinolones have been used with some success. Bordetellosis is prevented by isolating guinea pigs from infected animals and other species known to be carriers, providing good husbandry, and minimizing stress. Given the high prevalence of latent B. bronchiseptica infection in numerous laboratory animal species and man, establishment and maintenance of a Bordetella-free colony is difficult. Repeated vaccination has been used in the past to facilitate eventual clearing of the pathogen from a guinea pig colony (10, 17).

Chlamydophila psittaci

Agent
Chlamydophila psittaci (formerly Chlamydia psittaci), the causative agent of "guinea pig inclusion conjunctivitis" (GPIC), is an obligate intracellular "gram-negative" coccobacillus. The chlamydiae are incapable of obtaining energy by independent metabolic activity, and therefore rely entirely on their host for survival.

Epidemiology
The life cycle of C. psittaci is direct and consists of infectious nonproliferative elementary bodies, which enter host cells primarily through receptor-mediated endocytosis, and noninfectious proliferative reticulate bodies, which develop into the next generation of elementary bodies, to be released with cell lysis (2, 12, 20). Genetically and serologically distinct subgroups exist which differ in host species and sites of infection, with guinea pig strains constituting a distinct subgroup (5, 8, 11, 13). Transmission is primarily through inhalation of infectious secretions, although under laboratory conditions, flies have also been shown capable of transmitting the organism (6). Prevalence of C. psittaci-infected guinea pig colonies is low. Within a colony, however, prevalence can be high (4).

Clinical signs
C. psittaci most commonly presents as ocular or genital infections. When evident, clinical signs may therefore include mild chemosis (edema in the conjunctiva), conjunctivitis, and ocular discharge; vaginitis; urethritis; and cystitis (16, 22). Severity of infection may be influenced by immune status (25) and hormonal

status, e.g., estradiol treatment produces infections of greater intensity (15).

Pathology
Histopathologic findings include inclusion bodies, and lymphocytic and neutrophilic infiltrates (22). Both humoral and cellular immune responses are detectable in both ocular and genital infections. While protective immunity appears to be primarily cellular in both cases, humoral immunity appears to play a more significant role in genital versus ocular infections (1, 14, 19, 21, 23).

Interference with research
Chlamydiae are essentially energy parasites. Reticulate bodies import ATP and export ADP, using the "stolen" energy to manufacture peptides (2). While elementary bodies have little biochemical activity, they do produce soluble and cell-bound products that may damage macrophages, neutralize specific antibody (2), attract neutrophils (17), and modulate the host immune response (9, 24). *Chlamydia*-induced apoptosis of epithelial cells and macrophages results in secretion of pro-inflammatory cytokines (3, 10). In addition, heparin-like molecules secreted by *C. psittaci* act as adhesins (2). In the pregnant sheep model, *C. psittaci* elevates amniotic and allantoic fluid prostaglandin levels (7). Natural infection of guinea pigs with *C. psittaci* could alter research involving the lymphoreticular, reproductive, respiratory, and urinary systems.

Diagnosis and control
Diagnosis of *C. psittaci* infection is accomplished by staining conjunctival scrapings with special stains, including Gimenez, Machiavello's, and Giemsa (2). Treatment is with tetracycline antibiotics. Preventing entry of the pathogen into the colony is the ultimate key to control, and is accomplished by examination of health records and/or screening new animals prior to arrival. Guinea pig isolates of *C. psittaci* should be considered zoonotic, although most cases of zoonotic chlamydiosis (ornithosis) are acquired from birds.

Streptococcus pneumoniae

Agent
Streptococcus pneumoniae is a gram-positive diplococcus that may be found uncommonly in laboratory guinea pig colonies (14). Several strains or capsular serotypes have been identified. Serotype 19 has historically been considered the most common serotype isolated from guinea pigs (14, 16), although guinea pigs are susceptible to other serotypes (26).

Epidemiology
Transmission is primarily by aerosol and infections are thought to originate from infected humans. Multiplication within the respiratory tract, and therefore transmission, are enhanced by concurrent infection with Sendai virus (18). Additional aspects of the biology of *S. pneumoniae* have been presented in the section on pathogens of mice and rats.

Clinical signs
In guinea pigs, the organism is usually carried as a commensal, although guinea pig strains differ in susceptibility to infection (18). Clinical signs, when present, may include listlessness, ruffled fur, emaciation, dehydration, dyspnea, torticollis, nasal discharge, and variable mortality (10, 11, 17, 29). Young, pregnant, or otherwise stressed guinea pigs are more susceptible to disease (16).

Pathology
Hallmark pathologic changes include fibrino-purulent exudation or focal abscessation within several body cavities, including the pericardium (pericarditis), airways (pneumonia), thoracic cavity (pleuritis), abdomen (peritonitis), middle ear (otitis media), and elsewhere (10, 11, 15, 16, 17, 29). Experimentally, pneumolysin, a thiol-activated toxin of *S. pneumoniae*, causes ultrastructural cochlear damage (3, 28). Lastly, exposure of guinea pig lung homogenates to *S. pneumoniae* results in decreased numbers of β-adrenoceptors, suggesting a possible mechanism contributing to the pathogenesis of chronic bronchitis (19).

Immunity to *S. pneumoniae* is primarily humoral, although the complement (8) and mononuclear phagocytic systems also contribute substantially (9). In other hosts, C-reactive protein (20, 21), tumor necrosis factor alpha (TNF-α) (22), and pulmonary surfactant (24) also appear to play roles; while IL-10, induced following *S. pneumoniae* infection, attenuates the response within the lungs, hampering effective clearance of the infection and shortening survival (25). Findings from other host systems should however be considered cautiously since species differ in aspects of their response to *S. pneumoniae* (5).

Interference with research
Natural infections of laboratory rats and mice with *S. pneumoniae* have been shown to alter a variety of physiologic functions. These findings should be extrapolated to the guinea pig with caution. Use of the guinea pig-*S. pneumoniae* model in human auditory research (1, 2) has led to several reports of the effects of experimental *S. pneumoniae* infection on host physiology. For example, middle ear infection with *S. pneumoniae* induces localized lipid peroxide production (23) and causes ultrastructural damage to the organ of Corti (4, 27). Depending on organ systems involved, natural infection of guinea pigs with *S. pneumoniae* could compromise a variety of research efforts, most prominently those involving the cardiovascular, enterohepatic, nervous, and respiratory systems. It is likely that asymptomatic carriage of *S. pneumoniae* would have no deleterious effect on research efforts.

Diagnosis and control
Depending on site of infection, diagnosis of *S. pneumoniae* infection has historically been by Gram staining of direct smears of exudates, or cultivation of nasal swabs, which are highly reliable in revealing most symptomatic and asymptomatic infections (16, 17). ELISA technology has also been used experimentally (13). More recently, PCR fingerprinting analysis has proven useful (6). Diagnosis of otitis media is greatly facilitated by radiography. Treatment of infected guinea pigs is possible (7), although antibiotic resistance is common (12). Antibiotic resistance in some cases is due to the production of penicillin-binding protein 2a (30). A more sound approach to control is culling of known carriers. Preventive measures include prearrival testing of animals and education of caretakers in standards and methods of personal hygiene.

Streptococcus zooepidemicus

Agent
Streptococcus zooepidemicus is a gram-positive, encapsulated, β-hemolytic, Lancefield's group C coccus, which primarily affects horses, although other animals, including guinea pigs, may also be infected.

Epidemiology
Prevalence is low in modern laboratory animal facilities (5). Transmission is presumed to be by aerosol and/or contact.

Clinical signs
Females and certain strains of guinea pigs tend to be more susceptible to disease (6). Healthy guinea pigs may harbor the pathogen in the conjunctiva and/or nasal cavity (3).

Pathology
The pathogen may enter through abraded oral and other mucous membranes and through the intact conjunctiva (4). Affected animals may develop systemic infection with sepsis, fibrinopurulent bronchopneumonia, pleuritis, and pericarditis (6), or may develop more focal lesions such as otitis media, or submaxillary lymph node abscessation (3). The latter is also called cervical lymphadenitis and is a sequella to entry of the pathogen through abraded oral mucosa (4, 6). The fact that both pulmonary and middle ear infections sometimes occur simultaneously suggests that both ascending and descending infections occur and originate in the upper respiratory tract (1). Immunity is likely humoral, although this has not been thoroughly evaluated.

Interference with research

There is virtually no information available on the effects of *S. zooepidemicus* on guinea pig research. It can be assumed that infection could alter research involving the cardiovascular, lymphoreticular, and respiratory systems. In streptococcal infections of other hosts, bacterial toxins have been shown to alter host cell phagocytic activity (2, 8) and sperm motility (7). Caution is warranted before extrapolating these findings to *S. zooepidemicus* infections of guinea pigs.

Diagnosis and control

Diagnosis of *S. zooepidemicus* infection is easily accomplished by bacterial culture. Antibiotic treatment is unlikely to eradicate the pathogen from the colony entirely, although controlled studies are lacking. Until additional information is published, effective control is only accomplished by depopulation of infected colonies. Health screening conducted prior to receipt of guinea pigs should include testing for *S. zooepidemicus*.

PARASITES

Cryptosporidium wrairi

Agent

There is a growing number of members of the genus *Cryptosporidium*, as species previously thought to be common to multiple hosts are found to be sufficiently unique, using a variety of parameters, to warrant separate species designations (7, 8, 13, 18). Guinea pigs are host to *Cryptosporidium wrairi*, an opportunistic protozoon parasite in the phylum Apicomplexa.

Epidemiology

Prevalence may be high in conventional colonies, although published surveys are lacking. The prepatent period is 4 days and transmission is fecal-oral.

Clinical disease

Clinical disease is more common in young guinea pigs (10) and may be potentiated by *Escherichia coli* infection. Clinical signs may include diarrhea, weight loss, emaciation, and death (10).

Pathology

Gross findings of clinical disease include thin, "pot-bellied" guinea pigs with fluid-filled intestines (19). Acute histologic lesions include crypt epithelial hyperplasia, edema of the lamina propria, leukocytic infiltration, and villus tip necrosis and sloughing, followed chronically by villus atrophy and flattening (19). Lesions are generally worse in the jejunum, ileum, and cecum (19). The underlying pathogenesis in cryptosporidiosis appears to include malabsorption, intestinal injury, and prostaglandin-induced changes in NaCl transport mediated by the intestinal nervous system (1, 11, 12).

Immunity is primarily cell mediated (9, 15, 16, 20, 24, 25), is fully responsive about 3 weeks after infection (3), and is augmented by IL-12 induced interferon-γ (IFN-γ) production (21, 26). In addition, age-related immunity, unrelated to previous exposure, has been reported in sheep (17).

Interference with research

Little information is available on the effects of *C. wrairi* on guinea pig physiology, although a considerable body of literature is available from cryptosporidial infections of host species of greater economic importance, as well as from human infections. This information is reviewed here but should be extrapolated to the guinea pig with caution. Studies to confirm or dismiss similar effects in guinea pigs have not been reported. In avian systems, *Cryptosporidium baileyi* may potentiate disease caused by other pathogens, and may suppress immune responsiveness to vaccines and sheep red blood cells (sRBC) (22, 23). In vitro studies involving *Cryptosporidium parvum* infection of human cell cultures reveals that *C. parvum* modulates apoptosis in epithelial cells (6, 14), while in vivo studies reveal permanently stunted growth (4, 5). In rats, *C. parvum* inactivates intestinal phosphatases (2). Natural infection of laboratory guinea pigs with *C. wrairi* would likely alter results of studies involving the enterohepatic, lymphoreticular, and enteric nervous systems.

Diagnosis and control
Diagnosis of *C. wrairi* infection is based on identifying parasites in intestinal scrapings, either by phase-contrast microscopy or following acid-fast staining; and in hematoxylin-and-eosin-stained intestinal sections. More recently, PCR assays have also been used (18). A variety of treatments have been recommended for eliminating cryptosporidia of other host species, with limited success. Infected colonies are best depopulated and reestablished with *C. wrairi*-free stock.

Eimeria caviae

Agent
Guinea pigs may serve as hosts for a large number of parasitic protozoa (19). However, few of them are thought to alter host physiology, and fewer still are associated with clinical disease. *Eimeria caviae* is an Apicomplexan parasite capable of causing disease in guinea pigs.

Epidemiology
E. caviae was first identified as a cause of morbidity nearly 100 years ago. The parasite is a typical coccidium with a direct life cycle. Development occurs in the colonic epithelium, primarily in the proximal portions. The prepatent period is 11 to 12 days. Unsporulated oocysts are passed in the feces, sporulate, and thereby become infectious to another host. Transmission is naturally fecal-oral. While historically high (11), prevalence is now thought to be low in well-managed colonies.

Clinical signs
Clinical signs of *E. caviae* infection are usually absent in mature pigs. Clinical disease is more common in young pigs and in those with hypovitaminosis C (19), and when present, frequently occurs as explosive outbreaks following shipping (6, 8, 11). In addition, some have reported seasonal variation in disease incidence and mortality rates, with both parameters being elevated in the spring (10, 11). In heavy infections, clinical signs may include diarrhea followed by constipation, dehydration, anorexia, hunched posture, weight loss, and occasionally death (7, 10).

Pathology
Gross findings include colonic edema, mucosal hyperemia, petechial hemorrhages, and nodule formation. Colonic contents may be watery and fetid. Histologically, there is marked colonic mucosal hyperplasia, degeneration and desquamation of the epithelium, and neutrophilic and lymphocytic infiltration of the lamina propria. Developmental stages can be identified in colonic epithelium, which may slough in patches (10, 19). As with *Eimeria* infections of other animals, immunity is primarily cell mediated (9, 12).

Interference with research
There is little information concerning the effects of *E. caviae* on its host, other than what can be inferred from the clinical effects of the pathogen, such as alterations in protein metabolism due to anorexia (17). Information gleaned from studies of *Eimeria* sp. infections in other host species suggest that consideration at least be given to possible effects of *E. caviae* on guinea pig physiology, while recognizing that *Eimeria* species differ greatly in pathogenicity. The preponderance of information comes from studies of avian coccidiosis. For example, *Eimeria* sp. have been shown to affect cecal bacterial (5) and intestinal lymphocyte populations (2) in chickens, and levels of stress hormones in turkeys (1). In addition, *Eimeria magna* alters Na^+-stimulated glucose absorption in the parasitized rabbit ileum (16). There is a considerable body of literature describing the interactions of coccidia with other types of pathogens, including viruses (14), nematodes (4, 13, 15), and protozoa (3). These relationships have not been evaluated in guinea pigs. At the least, it is likely that heavy natural infection of guinea pigs with *E. caviae* would alter studies involving the

enterohepatic system. It is also likely that physiologic changes do not occur in mildly infected guinea pigs.

Diagnosis and control
Diagnosis of *E. caviae* infection is first attempted by examining feces for large numbers of oocysts, but may be confirmed by histologic examination of the colon. Strict attention to hygiene facilitates control of this infection. Both antibiotics (19) and cesarean rederivation (18) have been used to eliminate the infection. Prevention is through obtaining *E. caviae*-free guinea pigs, and adherence to strict husbandry standards.

Trixacarus caviae

Agent
Guinea pigs may be infested with several ectoparasite species. Most are uncommon in laboratory settings and their presentation here is therefore unwarranted. Among those still occurring in laboratory-quality guinea pigs is *Trixacarus caviae*, a sarcoptid (burrowing) mite, which may also transiently infest humans (4, 6).

Epidemiology
Transmission between hosts is by contact.

Clinical signs
Moderate to severe infestation presents as mange, mainly around the head, neck, and shoulders, but also extending to the back, ventral abdomen, flanks, and thighs (5, 7, 8). In very severe cases, the entire body may be involved (11). Clinical signs include alopecia (hair loss); "bran-like" or crusted, dried serum exudates on the skin; anorexia; frantic activity followed later by the lethargy accompanying debilitation; progressive emaciation; pruritus; and vocalizing (5, 11, 13).

Pathology
Infested animals may excoriate themselves by biting and scratching affected areas, often leading to localized skin trauma, secondary bacterial infections, and death. Histologically, the lesions consist of acanthosis, hyperkeratosis, and exfoliative dermatitis, with accumulation of lymphocytes, monocytes, and eosinophils (5, 7, 8, 11). Even mild infestations may result in reactive changes in local lymph nodes (10). Mites may be observed in epidermal tunnels (6). Hematologic changes may include neutrophilia, monocytosis, eosinophilia, and basophilia (10).

Immunity is likely cell mediated, as described for *Sarcoptes scabiei* infestation of swine (1). Interestingly, Rothwell and coworkers (9) reported that guinea pigs bred for resistance to the nematode parasite *Trichostrongylus colubriformis*, were more susceptible to severe infestation with *T. caviae*. This suggests that shifting of T-cell populations toward those indirectly associated with antibody production increases susceptibility to *T. caviae*.

Interference with research
There is a paucity of information concerning the behavioral and physiologic effects of *T. caviae* infestation on guinea pigs. Intense pruritus could be expected to affect results of behavioral studies and decrease food consumption. The latter would alter studies in which normal nutrition is important. Likewise, hematologic changes would interfere with studies in which those parameters are assessed. Obviously, dermatologic studies would also be severely compromised. While there is no information to directly support it, one should consider the possibility that products from *T. caviae* might modulate the host immune response in a manner similar to that reported for some other ectoparasites (2, 12).

Diagnosis and control
T. caviae may be diagnosed by careful examination of 10% KOH-treated skin scrapings, recognizing that guinea pigs may also be infested with other superficially similarly appearing sarcoptid mites, namely *Notoedres* sp. and *S. scabiei* (3, 8). Treatment is accomplished by ivermectin treatment, as described for acariasis of mice and rats. Diazepam may be indicated to ameliorate pruritic "fits" after ivermectin therapy. Guinea pigs should be free

TABLE 5-1. Body systems known or likely to be affected by pathogen indicated

Pathogen	Cardio-vascular	Dermal	Endocrine	Entero-hepatic	Hema-topoietic	Lympho-reticular	Musculo-skeletal	Nervous	Reproductive	Respiratory	Urinary
Cytomegalovirus				×	×	×		×	×	×	×
Lymphocytic choriomeningitis virus			×	×	×	×	×	×		×	×
Bordetella bronchiseptica	×					×		×		×	
Chlamydophila psittaci				×		×		×	×	×	×
Streptococcus pneumoniae	×	×						×			
Streptococcus zooepidemicus	×					×		×		×	
Cryptosporidium wrairi				×							
Eimeria caviae				×							
Trixacarus caviae		×			×	×					

of *T. caviae* prior to entering the animal facility, or should be quarantined and examined for mites prior to release into the colony.

REFERENCES
VIRUSES
Cytomegalovirus

1. **Arkonac, B., K. A. Mauch, S. Chou, and J. D. Hosenpud.** 1997. Low multiplicity of cytomegalovirus infection of human aortic smooth muscle cells increases levels of major histocompatibility complex class I antigens and induces a proinflammatory cytokine milieu in the absence of cytopathology. *J. Heart Lung Transplant.* **16:**1035–1045.
2. **Booss, J., and J. H. Kim.** 1989. Cytomegalovirus encephalitis: neuropathological comparison of the guinea pig model with the opportunistic infection in AIDS. *Yale J. Biol. Med.* **62:**187–195.
3. **Bratcher, D. F., N. Bourne, F. J. Bravo, M. R. Schleiss, M. Slaoui, M. G. Myers, and D. I. Berstein.** 1995. Effect of passive antibody on congenital cytomegalovirus infection in guinea pigs. *J. Infect. Dis.* **172:**944–950.
4. **Bu, F. R., and B. P. Griffith.** 1990. Immunoblot analysis of the humoral immune response to cytomegalovirus in non-pregnant and pregnant guinea pigs. *Arch. Virol.* **110:**247–254.
5. **Cinatl, J., Jr., R. Kotchetkov, M. Scholz, J. Cinatl, J. U. Vogel, P. H. Driever, and H. W. Doerr.** 1999. Human cytomegalovirus infection decreases expression of thrombospondin-1 independent of the tumor suppressor protein 53. *Am. J. Pathol.* **155:**285–292.
6. **Cook, J. E.** 1958. Salivary-gland virus disease of guinea pigs. *J. Natl. Cancer Inst.* **20:**905–909.
7. **Davis, L. E.** 1993. Viruses and vestibular neuritis: review of human and animal studies. *Acta Otolaryngol. Suppl.* **503:**70–73.
8. **Fong, C. K., F. Bia, and G. D. Hsiung.** 1980. Ultrastructural development and persistence of guinea pig cytomegalovirus in duct cells of guinea pig submaxillary gland. *Arch. Virol.* **64:**97–108.
9. **Geist, L. J., and L. Y. Dai.** 2000. Immediate early gene 2 of human cytomegalovirus increases interleukin 2 receptor-alpha gene expression. *J. Investig. Med.* **48:**60–65.
10. **Griffith, B. P., M. Chen, and H. C. Isom.** 1990. Role of primary and secondary maternal viremia in transplacental guinea pig cytomegalovirus infection. *J. Virol.* **64:**1991–1997.
11. **Griffith, B. P., and G. D. Hsiung.** 1980. Cytomegalovirus infection in guinea pigs. IV. Maternal infection at different stages of gestation. *J. Infect. Dis.* **141:**787–793.

12. Griffith, B. P., H. C. Isom, and J. T. Lavallee. 1990. Cellular localization of cytomegalovirus nucleic acids in guinea pig salivary glands by in situ hybridization. *J. Virol. Methods* **27:**145–157.
13. Harrison, C. J., and R. Burger. 1991. Low maternal CD4 count at inception of gestational cytomegalovirus (CMV) infection and impaired humoral response: effect on congenital CMV infection in the guinea pig. *Clin. Immunol. Immunopathol.* **60:**171–180.
14. Harrison, C. J., and N. Caruso. 2000. Correlation of maternal and pup NK-like activity and TNF responses against cytomegalovirus to pregnancy outcome in inbred guinea pigs. *J. Med. Virol.* **60:**230–236.
15. Harrison, C. J., and M. G. Myers. 1989. Maternal cell-mediated cytolysis of CMV-infected fetal cells and the outcome of pregnancy in the guinea pig. *J. Med. Virol.* **27:**66–71.
16. Harrison, C. J., and M. G. Myers. 1990. Relation of maternal CMV viremia and antibody response to the rate of congenital infection and intrauterine growth retardation. *J. Med. Virol.* **31:**222–228.
17. Holberg-Petersen, M., H. Rollag, S. Beck, and M. Degre. 1997. The effect of human cytomegalovirus on selected functions of peripheral blood monocytes. *APMIS* **105:**89–98.
18. Johnson, K. P., and W. S. Connor. 1976. Guinea pig cytomegalovirus: transplacental transmission. Brief report. *Arch. Virol.* **59:**263–267.
19. Kacica, M. A., C. J. Harrison, M. G. Myers, and D. I. Bernstein. 1990. Immune response to guinea pig cytomegalovirus polypeptides and cross reactivity with human cytomegalovirus. *J. Med. Virol.* **32:**155–159.
20. Miller, D. M., Y. Zhang, B. M. Rahill, K. Kazor, S. Rofagha, J. J. Eckel, and D. D. Sedmak. 2000. Human cytomegalovirus blocks interferon-gamma stimulated up-regulation of major histocompatibility complex class I expression and the class I antigen processing machinery. *Transplantation* **69:**687–690.
21. Motzel, S. L., and J. E. Wagner. 1989. Diagnostic Exercise: Fetal death in guinea pigs. *Lab. Anim. Sci.* **39:**342–344.
22. Penfold, M. E., D. J. Dairaghi, G. M. Duke, N. Saederup, E. S. Mocarski, G. W. Kemble, and T. J. Schall. 1999. Cytomegalovirus encodes a potent alpha chemokine. *Proc. Natl. Acad. Sci. USA* **96:**9839–9844.
23. Piazze, J., G. Nigro, M. Mazzocco, E. Marchiani, V. Brancato, M. M. Anceschi, and E. V. Cosmi. 1999. The effect of primary cytomegalovirus infection on fetal lung maturity indices. *Early Hum. Dev.* **54:**137–144.
24. Sindre, H., H. Rollag, M. Degre, and K. Hestadal. 2000. Human cytomegalovirus induced inhibition of hematopoietic cell line growth is initiated by events taking place before translation of viral gene products. *Arch. Virol.* **145:**99–111.
25. Strauss, M., and B. P. Griffith. 1991. Guinea pig model of transplacental congenital cytomegaloviral infection with analysis of labyrinthitis. *Am. J. Otol.* **12:**97–100.
26. Van Hoosier, G. L., Jr., W. E. Giddens, Jr., C. S. Gillett, and H. Davis. 1985. Disseminated cytomegalovirus disease in the guinea pig. *Lab. Anim. Sci.* **35:**81–84.
27. Van Hoosier, G. L., Jr., and L. R. Robinette. 1976. Viral and chlamydial diseases, p. 137–152. In J. E. Wagner and P. J. Manning (ed.), *The Biology of the Guinea Pig*. Academic Press, Inc., New York, N.Y.
28. Yourtee, E. L., F. J. Bia, B. P. Griffith, and R. K. Root. 1982. Neutrophil response and function during acute cytomegalovirus infection in guinea pigs. *Infect. Immun.* **36:**11–16.
29. Zheng, Z. M., J. T. Lavallee, F. J. Bia, and B. P. Griffith. 1987. Thymic hypoplasia, splenomegaly and immune depression in guinea pigs with neonatal cytomegalovirus infection. *Dev. Comp. Immunol.* **11:**407–418.

Lymphocytic choriomeningitis virus

1. Djavani, M., I. S. Lukashevich, and M. S. Salvato. 1998. Sequence comparison of the large genomic RNA segments of two strains of lymphocytic choriomeningitis virus differing in pathogenic potential for guinea pigs. *Virus Genes* **17:**151–155.
2. Kraft, V., and B. Meyer. 1990. Seromonitoring in small laboratory animal colonies. A five year survey: 1984–1988. *Z. Verstierkd.* **33:**29–35.
3. Martinez-Paralta, L. A., M. Laguens, C. Ponzinibbio, and R. P. Laguens. 1990. Infection of guinea pigs with two strains of lymphocytic choriomeningitis virus. *Medicina* **50:**225–229.
4. Riviere, Y., R. Ahmed, P. J. Southern, M. J. Buchmeier, and M. B. Oldstone. 1985. Genetic mapping of lymphocytic choriomeningitis virus pathogenicity: virulence in guinea pigs is associated with the L RNA segment. *J. Virol.* **55:**704–709.
5. Sato, H., and H. Miyata. 1986. Detection of lymphocytic choriomeningitis virus antibody in colonies of laboratory animals in Japan. *Jikken Dobutsu* **35:**189–192.
6. Van Hoosier, G. L., Jr., and L. R. Robinette. 1976. Viral and chlamydial diseases, p. 137–152. In J. E. Wagner and P. J. Manning (ed.), *The Biology of the Guinea Pig*. Academic Press, Inc., New York, N.Y.

7. **Webster, J. M., and B. E. Kirk.** 1974. Neutralizing antibody response of guinea pigs to lymphocytic choriomeningitis virus. *Infect. Immun.* **10:**516–519.

BACTERIA

Bordetella bronchiseptica
1. **Bemis, D. A., H. A. Greisen, and M. J. Appel.** 1977. Bacteriological variation among *Bordetella bronchiseptica* isolates from dogs and other species. *J. Clin. Microbiol.* **5:**471–480.
2. **Binns, S. H., A. J. Speakman, S. Dawson, M. Bennett, R. M. Gaskell, and C. A. Hart.** 1998. The use of pulsed-field gel electrophoresis to examine the epidemiology of *Bordetella bronchiseptica* isolated from cats and other species. *Epidemiol. Infect.* **120:**201–208.
3. **Boot, R., and H. C. Walvoort.** 1986. Otitis media in guinea pigs: pathology and bacteriology. *Lab. Anim.* **20:**242–248.
4. **Burns, E. H., Jr., J. M. Norman, M. D. Hatcher, and D. A. Bemis.** 1993. Fimbriae and determination of host species specificity of *Bordetella bronchiseptica*. *J. Clin. Microbiol.* **31:**1838–1844.
5. **Cotter, P. A., M. H. Yuk, S. Mattoo, B. J. Akerley, J. Boschwitz, D. A. Relman, and J. F. Miller.** 1998. Filamentous hemagglutinin of *Bordetella bronchiseptica* is required for efficient establishment of tracheal colonization. *Infect. Immun.* **66:**5921–5929.
6. **Endoh, M., M. Amitani, and Y. Nakase.** 1986. Effect of purified heat-labile toxin of *Bordetella bronchiseptica* on the peripheral blood vessels in guinea pigs or suckling mice. *Microbiol. Immunol.* **30:**1327–1330.
7. **Forde, C. B., X. Shi, J. Li, and M. Roberts.** 1999. *Bordetella bronchiseptica*-mediated cytotoxicity to macrophages is dependent on bvg-regulated factors, including pertactin. *Infect. Immun.* **67:**5972–5978.
8. **Gawin, A. Z., M. Kaliner, and J. N. Baraniuk.** 1998. Enhancement of histamine-induced permeability to guinea pigs infected with *Bordetella bronchiseptica*. *Am. J. Rhinol.* **12:**143–147.
9. **Hozbor, D., F. Fouque, and N. Guiso.** 1999. Detection of *Bordetella bronchiseptica* by the polymerase chain reaction. *Res. Microbiol.* **150:**333–341.
10. **Matherne, C. M., E. K. Steffen, and J. E. Wagner.** 1987. Efficacy of commercial vaccines for protecting guinea pigs against *Bordetella bronchiseptica* pneumonia. *Lab. Anim. Sci.* **37:**191–194.
11. **Mattoo, S., J. F. Miller, and P. A. Cotter.** 2000. Role of *Bordetella bronchiseptica* fimbriae in tracheal colonization and development of a humoral immune response. *Infect. Immun.* **68:**2024–2033.
12. **Nakagawa, M., M. Saito, E. Suzuki, K. Nakayama, J. Matsubara, and K. Matsuno.** 1986. A survey of *Streptococcus pneumoniae*, *Streptococcus zooepidemicus*, *Salmonella* spp., *Bordetella bronchiseptica* and Sendai virus in guinea pig colonies in Japan. *Jikken Dobutsu* **35:**517–520.
13. **Nakai, T., A. Sawata, and K. Kume.** 1985. Intracellular locations of dermonecrotizing toxins in *Pasteurella multocida* and in *Bordetella bronchiseptica*. *Am. J. Vet. Res.* **46:**870–874.
14. **Ohnishi, T., Y. Horiguchi, M. Masuda, N. Sugimoto, and M. Matsuda.** 1998. *Pasteurella multocida* toxin and *Bordetella bronchiseptica* dermonecrotizing toxin elicit similar effects on cultured cells by different mechanisms. *J. Vet. Med. Sci.* **60:**301–305.
15. **Percy, D. H., and S. W. Barthold.** 2001. *Pathology of Laboratory Rodents and Rabbits*, 2nd ed. Iowa State University Press, Ames.
16. **Register, K. B., A. Boisvert, and M. R. Ackermann.** 1997. Use of ribotyping to distinguish *Bordetella bronchiseptica* isolates. *Int. J. Syst. Bacteriol.* **47:**678–683.
17. **Stephenson, E. J., C. J. Trahan, J. W. Ezzell, W. C. Mitchell, T. G. Abshire, D. D. Oland, and G. O. Neson.** 1989. Efficacy of a commercial bacterin in protecting strain 13 guinea pigs against *Bordetella bronchiseptica* pneumonia. *Lab. Anim.* **23:**261–269.
18. **Trahan, C. J., E. H. Stephenson, J. W. Ezzell, and W. C. Mitchell.** 1987. Airborne-induced experimental *Bordetella bronchiseptica* pneumonia in strain 13 guinea pigs. *Lab. Anim.* **21:**226–232.
19. **Wagner, J. E., D. R. Owens, D. F. Kusewitt, and E. A. Corley.** 1976. Otitis media of guinea pigs. *Lab. Anim. Sci.* **26:**902–907.
20. **Wullenweber, M., and R. Boot.** 1994. Interlaboratory comparison of enzyme-linked immunosorbent assay (ELISA) and indirect immunofluorescence (IIF) for detection of *Bordetella bronchiseptica* antibodies in guinea pigs. *Lab. Anim.* **28:**335–339.
21. **Yuk, M. H., E. T. Harvill, P. A. Cotter, and J. F. Miller.** 2000. Modulation of host immune responses, induction of apoptosis and inhibition of NF-kappaB activation by the *Bordetella* type III secretion system. *Mol. Microbiol.* **35:**991–1004.

Chlamydophila psittaci
1. **Batteiger, B. E., and R. G. Rank.** 1987. Analysis of the humoral immune response to chlamydial genital infection in guinea pigs. *Infect. Immun.* **55:**1767–1773.
2. **Biberstein, E. L., and D. C. Hirsh.** 1999. *Chlamydiae*, p. 173–177. *In* D. C. Hirsh and

Y. C. Zee (ed.), *Veterinary Microbiology.* Blackwell Science, Inc., Malden, Mass.

3. **Darville, T., K. K. Laffoon, L. R. Kishen, and R. G. Rank.** 1995. Tumor necrosis factor alpha activity in genital tract secretions of guinea pigs infected with chlamydiae. *Infect. Immun.* **63:** 4675–4681.

4. **Deeb, B. J., R. F. DiGiacomo, and S. P. Wang.** 1989. Guinea pig inclusion conjunctivitis (GPIC) in a commercial colony. *Lab. Anim.* **23:** 103–106.

5. **Everett, K. D., and A. A. Andersen.** 1997. The ribosomal intergenic spacer and domain I of the 23S rRNA gene are phylogenetic markers for *Chlamydia* spp. *Int. J. Syst. Bacteriol.* **47:**461–473.

6. **Forsey, T., and S. Darougar.** 1981. Transmission of chlamydiae by the housefly. *Br. J. Ophthalmol.* **65:**147–150.

7. **Howie, A., H. A. Leaver, I. D. Aitken, L. A. Hay, I. E. Anderson, G. E. Williams, and G. Jones.** 1989. The effect of chlamydial infection on the initiation of premature labour: serial measurements of intrauterine prostaglandin E2 in amniotic fluid, allantoic fluid and utero-ovarian vein, using catheterised sheep experimentally infected with an ovine abortion strain of *Chlamydia psittaci. Prostaglandins Leukot. Essent. Fatty Acids* **37:**203–311.

8. **Kuroda-Kitagawa, Y., C. Suzuki-Muramatsu, T. Yamaguchi, H. Fukushi, and K. Hirai.** 1993. Antigenic analysis of *Chlamydia pecorum* and mammalian *Chlamydia psittaci* by use of monoclonal antibodies to the major outer membrane protein and a 56- to 64-kd protein. *Am. J. Vet. Res.* **54:**709–712.

9. **Lammert, J. K., and P. B. Wyrick.** 1982. Modulation of the host immune response as a result of *Chlamydia psittaci* infection. *Infect. Immun.* **35:**537–545.

10. **Ojcius, D. M., P. Souque, J. L. Perfettini, and A. Dautry-Varsat.** 1999. Apoptosis of epithelial cells and macrophages due to infection with the obligate intracellular pathogen *Chlamydia psittaci. J. Immunol.* **161:**4220–4226.

11. **Perez-Martinez, J. A., and J. Storz.** 1985. Antigenic diversity of *Chlamydia psittaci* of mammalian origin determined by microimmunofluorescence. *Infect. Immun.* **50:**905–910.

12. **Prain, C. J., and J. H. Pearce.** 1989. Ultrastructural studies on the intracellular fate of *Chlamydia psittaci* (strain guinea pig inclusion conjunctivitis) and *Chlamydia trachomatis* (strain lymphogranuloma venereum 434): modulation of intracellular events and relationship with endocytic mechanism. *J. Gen. Microbiol.* **135:**2107–2123.

13. **Pudjiatmoko, F. H., Y. Ochiai, T. Yamaguchi, and K. Hirai.** 1997. Phylogenetic analysis of the genus *Chlamydia* based on 16S rRNA gene expression. *Int. J. Syst. Bacteriol.* **47:**425–431.

14. **Rank, R. G., H. J. White, and A. L. Barron.** 1979. Humoral immunity in the resolution of genital infection in female guinea pigs infected with the agent of guinea pig inclusion conjunctivitis. *Infect. Immun.* **26:**573–579.

15. **Rank, R. G., H. J. White, A. J. Hough, Jr., J. N. Pasley, and A. L. Barron.** 1982. Effect of estradiol on chlamydial genital infection of female guinea pigs. *Infect. Immun.* **38:**699–705.

16. **Rank, R. G., H. J. White, B. L. Soloff, and A. L. Barron.** 1981. Cystitis associated with chlamydial infection of the genital tract in male guinea pigs. *Sex. Transm. Dis.* **8:**203–210.

17. **Register, K. B., P. A. Morgan, and P. B. Wyrick.** 1986. Interaction between *Chlamydia* spp. and human polymorphonuclear leukocytes in vitro. *Infect. Immun.* **52:**664–670.

18. **Rothermel, C. D., B. Y. Rubin, and H. W. Murray.** 1983. Gamma-interferon is the factor in lymphokine that activates human macrophages to inhibit intracellular *Chlamydia psittaci* replication. *J. Immunol.* **131:**2542–2544.

19. **Senyk, G., R. Kerlan, D. P. Stites, D. J. Schanzlin, H. B. Ostler, L. Hanna, H. Keshishyan, and E. Jawetz.** 1981. Cell-mediated and humoral immune responses to chlamydial antigens in guinea pigs infected ocularly with the agent of guinea pig inclusion conjunctivitis. *Infect. Immun.* **32:**304–310.

20. **Soloff, B. L., R. G. Rank, and A. L. Barron.** 1985. Electron microscopic observations concerning the in vivo uptake and release of the agent of guinea-pig inclusion conjunctivitis (*Chlamydia psittaci*) in guinea-pig exocervix. *J. Comp. Pathol.* **95:**335–344.

21. **Treharne, J. D., and A. Shallal.** 1991. The antigenic specificity of the humoral immune responses to primary and repeated ocular infections of the guinea pig with the GPIC agent (*Chlamydia psittaci*). *Eye* **5:**299–305.

22. **Van Hoosier, G. L., Jr., and L. R. Robinette.** 1976. Viral and chlamydial diseases, p. 137–152. *In* J. E. Wagner and P. J. Manning (ed.), *The Biology of the Guinea Pig.* Academic Press, Inc., New York, N.Y.

23. **Watkins, N. G., W. J. Hadlow, A. B. Moos, and H. D. Caldwell.** 1986. Ocular delayed hypersensitivity: a pathogenetic mechanism of chlamydial-conjunctivitis in guinea pigs. *Proc. Natl. Acad. Sci. USA* **83:**7480–7484.

24. **Westbay, T. D., C. C. Dascher, R. C. Hsia, M. Zauderer, and P. M. Bavoil.** 1995. De-

viation of immune response to *Chlamydia psittaci* outer membrane protein in lipopolysaccharide-hyporesponsive mice. *Infect. Immun.* **63**:1391–1393.
25. **White, H. J., R. G. Rank, B. L. Soloff, and A. L. Barron.** 1979. Experimental chlamydial salpingitis in immunosuppressed guinea pigs infected in the genital tract with the agent of guinea pig inclusion conjunctivitis. *Infect. Immun.* **26**:728–735.

Streptococcus pneumoniae
1. **Barry, B., M. Muttat-Joly, P. Gehanno, and J. J. Pocidalo.** 1993. Physiopathological and therapeutic values of experimental model of acute otitis media. *Ann. Otolaryngol. Chir. Cervicofac.* **110**:326–331.
2. **Blank, A. L., G. L. Davis, T. R. VanDeWater, and R. J. Ruben.** 1994. Acute *Streptococcus pneumoniae* meningogenic labyrinthitis. An experimental guinea pig model and literature review. *Arch. Otolaryngol. Head Neck Surg.* **120**:1342–1346.
3. **Comis, S. D., M. P. Osborne, J. Stephen, M. J. Tarlow, T. L. Hayward, T. J. Mitchell, P. W. Andrew, and G. J. Boulnois.** 1993. Cytotoxic effects on hair cells of guinea pig cochlea produced by pneumolysin, the thiol activated toxin of *Streptococcus pneumoniae*. *Acta Otolaryngol.* **113**:152–159.
4. **Cook, R. D., D. S. Postma, G. M. Brinson, J. Prazma, and H. C. Pillsbury.** 1999. Cytotoxic changes in hair cells secondary to pneumococcal middle-ear infection. *J. Otolaryngol.* **28**:325–331.
5. **Coonrod, J. D., R. Varble, and M. C. Jarrells.** 1990. Species variation in the mechanism of killing of inhaled pneumococci. *J. Lab. Clin. Med.* **116**:354–362.
6. **Gerardoa, S. H., D. M. Citron, and E. J. Goldstein.** 2000. PCR fingerprinting analysis for differentiation of *Streptococcus pneumoniae* reinfection versus relapse. *Diagn. Microbiol. Infect. Dis.* **36**:275–278.
7. **Hori, R., H. Araki, M. Yonezawa, S. Minami, and Y. Watanabe.** 2000. Therapeutic effects of parenteral beta-lactam antibiotics on experimental otitis media caused by penicillin-resistant *Streptococcus pneumoniae* in guinea-pigs. *J. Antimicrob. Chemother.* **45**:311–314.
8. **Hummell, D. S., R. W. Berninger, A. Tomasz, and J. A. Winkelstein.** 1981. The fixation of C3b to pneumococcal cell wall polymers as a result of activation of the alternative complement pathway. *J. Immunol.* **127**:1287–1289.
9. **Kaneda, N., H. Kawauchi, and G. Mogi.** 1991. Role of phagocytes in antimicrobial defense of the middle ear. *Auris Nasus Larynx* **18**:331–342.
10. **Keyhani, M., and R. Naghshineh.** 1974. Spontaneous epizootic of pneumococcus infection in guinea-pigs. *Lab. Anim.* **8**:47–49.
11. **Kohn, D. F.** 1974. Bacterial otitis media in the guinea pig. *Lab. Anim. Sci.* **24**:823–825.
12. **Mason, E. O., Jr., L. B. Lamberth, N. L. Kershaw, B. L. Prosser, A. Zoe, and P. G. Ambrose.** 2000. *Streptococcus pneumoniae* in the USA: in vitro susceptibility and pharmacodynamic analysis. *J. Antimicrob. Chemother.* **45**:623–631.
13. **Matsubara, J., T. Kamiyama, T. Miyoshi, H. Ueda, M. Saito, and M. Nakagawa.** 1988. Serodiagnosis of *Streptococcus pneumoniae* infection in guinea pigs by an enzyme-linked immunosorbent assay. *Lab. Anim.* **22**:304–308.
14. **Nakagawa, M., M. Saito, E. Suzuki, K. Nakayama, J. Matsubara, and K. Matsuno.** 1986. A survey of *Streptococcus pneumoniae*, *Streptococcus zooepidemicus*, *Salmonella* spp., *Bordetella bronchiseptica* and Sendai virus in guinea pig colonies in Japan. *Jikken Dobutsu* **35**:517–520.
15. **Parker, G. A., R. J. Russel, and A. Paoli.** 1977. Extrapulmonary lesions of *Streptococcus pneumoniae* infection in guinea pigs. *Vet. Pathol.* **14**:332–337.
16. **Percy, D. H., and S. W. Barthold.** 2001. *Pathology of Laboratory Rodents and Rabbits*, 2nd ed. Iowa State University Press, Ames.
17. **Saito, M., T. Muto, S. Haruzono, M. Nakagawa, and M. Sato.** 1983. An epizootic of pneumococcal infection occurred in inbred guinea pig colonies. *Jikken Dobutsu* **32**:29–37.
18. **Saito, M., K. Nakayama, J. Matsubara, K. Matsuno, and M. Nakagawa.** 1988. Enhanced multiplication and transmission of *Streptococcus pneumoniae* in guinea pigs by Sendai virus infection. *Jikken Dobutsu* **37**:59–65.
19. **Schreurs, A. J., J. Verhoef, and F. P. Nijkamp.** 1983. Bacterial cell wall components decrease the number of guinea-pig lung beta-adrenoceptors. *Eur. J. Pharmacol.* **87**:127–132.
20. **Szalai, A. J., D. E. Briles, and J. E. Volanakis.** 1995. Human C-reactive protein is protective against fatal *Streptococcus pneumoniae* infection in transgenic mice. *J. Immunol.* **155**:2557–2563.
21. **Szalai, A. J., D. E. Briles, and J. E. Volanakis.** 1996. Role of complement in C-reactive-protein-mediated protection of mice from *Streptococcus pneumoniae*. *Infect. Immun.* **64**:4850–4853.
22. **Takashima, K., K. Tateda, T. Matsumoto, Y. Iizawa, M. Nakao, and K. Yamaguchi.** 1997. Role of tumor necrosis factor alpha in pathogenesis of pneumococcal pneumonia in mice. *Infect. Immun.* **65**:257–260.

23. Takoudes, T. G., and J. Haddad, Jr. 2001. Free radical production by antibiotic-killed bacteria in the guinea pig middle ear. *Laryngoscope* **111**:283–289.
24. Tino, M. J., and J. R. Wright. 1996. Surfactant protein A stimulates phagocytosis of specific pulmonary pathogens by alveolar macrophages. *Am. J. Physiol.* **270**:L677–L688.
25. Van der Poll, T., A. Marchant, C. V. Keogh, M. Goldman, and S. F. Lowry. 1996. Interleukin-10 impairs host defense in murine pneumococcal pneumonia. *J. Infect. Dis.* **174**:994–1000.
26. Vinnik, A. L., and S. I. Elkina. 1984. Cross infection of guinea pigs with different pneumococcal serotypes in the presence of the carrier state. *Zh. Mikrobiol. Epidemiol. Immunobiol.* **2**:32–36.
27. Winter, A. J., S. D. Comis, M. P. Osborne, T. L. Hayward, J. Stephen, and M. J. Tarlow. 1998. Ototoxicity resulting from intracochlear perfusion of *Streptococcus pneumoniae* in the guinea pig is modified by cefotaxime or amoxycillin pretreatment. *J. Infect.* **36**:73–77.
28. Winter, A. J., S. D. Comis, M. P. Osborne, M. J. Tarlow, J. Stephen, P. W. Andrew, J. Hill, and T. J. Mitchell. 1997. A role for pneumolysin but not neuraminidase in the hearing loss and cochlear damage induced by experimental pneumococcal meningitis in guinea pigs. *Infect. Immun.* **65**:4411–4418.
29. Witt, W. M., G. B. Hubbard, and J. W. Fanton. 1988. *Streptococcus pneumoniae* arthritis and osteomyelitis with Vitamin C deficiency in guinea pigs. *Lab. Anim. Sci.* **38**:192–194.
30. Zhao, G., T. I. Meier, J. Hoskins, and K. A. McAllister. 2000. Identification and characterization of the Penicillin-Binding Protein 2a of *Streptococcus pneumoniae* and its possible role in resistance to beta-lactam antibiotics. *Antimicrob. Agents Chemother.* **44**:1745–1748.

Streptococcus zooepidemicus
1. Boot, R., and H. C. Walvoort. 1986. Otitis media in guinea pigs: pathology and bacteriology. *Lab. Anim.* **20**:242–248.
2. Chaussee, M. S., R. L. Cole, and J. P. van Putten. 2000. Streptococcal erythrogenic toxin B abrogates fibronectin-dependent internalization of *Streptococcus pyogenes* by cultured mammalian cells. *Infect. Immun.* **68**:3226–3232.
3. Ito, M., T. Nishihara, T. Magaribuchi, and K. Koshimizu. 1978. Three cases of hemolytic *Streptococcus* infection in guinea-pigs. *Jikken Dobutsu* **27**:177–181.
4. Murphy, J. C., J. I. Ackerman, R. P. Marini, and J. G. Fox. 1991. Cervical lymphadenitis in guinea pigs: infection via intact ocular and nasal mucosa by *Streptococcus zooepidemicus*. *Lab. Anim. Sci.* **41**:251–254.
5. Nakagawa, M., M. Saito, E. Suzuki, K. Nakayama, J. Matsubara, and K. Matsuno. 1986. A survey of *Streptococcus pneumoniae*, *Streptococcus zooepidemicus*, *Salmonella* spp., *Bordetella bronchiseptica* and Sendai virus in guinea pig colonies in Japan. *Jikken Dobutsu* **35**:517–520.
6. Percy, D. H., and S. W. Barthold. 2001. *Pathology of Laboratory Rodents and Rabbits*, 2nd ed. Iowa State University Press, Ames.
7. Rideout, M. I., S. J. Burns, and R. B. Simpson. 1982. Influence of bacterial products on the motility of stallion spermatozoa. *J. Reprod. Fertil. Suppl.* **32**:35–40.
8. Wibawan, I. W., F. H. Pasaribu, I. H. Utama, A. Abdulmawjood, and C. Lammler. 1999. The role of hyaluronic acid capsular material of *Streptococcus equi* subsp. *zooepidemicus* inmediating adherence to HeLa cells and in resisting phagocytosis. *Res. Vet. Sci.* **67**:131–135.

PARASITES
Cryptosporidium wrairi
1. Argenzio, R. A., M. Armstrong, and J. M. Rhoads. 1996. Role of the enteric nervous system in piglet cryptosporidiosis. *J. Pharmacol. Exp. Ther.* **279**:1109–1115.
2. Beier, T. V., N. V. Sidorenko, and N. V. Svezhova. 1995. Cellular interactions in the intracellular parasitism of cryptosporidia. I. The effect of *Cryptosporidium parvum* on the phosphatase activity in the small intestine of experimentally infected newborn rat pups. *Tsitologiia* **37**:829–837.
3. Chai, J. Y., S. M. Guk, H. K. Han, and C. K. Yun. 1999. Role of intraepithelial lymphocytes in mucosal immune responses of mice experimentally infected with *Cryptosporidium parvum*. *J. Parasitol.* **85**:234–239.
4. Checkley, W., L. D. Epstein, R. H. Gilman, R. E. Black, L. Cabrera, and C. R. Sterling. 1998. Effects of *Cryptosporidium parvum* infection in Peruvian children: growth faltering and subsequent catch-up growth. *Am. J. Epidemiol.* **148**:497–506.
5. Checkley, W., R. H. Gilman, L. D. Epstein, M. Suarez, J. F. Diaz, L. Cabrera, R. E. Black, and C. R. Sterling. 1997. Asymptomatic and symptomatic cryptosporidiosis: their acute effect on weight gain in Peruvian children. *Am. J. Epidemiol.* **145**:156–163.
6. Chen, X. M., G. J. Gores, C. V. Paya, and N. F. LaRusso. 1999. *Cryptosporidium parvum* induces apoptosis in biliary epithelia by a Fas/Fas ligand-dependent mechanism. *Am. J. Physiol.* **277**:G599–G608.

7. **Chrisp, C. E., P. Mason, and L. E. Perryman.** 1995. Comparison of *Cryptosporidium parvum* and *Cryptosporidium wrairi* by reactivity with monoclonal antibodies and ability to infect severe combined immunodeficient mice. *Infect. Immun.* **63:**360–362.
8. **Chrisp, C. E., M. A. Suckow, R. Fayer, M. J. Arrowood, M. C. Healey, and C. R. Sterling.** 1992. Comparison of the host ranges of *Cryptosporidium parvum* and *Cryptosporidium wrairi* from guinea pigs. *J. Protozool.* **39:**406–409.
9. **Eichelberger, M. C., P. Suresh, and J. E. Rehg.** 2000. Protection from *Cryptosporidium parvum* infection by gammadelta T cells in mice that lack alphabeta T cells. *Comp. Med.* **50:**270–276.
10. **Gibson, S. V., and J. E. Wagner.** 1986. Cryptosporidiosis in guinea pigs: A retrospective study. *J. Am. Vet. Med. Assoc.* **189:**1033–1034.
11. **Goodgame, R. W., K. Kimball, C. N. Ou, A. C. White, Jr., R. M. Genta, C. H. Lifschitz, and C. L. Chappell.** 1995. Intestinal function and injury in acquired immunodeficiency syndrome-related cryptosporidiosis. *Gastroenterology* **108:**1075–1082.
12. **Hornok, S., Z. Szell, T. A. Shibalova, and I. Varga.** 1999. Study on the course of *Cryptosporidium baileyi* infection in chickens treated with interleukin-1 or indomethacin. *Acta. Vet. Hung.* **47:**207–216.
13. **Kimbell, L. M., III, D. L. Miller, W. Chavez, and N. Altman.** 1999. Molecular analysis of the 18S rRNA gene of *Cryptosporidium serpentis* in a wild-caught corn snake (*Elapha guttata guttata*) and a five-species restriction fragment length polymorphism-based assay that can additionally discern *C. parvum* from *C. wrairi*. *Appl. Environ. Microbiol.* **65:**5345–5349.
14. **McCole, D. F., L. Eckmann, F. Laurent, and M. F. Kagnoff.** 2000. Intestinal epithelial cell apoptosis following *Cryptosporidium parvum* infection. *Infect. Immun.* **68:**1710–1713.
15. **McDonald, V., and G. J. Bancroft.** 1994. Mechanisms of innate and acquired resistance to *Cryptosporidium parvum* infection in SCID mice. *Parasite Immunol.* **16:**315–320.
16. **McDonald, V., H. A. Robinson, J. P. Kelly, and G. J. Bancroft.** 1994. *Cryptosporidium muris* in adult mice: adoptive transfer of immunity and protective roles of CD4 versus CD8 cells. *Infect. Immun.* **62:**2289–2294.
17. **Ortega-Mora, L. M., and S. E. Wright.** 1994. Age-related resistance in ovine cryptosporidiosis: patterns of infection and humoral immune response. *Infect. Immun.* **62:**5003–5009.
18. **Patel, S., S. Pedraza-Diaz, and J. McLauchlin.** 1999. The identification of *Cryptosporidium* species and *Cryptosporidium parvum* directly from whole faeces by analysis of a multiplex PCR of the 18S rRNA gene and by PCR/RFLP of the *Cryptosporidium* outer wall protein (COWP) gene. *Int. J. Parasitol.* **29:**1241–1247.
19. **Percy, D. H., and S. W. Barthold.** 2001. *Pathology of Laboratory Rodents and Rabbits,* 2nd ed. Iowa State University Press, Ames.
20. **Perryman, L. E., P. H. Mason, and C. E. Chrisp.** 1994. Effect of spleen cell populations on resolution of *Cryptosporidium parvum* infection in SCID mice. *Infect. Immun.* **62:**1474–1477.
21. **Rehg, J. E.** 1996. Effect of interferon-gamma in experimental *Cryptosporidium parvum* infection. *J. Infect. Dis.* **174:**229–232.
22. **Rhee, J. K., H. C. Kim, and B. K. Park.** 1998. Effect of *Cryptosporidium baileyi* infection on antibody response to sRBC in chickens. *Korean J. Parasitol.* **36:**33–36.
23. **Rhee, J. K., H. J. Yang, S. Y. Yook, and H. C. Kim.** 1998. Immunosuppressive effect of *Cryptosporidium baileyi* infection on vaccination against avian infectious bronchitis in chicks. *Korean J. Parasitol.* **36:**203–206.
24. **Smith, L. M., M. T. Bonafonte, and J. R. Mead.** 2000. Cytokine expression and specific lymphocyte proliferation in two strains of *Cryptosporidium parvum*-infected gamma-interferon knockout mice. *J. Parasitol.* **86:**300–307.
25. **Tatalick, L. M., and L. E. Perryman.** 1995. Effect of surface antigen-1 (SA-1) immune lymphocyte subsets and naive cell subsets in protecting scid mice from initial and persistent infection with *Cryptosporidium parvum*. *Vet. Immunol. Immunopathol.* **47:**43–55.
26. **Urban, J. F., Jr., R. Fayer, S. J. Chen, W. C. Gause, M. K. Gately, and F. D. Finkelman.** 1996. IL-12 protects immunocompetent and immunodeficient neonatal mice against infection with *Cryptosporidium parvum*. *J. Immunol.* **156:**263–268.

Eimeria caviae

1. **Augustine, P. C., and D. M. Denbow.** 1991. Effect of coccidiosis on plasma epinepherine and norepinepherine levels in turkey poults. *Poult. Sci.* **70:**785–789.
2. **Bessay, M., Y. Le Vern, D. Kerboeuf, P. Yvore, and P. Quere.** 1996. Changes in intestinal intra-epithelial and systemic T-cell subpopulations after an *Eimeria* infection in chickens: comparative study between *E. acervulina* and *E. tenella*. *Vet. Res.* **27:**503–514.
3. **Chinchilla, C. M., B. O. M. Guerrero, and R. R. Marin.** 1986. Effect of *Eimeria falciformis*

infection on the development of toxoplasmosis in mice. *Rev. Biol. Trop.* **34:**1–6.
4. **de la Fuente, C., M. Cuquerella, L. Carrera, and J. M. Alunda.** 1993. Effect of subclinical coccidiosis in kids on subsequent trichostrongylid infection after weaning. *Vet. Parasitol.* **45:**177–183.
5. **Fukata, T., A. Fageyama, E. Baba, and A. Arakawa.** 1987. Effect of infection with *Eimeria tenella* upon the cecal bacterial population in monoflora chickens. *Poult. Sci.* **66:**841–844.
6. **Hankinson, G. J., J. C. Murphy, and J. G. Fox.** 1982. Diagnostic exercise. *Lab. Anim. Sci.* **32:**35–36.
7. **Henry, D. P.** 1932. Coccidiosis of the guinea pig. *Univ. Calif. Publ. Zool.* **37:**211–268.
8. **Hurley, R. J., J. C. Murphy, and N. S. Lipman.** 1995. Diagnostic exercise: Depression and anorexia in recently shipped guinea pigs. *Lab. Anim. Sci.* **45:**305–308.
9. **McDonald, V.** 1999. Gut intraepithelial lymphocytes and immunity to Coccidia. *Parasitol. Today* **15:**483–487.
10. **Muto, T., M. Sugisaki, T. Yusa, and Y. Noguchi.** 1985. Studies on coccidiosis in guinea pigs. 1. Clinico-pathological observation. *Jikken Dobutsu* **34:**23–30.
11. **Muto, T., T. Yusa, M. Sugisaki, K. Tanaka, Y. Noguchi, and K. Taguchi.** 1985. Studies on coccidiosis in guinea pigs. 2. Epizootiological survey. *Jikken Dobutsu* **34:**31–39.
12. **Rose, M. E., P. Hesketh, and D. Wakelin.** 1992. Immune control of murine coccidiosis: CD4$^+$ and CD8$^+$ T lymphocytes contribute differentially in resistance to primary and secondary infections. *Parasitology* **105:**349–354.
13. **Rose, M. E., D. Wakelin, and P. Hesketh.** 1994. Interactions between infections with *Eimeria* spp. and *Trichinella spiralis* in inbred mice. *Parasitology* **108:**69–75.
14. **Ruff, M. D., and J. K. Rosenberger.** 1985. Interaction of low-pathogenicity reoviruses and low levels of infection with several coccidial species. *Avian Dis.* **29:**1057–1065.
15. **Sambrano, G. R., L. F. Mayberry, and J. R. Bristol.** 1992. Effect of *Eimeria nieschulzi* on *Nippostrongylus brasiliensis*-induced IgE. *Parasitol. Res.* **78:**172–174.
16. **Sundaram, U., S. Wisel, V. M. Rajendren, and A. B. West.** 1997. Mechanism of inhibition of Na$^+$-glucose cotransport in the chronically inflamed rabbit ileum. *Am. J. Physiol.* **273:**G913–G919.
17. **Symons, L. E., and W. O. Jones.** 1977. Protein Metabolism. IV. Altered protein synthesis in hosts infected with *Eimeria tenella* or bacteria compared to synthesis in hosts infected with intestinal nematodes. *Exp. Parasitol.* **42:**194–202.
18. **Syukuda, Y.** 1979. Rearing of germfree guinea pigs and establishment of an SPF guinea pig colony. *Jikken Dobutsu* **28:**49–56.
19. **Vetterling, J. M.** 1976. Protozoan parasites, p. 163–196. *In* J. E. Wagner and P. J. Manning (ed.), *The Biology of the Guinea Pig*. Academic Press, Inc., New York, N.Y.

Trixacarus caviae
1. **Baker, D. G., J. D. Bryant, J. F. Urban, Jr., and J. K. Lunney.** 1994. Swine immunity to selected parasites. *Vet. Immunol. Immunopathol.* **43:**127–133.
2. **Bergman, D. K., R. N. Ramachandra, and S. K. Wikel.** 1998. Characterization of an immunosuppressant protein from *Dermacentor andersoni* (Acari: Ixodidae) salivary glands. *J. Med. Entomol.* **35:**505–509.
3. **Dorrestein, G. M., and J. E. M. H. Van Bronswijk.** 1977. Mange caused by *Trixacarus caviae* in guinea pigs. *Tijdschr. Diergeneeskd.* **102:**748–753.
4. **Dorrestein, G. M., and J. E. M. H. Van Bronswijk.** 1979. *Trixacarus caviae* Fain, Howell and Hyatt, 1972 (Acari: Sarcoptidae) as a cause of mange in guinea pigs and papular urticaria in man. *Vet. Parasitol.* **5:**389–398.
5. **Fuentealba, C., and P. Hanna.** 1996. Mange induced by *Trixacarus caviae* in a guinea pig. *Can. Vet. J.* **37:**749–750.
6. **Kummel, B. A., S. A. Estes, and L. G. Arlian.** 1980. *Trixacarus caviae* infestation of guinea pigs. *J. Am. Vet. Med. Assoc.* **177:**903–908.
7. **Manning, P. J., J. E. Wagner, and J. E. Harkness.** 1984. Biology and diseases of guinea pigs, p. 149–181. *In* J. G. Fox, B. J. Cohen, and F. M. Loew (ed.), *Laboratory Animal Medicine*. Academic Press, Inc., New York, N.Y.
8. **McDonald, S. E., and M. M. Lavoipierre.** 1980. *Trixacarus caviae* infestation in two guinea pigs. *Lab. Anim. Sci.* **30:**67–70.
9. **Rothwell, T. L., S. E. Pope, and G. H. Collins.** 1989. *Trixacarus caviae* infection of guinea pigs with genetically determined differences in susceptibility to *Trichostrongylus colubriformis* infection. *Int. J. Parasitol.* **19:**347–348.
10. **Rothwell, T. L., S. E. Pope, Z. K. Rajczyk, and G. H. Collins.** 1991. Haematological and pathological responses to experimental *Trixacarus caviae* infection in guinea pigs. *J. Comp. Pathol.* **104:**179–185.
11. **Thoday, K. L., and W. P. Beresford-Jones.** 1977. The diagnosis and treatment of mange in the guinea-pig caused by *Trixacarus (Caviacoptes) caviae* (Fain, Hovell & Hyatt, 1972). *J. Small Anim. Pract.* **18:**591–595.

12. **Wikel, S. K., R. N. Ramachandra, and D. K. Bergman.** 1994. Tick-induced modulation of the host immune response. *Int. J. Parasitol.* 24:59–66.

13. **Zajac, A., J. F. Williams, and C. S. Williams.** 1980. Mange caused by *Trixacarus caviae* in guinea pigs. *J. Am. Vet. Med. Assoc.* **177**:900–903.

PATHOGENS OF RABBITS

6

INTRODUCTION

The rabbit continues to serve a valuable role in biomedical research. Rabbits serve as animal models for studies in orthopedics, ophthalmology, physiology, infectious diseases, and many other areas of study. In addition, they are commonly used in the production of polyclonal antiserum. The New Zealand white rabbit is the breed most often used in biomedical research. However, the Angora, New Zealand red, Californian, American Dutch, Flemish Giant, Rex, and others, also serve as useful models of specific conditions and diseases. While most rabbits are obtained from commercial vendors of laboratory animals, or from in-house breeding programs, small numbers of rabbits may still be obtained from small, "backyard" production units. These operations vary widely in the quality of rabbits produced. Therefore, the biomedical research community may continue to encounter the pathogens discussed in this chapter. In addition, even the best commercial operations occasionally encounter some of these pathogens. These circumstances require the laboratory animal veterinarian and others working with rabbits in a biomedical setting to be familiar with the pathogens of rabbits, and the effects they have on research with rabbits.

VIRUSES

Adenovirus

Agent
Adenoviruses are double-stranded DNA (dsDNA) viruses in the family *Adenoviridae*.

Epidemiology
Adenoviruses are known to infect many animal species. However, adenovirus infection is uncommon in rabbits, and has only been reported in Europe. It is likely that transmission is through direct contact, similar to adenoviruses of other host species.

Clinical signs
In the only report of an apparently natural infection, an adenovirus was isolated from the spleen, kidney, lungs, and intestines of 6- to 8-week-old rabbits. The only clinical sign was profuse diarrhea (2). The virus agglutinated rabbit erythrocytes.

Pathology
Natural infection of rabbits results in fluid accumulation in the cecum and increased numbers of *Escherichia coli* in the cecum and small intestine (2). Experimental inoculation of rabbits with human adenovirus type 5 results in persistent viral infection of lymphoid tissues

(7). It is unknown whether this also occurs in natural cases of rabbit adenovirus infection. Immunity to adenovirus infection of rabbits is likely humoral, similar to that reported for other host species.

Interference with research
Other than the information cited above, essentially nothing is known of the physiologic effects of natural infection of rabbits with adenovirus. Lippe and coworkers demonstrated binding of the E3/19K protein component of adenovirus type 2 to newly synthesized human cell line MHC Class I molecules, with inhibition of MHC molecule phosphorylation and trafficking to the cell surface (6). It is not currently known whether similar interference occurs in rabbits naturally infected with rabbit strains of adenovirus. Recombinant adenoviruses have successfully infected rabbit hepatocytes (4), autologous rabbit vascular interposition grafts (5), and cultured rabbit corneal epithelial cells (1). An in vivo rabbit model system was developed for testing the efficacy of antiviral drugs against human adenovirus type 5 infections (3). These studies illustrate the utility of the rabbit as a model for adenovirus infection. Endogenous infections with adenovirus would interfere with such studies. In this regard, natural infection of laboratory rabbits with adenovirus would compromise research involving the enterohepatic, respiratory, and urinary systems.

Diagnosis and control
Diagnosis of adenovirus infection should be easily accomplished serologically. However, due to the infrequent occurrence of this pathogen, the author is unaware of a commercial source of such a service. Because the extent of infection is unknown, methods of controlling natural adenovirus infections in rabbits have not been established.

Cottontail rabbit papillomavirus

Agent
Cottontail rabbit papillomavirus (CRP) is a dsDNA virus of the family *Papovaviridae*.

Epidemiology
Infection with CRP is common in wild rabbits in the midwestern and western United States, but uncommon in laboratory rabbits. Wild rabbits therefore are the likely initial source of infection for a laboratory rabbit colony. Once introduced, virus may persist in lesions on domestic rabbits, although at much lower copy numbers than in lesions of wild rabbits (17). Transmission is by arthropod vectors such as mosquitoes and ticks (2).

Clinical signs
In domestic rabbits, wart-like growths (papillomas) occur most commonly on the eyelids and ears (5). These frequently progress to squamous cell carcinomas that may metastasize to regional lymph nodes and/or the lungs (9).

Pathology
Progression from papilloma to carcinoma is virus strain dependent (13), and is accompanied by alterations in antibody profiles, and increased T-cell response to structural proteins, suggestive of increased interaction between virus-infected host cells and the immune system (10, 14). In some cases, lesions spontaneously regress due to cell-mediated immunity (7, 8, 11, 15), which primarily involves $CD-8^+$ cells, tumor necrosis factor α (TNF-α), and apoptosis of papilloma cells (4, 16). Amyloid deposition in the kidneys, liver, and spleen is common (2).

Interference with research
Cottontail rabbit papillomavirus was the first oncogenic virus recognized from mammals. It has been used extensively as a model of oncogenesis (10, 12). Natural infection of laboratory rabbits could compromise several types of studies, most obviously involving the dermal system. Likewise, tumor formation or metastasis of squamous cell carcinomas would compromise long-term carcinogenicity studies and studies involving the lymphoreticular and respiratory systems. Lastly, amyloid deposition could compromise studies involving the enterohepatic and urinary systems.

Diagnosis and control
Diagnosis is based on the presence of papillomas, which never appear in the mouth (2). Control measures include exclusion of wild rabbits and arthropod vectors from the rabbit colony. While growth of warts has been suppressed with vaccination (6) or antiviral treatment (1, 3), these treatments are not advisable since infected colonies would be unsuitable for most types of research and would represent a source of infection for other rabbits. Infected colonies should therefore be eliminated.

Lapine parvovirus

Agent
Lapine parvovirus is a single-stranded DNA (ssDNA) virus in the family *Parvoviridae*. It is biologically similar to other members of the family.

Epidemiology
Infection has been identified in commercial rabbitries in the United States, Europe, and Japan. In one report, virus was initially found contaminating rabbit kidney cell cultures (3). Seroprevalence rates range from 60 to 75% in infected rabbit colonies (2, 3). Like other parvoviruses, transmission is fecal-oral. It is likely that following recovery from infection, rabbits remain as asymptomatic virus excretors.

Clinical signs
Complete studies investigating the clinical response to infection in rabbits of varying ages are lacking. However, clinical signs in one-month-old rabbits consist of anorexia and listlessness (1).

Pathology
Pathologic changes consist of catarrhal enteritis with hyperemia of the small intestine, hypersecretion of intestinal mucus, and exfoliation of small intestinal epithelial cells. Virus can be detected in most visceral organs (1).

Interference with research
Little is known of the effects of lapine parvovirus on host physiology. Natural infection of laboratory rabbits could interfere with research involving the enterohepatic system, studies in which rabbit cell cultures or in vitro immunologic assays are used, and in research in which cytoarchitectural changes in visceral organs would be confounding.

Diagnosis and control
In experimental infections, diagnosis has been accomplished serologically and through virus isolation. Because of the rarity of this infection, screening prior to procurement is not routinely practiced. However, there may be circumstances in which testing is warranted, such as prior to beginning studies on intestinal physiology.

Myxoma virus

Agent
Myxoma virus is a dsDNA virus of the family *Poxviridae*.

Epidemiology
Myxoma virus has a nearly worldwide distribution in wild rabbit populations (18). In contrast, infection is uncommon in laboratory rabbits. The virus can be introduced into a laboratory rabbit colony by arthropod vectors such as mosquitoes and fleas. These enter unscreened areas of animal facilities (21, 30).

Clinical signs
Clinical signs of infection (myxomatosis) vary greatly depending on the strain of virus (nodular versus amyxomatous and virulent versus attenuated) and breed of host (4, 20, 23). In general, clinical disease is more severe in laboratory breeds such as the New Zealand white rabbit, which have not been selected for viral resistance (3). Virulent viral strains, such as those found in California, frequently cause sudden death. Rabbits often develop conjunctivitis, and edema and inflammation of the eyelids and the nasal, anal, genital, and oral orifices. The periocular signs can be striking, if not pathognomonic. Skin nodules, while characteristic of the disease caused by strains elsewhere in the world, are not observed in

the western United States. Myxoma virus is not considered zoonotic, in part, because of a report in which attendees at a boys' camp did not seroconvert during a summer of working with myxoma-infected rabbits (13).

Pathology
Due to the generalized nature of the infection, strain-dependent pathology may be observed in many organs. When present, localized skin tumors consist of masses of stellate mesenchymal cells ("myxoma cells") and occasional inflammatory cells, interspersed within a matrix of mucin-like material (28). Other pathologic changes include cutaneous edema and hemorrhage of the skin, heart, and gastrointestinal subserosa. In addition, proliferative and/or hemorrhagic lesions, followed by degeneration and necrosis, may be observed in the lungs, liver, spleen, vasculature, kidneys, lymph nodes, and testes (7, 22). Experimental infections with an attenuated strain of myxoma virus caused interstitial orchitis and epididymitis, with degeneration of the seminiferous epithelium, decreased serum testosterone concentrations, increased serum-luteinizing hormone, and transient detection of antisperm antibodies (9, 23). Immunofluorescence studies have demonstrated progressive localization of the virus in dendritic cells of the dermis, epidermis, and the lymph nodes, with viral replication in T lymphocytes (3).

Interference with research
Myxoma virus, like other Leporipoxviruses, may be immunosuppressive (12), with both extracellular and intracellular disruption of immune functions (27). Myxoma virus produces various immunosubversive proteins (16, 24), including: myxoma growth factor; SERP-1, a serine proteinase inhibitor that ameliorates chronic inflammation (19); SERP-2, an inhibitor of interleukin 1β (IL-1β)-converting enzyme activity (25, 29); M11L, a receptor-like surface protein modulating apoptosis (8); M-T1, a chemokine-binding protein that may inhibit monocyte influx during the acute phase of infection (11, 15); M-T2, an inhibitor of TNF activity and $CD4^+$ T-lymphocyte apoptosis (32); M-T4, an intracellular virulence factor necessary for the productive infection of lymphocytes, which is retained within the endoplasmic reticulum (1); and M-T7, which modifies leukocyte traffic and inhibits interferon gamma (IFN-γ) activity (14, 26), binds to the heparin-binding domains of members of the chemokine superfamily (16), and reduces vascular intimal hyperplasia (17). Immune suppression is evidenced by downregulation of class I-mediated presentation of viral antigen (5) and of $CD4^+$ T cells (2). Interestingly, in one study apoptosis occurred in uninfected cells adjacent to infected cells (4). Lastly, virus-virus interactions may result in compromise of viral studies, in rabbits naturally infected with myxoma virus (6). Given the generalized nature of infection, natural infection of laboratory rabbits could compromise research involving the cardiovascular, dermal, endocrine, enterohepatic, hematopoietic, lymphoreticular, reproductive, respiratory, and urinary systems.

Diagnosis and control
Diagnosis of the nodular form of the disease, and of the more virulent amyxomatous forms, is accomplished by clinical and histopathologic findings, whereas serologic assays such as enzyme-linked immunosorbent assay (ELISA), immunofluorescence assay (IFA), and the complement fixation (CF) test may facilitate diagnosis of less virulent amyxomatous disease (10, 21). Virus isolation may also be performed but is more labor intensive. Rabbits coming from areas in which myxomatosis is endemic should be quarantined and treated for external parasites on entry into the facility. Epidemiologic studies have shown that rabbits housed outdoors have higher seropositivity than those housed indoors (21). Infected rabbits should be isolated or destroyed, since there is evidence of a carrier state, possibly accounting for recurring outbreaks in closed colonies (9, 23, 31).

Pleural effusion disease virus

Agent
Pleural effusion disease virus (PEDV), also known as cardiomyopathy virus, is an ssRNA virus of the family *Coronaviridae*. Antisera to PEDV cross-reacts with other members of the mammalian group I coronaviruses, including feline infectious peritonitis (FIP) virus, canine coronavirus, porcine transmissible gastroenteritis virus, and human coronavirus (14).

Epidemiology
During the 1960s in Scandinavia, and subsequently elsewhere in the world, a coronavirus was found contaminating stocks of *Treponema pallidum* used experimentally in rabbits (7, 11, 12). Whether the agent is a natural pathogen of rabbits is uncertain. The lack of reports of natural infection suggests that the virus may be from another species (3). PEDV appears to be biologically similar to other members of the family, except that transmission by direct contact is uncommon (9).

Clinical signs
Manifestations of pleural effusion disease are multisystemic and are similar to those observed in cats with FIP (5). However, clinical signs of PEDV infection depend on strain and culture passage of the agent. Following infection, fever is common, develops within 1 to 4 days, and persists for 5 to 10 days. Other signs include anorexia and weight loss. More variable signs include iridocyclitis, atony, muscular weakness, tachypnea, and circulatory insufficiency. Mortality is high following infection with virulent strains (3).

Pathology
The major target organ of PEDV is the heart (4, 10, 12). Pathologic findings of infection depend on the stage of disease, and include pulmonary edema, pleural effusion, and right ventricular dilation in the acute phase. Rabbits dying after the first week may have ascites and subepicardial and subendocardial hemorrhages. Other pathologic findings include myocarditis, with myocardial degeneration and necrosis; hepatosplenomegaly with reduction of splenic white pulp; focal hepatic necrosis; congestion and focal degeneration of lymph nodes followed by proliferation; focal degenerative changes of the thymus; mild proliferative changes of renal glomeruli; and mild nonsuppurative, nongranulomatous anterior uveitis (3). Clinicopathologic changes include transient lymphopenia, heterophilia, transient hypoalbuminemia, increased serum potassium and lactate dehydrogenase, and elevated γ-globulins (6, 8, 10).

Interference with research
There is little information on the physiologic effects of PEDV infection in rabbits. Sera from an infected animal produced cytopathic effects in primary rabbit kidney and newborn human intestine cells (13). Natural infection of laboratory rabbits with PEDV has been shown to alter electrocardiographic profiles (1, 2), and may also result in pathologic changes in multiple body systems, including the enterohepatic, hematopoietic, lymphoreticular, musculoskeletal, respiratory, and urinary systems.

Diagnosis and control
Sufficient cross-reactivity exists between PEDV and other coronaviruses. Therefore, diagnosis of PEDV infection may be accomplished serologically by using other coronavirus antigens. Because it is unknown whether PEDV is a natural pathogen of rabbits, recommendations for control are lacking. Isolates of *T. pallidum* should be determined to be free of virus prior to their use in rabbits.

Rabbit enteric coronavirus

Agent
Rabbit enteric coronavirus (REC) is an ssRNA virus in the family *Coronaviridae*. There is a high level of serologic cross-reactivity between REC and other mammalian group 1 coronaviruses (8).

Epidemiology
REC was first detected in rabbits in Canada and Europe (4, 5, 6). Serologic surveys have extended the range of infected rabbitries to those in the United States (1). However, only one natural outbreak of disease has been reported in laboratory rabbits. That outbreak occurred in Germany (4).

Clinical signs
Natural infection with REC results in clinical signs in 3- to 8-week-old rabbits. Signs include lethargy, diarrhea, abdominal distension, and up to 100% mortality (4). Death generally occurs within 24 h of the onset of clinical signs.

Pathology
Natural infection with REC resulted in cachexia, distension of the cecum with watery fluid, diffuse inflammation and mucosal edema throughout the intestinal tract, and mild multifocal intestinal epithelial necrosis (4). The thymus also contained focal areas of hemorrhaging, without evidence of inflammation. Rabbits were concurrently infected with enteric coccidia, but coccidial infections were considered mild. Rabbits in that study were also found infected with a range of bacteria, including *E. coli, Clostridium perfringens* type A, α-hemolytic streptococci, *Bordetella bronchiseptica,* and others (4). Because the clinical signs observed during natural infection differed from, and were more severe than, those in rabbits infected experimentally, it is possible that concurrent microbial infection may have contributed to disease. Antibiotic treatment did not reduce the mortality rate. The author noted that 19% of fecal samples contained reovirus-like particles (4). Clinical signs of experimental infection are limited to variably watery feces without mortality (2, 6). In one report, the small intestines were congested, with transient evidence of villus tip and M-cell necrosis, atrophy, crypt hyperplasia, and the cecal contents were watery (2, 6). Because coronavirus infections are uniformly self-limiting, it is likely that rabbits infected with REC clear the virus. REC hemagglutinates rabbit erythrocytes, but has not been shown to be cytopathic for a variety of cell lines (3, 5).

Interference with research
Natural infection of laboratory rabbits with REC would interfere with research involving the enterohepatic and lymphoreticular systems. In addition, infection would confound research using polyclonal antimammalian coronavirus serum produced in rabbits. The self-limiting nature of coronavirus infection should allow for the eventual experimental use of affected rabbits, following clearing of the virus.

Diagnosis and control
Diagnosis of REC should be accomplished serologically, although to this author's knowledge, commercial tests are not available. Immunoelectron microscopic demonstration of coronaviral particles in the intestine would also support diagnosis (7). Simultaneous screening for copathogens should also be undertaken. Given the rarity of this pathogen in rabbits, it is not commonly screened for prior to procurement. Control measures have not been described.

Rabbit hemorrhagic disease virus

Agent
Rabbit hemorrhagic disease virus (RHDV) is an ssRNA virus of the family *Caliciviridae* (8, 25), and is closely related to European brown hare syndrome (EBHS) virus (38). Antigenic relationships between these viruses have complicated past efforts at serodiagnosis (23).

Epidemiology
Based both on outbreaks and serologic studies, distribution appears to be worldwide (6, 13, 18, 27, 28, 37). While new variants have been reported (7, 16, 35), most isolates collected from multiple sites around the world are similar in the epidemiologic features, clinical signs, and pathologic lesions produced (4). Transmission is horizontal, and occurs through a variety of means, including aerosol, direct contact, fomites, and contaminated car-

casses (28), although apparently not by feces or urine (10). Arthropod vectors, including flies, mosquitoes, and fleas, have been proven or implicated in transmission (2, 19). Young rabbits in endemic areas are susceptible, after maternal antibodies have disappeared, although the incidence is seasonal, and is greatest in the autumn (11).

Clinical signs
Sudden death, observed most commonly in adult naive rabbits, may preclude observation of additional clinical signs. Experimentally infected rabbits may die within 2 to 4 days (26). When observed, clinical signs may be referable to nearly any body system, and may include incoordination, shaking, and other nervous signs (28). Morbidity can reach 100% (26).

Pathology
The pathogenesis of infection involves viral replication in the liver, small intestine, and spleen, followed by viremia, disseminated intravascular coagulation, and multiple organ system failure. Virus is first detected in the liver and spleen (10, 14, 28, 29). Pathologic changes are observed in multiple organs. One of the hallmarks of the disease is acute hepatic necrosis, beginning periportally and spreading to the rest of the lobule (26), with apoptosis of hepatocytes, macrophages, and endothelial cells (1, 15, 21). There is congestion, hemorrhage, and thrombosis in the lungs. Many other organs may have pathologic changes due to microinfarction (20) and hemorrhage (28).

Interference with research
Hematologic alterations include lymphopenia, thrombocytopenia, and prolongation of clotting times (12), possibly associated with apoptosis of intravascular monocytes (1, 30). Virus binds to blood group antigens in the upper respiratory and digestive tracts (34). The effects of natural RHDV infection on research could vary from mild to catastrophic, depending on the virulence of the infecting strain. Natural infection of laboratory rabbits with RHDV could compromise studies involving the enterohepatic, hematopoietic, musculoskeletal, reproductive, and respiratory systems.

Diagnosis and control
Several immunologically based assays have been developed for detecting RHDV, including ELISA (9, 11, 22, 31), immunoblotting (33), and hemagglutination inhibition (4), although cross-reactions with EBHS virus have been observed (24). PCR assay of liver has been used to identify infected rabbits (28, 32, 36), without the problem of serologic cross-reactivity with other, closely related viruses. Because RHDV is uncommon, rabbits are generally not screened for this agent prior to entry into an animal facility. Although vaccines have been developed for use under special circumstances (3, 5, 17), there are few scenarios of natural infection of laboratory rabbits for which they would be practical. Infected rabbits should be isolated and culled.

Rabbit oral papillomavirus

Agent
Rabbit oral papillomavirus (ROP) is a dsDNA virus of the family *Papovaviridae*.

Epidemiology
The prevalence of ROP infection is generally low in laboratory rabbit colonies, although outbreaks have been reported (7). Transmission is by direct contact.

Clinical signs
When present, lesions are usually found on the ventral surface of the tongue but may also be found on the mucosal surface of the buccal cavity (6), and consist of small whitish pedunculated growths which may eventually ulcerate (3) before disappearing (1, 2, 5). Development of lesions may be facilitated by damage to oral mucosa (8).

Pathology
Histologically the lesions appear as papillomas, with basophilic intranuclear inclusions (6, 8). Other mucosal sites, such as the genital mucosa, may be infected experimentally (4).

Interference with research

Natural infection of laboratory rabbits with rabbit oral papillomavirus could interfere with feeding, and studies in which feed intake and/or weight gain are measured. Therefore, studies involving the enterohepatic system would be compromised.

Diagnosis and control

Diagnosis of ROP infection is based on clinical and histologic findings. Screening for this virus prior to entry of rabbits into an animal facility is not commonly practiced. Because this is a chronic infection, infected rabbits should be eliminated from the colony.

Rotavirus

Agent

Rotaviruses are dsRNA viruses of the family *Reoviridae,* and are classified into groups and subgroups (7). The virus infecting rabbits (group A, serotype 3) also infects humans and other animals. Multiple strains have been reported (12, 16, 19).

Epidemiology

Rotavirus infection is common in wild and laboratory rabbits (8, 18). The virus is extremely contagious and transmission is fecal-oral. In endemically infected colonies, outbreaks are most common in recently weaned rabbits, and coincide with waning passively transferred maternal antibodies (9). Many of these infections may be subclinical.

Clinical signs

Clinical signs of rotavirus infection vary depending on host age, exposure history, and presence of other synergistic organisms (7). In naive colonies or experimentally infected rabbits, disease is most severe in preweanlings (4). Clinical signs include severe diarrhea, anorexia, dehydration, and high mortality (7, 18).

Pathology

Virus replication occurs in the mature enterocytes of the small intestine (15). Gross pathologic findings include marked congestion, distension, and petechiation in the colon (17); small intestinal distension with mucosal hemorrhages; and a fluid-filled cecum. Microscopically, intestinal villi are blunted and fused, with attenuated villous enterocytes (2). However, in most reports of outbreaks, attempts to demonstrate the presence of other pathogens have not been made. In general, it is thought that pure rotavirus infections are mild, and that lesions are limited to a fluid-filled cecum, swollen mesenteric lymph nodes, small intestinal villous atrophy most pronounced in the ileum, increased crypt depth, and lymphocytic infiltrates in the lamina propria, without involvement of the large intestine (7, 13, 14, 18, 21). Experimentally, a synergistic effect between rotavirus and *E. coli,* whereby weanling rabbits developed more severe diarrheal disease than that resulting from either pathogen alone, has been reported (20).

Interference with research

Rotavirus infection impairs intestinal brush-border membrane ion transport (10), indicating that cell dysfunction, rather than mucosal cell damage, is the likely mechanism of diarrhea. Infection is self-limiting, and immunity is long lasting (6, 7, 11) and primarily humoral (5, 8). Therefore, natural infection of laboratory rabbits with rotavirus would have at least temporary adverse effects on studies involving the enterohepatic system, and on those studies in which nutritional parameters are monitored.

Diagnosis and control

Diagnosis of rotavirus is based on clinical presentation; histologic changes; identification of virus in the feces, either by electron microscopy or the more sensitive ELISA-based tests; virus isolation; and demonstration of anti-rotavirus antibodies (1, 8, 9, 15). However, copathogens may have an important role in pathogenesis. Infected rabbits should be isolated. Because there is no carrier state, it may be possible to allow the infection to "die out" in valuable colonies, although the highly contagious nature of the organism, and interference by maternal antibodies, may complicate such an approach. While a vaccine has been developed and used experimentally (3), it is not available for routine use, nor would its use be practical.

BACTERIA

Bordetella bronchiseptica

Agent
Bordetella bronchiseptica is a gram-negative rod commonly found in the respiratory tracts of rabbits and other animals (3, 12, 16). These isolates can be grouped by using restriction enzyme analysis and ribotyping (12).

Epidemiology
The prevalence of B. bronchiseptica is high in laboratory rabbit colonies (11). Transmission is by aerosol, fomites, and contact, and it occurs early in life.

Clinical signs
Most infections are asymptomatic and only become clinical in association with Pasteurella multocida infection (4). In those cases, clinical signs include oculonasal discharge ("snuffles"), lethargy, anorexia, dyspnea, and occasionally death. However, in some clinical cases of snuffles, no other pathogens can be detected, or a primary infection with P. multocida is eliminated with antibiotics only to have clinical signs resume with overgrowth of B. bronchiseptica. Rabbits may also occasionally develop abscesses due to B. bronchiseptica. Following experimental inoculation, some rabbits eliminated the infection from the lungs and trachea 40 days after inoculation, but retained the organism in the nasal cavity, without clinical signs of infection (15).

Pathology
Typical pathologic changes of the lower respiratory tract include suppurative bronchopneumonia and interstitial pneumonitis (7, 10). Microscopically, there may be prominent peribronchial lymphocytic cuffing (10).

Interference with research
B. bronchiseptica colonizes tracheal epithelial cell cilia in rabbits (9), and causes ciliostasis in primary canine tracheal cell cultures (1). These alterations to normal ciliary function may facilitate infection and disease caused by copathogens such as P. multocida (10). Rabbits with B. bronchiseptica infection have defective alveolar macrophage function (17), supporting the hypothesis that infection with B. bronchiseptica facilitates infection with other pathogens. In addition to the pulmonary changes, experimentally infected rabbits develop acute serous rhinitis and mild pleuritis (7). Clinical bordetellosis would compromise the usefulness of laboratory rabbits used in respiratory, and possibly other, studies.

Diagnosis and control
Diagnosis is based on clinical signs and recovery of the organism on standard or modified blood agar plates (5). Serological methods are useful (2), although results should be interpreted with caution in nursing or recently weaned rabbits (6). Cesarean section or embryo transfer can be used to derive rabbits free of B. bronchiseptica (13, 14). However, given the high prevalence of latent B. bronchiseptica infection in rabbits; the large number of reservoir hosts, including humans (8); and the highly infectious nature of the organism, it is unlikely that a laboratory rabbit colony can remain free of infection without strict attention to barrier housing procedures. Clinically affected rabbits should be treated immediately or, preferably, culled.

Cilia-associated respiratory bacillus

Agent
Cilia-associated respiratory (CAR) bacillus is a gram-negative, filamentous, rod-shaped, gliding bacterium. Analysis of 16S rRNA gene sequences from CAR bacillus of rabbits suggests close relationship to members of the ge-

nus *Helicobacter* (3), although there are few biological correlates. Monoclonal antibodies have been used to distinguish rabbit CAR bacillus isolates from those of rodents (4).

Epidemiology
Infection of laboratory rabbits has been reported in the United States, Japan, and Europe (1, 2, 5, 7). Prevalence of infection ranges from 30 to 100% within a colony (1).

Clinical signs
Clinical disease has not been demonstrated in naturally or experimentally infected rabbits (1, 5, 7).

Pathology
Following infection, organisms primarily colonize the apices of cells lining the larynx, trachea, and bronchi (1, 5, 7). Lesions consist of mild hypertrophy and hyperplasia of ciliated upper respiratory epithelium, with occasional loss of cilia and mild inflammation of the lamina propria (1). Seroconversion, without the development of either clinical disease or lesions, following experimental inoculation of rabbits with CAR bacillus from rats (6), or mice (8), have been reported.

Interference with research
Natural infection of rabbits may confound studies involving the respiratory system, especially those studies in which upper airway cytoarchitecture is evaluated.

Diagnosis and control
Diagnosis is more thoroughly described in the chapter on pathogens of mice and rats. In brief, diagnosis consists principally of examination of immunoperoxidase or silver-stained sections of the upper airways (7), combined with standard hematoxylin and eosin staining for evidence of airway inflammation (1). Control measures are not usually practiced. However, there may be circumstances in which it is desirable to eliminate CAR bacillus from a rabbit colony (7). Control measures have yet to be adequately developed. There is no completely effective therapy for eradicating CAR bacillus from a rabbit colony. Introduction of the organism may be prevented through purchase of pathogen-free rabbits from reputable vendors, followed by husbandry practices that preclude opportunity for infection.

Clostridium piliforme

Agent
Clostridium piliforme (formerly *Bacillus piliformis*) is a gram-negative, filamentous bacterium that infects a wide range of animals, including rabbits, and is the cause of Tyzzer's disease.

Epidemiology
Prevalence of infection is high in domestic rabbits supplied for research (3). Transmission is by ingestion of infectious endospores.

Clinical signs
Young rabbits are most susceptible, although rabbits of all ages may develop clinical signs. The organism may exist enzootically within a rabbit colony; that is, it may be present in many animals yet cause disease in only a few rabbits. Alternatively, *C. piliforme* infections may occur in epizootic form; that is, occur as a traditional outbreak in a susceptible population (2). Clinical signs include profuse, watery diarrhea, lethargy, anorexia, dehydration, and death. Surviving rabbits may become chronically infected and serve as a source of contamination for other rabbits. Enzootic infections may be revealed following immune suppression or other stressors (1).

Pathology
Lesions of Tyzzer's disease consist primarily of necrotic foci in the cecum and adjacent intestinal segments, liver, and rarely the myocardium. There are petechial and ecchymotic hemorrhages on the serosal surface of the cecum and adjacent intestinal segments. Intestinal stenosis may follow fibrotic healing of necrotic foci (1, 2, 4).

Interference with research
While no publications were found specifically addressing the effect of *C. piliforme* on research

involving rabbits, natural infection would compromise studies involving the cardiovascular and enterohepatic systems even if no deaths occurred.

Diagnosis and control
Diagnosis of *C. piliforme* infection is complicated by the inability to culture the organism on artificial media. Growth does occur in embryonated chicken eggs and in some cell lines, and these have been used diagnostically. Serologic assays have been developed, and special stains of impression smears (Giemsa) or histologic sections (Warthin-Starry) facilitate diagnosis (4). There is a dearth of information on control of *C. piliforme* in rabbit colonies. Pending some information, prevention should begin with procurement of *C. piliforme*-free rabbits and adherence to standard operating procedures for good hygiene.

Clostridium spiroforme

Agent
Enteric diseases, in general, and enterotoxemic conditions, in particular, are common in laboratory rabbits. *Clostridium spiroforme*, a gram-positive, helically coiled, endospore-forming anaerobe, is the predominant cause of enterotoxemia in rabbits (11). Multiple strains have been identified (2).

Epidemiology
Occasionally, other bacterial species, such as *C. perfringens, C. difficile,* and *E. coli,* as well as viral and parasitic agents, are involved with *C. spiroforme* (6, 8, 11, 12). In general, rabbits do not normally harbor *C. spiroforme,* although it has been shown that occasional asymptomatic carriers may be detected (3). The latter may explain the occurrence of outbreaks in closed colonies. Transmission is fecal-oral.

Clinical signs
Recently weaned rabbits are most susceptible to enterotoxemia (5, 16). Overgrowth of *C. spiroforme* is facilitated by, but does not require, some local or systemic stress such as shipping, weaning, antibiotic administration, or change of feed to a high-energy, low-fiber diet (1). Disease also occurs in adults following disruption of the normal flora by antibiotics, co-pathogens, or stressors, including lactation or dietary changes (5, 6). The hallmark of enterotoxemia is acute onset of watery diarrhea accompanied by anorexia and lethargy, which may end in death (9). Peracute cases with no premonitory signs, and chronic cases presenting as anorexia and weight loss, also occur.

Pathology
Pathologic findings include petechial and ecchymotic hemorrhages of the serosal surface of the cecum and, occasionally, other segments of the large intestine. The cecum is usually filled with fluid and gas (9), and is the organ of choice for diagnosis (3). Mucosal lesions consist of inflammation, focal necrosis, and formation of erosions and ulcers. Most rabbit isolates of *C. spiroforme* produce a binary cytotoxin similar to *C. perfringens* type E iota toxin (1, 14, 15), although it is not always possible to detect in *C. spiroforme*-infected rabbits (11).

Interference with research
Little information exists on the effects of *C. spiroforme* on research. Three- to eight-week-old rabbits with natural *C. spiroforme* infection had decreased volatile fatty acid production (13). Natural infection of laboratory rabbits would interfere with many types of studies, most notably those involving the enterohepatic system.

Diagnosis and control
Yonushonis and coworkers (16) recommended the following criteria for establishing a diagnosis of *C. spiroforme* enteritis: "(a) identification of coiled gram-positive organisms on thin layered gram stained smears; (b) gross and histopathologic examination of the cecum and colon showing typhlitis or hemorrhagic typhlitis; (c) isolation and identification of *C. spiroforme* under strict anaerobic conditions; and (d) demonstration of *C. spiroforme* iota toxin in cecal and colonic filtrates." Holmes and coworkers (10) reported success in isolat-

ing *C. spiroforme* by sampling the supernatant-pellet interface of centrifuged intestinal contents. Others have reported using a cytotoxicity assay for *C. spiroforme* toxin in cecal fluid (4). It is likely that the PCR assay may soon be routinely used for diagnosis (1). Screening of rabbits for *C. spiroforme* is generally not practiced, since so few healthy rabbits are carriers. While a toxoid vaccine has proven effective in protecting rabbits from challenge with *C. spiroforme* (7), its use in laboratory rabbits is unwarranted under most conditions. To help prevent establishment of the infection in a laboratory colony, stress on rabbits should be minimized.

Francisella tularensis

Agent
Francisella tularensis is a gram-negative coccobacillus causing acute septicemic disease (tularemia) in a wide range of mammalian hosts, including humans (9, 29).

Epidemiology
Infection with *F. tularensis* is common in wild leporids (1, 16) but rare in laboratory rabbits. Multiple subspecies of *F. tularensis* infect rabbits, with *F. tularensis* subsp. *tularensis* the most pathogenic (18). This subspecies was originally thought to exist only in the United States and Canada, but has recently also been found in Europe (10). Transmission is by multiple routes, including aerosol, contact, and arthropod vectors (4, 13, 14, 21).

Clinical signs
Clinical signs, when present, may include anorexia, depression, and ataxia, or sudden death without premonitory signs.

Pathology
Pathologic changes include focal coagulative necrosis and congestion of the liver, spleen, and bone marrow (5). Experimental aerosol exposure of rabbits resulted in bronchointerstitial pneumonia, in addition to pyogranulomatous lesions in the liver, spleen, and lymph nodes (3). Pathologic responses to intravenous injection of *F. tularensis* inactivated by ionizing radiation in rabbits are not abolished, indicating mediation by endotoxin release (8). Virulence appears to be associated with capsulation (12, 22), catalase activity, cytochrome b_1 levels (7), and the presence of an envelope antigen C (28). Virulent strains are lethal to peritoneal macrophages (17). Studies in rabbits and rodents indicate that immunity is similar to that induced by other intracellular pathogens, being primarily cellular, with participation of neutrophils (6), and the classical pathway of complement activation (2, 15, 24). In the cellular response, $\alpha\beta$ T-cell receptor$^+$ ($\alpha\beta$ TCR$^+$) cells are required for protection, but either CD4$^+$ or CD8$^+$ T cells are individually sufficient for eliminating infection (30).

Interference with research
In rabbits experimentally infected with *F. tularensis,* there were changes in serum levels of trace metals, neutral fat, alkaline phosphatase activity, reduced serum amino acids, and a marked early leukopenia (11). In natural or experimental infections in rats, *F. tularensis* induces synthesis of acute-phase globulins (23); alters blood ketone levels, likely due to decreased lipolysis (19); slows tumor growth and reduces chromosomal aberrations caused by 3,4-benz(a)pyrene (20, 31); and increases radioresistance (32). In vitro, specific antigens of *F. tularensis* may increase or decrease adhesion, ingestion and presentation of antigens by peritoneal macrophages (26, 27). Hence, natural infection of laboratory rabbits, besides being fatal, could alter research involving many body systems, including the enterohepatic, hematopoietic, lymphoreticular, nervous, and respiratory systems.

Diagnosis and control
Diagnosis is based on pathology, immunohistochemistry, and isolation of the organism. Serology is of limited value, since chronic infection does not seem to occur (25). Infected rabbits should be eliminated because

they represent a source of infection for other rabbits, as well as for laboratory personnel.

Listeria monocytogenes

Agent
Listeria monocytogenes is a gram-positive, rod-shaped, intracellular bacterium that uncommonly causes disease in rabbits.

Epidemiology
Infection may be common in large commercial facilities raising rabbits for human consumption (19, 26). Because some research institutions purchase rabbits from these sources, rather than specifically from vendors of laboratory-quality rabbits, the pathogen may occur in laboratory rabbits. Infection is acquired with contaminated feed (26). There is concern for human exposure since *L. monocytogenes* is zoonotic.

Clinical signs
Clinical signs are generally absent in males and nonpregnant females, although under experimental conditions, pathogenicity may increase with repeated passage (30). Asymptomatic carriers may excrete the agent in the feces (8). When present, clinical signs may be nonspecific and include anorexia, ascites, depression, weight loss, and sudden death. Pregnant does are more susceptible to infection, either because of physiologic stress or a uterine microenvironment more conducive to survival of the organism and may abort (8, 26).

Pathology
Pathologic findings are most prominent in the liver and consist of multifocal hepatic necrosis. Similar microabscesses occur in the spleen and adrenal glands. There may be straw-colored fluid in the peritoneal cavity with fibrinous exudate and ecchymosis on the surface of the uterus (25). Septicemic spread is facilitated by phagocytosis and transport by macrophages. Pregnant does may develop acute necrotizing suppurative metritis. Pathogenesis is dependent on hemolysin production (5, 31). Abortion may also be related to the ability of pathogenic strains of *L. monocytogenes* to cause contraction of human uterine muscle (21). Hematologic changes include a marked monocytosis (22). While protection is primarily cell mediated (24), and is in part stimulated by *Listeria* factor Ei (16), serologic responses also develop and are greater in rabbits infected orally rather than intragastrically (6). In this regard, as immunity develops, specific antibodies enhance neutrophil response against *L. monocytogenes* by promoting opsonization (29). In addition, activated macrophages participate in clearing infection (18).

Interference with research
Hemolysins and other products from *L. monocytogenes* have been shown to have deleterious effects on several organs and/or physiologic functions in the rabbit, including the ileum (27), heart (32), blood cell formation (28), and spleen cell migration (17). *L. monocytogenes* may also interfere with resistance to other pathogens, including pneumococci (23). In addition, there are several reports of physiologic effects from experimental studies of *L. monocytogenes* in a variety of other hosts. In rodents, *L. monocytogenes* suppressed growth of transplanted tumors. Killed organisms were less effective (3, 4). In mice, lipids extracted from *L. monocytogenes* increased resistance to infection with fungal, parasitic, and other bacterial agents (12, 14), through augmentation of nonspecific immune responses (1, 13), principally macrophage activation (10, 15). This has also been demonstrated in cattle (2). In mice, *L. monocytogenes* suppressed production of all blood cells, most markedly erythropoiesis (11). In goats, *L. monocytogenes* may colonize the placenta, and alter levels of hormones associated with pregnancy, including progesterone and 15-ketodihydroprostaglandin $F_{2\alpha}$ (PGF2α), resulting in abortion (9). Laboratory rabbits are frequently used to produce anti-*Listeria* antiserum, and rabbits have been used to study keratitis induced by *L. monocytogenes* (33). Natural infection of laboratory rabbits could interfere with

Diagnosis and control

Diagnosis of *L. monocytogenes* infection is by clinical presentation; histopathologic findings; Gram staining of affected tissues; and recovery of the organism from uterine wall, placenta, fetuses, blood, liver, and spleen (20, 25). Serology is of lesser value, since a high percentage of normal rabbits may be seropositive (7). In the event of an outbreak, or even with isolated cases, all other rabbits in direct or indirect contact should be removed from the colony. Due to the low prevalence of infection with this pathogen, testing rabbits prior to entry into the facility is not practiced. It should be remembered, however, that institutions purchasing rabbits from other than specific-pathogen-free (SPF) commercial vendors, risk introducing *L. monocytogenes* into the facility, where infection may spread among colony animals and personnel.

Pasteurella multocida

Agent

Pasteurella multocida is a gram-negative, bipolarly staining rod. It is the most common pathogen of laboratory rabbits.

Epidemiology

Infection is nearly ubiquitous among rabbit colonies. Within a colony, infection is common, generally does not occur prior to 12 weeks of age, and increases with age (15, 22, 24, 27, 32, 35, 39). The organism can often be recovered from deep nasal swabs of asymptomatic rabbits (35). Transmission is by direct contact, and to a lesser extent, by fomite, aerosol, and sexual exposure (23).

Clinical signs

Disease susceptibility depends on host, environmental, and bacterial factors. Differences in susceptibility have been reported among bacterial strains recovered from rabbits (26, 41). Type A strains of *P. multocida* are the most commonly isolated (14). Environmental factors such as shipping, experimentation, wide temperature fluctuations, and high ammonia levels increase susceptibility (17). Lastly, bacterial strains differ in many aspects, including growth characteristics (7, 25, 35) and colonization site. The site of colonization may indirectly affect pathogenicity, likely because of production of specific adhesion molecules (2, 6, 18, 29). Bacterial strains also differ in endotoxin and exotoxin production, and in ability to resist phagocytosis and killing by neutrophils (3). However, these latter factors have not been absolutely correlated with virulence (20, 48). Bacterial strains have been grouped on the basis of an indirect hemagglutination assay or gel-diffusion precipitin test (17). The majority of rabbits infected with *P. multocida* are asymptomatic carriers. Transition from asymptomatic to symptomatic infection is related to factors discussed previously. When present, clinical signs can occur in nearly any organ, likely due to hematogenous spread of the organism. The most common presentations, in descending order of occurrence, are rhinitis (snuffles), conjunctivitis, pneumonia, otitis media or interna with or without torticollis (head tilt), abscesses, genital tract infections, osteomyelitis, septicemia, meningoencephalomyelitis, and peritonitis (4, 5, 10, 19, 21, 22, 24, 27, 31, 34, 38, 47).

Pathology

Colonization often occurs initially in the pharynx. The infection quickly spreads to the nasal cavity from which it disseminates by direct or hematogenous spread to the lungs, middle ear, conjunctival sac, subcutaneous tissues, and visceral organs (17, 24). Regardless of the organ system affected, the hallmark of *P. multocida* infection is suppurative inflammation. The accompanying exudate is most often purulent. Microscopically, affected tissues may be edematous, hyperemic, congested, and necrotic (40). Ultrastructural changes include ciliary destruction and deciliation of the ciliated epithelial cells, cellular swelling, goblet cell hyperplasia, and endothelial cell damage (1). As alluded to above, the factors responsible for tissue damage are incompletely known but may include the production of toxins, antiphagocytic substances, or adhesions (11, 17). Large abscesses may also place direct pressure on adjacent tissues, such as in the lungs, and further compromise organ function. Immunity is largely humoral, with limited cross-immunity between strains of *P. multocida* (8). In endemically infected colonies, passively acquired maternal antibodies tend to decline shortly after weaning, and actively acquired antibodies appear with infection at 2 to 3 months of age (15, 28). Other nonspecific immune mechanisms may also contribute to immunity, such as serum bactericidins and neutrophils (45).

Interference with research
In rabbits, *P. multocida* infection has been shown to increase expression of vascular cell adhesion molecule-1 by aortic endothelium (43), alter sleep patterns (51), lower serum iron concentration (33), elevate serum cortisol (42, 51), and alter hematologic parameters such as leukocyte distribution (44, 51). Eventual infection of laboratory rabbits with *P. multocida* is nearly unavoidable without the use of at least some form of barrier housing (46). While latent nasal colonization will likely have no impact on experimental studies, clinical pasteurellosis could invalidate several types of studies, in particular, those involving the endocrine, hematopoietic, musculoskeletal, nervous, reproductive, respiratory, and urinary systems.

Diagnosis and control
Diagnosis of infection has historically been accomplished by isolating the organism from nasal swabs (39). Serology has also been used (50, 52), although caution is warranted when using ELISA-based technology where lipopolysaccharide is used as antigen, since not all rabbit isolates cross-react (9). Recently, a PCR assay has been developed for rapid diagnosis of infection (13). Some success in eliminating *P. multocida* from infected colonies with antibiotics has been reported. For example, Suckow and coworkers (49) interrupted the transmission cycle from does to their litters by treating does with enrofloxacin in the periparturient period, resulting in *Pasteurella*-free offspring. Hanan and coworkers (30) reported elimination of *P. multocida* by use of ciprofloxacin. However, most attempts have failed to completely eliminate the pathogen from adult rabbits, using a variety of antibiotics (36, 37, 49). While respiratory infections are relatively easy to treat with antibiotics, once torticollis has occurred, the head tilt rarely if ever completely resolves, even after elimination of the pathogen. This generally does not seem to compromise the overall health and well-being of the rabbit. Also, *P. multocida* abscesses may be extremely invasive and difficult to treat, especially when present on the rabbit's head. An efficacious vaccine has recently been developed which may have practical use in specific circumstances (12). It is recommended that all rabbits showing clinical signs be culled, unless the value of the rabbit warrants treatment. In this way, the overall environmental burden of, and therefore the exposure to, the pathogen is minimized. In addition, stress reduction is essential to prevent outbreaks. In this regard, where rabbits are housed in a manner that allows them to experience changes in outside temperature, large daily swings in ambient temperature, such as occur in the spring, often precipitate outbreaks. Similarly, outbreaks may be precipitated by high humidity (16). *P. multocida*-free rabbits are commercially available, and may be necessary for specific research applications. However, given the inevitability of infection, it is difficult to justify their increased purchase price.

Staphylococcus aureus

Agent
Staphylococcus aureus is a gram-positive, coagulase-positive coccus that commonly inhabits the skin, upper respiratory tract, and lower digestive tract of many animals, including lab-

oratory rabbits. Multiple strains of *S. aureus* have been reported in rabbits (10).

Epidemiology
S. aureus is common in laboratory rabbit colonies. Transmission is by breaks in normal skin or mucosal barriers and may also occur following ingestion of mastitic milk.

Clinical signs
In general, infection occurs in the skin and subcutaneous tissues, but may also be found in the upper airways, lungs, conjunctiva, middle ears, feet, and mammary glands (4, 9, 16). In kits, staphylococcal septicemia occasionally occurs, initiating disseminated abscessation (9, 16).

Pathology
S. aureus colonizes tissues following a break in normal skin or mucosal barriers. Suppurative inflammation consists primarily of neutrophils and necrotic cellular debris, and may be accompanied by edema, hemorrhage, and fibrin deposition (16). Biologically active products of *S. aureus* may have profound effects on the host. Specific effects reported in experimentally exposed rabbit tissues include vasoconstriction (19), inhibition of developed myocardial force (systolic function) (7, 15), structural and functional shifts of hepatic subcellular structures (12), vascular leakage (17), accumulation of fluid within the ileum (13), T-lymphocyte stimulation (5), localized inflammation (18), and decreased neutrophil function (2).

Interference with research
Rabbits are highly susceptible to staphylococcal infections, and are therefore used extensively in *S. aureus* research (1, 3, 6, 7, 8, 11, 14). While asymptomatic colonization is of no concern, and is indeed unavoidable outside of strict barrier containment, active infection would interfere with nearly any studies utilizing rabbits. Studies most likely to be affected involve the cardiovascular, dermal, enterohepatic, lymphoreticular, reproductive, and respiratory systems.

Diagnosis and control
Diagnosis of staphylococcus infection is easily made by identifying the gram-positive organism in tissue sections or exudates, with confirmation after bacterial culture. Isolated cases can be treated with a variety of antibiotics, the optimal choice depending on clinical presentation. Considering the ubiquitous nature of the organism, culling whole colonies of rabbits because of a few cases is not recommended.

Treponema paraluis-cuniculi

Agent
Treponema paraluis-cuniculi is a gram-negative spirochete, and the causative agent of rabbit syphilis.

Epidemiology
Infection is uncommon in wild hares (15, 21), and occurs only occasionally in rabbits produced for research facilities (11). Transmission is primarily sexual, by penetration of mucous membranes. Seroprevalence tends to increase with parity, with most does seropositive after six litters (11). Transmission may also occur by direct and indirect contact (8). Susceptibility is rabbit age and breed dependent. Adult rabbits are more susceptible to infection (6). Rabbits of the X/J and WH/J strains appear particularly susceptible (6).

Clinical signs
The course of the disease is relatively lengthy. Erythematous macules or papules develop 3 to 6 weeks following exposure, and are most apparent on and around the mucocutaneous junctions of the face, anus, and genitalia. Lesions progress to erosions, ulcers, and crusts (5).

Pathology
Grossly, lesions begin as areas of erythema and edema, with or without vesicles, and as pre-

viously noted, progress to ulcers and crusts. Lesions generally resolve after several weeks (5). Histologically, advanced lesions consist of epidermal ulceration, hyperkeratosis, hyperplasia, and acanthosis overlain by crusts (8). Dermal inflammation consists primarily of macrophages and plasma cells. Serologic responses are also slow to develop, occurring 2 to 3 months after infection (6, 10). In unmedicated rabbits, in contrast to rabbits treated with antibiotics, antibodies may persist (9), suggesting a carrier state, possibly in regional lymph nodes (8, 10).

Interference with research
Because most treponemes cannot be grown in vitro, and because *Treponema pallidum,* the causative agent of human syphilis, is known to infect rabbits (13), the laboratory rabbit has been used extensively as a model of human syphilis (1, 4, 16, 19, 20). Consequently, a considerable body of information has accumulated on *T. pallidum* infections of rabbits, and cautious extrapolation to *T. paraluis-cuniculi* is possible. In this model, it has been demonstrated that the development of immunity is extremely complex and involves both stimulation and down-regulation of macrophage and T-lymphocyte function (12, 22). Stimulation of dendritic cells, the first immune-competent cells to encounter treponemal antigens in the skin and mucous membranes, drives the cellular immune response to *Treponema* spp. (3). Mononuclear cells from rabbits chronically infected with *T. pallidum* may lose the ability to produce or bind IL-2 (19), while spleen cells of rabbits infected with *T. pallidum* produce antitreponemal lymphotoxins (ATLs). This ability was disturbed when circulating immune complexes and autolymphocytotoxins were present, suggesting that the impairment of the cells' ability to produce ATLs may facilitate the survival of treponemes in the host despite the presence of immunologically competent cells (18). Lastly, defensins produced by rabbit alveolar macrophages and neutrophils may contribute to the control of local *T. pallidum* infection and suggest a role for acute inflammatory processes in the resolution of early experimental syphilis (2). Natural infection of laboratory rabbits would interfere with several types of studies, such as those involving the dermal, lymphoreticular, and reproductive systems.

Diagnosis and control
Diagnosis of infection can be accomplished by several means. Wet mounts of lesion scrapings can be directly examined for spirochetes by using dark-field microscopy. This is the screening test of choice (8). Fixed tissues may also be examined following silver staining (17). Several serologic tests have also been used. The microhemagglutination test was considered the best overall serologic screening and verification test, while the nontreponemal antigen tests, including the Venereal Disease Research Laboratory slide (VDRL) test and the rapid plasma reagin card (RPR) test were less sensitive (11). Seroconversion is slow to occur. Elimination of the organism from a rabbit colony is desirable for the benefit of the rabbits, research, and lastly, because *T. paraluis-cuniculi* is capable, at least experimentally, of temporarily infecting humans (14). Rabbit colonies can be rendered free of infection with *T. paraluis-cuniculi* by parenteral administration of penicillin G (7), or by cesarean rederivation (6).

FUNGI

Dermatomycosis

Agent
Rabbits are susceptible to infection with dermatophytes, including *Trichophyton mentagrophytes, Microsporum gypseum,* and *Microsporum canis* (1, 8).

Epidemiology
Dermatophytes are common in rabbitries in many parts of the world (2, 3, 4, 6, 7). How-

ever, incidence of infection and clinical disease (dermatophytosis, dermatomycosis, ringworm, flavus) are low in well-managed animal facilities.

Clinical signs
Young or immunocompromised rabbits are thought to be more susceptible (1). Dermatophytes infect the epidermis and adnexal structures, including hair follicles and shafts, usually on or around the head, and cause pruritus, patchy alopecia, erythema, and crusting.

Pathology
Following infection, histopathologic changes in underlying skin include neutrophilic and lymphoplasmacytic dermatitis, hyperkeratosis, folliculitis, and acanthosis. Abscessation of hair follicles may occur secondarily (1, 5).

Interference with research
Natural infection of laboratory rabbits may result in histopathologic changes that could confound studies involving the dermal system. In addition, moderate to severe pruritus could affect food intake and thereby compromise studies in which growth rate or feed intake was measured.

Diagnosis and control
Diagnosis of dermatomycosis is relatively easily accomplished and is based on clinical signs and confirmation of growth of the organism on dermatophyte test media. Localized infections are readily treated with topical application of antifungal agents such as miconazole. Additional information pertaining to treatment options can be obtained in general veterinary medical texts. Because dermatophytes readily infect humans, personnel handling infected rabbits should utilize personal protective clothing and practice excellent personal hygiene.

PARASITES
Cheyletiella parasitivorax

Agent
Cheyletiella parasitivorax is a nonburrowing mite with widespread distribution (5, 6).

Epidemiology
The life cycle consists of egg, larva, nymph, and adult. The entire life cycle is completed on the rabbit host. Mites attach to the host, primarily in the interscapular region, and obtain tissue fluids.

Clinical signs
Clinical signs may be absent, or may consist of skin lesions (2). Affected areas may be alopecic and erythematous, with a finely granular material (dried exudate), or scale covering the skin (3). Lesions are nonpruritic (4, 7).

Pathology
Histopathologic changes associated with mite infestation include subacute dermatitis with mild hyperkeratosis, accompanied by an inflammatory exudate.

Interference with research
While infested rabbits appear largely unaffected by the parasite, histopathologic changes in the skin could compromise dermal studies conducted in affected rabbits. In addition, the mites can infest animal technicians and while infestation is temporary, the mite causes skin irritation and pruritus (1).

Diagnosis and control
Mite infestation can be diagnosed by microscopic examination of skin scrapings for mites. On occasion, mites may also be observed grossly. Effective acaricides are readily available. Therefore, culling of an infested colony is neither necessary nor recommended.

Cryptosporidium parvum

Agent
Rabbits, like other mammals, may become infected with a *Cryptosporidium* sp., an intra-

cellular, extracytoplasmic, apicomplexan parasitic protozoan inhabiting the epithelial lining of the ileum and jejunum. Because it was thought that *Cryptosporidium* spp. were host specific, the name *Cryptosporidium cuniculus* was applied to the organism found naturally in the rabbit (14). However, results of cross-infectivity studies suggest that the organism is actually *C. parvum* (9, 12).

Epidemiology
The prevalence of infection is assumed to be low in laboratory rabbits. The life cycle is direct. Sporulated, infectious oocysts are released in the feces. Following ingestion by a suitable host, the oocysts break down, releasing the infectious sporozoites, which penetrate the intestinal mucosal epithelium. There, both asexual and sexual replication occur, culminating in the release of sporulated oocysts into the feces.

Clinical signs
In most mammals, infection with *Cryptosporidium* spp. results in severe enteritis, even in adult animals. In contrast, neither diarrheal disease or clinicopathologic changes occur with either natural or experimental infections of adult rabbits (5, 8, 14). However, naturally infected, recently weaned rabbits develop inappetency, apathy, lethargy, lowered body weight, and dehydration (13). Similarly, experimentally infected neonatal rabbits develop diarrheal disease (10).

Pathology
Histologic examination of the intestines of infected rabbits reveals alterations in villus cytoarchitecture, including a decrease in villus-to-crypt ratio, disruption of microvilli, mild edema of the lamina propria, and dilation of intestinal lacteals (8, 13, 14).

Interference with research
Little information is available dealing with the effects of *C. parvum* on rabbit physiology. In other species, *Cryptosporidium* sp. infection causes lymphocytopenia in rats (1), decreased responsiveness to vaccination against viral pathogens in chickens (16, 17), reduced weight gain (4), inactivation of phosphatases and altered ion balance in rat intestinal enterocytes (2, 7), altered electroencephalographic patterns following antigen exposure in rats (6), and induced apoptosis in human biliary epithelia (3). Rabbits are used extensively in studies of cryptosporidiosis. Near-term fetal rabbit small intestinal xenografts are suitable for study of early events of cryptosporidial infection (18). Lastly, laboratory rabbits are used to produce polyclonal anticryptosporidial antiserum (11, 15). Natural infection of rabbits with *C. parvum* would interfere with these efforts; it might complicate interpretation of histologic changes in the intestines of rabbits in studies in which intestinal mucosal cytoarchitecture is evaluated, and interfere with studies involving the enterohepatic and lymphoreticular systems. It is unknown whether natural infection with *C. parvum* influences studies involving the nervous system.

Diagnosis and control
Diagnosis of infection is based on finding cryptosporidial oocysts in feces. This may be difficult, unless there is a high level of suspicion, since oocysts are small, and special stains are required to facilitate their identification in fecal samples. Various developmental stages are readily identified in histologic examination. Currently there is no completely effective therapy for eliminating the organism. Infected rabbits should be culled. The zoonotic potential of *C. parvum* should be considered and appropriate sanitary measures practiced to prevent infection of persons handling infected rabbits.

Encephalitozoon cuniculi

Agent
Encephalitozoon cuniculi is an obligate intracellular microsporidian protozoan parasite capable of infecting a wide range of hosts, including rabbits and humans (10, 24, 33).

Epidemiology
Prevalence of *E. cuniculi* infection is high in wild rabbits (34), and remains high in some rabbitries (15, 16, 23, 37), ensuring that at least some laboratory rabbits are infected. Prevalence of infection increases with age up to about 5 months (5). *E. cuniculi* is excreted in the urine within 6 weeks after infection (9) but is poorly contagious (4). There is no transplacental transmission (39).

Clinical signs
Infection is usually asymptomatic. When clinical signs do appear, they are generally referable to the nervous system, and include torticollis, convulsions, tremors, paresis, and coma (20, 30). Involvement of other systems may result in muscular weakness, polydipsia, polyuria, and death (18). Infection of rabbits has also been implicated in cases of cataract (2) and phacoclastic uveitis (40).

Pathology
Following ingestion, sporoplasm from infectious spores gains entrance to host intestinal epithelium, where multiplication occurs. Continued multiplication results in eventual host cell rupture, with dissemination to other organs, including liver, lungs, brain, heart, and kidneys (9). Lesions are most commonly found in the kidneys and brain. Multiple pinpoint depressions may be observed on the surface of the kidneys. Microscopically, these represent areas of granulomatous nephritis or lymphoplasmacytic infiltration, with fibrosis, tubular degeneration, and eventual focal and segmental hyalinosis and sclerosis (12, 25, 27). Organisms may be observed, following special staining, within renal tubule cells. In the brain, lesions consist of randomly distributed, multifocal granulomas (granulomatous encephalitis), characterized by areas of necrosis, often containing organisms, and usually surrounded by mixed leukocytes. Lesions are often perivascular and periventricular. Multifocal mineralization may be present. Lymphoplasmacytic perivascular cuffing, vasculitis, nonsuppurative meningitis, and focal radiculoneuritis may also be noted (25, 28). Although less common, cardiac, pulmonary, splenic, and hepatic lesions have also been reported (13, 19, 25, 38). Immunity to *E. cuniculi* consists of specific antibody-mediated phagocytosis by macrophages (26). *E. cuniculi* infection of mice is used as a model of human microsporidiosis, and it may be possible to cautiously extrapolate pathophysiologic and/or immune mechanisms observed in the mouse to the rabbit. For example, Didier (11) demonstrated that reactive nitrogen intermediates contribute to the killing of *E. cuniculi* by lipopolysaccharide (LPS) plus IFN-γ-activated murine peritoneal macrophages in vitro.

Interference with research
E. cuniculi has been reported to interfere with viral research when contaminated rabbit kidney cell cultures were used (1), and to alter humoral immune responsiveness (7), possibly through alterations in circulating catecholamine levels (22). Antibodies against *E. cuniculi* cross-react with antigens of other microsporidia, including *Encephalitozoon bieneusi* (36). Furthermore, antibodies have been found in commercially available rabbit sera (6). Lastly, immune suppression of laboratory rabbits may result in lethal encephalitozoonosis of previously infected but asymptomatic rabbits (17). Natural infection of laboratory rabbits could compromise studies involving the cardiovascular, enterohepatic, lymphoreticular, musculoskeletal, nervous, respiratory, and urinary systems. In addition, infection of rabbits used directly in microsporidial research (38), or for antibody production, may compromise such studies.

Diagnosis and control
E. cuniculi infections are currently diagnosed serologically (3, 8, 21, 29, 35). For colony surveillance, an adequate sample size is important, and may need to approach 100%, since prevalence may be as low as 5% (4). Other methods include direct staining and examination of urine, histologic examination, and identification in tissue culture following ex-

posure of the culture to the urine of infected rabbits (14, 32). It is anticipated that PCR techniques, developed for experimental use (14), will also become available for colony screening. Control of *E. cuniculi* infections is accomplished by serologic testing followed by elimination of reactors (31). Eradication of the infection is recommended not only for the integrity of the research and the health of the rabbits, but also because *E. cuniculi* is transmissible to humans (10, 24, 33).

Hepatic coccidiosis

Agent
Eimeria stiedai, an apicomplexan parasitic protozoan, is the causative agent of hepatic coccidiosis in rabbits.

Epidemiology
While infection may be common in some commercial rabbitries (12, 16), modern laboratory animal husbandry methods and effective chemotherapeutics have considerably reduced the prevalence of infection in laboratory rabbits. The life cycle is direct, with unsporulated oocysts released in the bile and exiting the rabbit via the feces. Sporulation to the infective stage occurs in less than 3 days under optimal conditions (14). Sporozoites penetrate the small intestinal mucosa and arrive in the liver. The exact means of transport from intestine to liver is uncertain, although evidence exists for both hematogenous and lymphatic migration (10). Once in the liver, sporozoites invade the bile duct epithelium and undergo asexual replication (schizogony), followed by production of sexual stages (gametogony) which unite to form oocysts. Virus-like RNA particles were found in sporozoites of all isolates of *E. stiedai* examined; however, their significance remains unknown (13).

Clinical signs
Mild infections are frequently asymptomatic. Severe infections usually occur in young rabbits from weaning to about 2 months of age (2, 16). The infection proceeds through four pathophysiologic events: (i) hepatic damage during schizogony, (ii) cholestasis, (iii) metabolic dysfunction, and (iv) "immunodepression" (3). When present, clinical signs are referable to hepatic dysfunction and biliary blockage and include anorexia, icterus, diarrhea or constipation, weight loss, failure to thrive, a "pot-bellied" appearance, and rarely, death.

Pathology
Gross necropsy findings include hepatomegaly with dilated bile ducts appearing as yellowish lesions throughout the liver. The gallbladder may also be enlarged and contain exudate. Microscopically, there is destruction and regeneration of the bile duct epithelium resulting in bile duct hyperplasia, fibrosis, distension, and lymphoplasmacytic infiltration. Rupture of enlarged bile ducts results in a severe granulomatous response, while compression of adjacent liver tissue results in ischemic hepatic necrosis (10, 11). Mildly infected rabbits mount both cellular and humoral immune responses (9, 10). However, Barriga and Arnoni (3) reported that the final pathophysiologic event of overwhelming hepatic coccidiosis is "immunodepression," so called because young rabbits were unable to control the production of sexual stages of the parasite. Caution is warranted in using the term "immunodepression," since no immune function tests were conducted. Rabbits may have been unable to control the infection due to immunosuppression, clonal exhaustion, anergy, or clinicopathologic changes. Further studies are needed to explain apparent unresponsiveness in terminal hepatic coccidiosis.

Interference with research
Physiologic effects of *E. stiedai* that could markedly alter research findings in infected rabbits have been reported. Clinicopathologic changes in natural and/or experimental infections include increases in serum β- and γ-globulin, β-lipoprotein, succinate dehydrogenase activity (which later declines), sorbitol dehydrogenase, glutamate dehydrogen-

ase, bilirubin, alanine transaminase, glutamic oxaloacetic transaminase, glutamic pyruvic transaminase, and aspartate transaminase. Decreases in serum α-lipoprotein and glucose; and liver alkaline phosphatase activity have also been noted (1, 2, 3, 8, 10). Increased γ-globulins and decreased albumin alter the albumen/globulin ratio (6). Two-month-old rabbits were affected to a greater degree than 4-month-old rabbits (7). In addition, pharmacokinetics, hepatic biotransformation, biliary and urinary excretion of conjugated bromosulfophthalein, and weight gains are markedly altered following experimental infection (2, 4). Finally, experimental infection results in acid-base imbalances indicative of an uncompensated metabolic acidosis (5). *E. stiedai* has been used to establish a model of liver disease mimicking biliary cirrhosis (4). Natural infection of laboratory rabbits with *E. stiedai* could interfere with such studies, and may confound other studies involving the enterohepatic system and/or evaluation of clinical chemistry profiles. Studies in which weight gain was important would also be affected. Light, asymptomatic infections are of little concern, but specific research needs may warrant eradication of the infection.

Diagnosis and control
E. stiedai infection can be diagnosed histologically, or by examining bile for oocysts (11). In the feces, oocysts of *E. stiedai* cannot be differentiated from those of some intestinal *Eimeria* spp. Because it is nearly impossible to find rabbits completely free of an *Eimeria* sp. infection, control should be centered around adequate cage sanitation to reduce the likelihood of overwhelming infection, since sanitation of cages removes infectious oocysts. Diclazuril, at one part per million in the feed, is effective at interrupting the life cycle and restoring normal growth (15), and can be used during outbreaks. However, sanitation remains the foundation of control.

Intestinal coccidiosis

Agent
Coccidia of several species of the genus *Eimeria* are known to infect laboratory rabbits.

The most pathogenic species are *E. intestinalis* and *E. flavescens,* followed by *E. magna, E. irresidua, E. piriformis, E. perforans, E. neoleporis* (*E. coecicola*), and *E. media* (3, 4, 20, 21). Both mixed and single species infections are common (14, 16, 18), although the prevalence has declined with improvements in facility management.

Epidemiology
The life cycles of intestinal coccidia are similar to that of *E. stiedai,* except that all stages occur in the intestine (8), the exact location depending on the species of *Eimeria*. Sporozoites invade intraepithelial lymphocytes (11, 12), both B and T cells (17), and in this way may be transported to their specific sites of multiplication.

Clinical signs
Clinical signs of infection are variable, and are usually present only in young animals from a few weeks to a few months of age. After weaning, infections tend to stabilize at a modest level (6) and with fewer coccidial species (16). When present, clinical signs include weight loss, diarrhea with or without blood, intussusception, and death (13, 22).

Pathology
Diarrhea occurs as a result of changes in Na^+ and K^+ transport (9). The cecum and colon contain dark, watery, foul-smelling fluid. Histopathologic changes in heavily infected intestinal segments include epithelial necrosis; mucosal ulceration, congestion, edema, and occasionally, hemorrhages; villous atrophy; and leukocytic exudate. Clinicopathologic changes reported in cases of experimental coccidiosis included hemodilution and hypokalemia (15). As with *E. stiedai,* even mild infections result in development of protective immunity (4, 10). However, immunity is not cross protective among intestinal coccidia.

Interference with research
Other than the physiologic effects noted previously, little information is available to indicate what effects *Eimeria* spp. could have on

research. Fioramonti and coworkers (5) reported gastric and small intestinal hypomotility, accompanied by increased rate of flow of digesta in rabbits, following experimental infection with E. magna. Decreased transepithelial conductance and increased paracellular permeability in inflamed ileum have been reported (7). Mild infections of laboratory rabbits with intestinal coccidia will probably not compromise most studies. In contrast, heavy infections will confound studies of the enterohepatic system.

Diagnosis and control
Historically, diagnosis of infection has been based on finding large numbers of coccidial oocysts in the feces. The site of infection in the intestine combined with oocyst morphology can often, although not always, allow identification to the species level. However, mixed infections are common. More recently, species-specific DNA probes for use in PCR assays have been developed (1, 2). The infection can be minimized with caging systems that render the feces unavailable to rabbits (14), and can be eradicated through strict adherence to sanitation protocols combined with the use of anticoccidial agents (16, 19). If maintenance of a coccidia-free colony is essential, all incoming rabbits should be treated before arrival, or should be quarantined and treated prophylactically after arrival.

Passalurus ambiguus

Agent
Passalurus ambiguus is an oxyurid nematode parasite of rabbits.

Epidemiology
P. ambiguus, the rabbit pinworm, is common in lagomorphs from many parts of the world. The life cycle is direct, with adult worms found principally in the anterior cecum and colon. Embryonated eggs are passed in the feces and are immediately infective (7). Larval stages are found in the mucosa of the small intestine and cecum. Infection is established following ingestion of infective eggs. The prepatent period is 56 to 64 days (5, 7). Levels of infection increase with age in naturally infected rabbits (2). While some researchers report no influence of host sex on parasite egg excretion (4), others report higher adult parasite loads in female rabbits (1). Clearly, additional studies are needed to clarify this issue.

Clinical signs
Rabbit pinworms rarely cause clinical disease. Taffs (7) cites earlier workers that ascribed signs of enteric disease to P. ambiguus infection. However, other possible causes of the clinical signs were not entirely ruled out. Declines in general condition and breeding performance of rabbits coinfected with P. ambiguus and Obeliscoides cuniculi, a trichostrongylid nematode parasite commonly found in the stomachs of wild rabbits, have been reported (3).

Pathology
Many consider rabbit pinworms harmless, while others have reported microstructural inflammatory and dystrophic changes in the cecum, and vacuolar dystrophy in the livers and kidneys of infected rabbits, accompanied by general immune stimulation (6).

Interference with research
More sophisticated studies may reveal subtle effects of these parasites on rabbit health and suitability as research subjects. Natural infection of laboratory rabbits with P. ambiguus may compromise studies involving the enterohepatic, lymphoreticular, and urinary systems.

Diagnosis and control
Pinworms are easily diagnosed by examining fecal samples for the characteristic eggs. Eradication can be accomplished by adding fenbendazole to the feed (3), in association with proper husbandry.

Psoroptes cuniculi

Agent
Psoroptes cuniculi is an obligate, nonburrowing parasite causing otoacariasis in domestic rabbits.

Epidemiology
Prevalence of infestation is high and worldwide. Mites are found almost exclusively on the inner surface of the pinnae, although ectopic infestations occur (3). The entire life cycle is completed on the rabbit.

Clinical signs
Clinical signs include intense pruritus, scratching, and head shaking with subsequent serum exudation and crusting on the pinnae, which are painful. Self-excoriation may lead to secondary bacterial infections (2). Initially, mites feed on skin detritus and later on serum exudates (6), although there is evidence that mites penetrate capillaries to feed (12).

Pathology
Following infestation, gross observations include inflammation and serum crusting of the inner surfaces of the pinnae. Histologically, the pinnae become chronically inflamed with hypertrophy of the malpighian layer, parakeratosis of the horny layer, and epithelial sloughing (5). Clinical signs and histopathology of *P. cuniculi* infestation are suggestive of an immunoglobulin E (IgE)-mediated type 1 hypersensitivity response. Lymphocyte responsiveness and antibody production have been observed to be suppressed in heavily infested rabbits (9), and immunogenic parasite glycoprotein antigens have been identified (10).

Interference with research
While mild infestations may not alter immune responsiveness (9), heavy infestations could alter immune function of laboratory rabbits. Alterations in immune response patterns may also occur when large numbers of mites die, releasing antigen, subsequent to ivermectin treatment (11). Therefore, natural infestation of rabbits with *P. cuniculi* may confound studies involving the dermal and lymphoreticular systems. Additionally, studies involving thermoregulation may be affected by infestation with *P. cuniculi* (7). Lastly, behavioral changes in pruritic rabbits could alter a variety of studies, including those depending on adequate feed intake.

Diagnosis and control
Diagnosis is based on finding mites during examination of gel swabs of the ear canal. On occasion, mites may be observed moving along the inner surface of the pinnae, if observation is made using a hand-held magnifying glass. Laboratory rabbits are routinely treated prophylactically with ivermectin (400 μg/kg subcutaneously [s.c.] or intramuscularly [i.m.]) to prevent clinical infestations (13). Other members of the avermectin class of compounds are also effective (4). Since animal room temperature and relative humidity profoundly influence longevity of mites in the environment (1, 8), these parameters could be modified to eliminate any free-living mites prior to introduction of uninfested rabbits.

Sarcoptes scabiei

Agent
Sarcoptes scabiei is an obligate, burrowing parasitic mite of the family *Sarcoptidae*. It is easily recognized as such by the possession of short, stumpy legs that extend only a short distance beyond the margins of the body. Subspecies or strains differ in their degree of host preference and specificity, with *S. scabiei* var. *canis* from the dog, completely cross infestive to rabbits (6).

Epidemiology
Prevalence of *S. scabiei* is low in well-managed rabbit colonies. The life cycle of *S. scabiei* consists of egg, larva, nymph, and adult. All these permanently inhabit the epidermis. Female mites burrow into the epidermis by digesting away and feeding on epidermal cells. Eggs and young larvae are also found in these tunnels, while older larvae, nymphs, and adult males are found on the surface (10). Mites feed on epithelial cells and serum exudates. The entire life cycle in completed on the rabbit and requires 10 to 25 days. Transmission is by direct contact, as well as indirect, through fomites.

TABLE 6-1. Body systems known or likely to be affected by pathogen indicated

Pathogen	Cardio-vascular	Dermal	Endocrine	Entero-hepatic	Hema-topoietic	Lympho-reticular	Musculo-skeletal	Nervous	Reproductive	Respiratory	Urinary
Adenovirus				X						X	X
Cottontail rabbit papillomavirus		X		X		X				X	X
Lapine parvovirus				X							
Myxoma virus	X	X	X	X	X	X			X	X	X
Pleural effusion disease virus	X			X	X	X	X			X	X
Rabbit enteric coronavirus				X		X					
Rabbit hemorrhagic disease virus				X	X	X		X		X	
Rabbit oral papillomavirus				X							
Rotavirus				X							
Bordetella bronchiseptica										X	
Cilia-associated respiratory bacillus										X	
Clostridium piliforme	X			X							
Clostridium spiroforme				X							
Francisella tularensis			X	X	X	X		X		X	
Listeria monocytogenes	X		X	X			X	X	X		
Pasteurella multocida				X		X			X	X	
Staphylococcus aureus	X	X				X			X	X	
Treponema paraluis-cuniculi		X							X		
Dermatomycosis		X									
Cheyletiella parasitivorax		X									
Cryptosporidium parvum				X		X					
Encephalitozoon cuniculi				X			X	X		X	X
Hepatic coccidiosis				X							
Intestinal coccidiosis				X							
Passalurus ambiguus						X					
Psoroptes cuniculi		X				X					X
Sarcoptes scabiei		X		X	X	X					X

Clinical signs
Infestations usually begin on the muzzle and extend to the remainder of the head. Pruritus associated with scabies is considered among the most intense known in veterinary or human medicine. Some animals, including swine, will forego feeding in favor of scratching, in an attempt to obtain some relief (9). Similar behavior is likely in other infested animal species. Self-excoriation often leads to secondary bacterial infections. In addition to pruritus, clinical signs in rabbits may include general debility, emaciation, and death (10).

Pathology
Pathologic findings include alopecia and dermatitis with serum exudation (11). It appears that rabbits proceed through stages of cutaneous hypersensitivity, and develop immune responses similar to those described for swine with sarcoptic mange (3, 5, 8), but reactions in the two species have not been directly compared.

Interference with research
Heavy infestations may result in anemia, leukopenia, and serum biochemical changes (1, 2). In addition, infestation may result in amyloidosis, particularly in the liver, renal glomerulus, splenic red pulp, intestines, and tongue (2). Serum antibody profiles of infested rabbits have been reported (3, 12). Antigens from *S. scabiei* cross react with antigens of the house dust mite, *Dermatophagoides pteronyssinus* (7), and *Dermatophagoides* sp. antigens can sensitize rabbits to scabies mites and induce protective immunity (4). Due to parasite-induced histologic changes and cross-reacting antibodies, natural infestation renders laboratory rabbits unusable for studies involving the dermal, enterohepatic, hematopoietic, lymphoreticular, and urinary systems.

Diagnosis and control
Diagnosis of infestation is achieved by finding mites in deep skin scrapings or histologic sections. Definitive diagnosis requires cleared specimens, although for the inexperienced, even these can be difficult to distinguish from other species of burrowing mites (11). Infestations can be eliminated by treatment with ivermectin or other acaricides. Because *S. scabiei* is a zoonosis, personnel working in the animal facility should wear protective clothing when handling infested rabbits.

REFERENCES
VIRUSES
Adenovirus
1. Araki, K., Y. Ohashi, T. Sasabe, S. Kinoshita, K. Hayashi, X. Z. Yang, Y. Hosaka, S. Aizawa, and H. Handa. 1993. Immortalization of rabbit corneal epithelial cells by a recombinant SV40-adenovirus vector. *Investig. Ophthalmol. Vis. Sci.* **34**:2665–2671.
2. Bodon, L., and L. Prohaszka. 1980. Isolation of adenovirus from rabbits with diarrhea. *Acta Vet. Acad. Sci. Hung.* **28**:247–255.
3. Gordon, Y. J., T. Araullo-Cruz, and E. G. Romanowski. 1998. The effects of topical non-steroidal anti-inflammatory drugs on adenoviral replication. *Arch. Ophthalmol.* **116**:900–905.
4. Kozarsky, K. F., D. K. Bonen, F. Giannoni, T. Funahashi, J. M. Wilson, and N. O. Davidson. 1996. Hepatic expression of the catalytic subunit of the apolipoprotein B mRNA editing enzyme (apobec-1) ameliorates hypercholesterolemia in LDL receptor-deficient rabbits. *Hum. Gene Ther.* **7**:943–957.
5. Kupfer, J. M., X. M. Ruan, G. Liu, J. Matloff, J. Forrester, and A. Chaux. 1994. High-efficiency gene transfer to autologous rabbit jugular vein grafts using adenovirus-transferrin/polylysine-DNA complexes. *Hum. Gene Ther.* **5**:1437–1443.
6. Lippe, R., E. Luke, Y. T. Kuah, C. Lomas, and W. A. Jefferies. 1991. Adenovirus infection inhibits the phosphorylation of major histocompatibility complex class I proteins. *J. Exp. Med.* **174**:1159–1166.
7. Reddick, R. A., and S. S. Lefkowitz. 1969. In vitro immune responses of rabbits with persistent adenovirus type 5 infection. *J. Immunol.* **103**:687–694.

Cottontail rabbit papillomavirus
1. Christensen, N. D., M. D. Pickel, L. R. Budgeon, and J. W. Kreider. 2000. In vivo anti-papillomavirus activity of nucleoside analogues including cidofovir on CRPV-induced rabbit papillomas. *Antivir. Res.* **48**:131–142.
2. DiGiacomo, R. F., and C. J. Maré. 1994. Viral diseases, p. 171–204. *In* P. J. Manning, D. H.

Ringler, and C. E. Newcomer (ed.), *The Biology of the Laboratory Rabbit*, 2nd ed. Academic Press, Inc., San Diego, Calif.
3. Duan, J., W. Paris, J. De Marte, D. Roopchand, T. L. Fleet, and M. G. Cordingley. 2000. Topical effects of cidofovir on cutaneous rabbit warts: treatment regimen and inoculum dependence. *Antivir. Res.* **46:**135–144.
4. Hagari, Y., L. R. Budgeon, M. D. Pickel, and J. W. Kreider. 1995. Association of tumor necrosis factor-a gene expression and apoptotic cell death with regression of Shope papillomas. *J. Investig. Dermatol.* **104:**526–529.
5. Hagen, K. W. 1966. Spontaneous papillomatosis in domestic rabbits. *Bull. Wildl. Dis. Assoc.* **2:**108–110.
6. Han, R., N. M. Cladel, C. A. Reed, X. Peng, L. R. Budgeon, M. Pickel, and N. D. Christensen. 2000. DNA vaccination prevents and/or delays carcinoma development of papillomavirus-induced skin papillomas on rabbits. *J. Virol.* **74:**9712–9716.
7. Hopfl, R. M., N. D. Christensen, M. G. Angell, and J. W. Kreider. 1993. Skin test to assess immunity against cottontail rabbit papillomavirus antigens in rabbits with progressing papillomas or after papilloma regression. *J. Investig. Dermatol.* **101:**227–231.
8. Hopfl, R., N. D. Christensen, M. G. Angell, and J. W. Kreider. 1995. Leukocyte proliferation in vitro against cottontail rabbit papillomavirus in rabbits with persisting papillomas/cancer or after regression. *Arch. Dermatol. Res.* **287:**652–658.
9. Kreider, J., and G. Bartlett. 1981. The Shope papilloma-carcinoma complex of rabbits: A model system of neoplastic progression and spontaneous regression. *Adv. Cancer Res.* **35:**81–109.
10. Lin, Y. L., L. A. Borenstein, R. Selvakumar, R. Ahmed, and F. O. Wettstein. 1993. Progression from papilloma to carcinoma is accompanied by changes in antibody response to papillomavirus proteins. *J. Virol.* **67:**382–389.
11. Okabayashi, M., M. G. Angell, N. D. Christensen, and J. W. Kreider. 1991. Morphometric analysis and identification of infiltrating leucocytes in regressing and progressing Shope rabbit papillomas. *Int. J. Cancer* **49:**919–923.
12. Roth, E. J., B. Kurz, L. Liang, C. L. Hansen, C. T. Dameron, D. R. Winge, and D. Smotkin. 1992. Metal thiolate coordination in the E7 proteins of human papilloma virus 16 and cottontail rabbit papilloma virus as expressed in *Escherichia coli*. *J. Biol. Chem.* **267:**16390–16395.
13. Salmon, J., N. Ramoz, P. Cassonnet, G. Orth, and F. Breitburd. 1997. A cottontail rabbit papillomasvirus strain (CRPVb) with strikingly divergent E6 and E7 oncoproteins: An insight in the evolution of papillomaviruses. *Virology* **235:**228–234.
14. Selvakumar, R., L. A. Borenstein, Y. L. Lin, R. Ahmed, and F. O. Wettstein. 1994. T-cell response to cottontail rabbit papillomavirus structural proteins in infected rabbits. *J. Virol.* **68:**4043–4048.
15. Selvakumar, R., L. A. Borenstein, Y. L. Lin, R. Ahmed, and F. O. Wettstein. 1995. Immunization with nonstructural proteins E1 and E2 of cottontail rabbit papillomavirus stimulates regression of virus-induced papillomas. *J. Virol.* **69:**602–605.
16. Selvakumar, R., A. Schmitt, T. Iftner, R. Ahmed, and F. O. Wettstein. 1997. Regression of papillomas induced by cottontail rabbit papillomavirus is associated with infiltration of $CD8^+$ cells and persistence of viral DNA after regression. *J. Virol.* **71:**5540–5548.
17. Watts, S. L., R. S. Ostrow, W. C. Phelps, J. T. Prince, and A. J. Faras. 1983. Free cottontail rabbit papillomavirus DNA persists in warts and carcinomas of infected rabbits and in cells in culture transformed with virus of viral DNA. *Virology* **125:**127–138.

Lapine parvovirus
1. Matsunaga, Y., and F. Chino. 1981. Experimental infection of young rabbits with rabbit parvovirus. *Arch. Virol.* **68:**257–264.
2. Matsunaga, Y., S. Matsumo, and J. Mukoyama. 1977. Isolation and characterization of a parvovirus of rabbits. *Infect. Immun.* **18:**495–500.
3. Metcalf, J. B., M. Lederman, E. R. Stout, and R. C. Bates. 1989. Natural parvovirus infection in laboratory rabbits. *Am. J. Vet. Res.* **50:**1048–1051.

Myxoma virus
1. Barry, M., S. Hnatiuk, K. Mossman, S. F. Lee, L. Boshkov, and G. McFadden. 1997. The myxoma virus M-T4 gene encodes a novel RDEL-containing protein that is retained within the endoplasmic reticulum and is important for the productive infection of lymphocytes. *Virology* **239:**360–377.
2. Barry, M., S. F. Lee, L. Boshkov, and G. McFadden. 1995. Myxoma virus induces extensive CD4 downregulation and dissociation of p56lck in infected rabbit $CD4^+$ T lymphocytes. *J. Virol.* **69:**5243–5251.
3. Best, S. M., S. V. Collins, and P. J. Kerr. 2000. Coevolution of host and virus: cellular localization of virus in myxoma virus infection of resistant and susceptible European rabbits. *Virology* **277:**76–91.

4. **Best, S. M., and P. J. Kerr.** 2000. Coevolution of host and virus: the pathogenesis of virulent and attenuated strains of myxoma virus in resistant and susceptible European rabbits. *Virology* **267:** 36–48.
5. **Boshkov, L. K., J. L. Macen, and G. McFadden.** 1992. Virus-induced loss of class I MHC antigens from the surface of cells infected with myxoma virus and malignant rabbit fibroma virus. *J. Immunol.* **148:**881–887.
6. **Csatary, L. K., J. Romvary, L. Kasza, S. Schaff, and R. J. Massey.** 1985. In vivo interference between pathogenic and non-pathogenic viruses. *J. Med.* **16:**563–573.
7. **DiGiacomo, R. F., and C. J. Maré.** 1994. Viral diseases, p. 171–204. *In* P. J. Manning, D. H. Ringler, and C. E. Newcomer (ed.), *The Biology of the Laboratory Rabbit,* 2nd ed. Academic Press, Inc., San Diego, Calif.
8. **Everett, H., M. Barry, S. F. Lee, X. Sun, K. Graham, J. Stone, R. C. Bleackley, and G. McFadden.** 2000. M11L: a novel mitochondria-localized protein of myxoma virus that blocks apoptosis of infected leukocytes. *J. Exp. Med.* **191:**1487–1498.
9. **Fountain, S., M. K. Holland, L. A. Hinds, P. A. Janssens, and P. J. Kerr.** 1997. Interstitial orchitis with impaired steroidogenesis and spermatogenesis in the testes of rabbits infected with an attenuated strain of myxoma virus. *J. Reprod. Fertil.* **110:**161–169.
10. **Gelfi, J., J. Chantal, T. T. Phong, R. Py, and C. Boucraut-Baralon.** 1999. Development of an ELISA for detection of myxoma virus-specific rabbit antibodies: test evaluation for diagnostic applications on vaccinated and wild rabbit sera. *J. Vet. Diagn. Invest.* **11:**240–245.
11. **Graham, K. A., A. S. Lalani, J. L. Macen, T. L. Ness, M. Barry, L. Y. Liu, A. Lucas, I. Clark-Lewis, R. W. Moyer, and G. McFadden.** 1997. The T1/35kDa family of poxvirus-secreted proteins bind chemokines and modulate leukocyte influx into virus-infected tissues. *Virology* **229:**12–24.
12. **Heard, H. K., K. O'Connor, and D. S. Strayer.** 1990. Molecular analysis of immunosuppression induced by virus replication in lymphocytes. *J. Immunol.* **144:**3992–3999.
13. **Jackson, E. W., C. R. Dorn, J. K. Saito, and D. G. McKercher.** 1966. Absence of serological evidence of myxoma virus infection in humans exposed during an outbreak of myxomatosis. *Nature* **211:**313–314.
14. **Lalani, A. S., K. Graham, K. Mossman, K. Rajarathnam, I. Clark-Lewis, D. Kelvin, and G. McFadden.** 1997. The purified myxoma virus gamma interferon receptor homolog M-T7 interacts with the heparin-binding domains of chemokines. *J. Virol.* **71:**4356–4363.
15. **Lalani, A. S., J. Masters, K. Graham, L. Liu, A. Lucas, and G. McFadden.** 1999. Role of the myxoma virus soluble CC-chemokine inhibitor glycoprotein, M-T1, during myxoma virus pathogenesis. *Virology* **256:**233–245.
16. **Lalani, A. S., and G. McFadden.** 1997. Secreted poxvirus chemokine binding proteins. *J. Leukoc. Biol.* **62:**570–576.
17. **Liu, L., A. Lalani, E. Dai, B. Seet, C. Macauley, R. Singh, L. Fan, G. McFadden, and A. Lucas.** 2000. The viral anti-inflammatory chemokine-binding protein M-T7 reduces intimal hyperplasia after vascular injury. *J. Clin. Investig.* **105:**1613–1621.
18. **Luna, R. M.** 2000. First report of myxomatosis in Mexico. *J. Wildl. Dis.* **36:**580–583.
19. **Maksymowych, W. P., N. Nation, P. Nash, J. Macen, A. Lucas, G. McFadden, and A. S. Russell.** 1996. Amelioration of antigen induced arthritis in rabbits treated with a secreted viral serine proteinase inhibitor. *J. Rheumatol.* **23:**878–882.
20. **Marlier, D., D. Cassart, C. Boucraut-Baralon, F. Coignoul, and H. Vindevogel.** 1999. Experimental infection of specific pathogen-free New Zealand White rabbits with five strains of amyxomatous myxoma virus. *J. Comp. Pathol.* **121:**369–384.
21. **Marlier, D., J. Herbots, J. Detilleux, M. Lemaire, E. Thiry, and H. Vindevogel.** 2001. Cross-sectional study of the association between pathological conditions and myxoma-virus seroprevalence in intensive rabbit farms in Europe. *Prev. Vet. Med.* **48:**55–64.
22. **Marlier, D., J. Mainil, A. Linden, and H. Vindevogel.** 2000. Infectious agents associated with rabbit pneumonia: isolation of amyxomatous myxoma virus strains. *Vet. J.* **159:**171–178.
23. **Marlier, D., J. Mainil, J. Sulon, J. F. Beckers, A. Linden, and H. Vindevogel.** 2000. Study of the virulence of five strains of amyxomatous myxoma virus in crossbred New Zealand White/Californian conventional rabbits, with evidence of long-term testicular infection in recovered animals. *J. Comp. Pathol.* **122:**101–113.
24. **McFadden, G., K. Graham, K. Ellison, M. Barry, J. Macen, M. Schreiber, K. Mossman, P. Nash, A. Lalani, and H. Everett.** 1995. Interruption of cytokine networks by poxviruses: lessons from myxoma virus. *J. Leukoc. Biol.* **57:** 731–738.
25. **Messud-Petit, F., J. Gelfi, M. Delverdier, M. F. Amardeilh, R. Py, G. Sutter, and S. Bertagnoli.** 1998. Serp2, an inhibitor of the interleukin-1β–converting enzyme, is critical in

the pathobiology of myxoma virus. *J. Virol.* **72:** 7830–7839.
26. **Mossman, K., P. Nation, J. Macen, M. Garbutt, A. Lucas, and G. McFadden.** 1996. Myxoma virus M-T7, a secreted homolog of the interferon-γ receptor, is a critical virulence factor for the development of myxomatosis in European rabbits. *Virology* **215:**17–30.
27. **Nash, P., J. Barrett, J. X. Cao, S. Hota-Mitchell, A. S. Lalani, H. Everett, X. M. Xu, J. Robichaud, S. Hnatiuk, C. Ainslie, B. T. Seet, and G. McFadden.** 1999. Immunomodulation by viruses: the myxoma virus story. *Immunol. Rev.* **168:**103–120.
28. **Percy, D. H., and S. W. Barthold.** 2001. *Pathology of Laboratory Rodents and Rabbits,* 2nd ed. Iowa State University Press, Ames.
29. **Petit, F., S. Bertagnoli, J. Gelfi, F. Fassy, C. Boucraut-Baralon, and A. Milon.** 1996. Characterization of a myxoma virus-encoded serpin-like protein with activity against interleukin-1β-converting enzyme. *J. Virol.* **70:**5860–5866.
30. **Sellers, R. F.** 1987. Possible windborne spread of myxomatosis to England in 1953. *Epidemiol. Infect.* **98:**119–125.
31. **Williams, R. T., J. D. Dunsmore, and I. Parer.** 1972. Evidence for the existence of latent myxoma virus in rabbits (*Oryctolagus cuniculus*). *Nature* **238:**99–101.
32. **Xu, X., P. Nash, and G. McFadden.** 2000. Myxoma virus expresses a TNF receptor homolog with two distinct functions. *Virus Genes* **21:** 97–109.

Pleural effusion disease virus
1. **Alexander, L. K., B. W. Keene, and R. S. Baric.** 1995. Echocardiographic changes following rabbit coronavirus infection. *Adv. Exp. Med. Biol.* **380P:**113–115
2. **Alexander, L. K., B. W. Keene, B. L. Yount, J. D. Geratz, J. D. Small, and R. S. Baric.** 1999. ECG changes after rabbit coronavirus infection. *J. Electrocardiol.* **32:**21–32.
3. **DiGiacomo, R. F., and C. J. Maré.** 1994. Viral diseases, p. 171–204. *In* P. J. Manning, D. H. Ringler, and C. E. Newcomer (ed.), *The Biology of the Laboratory Rabbit,* 2nd ed, Academic Press, Inc., San Diego, Calif.
4. **Edwards, S., J. D. Small, J. D. Geratz, L. K. Alexander, and R. S. Baric.** 1992. An experimental model for myocarditis and congestive heart failure after rabbit coronavirus infection. *J. Infect. Dis.* **165:**134–140.
5. **Evermann, J. F., C. J. Henry, and S. L. Marks.** Feline infectious peritonitis. 1995. *J. Am. Vet. Med. Assoc.* **206:**1130–1134.
6. **Fennestad, K. L.** 1985. Pathogenetic observations on pleural effusion disease in rabbits. *Arch. Virol.* **84:**163–174.
7. **Fennestad, K. L., L. Bruun, and E. Wedo.** 1980. Pleural effusion disease agent as passenger of *Treponema pallidum* suspensions from rabbits. Survey of laboratories. *Br. J. Vener. Dis.* **56:**198–203.
8. **Fennestad, K. L., B. Mansa, N. Christensen, S. Larsen, and S. V. E. Svehag.** 1986. Pathogenicity and persistence of pleural effusion disease virus isolates in rabbits. *J. Gen. Virol.* **67:** 993–1000.
9. **Fennestad, K. L., B. Mansa, and S. Larsen.** 1981. Pleural effusion disease in rabbits. Observations on viraemia, immunity, and transmissibility. *Arch. Virol.* **70:**11–19.
10. **Fennestad, K. L., H. J. Skovgaard Jensen, S. Moller, and M. W. Bentzon.** 1975. Pleural effusion disease in rabbits. Clinical and post mortem observations. *Acta Pathol. Microbiol. Scand. B* **83:**541–548.
11. **Gudjonsson, H., B. Newman, and T. B. Turner.** 1970. Demonstration of a virus-like agent contaminating material containing the Stockholm substrain of the Nichols pathogenic *Treponema pallidum. Br. J. Vener. Dis.* **46:**435–440.
12. **Jorgensen, B. B.** 1968. Spontaneous deaths among rabbits inoculated with *Treponema pallidum* less than 2 weeks before abnormal susceptibility in apparently normal laboratory rabbits indicated by serological tests for human syphilis. *Z. Verstierkd.* **10:**46–54.
13. **Small, J. D., L. Aurelian, R. A. Squire, J. D. Strandberg, E. C. Melby, Jr., T. B. Turner, and B. Newman.** 1979. Rabbit cardiomyopathy associated with a virus antigenically related to human coronavirus strain 229E. *Am. J. Pathol.* **95:**709–730.
14. **Small, J. D., and R. D. Woods.** 1987. Relatedness of rabbit coronavirus to other coronaviruses. *Adv. Exp. Med. Biol.* **218:**521–527.

Rabbit enteric coronavirus
1. **Deeb, B. J., R. F. DiGiacomo, J. F. Evermann, and M. E. Thouless.** 1993. Prevalence of coronavirus antibodies in rabbits. *Lab. Anim. Sci.* **43:**431–433.
2. **Descoteaux, J. P., and G. Lussier.** 1990. Experimental infection of young rabbits with a rabbit enteric coronavirus. *Can. J. Vet. Res.* **54:**473–476.
3. **Descoteaux, J. P., G. Lussier, L. Berthiaume, R. Alain, C. Seguin, and M. Trudel.** 1985. An enteric coronavirus of the rabbit: Detection by immunoelectron microscopy and identification of the structural polypeptides. *Arch. Virol.* **84:**241–250.
4. **Eaton, P.** 1984. Preliminary observations on enteritis associated with a coronavirus-like agent in rabbits. *Lab. Anim.* **18:**71–74.

5. **La Pierre, J., G. Marsolais, P. Pilon, and J. P. Descoteaux.** 1980. Preliminary report on the observation of a coronavirus in the intestine of the laboratory rabbit. *Can. J. Microbiol.* **26:**1204–1208.
6. **Osterhaus, A. D. M. E., J. S. Teppema, and G. Van Steenis.** 1982. Coronavirus-like particles in laboratory rabbits with different syndromes in the Netherlands. *Lab. Anim. Sci.* **32:**663–665.
7. **Percy, D. H., and S. W. Barthold.** 2001. *Pathology of Laboratory Rodents and Rabbits*, 2nd ed. Iowa State University Press, Ames.
8. **Small, J. D., and R. D. Woods.** 1987. Relatedness of rabbit coronavirus to other coronaviruses. *Adv. Exp. Med. Biol.* **218:**521–527.

Rabbit hemorrhagic disease virus
1. **Alonso, C., J. M. Oviedo, J. M. Martin-Alonso, E. Diaz, J. A. Boga, and F. Parra.** 1998. Programmed cell death in the pathogenesis of rabbit hemorrhagic disease. *Arch. Virol.* **143:**321–332.
2. **Asgari, S., J. R. Hardy, R. G. Sinclair, and B. D. Cooke.** 1998. Field evidence for mechanical transmission of rabbit haemorrhagic disease virus (RHDV) by flies (Diptera: Calliphoridae) among wild rabbits in Australia. *Virus Res.* **54:**123–132.
3. **Barcena, J., M. Morales, B. Vazquez, J. A. Boga, F. Parra, J. Lucientes, A. Pages-Mante, J. M. Sanchez-Vizcaino, R. Blasco, and J. M. Torres.** 2000. Horizontal transmissible protection against myxomatosis and rabbit hemorrhagic disease by using a recombinant myxoma virus. *J. Virol.* **74:**1114–1123.
4. **Berninger, M. L., and C. House.** 1995. Serologic comparison of four isolates of rabbit hemorrhagic disease virus. *Vet. Microbiol.* **47:**157–165.
5. **Boga, J. A., J. M. Martin Alonso, R. Casais, and F. Parra.** 1997. A single dose immunization with rabbit hemorrhagic disease virus major capsid protein produced in *Saccharomyces cerevisiae* induces protection. *J. Gen. Virol.* **78:**2315–2318.
6. **Bouslama, A., G. M. De Mia, S. Hammami, T. Aouina, H. Soussi, and T. Frescura.** 1996. Identification of the virus of rabbit haemorrhagic disease in Tunisia. *Vet. Rec.* **138:**108–110.
7. **Capucci, L., F. Fallacara, S. Grazioli, A. Lavazza, M. L. Pacciarini, and E. Brocchi.** 1998. A further step in the evolution of rabbit hemorrhagic disease virus: the appearance of the first consistent antigenic variant. *Virus Res.* **58:**115–126.
8. **Capucci, L., P. Fusi, A. Lavazza, M. L. Pacciarini, and C. Rossi.** 1996. Detection and preliminary characterization of a new rabbit calicivirus related to rabbit hemorrhagic disease virus but nonpathogenic. *J. Virol.* **70:**8614–8623.
9. **Collins, B. J., J. R. White, C. Lenghaus, V. Boyd, and H. A. Westbury.** 1995. A competition ELISA for the detection of antibodies to rabbit haemorrhagic disease virus. *Vet. Microbiol.* **43:**85–96.
10. **Collins, B. J., J. R. White, C. Lenghaus, C. J. Morrissy, and H. A. Westbury.** 1996. Presence of rabbit haemorrhagic disease virus antigen in rabbit tissues as revealed by a monoclonal antibody dependent capture ELISA. *J. Virol. Methods* **58:**145–154.
11. **Cooke, B. D., A. J. Robinson, J. C. Merchant, A. Nardin, and L. Capucci.** 2000. Use of ELISA in field studies of rabbit haemorrhagic disease (RHD) in Australia. *Epidemiol. Infect.* **124:**563–576.
12. **DiGiacomo, R. F., and C. J. Maré.** 1994. Viral diseases, p. 171–204. *In* P. J. Manning, D. H. Ringler, and C. E. Newcomer (ed.), *The Biology of the Laboratory Rabbit*, 2nd ed. Academic Press, Inc., San Diego, Calif.
13. **Graham, D. A., J. Cassidy, N. Beggs, W. L. Curran, I. E. McLaren, T. J. Connor, and S. Kennedy.** 1996. Rabbit viral haemorrhagic disease in Northern Ireland. *Vet. Rec.* **138:**47.
14. **Guittre, C., N. Ruvoen-Clouet, L. Barraud, Y. Cherel, I. Baginski, M. Prave, J. P. Ganiere, C. Trepo, and L. Cova.** 1996. Early stages of rabbit haemorrhagic disease virus infection monitored by polymerase chain reaction. *Zentbl. Vetmed. Reihe B* **43:**109–118.
15. **Jung, J. Y., B. J. Lee, J. H. Tai, J. H. Park, and Y. S. Lee.** 2000. Apoptosis in rabbit haemorrhagic disease. *J. Comp. Pathol.* **123:**135–140.
16. **Kesy, A., A. Fitzner, W. Niedbalski, G. Paprocka, and B. Walkowiak.** 1996. A new variant of the viral hemorrhagic disease of rabbits virus. *Rev. Sci. Tech.* **15:**1029–1035.
17. **Kpodekon, M., and T. Alogninouwa.** 1998. Control of rabbit haemorrhagic disease in Benin by vaccination. *Vet. Rec.* **143:**693–694.
18. **Leighton, A.** 1995. Surveillance of wild animal diseases in Europe. *Rev. Sci. Tech.* **14:**819–830.
19. **Lugton, I. W.** 1999. A cross-sectional study of risk factors affecting the outcome of rabbit haemorrhagic disease virus releases in New South Wales. *Aust. Vet. J.* **77:**322–328.
20. **Marcato, P. S., C. Benazzi, G. Vecchi, M. Galeotti, L. Della Salda, G. Sarli, and P. Lucidi.** 1991. Clinical and pathological features of viral haemorrhagic disease of rabbits and the European brown hare syndrome. *Rev. Sci. Tech. Off. Int. Epizoot.* **10:**371–392.
21. **Mikami, O., J. H. Park, T. Kimura, K. Ochiai, and C. Itakura.** 1999. Hepatic lesions in young rabbits experimentally infected with

rabbit haemorrhagic disease virus. *Res. Vet. Sci.* **66:**237–242.
22. Motha, M. X., and R. Kittelberger. 1998. Evaluation of three tests for the detection of rabbit haemorrhagic disease virus in wild rabbits. *Vet. Rec.* **143:**627–629.
23. Nagesha, H. S., K. A. McColl, B. J. Collins, C. J. Morrissy, L. F. Wang, and H. A. Westbury. 2000. The presence of cross-reactive antibodies to rabbit haemorrhagic disease virus in Australian wild rabbits prior to the escape of virus from quarantine. *Arch. Virol.* **145:**749–757.
24. Nardelli, S., F. Agnoletti, F. Costantini, and R. Parajola. 1996. Diagnosis of rabbit hemorrhagic disease (RHD) by indirect sandwich polyclonal ELISA. *Zentbl. Vetmed Reihe B* **43:**393–400.
25. Ohlinger, V. F., H. Bernd, G. Meyers, F. Weiland, and H.-J. Thiel. 1990. Identification and characterization of the virus causing rabbit hemorrhagic disease. *J. Virol.* **64:**3331–3336.
26. Park, J. H., Y. S. Lee, and C. Itakura. 1995. Pathogenesis of acute necrotic hepatitis in rabbit hemorrhagic disease. *Lab. Anim. Sci.* **45:**445–449.
27. Patterson, I. A., and F. E. Howie. 1995. Rabbit haemorrhagic disease in Scotland. *Vet. Rec.* **137:**523.
28. Percy, D. H., and S. W. Barthold. 2001. *Pathology of Laboratory Rodents and Rabbits*, 2nd ed. Iowa State University Press, Ames.
29. Prieto, J. M., F. Ferndndez, V. Alvarez, A. Espi, J. F. Garcia Marin, M. Alvarez, J. M. Martin, and F. Parra. 2000. Immunohistochemical localisation of rabbit haemorrhagic disease virus VP-60 antigen in early infection of young and adult rabbits. *Res. Vet. Sci.* **68:**181–187.
30. Ramiro-Ibanez, F., J. M. Martin-Alonso, P. Garcia Palencia, F. Parra, and C. Alonso. 1999. Macrophage tropism of rabbit haemorrhagic disease virus is associated with vascular pathology. *Virus Res.* **60:**21–28.
31. Rodák, L., B. Šmíd, L. Valícek, T. Veselý, J. Štěpánek, J. Hampl, and E. Jurák. 1990. Enzyme-linked immunosorbent assay of antibodies to rabbit haemorrhagic disease virus and determination of its major structural proteins. *J. Gen. Virol.* **71:**1075–1080.
32. Ros Bascunana, C., N. Nowotny, and S. Belak. 1997. Detection and differentiation of rabbit hemorrhagic disease and European brown hare syndrome viruses by amplification of VP60 genomic sequences from fresh and fixed tissue specimens. *J. Clin. Microbiol.* **35:**2492–2495.
33. Ruvoen-Clouet, N., D. Blanchard, G. Andre-Fontaine, B. Song, and J. P. Ganiere. 1995. Detection of antibodies to rabbit haemorrhagic disease virus: an immunoblotting method using virus-coated human erythrocyte membranes. *Zentbl. Vetemed. Reihe B* **42:**197–204.
34. Ruvoen-Clouet, N., J. P. Ganiere, G. Andre-Fontaine, D. Blanchard, and J. Le Pendu. 2000. Binding of rabbit hemorrhagic disease virus to antigens of the ABH histo-blood group family. *J. Virol.* **74:**11950–11954.
35. Schirrmeier, H., I. Reimann, B. Kollner, and H. Granzow. 1999. Pathogenic, antigenic and molecular properties of rabbit haemorrhagic disease virus (RHDV) isolated from vaccinated rabbits: detection and characterization of antigenic variants. *Arch. Virol.* **144:**719–735.
36. Shien, J. H., H. K. Shieh, and L. H. Lee. 2000. Experimental infections of rabbits with rabbit haemorrhagic disease virus monitored by polymerase chain reaction. *Res. Vet. Sci.* **68:**255–259.
37. Villafuerte, R., C. Calvete, C. Gortazar, and S. Moreno. 1994. First epizootic of rabbit hemorrhagic disease in free living populations of *Oryctolagus cuniculus* at Doñana National Park, Spain. *J. Wildl. Dis.* **30:**176–179.
38. Wirblich, C., G. Meyers, V. F. Ohlinger, L. Capucci, U. Eskens, B. Haas, and H. J. Thiel. 1994. European brown hare syndrome virus: relationship to rabbit hemorrhagic disease virus and other caliciviruses. *J. Virol.* **68:**5164–5173.

Rabbit oral papillomavirus

1. Christensen, N. D., N. M. Cladel, C. A. Reed, and R. Han. 2000. Rabbit oral papillomavirus complete genome sequence and immunity following genital infection. *Virology* **269:**451–461.
2. Christensen, N. D., M. D. Pickel, L. R. Budgeon, and J. W. Kreider. 2000. In vivo antipapillomavirus activity of nucleoside analogues including cidofovir on CRPV-induced rabbit papillomas. *Antivir. Res.* **48:**131–142.
3. DiGiacomo, R. F., and C. J. Maré. 1994. Viral diseases, p. 171–204. *In* P. J. Manning, D. H. Ringler, and C. E. Newcomer (ed.), *The Biology of the Laboratory Rabbit*, 2nd ed. Academic Press, Inc., San Diego, Calif.
4. Harvey, S. B., N. M. Cladel, L. R. Budgeon, P. A. Welsh, J. W. Griffith, C. M. Lang, and N. D. Christensen. 1998. Rabbit genital tissue is susceptible to infection by rabbit oral papillomavirus: an animal model for a genital tissue-targeting papillomavirus. *J. Virol.* **72:**5239–5244.
5. Parsons, R. J., and J. G. Kidd. 1936. A virus causing oral papillomatosis in rabbits. *Proc. Soc. Exp. Biol. Med.* **35:**441–443.
6. Percy, D. H., and S. W. Barthold. 2001. *Pathology of Laboratory Rodents and Rabbits*, 2nd ed. Iowa State University Press, Ames.

7. **Sundberg, J. P., R. E. Junge, and M. O. el Shazly.** 1985. Oral papillomatosis in New Zealand White rabbits. *Am. J. Vet. Res.* **46:**664–668.
8. **Weisbroth, S. H., and S. Scher.** 1970. Spontaneous oral papillomatosis in rabbits. *J. Am. Vet. Med. Assoc.* **157:**1940–1944.

Rotavirus

1. **Beards, G. M., A. D. Campbell, N. R. Cottrell, J. S. Peiris, N. Rees, R. C. Sanders, J. A. Shirley, H. C. Wood, and T. H. Flewett.** 1984. Enzyme-linked immunosorbent assays based on polyclonal and monoclonal antibodies for rotavirus detection. *J. Clin. Microbiol.* **19:**248–254.
2. **Castrucci, G., M. Ferrari, F. Frigeri, V. Cilli, L. Perucca, and G. Donelli.** 1985. Isolation and characterization of cytopathic strains of rotavirus from rabbits. *Arch. Virol.* **83:**99–104.
3. **Ciarlet, M., S. E. Crawford, C. Barone, A. Bertolotti-Ciarlet, R. F. Ramig, M. K. Estes, and M. E. Conner.** 1998. Subunit rotavirus vaccine administered parenterally to rabbits induces active protective immunity. *J. Virol.* **72:**9233–9246.
4. **Ciarlet, M., M. A. Gilger, C. Barone, M. McArthur, M. K. Estes, and M. E. Conner.** 1998. Rotavirus disease, but not infection and development of intestinal histopathological lesions, is age restricted in rabbits. *Virology* **251:**343–360.
5. **Conner, M. E., M. K. Estes, and D. Y. Graham.** 1988. Rabbit model of rotavirus infection. *J. Virol.* **62:**1625–1633.
6. **Conner, M. E., M. A. Gilger, M. K. Estes, and D. Y. Graham.** 1991. Serologic and mucosal immune response to rotavirus infection in the rabbit model. *J. Virol.* **65:**2562–2571.
7. **DiGiacomo, R. F., and C. J. Maré.** 1994. Viral diseases, p. 171–204. *In* P. J. Manning, D. H. Ringler, and C. E. Newcomer (ed.), *The Biology of the Laboratory Rabbit,* 2nd ed., Academic Press, Inc., San Diego, Calif.
8. **DiGiacomo, R. F., and M. F. Thouless.** 1984. Age-related antibodies to rotavirus in New Zealand rabbits. *J. Clin. Microbiol.* **19:**710–711.
9. **DiGiacomo, R. F., and M. F. Thouless.** 1986. Epidemiology of naturally occurring rotavirus infection in rabbits. *Lab. Anim. Sci.* **36:**153–156.
10. **Halaihel, N., V. Lievin, F. Alvarado, and M. Vasseur.** 2000. Rotavirus infection impairs intestinal brush-border membrane Na^+-solute cotransport activities in young rabbits. *Am. J. Physiol.* **279:**G587–G596.
11. **Hambraeus, B. A., L. E. Hambraeus, and G. Wadell.** 1989. Animal model of rotavirus infection in rabbits-protection obtained without shedding of viral antigen. *Arch. Virol.* **107:**237–251.
12. **Legrottaglie, R., A. Mannelli, V. Rizzi, A. Cini, and P. Agrimi.** 1997. Isolation and characterization of cytopathic strains of rotavirus from hares (*Lepus europaeus*). *New Microbiol.* **20:**135–140.
13. **Leichus, L. S., J. M. Goldhill, J. D. Long, W. H. Percy, R. D. Shaw, V. Donovan, and R. Burakoff.** 1994. Effects of rotavirus on epithelial transport in rabbit small intestine. *Dig. Dis. Sci.* **39:**2202–2208.
14. **Peeters, J. E., P. Pohl, and G. Charlier.** 1984. Infectious agents associated with diarrhoea in commercial rabbits: A field study. *Ann. Rech. Vet.* **15:**335–340.
15. **Percy, D. H., and S. W. Barthold.** 2001. *Pathology of Laboratory Rodents and Rabbits,* 2nd ed. Iowa State University Press, Ames.
16. **Rizzi, V., R. Legrottaglie, A. Cini, and P. Agrimi.** 1995. Electrophoretic typing of some strains of enteric viruses isolated in rabbits suffering from diarrhoea. *New Microbiol.* **18:**77–81.
17. **Sato, K., Y. Inaba, Y. Miura, S. Tokuhisa, and M. Matumoto.** 1982. Isolation of lapine rotaviruses in cell cultures. *Arch. Virol.* **71:**267–271.
18. **Schoeb, T. R., D. B. Casebolt, V. E. Walker, L. N. Potgieter, M. E. Thouless, and R. F. DiGiacomo.** 1986. Rotavirus-associated diarrhea in a commercial rabbitry. *Lab. Anim. Sci.* **36:**149–152.
19. **Tanaka, T. N., M. E. Conner, D. Y. Graham, and M. K. Estes.** 1988. Molecular characterization of three rabbit rotavirus strains. *Arch. Virol.* **98:**253–265.
20. **Thouless, M. E., R. F. DiGiacomo, and B. J. Deeb.** 1996. The effect of combined rotavirus and *Escherichia coli* infections in rabbits. *Lab. Anim. Sci.* **46:**381–385.
21. **Thulin, J. D., M. S. Kuhlenschmidt, and H. B. Gelberg.** 1991. Development, characterization, and utilization of an intestinal xenograft model for infectious disease research. *Lab. Invest.* **65:**719–731.

BACTERIA

Bordetella bronchiseptica

1. **Bemis, D. A., and S. A. Wilson.** 1985. Influence of potential virulence determinants on *Bordetella bronchiseptica*-induced ciliostasis. *Infect. Immun.* **50:**35–42.
2. **Boot, R., R. H. Bakker, H. Thuis, and J. L. Veenema.** 1993. An enzyme-linked immunosorbent assay (ELISA) for monitoring guinea pigs and rabbits for *Bordetella bronchiseptica* antibodies. *Lab. Anim.* **27:**342–349.

3. Boot, R., H. Thuis, and G. Wieten. 1995. Multifactorial analysis of antibiotic sensitivity of *Bordetella bronchiseptica* isolates from guinea pigs, rabbits and rats. *Lab. Anim.* **29**:45–49.
4. Deeb, B. J., R. F. DiGiacomo, B. L. Bernard, and S. M. Silbernagel. 1990. *Pasteurella multocida* and *Bordetella bronchiseptica* infections in rabbits. *J. Clin. Microbiol.* **28**:70–75.
5. Garlinghouse, L. E., Jr., R. F. DiGiacomo, G. L. Van Hoosier, Jr., and J. Condon. 1981. Selective media for *Pasteurella multocida* and *Bordetella bronchiseptica*. *Lab. Anim. Sci.* **31**:39–42.
6. Glass, L. S., and J. N. Beasley. 1989. Infection with and antibody response to *Pasteurella multocida* and *Bordetella bronchiseptica* in immature rabbits. *Lab. Anim. Sci.* **39**:406–410.
7. Glavits, R., and T. Magyar. 1990. The pathology of experimental respiratory infection with *Pasteurella multocida* and *Bordetella bronchiseptica* in rabbits. *Acta. Vet. Hung.* **38**:211–215.
8. Gueirard, P., C. Weber, A. Le Coustumier, and N. Guiso. 1995. Human *Bordetella bronchiseptica* infection related to contact with infected animals: persistence of bacteria in host. *J. Clin. Microbiol.* **33**:2002–2006.
9. Matsuyama, T., and T. Takino. 1980. Scanning electronmicroscopic studies of *Bordetella bronchiseptica* on the rabbit tracheal mucosa. *J. Med. Microbiol.* **13**:159–161.
10. Percy, D. H., and S. W. Barthold. 2001. *Pathology of Laboratory Rodents and Rabbits*, 2nd ed. Iowa State University Press, Ames.
11. Percy, D. H., N. Karrow, and J. L. Bhasin. 1988. Incidence of *Pasteurella* and *Bordetella* infections in fryer rabbits: An abattoir survey. *J. Appl. Rabbit Res.* **11**:245–246.
12. Sacco, R. E., K. B. Register, and G. E. Nordholm. 2000. Restriction endonuclease analysis discriminates *Bordetella bronchiseptica* isolates. *J. Clin. Microbiol.* **38**:4387–4393.
13. Suzuki, H., M. Togashi, E. Kumagai, M. Miwa, T. Tatsumi, M. Nakura, T. Nakagawa, N. Tanaka, and J. Adachi. 1990. An attempt at embryo transfer as a means of controlling *Bordetella bronchiseptica* infection in the rabbit. *Jikken Dobutsu* **39**:397–400.
14. Syukuda, Y. 1979. Rearing of germfree rabbits and establishment of an SPF rabbit colony. *Jikken Dobutsu* **28**:39–48.
15. Yoda, H., K. Nakayama, and M. Nakagawa. 1982. Experimental infection of *Bordetella bronchiseptica* to rabbits. *Jikken Dobutsu* **31**:113–118.
16. Yoda, H., K. Nakayama, T. Yusa, S. Sato, and S. Fukuda. 1976. Bacteriological survey on *Bordetella bronchiseptica* in various animal species. *Jikken Dobutsu* **25**:7–11.
17. Zeligs, B. J., J. D. Zeligs, and J. A. Bellanti. 1986. Functional and ultrastructural changes in alveolar macrophages from rabbits colonized with *Bordetella bronchiseptica*. *Infect. Immun.* **53**:702–706.

Cilia-associated respiratory bacillus
1. Caniatti, M., L. Crippa, G. Giusti, S. Mattiello, G. Grilli, R. Orsenigo, and E. Scanziani. 1998. Cilia-associated respiratory (CAR) bacillus infection in conventionally reared rabbits. *Zentbl. Vetmed. Reihe B* **45**:363–371.
2. Cundiff, D. D., C. L. Besch-Williford, R. R. Hook, Jr., C. L. Franklin, and L. K. Riley. 1994. Characterization of cilia-associated respiratory bacillus isolates from rats and rabbits. *Lab. Anim. Sci.* **44**:305–312.
3. Cundiff, D. D., C. L. Besch-Williford, R. R. Hook, Jr., C. L. Franklin, and L. K. Riley. 1995. Characterization of cilia-associated respiratory bacillus in rabbits and analysis of the 16S rRNA gene sequence. *Lab. Anim. Sci.* **45**:22–26.
4. Hook, R. R., Jr., C. L. Franklin, L. K. Riley, B. A. Livingston, and C. L. Besch-Williford. 1998. Antigenic analyses of cilia-associated respiratory (CAR) bacillus isolates by use of monoclonal antibodies. *Lab. Anim. Sci.* **48**:234–239.
5. Kurisu, K., S. Kyo, Y. Shiomoto, and S. Matsushita. 1990. Cilia-associated respiratory bacillus infection in rabbits. *Lab. Anim. Sci.* **40**:413–415.
6. Matsushita, S., J. Joshima, T. Matsumoto, and K. Fukutsu. 1989. Transmission experiments of cilia-associated respiratory bacillus in mice, rabbits, and guinea pigs. *Lab. An.* **23**:96–102.
7. Oros, J., Poveda, J. B., Rodriguez, J. L., Franklin, C. L. and Fernandez, A. 1997. Natural cilia-associated respiratory bacillus infection in rabbits used for elaboration of hyperimmune serum against *Mycoplasma* sp. *Zentbl. Vetmed. Reihe B* **44**:313–317.
8. Shoji-Darkye, Y., T. Itoh, and N. Kagiyama. 1991. Pathogenesis of CAR bacillus in rabbits, guinea pigs, Syrian hamsters, and mice. *Lab. Anim. Sci.* **41**:567–571.

Clostridium piliforme
1. Allen, A. M., J. R. Ganaway, T. D. Moore, and R. F. Kinard. 1965. Tyzzer's disease syndrome in laboratory rabbits. *Am. J. Pathol.* **46**:859–882.
2. DeLong, D., and P. J. Manning. 1994. Bacterial Diseases, p. 131–170. *In* P. J. Manning, D. H. Ringler, and C. E. Newcomer (ed.), *The Biology of the Laboratory Rabbit*, 2nd ed. Academic Press, Inc., San Diego, Calif.
3. Goto, K., T. Itoh, A. Takakura, S. Kunita, E. Terada, and N. Kagiyama. 1991. A serological

survey on *Bacillus piliformis* infection in laboratory rabbits in Japan. *Jikken Dobutsu* **40:**231–233.
4. **Percy, D. H., and S. W. Barthold.** 2001. *Pathology of Laboratory Rodents and Rabbits,* 2nd ed. Iowa State University Press, Ames.

Clostridium spiroforme
1. **Bain, M. S., R. D. Naylor, and N. J. Griffiths.** 1998. *Clostridium spiroforme* infection in rabbits. *Vet. Rec.* **142:**47.
2. **Baldassarri, L., A. Pantosti, A. Caprioli, P. Mastrantonio, and G. Donelli.** 1989. Haemagglutination and surface structures in strains of *Clostridium spiroforme*. *FEMS Microbiol. Lett.* **51:**1–4.
3. **Borriello, S. P., and R. J. Carman.** 1983. Association of iota-like toxin and *Clostridium spiroforme* with both spontaneous and antibiotic-associated diarrhea and colitis in rabbits. *J. Clin. Microbiol.* **17:**414–418.
4. **Butt, M. T., R. E. Papendick, L. G. Carbone, and F. W. Quimby.** 1994. A cytotoxicity assay for *Clostridium spiroforme* enterotoxin in cecal fluid of rabbits. *Lab. Anim. Sci.* **44:**52–54.
5. **Carman, R. J., and S. P. Borriello.** 1984. Infectious nature of *Clostridium spiroforme*-mediated rabbit enterotoxaemia. *Vet. Microbiol.* **9:**497–502.
6. **DeLong, D., and P. J. Manning.** 1994. Bacterial Diseases, p. 131–170. *In* P. J. Manning, D. H. Ringler, and C. E. Newcomer (ed.), *The Biology of the Laboratory Rabbit,* 2nd ed. Academic Press, Inc., San Diego, Calif.
7. **Ellis, T. M., A. R. Gregory, and G. D. Logue.** 1991. Evaluation of a toxoid for protection of rabbits against enterotoxaemia experimentally induced by trypsin-activated supernatant of *Clostridium spiroforme*. *Vet. Microbiol.* **28:**93–102.
8. **Hara-Kudo, Y., Y. Morishita, Y. Nagaoka, F. Kasuga, and S. Kumagai.** 1996. Incidence of diarrhea with antibiotics and the increase of clostridia in rabbits. *J. Vet. Med. Sci.* **58:**1181–1185.
9. **Harris, I. E., and B. H. Portas.** 1985. Enterotoxaemia in rabbits caused by *Clostridium spiroforme*. *Aust. Vet. J.* **62:**342–343.
10. **Holmes, H. T., R. J. Sonn, and N. M. Patton.** 1988. Isolation of *Clostridium spiroforme* from rabbits. *Lab. Anim. Sci.* **38:**167–168.
11. **Peeters, J. E., R. Geeroms, R. J. Carman, and T. D. Wilkins.** 1986. Significance of *Clostridium spiroforme* in the enteritis-complex of commercial rabbits. *Vet. Microbiol.* **12:**25–31.
12. **Peeters, J. E., P. Pohl, and G. Charlier.** 1984. Infectious agents associated with diarrhoea in commercial rabbits: A field study. *Ann. Rech. Vet.* **15:**335–340.
13. **Piattoni, F., D. I. Demeyer, and L. Maertens.** 1996. In vitro study of the age-dependent caecal fermentation pattern and methanogenesis in young rabbits. *Reprod. Nutr. Dev.* **36:**253–261.
14. **Popoff, M. R., F. W. Milward, B. Bancillon, and P. Boquet.** 1989. Purification of the *Clostridium spiroforme* binary toxin and activity of the toxin on Hep-2 cells. *Infect. Immun.* **57:**2462–2469.
15. **Wilkins, T., H. Krivan, B. Stiles, R. Carman, and D. Lyerly.** 1985. Clostridial toxins active locally in the gastrointestinal tract. *Ciba Found. Symp.* **112:**230–241.
16. **Yonushonis, W. P., M. J. Roy, R. J. Carman, and R. E. Sims.** 1987. Diagnosis of spontaneous *Clostridium spiroforme* iota enterotoxemia in a barrier rabbit breeding colony. *Lab. Anim. Sci.* **37:**69–71.

Francisella tularensis
1. **Akerman, M. B., and J. A. Embil.** 1982. Antibodies to *Francisella tularensis* in the snowshoe hare (*Lepus americanus struthopus*) populations of Nova Scotia and Prince Edward Island and in the moose (*Alces alces americana* Clinton) population of Nova Scotia. *Can. J. Microbiol.* **28:**403–405.
2. **Anthony, L. S., P. J. Morrissey, and F. E. Nano.** 1992. Growth inhibition of *Francisella tularensis* live vaccine strain by IFN-γ-activated macrophages is mediated by reactive nitrogen intermediates derived from L-arginine metabolism. *J. Immunol.* **148:**1829–1834.
3. **Baskerville, A., and P. Hambleton.** 1976. Pathogenesis and pathology of respiratory tularaemia in the rabbit. *Br. J. Exp. Pathol.* **57:**339–347.
4. **Dahlstrand, S., O. Ringertz, and B. Zetterberg.** 1971. Airborne tularemia in Sweden. *Scand. J. Infect. Dis.* **3:**7–16.
5. **DeLong, D., and P. J. Manning.** 1994. Bacterial diseases, p. 131–170. *In* P. J. Manning, D. H. Ringler, and C. E. Newcomer (ed.), *The Biology of the Laboratory Rabbit,* 2nd ed. Academic Press, Inc., San Diego, Calif.
6. **Dunaeva, T. N., and K. N. Shlygina.** 1975. Phagocytic activity of the neutrophils in tularemia in animals with varying infective sensitivity. *Zh. Mikrobiol. Epidemiol. Immunobiol.* **10:**22–26.
7. **Eigelsbach, H. T., and V. G. McGann.** 1984. Genus *Francisella,* p. 394–399. *In* J. G. Holt and N. R. Kreig (ed.), *Bergey's Manual of Systematic Bacteriology,* Williams & Wilkins, Baltimore, Md.
8. **Finegold, M., J. D. Pulliam, M. E. Landay, and G. G. Wright.** 1969. Pathological changes in rabbits injected with *Pasteurella tularensis* killed by ionizing radiation. *J. Infect. Dis.* **119:**635–640.
9. **Gill, V., and B. A. Cunha.** 1997. Tularemia pneumonia. *Semin. Respir. Infect.* **12:**61–67.
10. **Gurycova, D.** 1998. First isolation of *Francisella tularensis* subsp. *tularensis* in Europe. *Eur. J. Epidemiol.* **14:**797–802.

11. Hambleton, P., P. W. Harris-Smith, N. E. Bailey, and R. E. Strange. 1977. Changes in whole blood and serum components during *Francisella tularensis* and rabbit pox infections of rabbits. *Br. J. Exp. Pathol.* **58**:644–652.
12. Hood, A. M. 1977. Virulence factors of *Francisella tularensis*. *J. Hyg.* **79**:47–60.
13. Hubalek, Z., F. Treml, J. Halouzka, Z. Juricova, M. Hunady, and V. Janik. 1996. Frequent isolation of *Francisella tularensis* from *Dermacentor reticulatus* ticks in an enzootic focus of tularemia. *Med. Vet. Entomol.* **10**:241–246.
14. Klock, L. E., P. E. Olsen, and T. Fukushima. 1973. Tularemia epidemic associated with the deerfly. *JAMA* **226**:149–152.
15. Kovarova, H., A. Marcela, and J. Stulik. 1992. Macrophage activating factors produced in the course of murine tularemia: effect on multiplication of microbes. *Arch. Immunol. Ther. Exp.* **40**:183–190.
16. Lepitzki, D. A., A. Woolf, and M. Cooper. 1990. Serological prevalence of tularemia in cottontail rabbits of southern Illinois. *J. Wildl. Dis.* **26**:279–282.
17. Maslova, T. N., and R. A. Savel'eva. 1977. Cytopathic effect of the tularemia microbe on a culture of peritoneal macrophages. *Zh. Mikrobiol. Epidemiol. Immunobiol.* **10**:104–107.
18. Morner, T., R. Mattsson, M. Forsman, K. E. Johansson, and G. Sandstrom. 1993. Identification and classification of different isolates of *Francisella tularensis*. *Zentbl. Vetmed. Reihe B* **40**:613–620.
19. Neufeld, H. A., J. A. Pace, and F. E. White. 1976. The effect of bacterial infections on ketone concentrations in rat liver and blood and on free fatty acid concentrations in rat blood. *Metabolism* **25**:877–884.
20. Nersesian, A. K. 1985. Effect of immunization with tularemia vaccine on 3,4-benz(a)pyrene-induced blastomogenesis and mutagenesis in rats. *Eksp. Onkol.* **7**:38–40.
21. Olin, G. 1942. The occurrence and mode of transmission of tularemia in Sweden. *Acta Pathol. Microbiol. Scand.* **19**:220–247.
22. Pavlovich, N. V., V. M. Sorokin, and N. S. Blagorodova. 1996. The resistance of *Francisella tularensis* to the bactericidal action of normal serum as a criterion for evaluating the virulence of the bacterium. *Zh. Mikrobiol. Epidemiol. Immunobiol.* **1**:7–10.
23. Pekarek, R. S., and M. C. Powanda. 1976. Protein synthesis in zinc deficient rats during tularemia. *J. Nutr.* **106**:905–912.
24. Sandstrom, G., S. Lofgren, and A. Tarnvik. 1988. A capsule-deficient mutant of *Francisella tularensis* LVS exhibits enhanced sensitivity to killing by serum but diminished sensitivity to killing by polymorphonuclear leukocytes. *Infect. Immun.* **56**:1194–1202.
25. Shoemaker, D., A. Woolf, R. Kirkpatrick, and M. Cooper. 1997. Humoral immune response of cottontail rabbits naturally infected with *Francisella tularensis* in southern Illinois. *J. Wildl. Dis.* **33**:733–737.
26. Skatov, D. V., V. G. Galaktionov, L. N. Semenkova, and V. S. Khlebnikov. 1994. The effect of the antigenic fractions of the outer membrane of *Francisella tularensis* on the T-cell immunity indices. *Zh. Mikrobiol. Epidemiol. Immunobiol.* **May-June**:100–103.
27. Skatov, D. V., V. S. Khlebnikov, R. N. Vasilenko, K. E. Kondakov, and V. G. Galaktionov. 1993. The effect of antigenic fractions of the outer membrane in *Francisella tularensis* on the functional activity of macrophages. *Zh. Mikrobiol. Epidemiol. Immunobiol.* **July-Aug.**:87–92.
28. Sukhar, V. V., and V. S. Uraleva. 1992. The C antigen of *Francisella tularensis* (in Russian). *Mikrobiol. Zh.* **54**:42–46.
29. Thompson, S., L. Omphroy, and T. Oetting. 2001. Parinaud's oculoglandular syndrome attributable to an encounter with a wild rabbit. *Am. J. Ophthalmol.* **131**:283–284.
30. Yee, D., T. R. Rhinehart-Jones, and K. L. Elkins. 1996. Loss of either $CD4^+$ or $CD8^+$ T cells does not affect the magnitude of protective immunity to an intracellular pathogen, *Francisella tularensis* strain LVS. *J. Immunol.* **157**:5042–5048.
31. Zil'fian, V. N., V. A. Kumkumadzhian, A. K. Nersesian, and B. S. Fichidzhian. 1985. Effect of immunization with live tularemia vaccine on the growth of various tumor strains in rats. *Vopr. Onkol.* **31**:66–70.
32. Zil'fian, V. N., V. A. Kumkumadzhian, A. K. Nersesian, and K. A. Tonapetian. 1989. The effect of tularemia vaccine on the radioresistance of white rats exposed to x-irradiation. *Radiobiologiia* **29**:113–116.

Listeria monocytogenes
1. Badmajew, W., P. Jakoniuk, and J. Borowski. 1980. The effect of *Listeria monocytogenes* lipids on immune response to T-dependent and T-independent antigens. *Experimentia* **36**:1321–1323.
2. Barbuddhe, S. B., S. V. Malik, and L. K. Gupta. 1998. Effect of in vitro monocyte activation by *Listeria monocytogenes* antigens on phagocytosis and production of reactive oxygen and nitrogen radicals in bovines. *Vet. Immunol. Immunopathol.* **64**:149–159.
3. Bast, R. C., Jr., B. Zbar, G. B. Mackaness, and H. J. Rapp. 1975. Antitumor activity of

bacterial infection. I. Effect of *Listeria monocytogenes* on growth of a murine fibrosarcoma. *J. Natl. Cancer Inst.* **54:**749–756.

4. **Bast, R. C., Jr., B. Zbar, T. E. Miller, G. B. Mackaness, and H. J. Rapp.** 1975. Antitumor activity of bacterial infection. II. Effect of *Listeria monocytogenes* on growth of a guinea pig hepatoma. *J. Natl. Cancer Inst.* **54:**757–761.

5. **Beattie, I. A., B. Swaminathan, and H. K. Ziegler.** 1990. Cloning and characterization of T-cell-reactive protein antigens from *Listeria monocytogenes*. *Infect. Immun.* **58:**2792-2803.

6. **Belen-Lopez, M., V. Briones, J. F. Fernandez-Garayzabal, J. A. Vazquez-Boland, J. A. Garcia, M. M. Blanco, G. Suarez, and L. Dominguez.** 1993. Serological response in rabbits to *Listeria monocytogenes* after oral or intragastric inoculation. *FEMS Immunol. Med. Microbiol.* **7:**131–134.

7. **Briones, V., L. Dominguez, M. Domingo, A. Marco, J. A. Ramos, J. A. Garcia, and G. Suarez.** 1989. Serological diagnosis of listeriosis in man, sheep, and rabbit by immunoperoxidase technique. *Acta Microbiol. Hung.* **36:**315–319.

8. **DeLong, D., and P. J. Manning.** 1994. Bacterial diseases, p. 131–170. *In* P. J. Manning, D. H. Ringler, and C. E. Newcomer (ed.), *The Biology of the Laboratory Rabbit,* 2nd ed. Academic Press, Inc., San Diego, Calif.

9. **Engeland, I. V., H. Waldeland, E. Ropstad, H. Kindahl, and O. Andresen.** 1997. Effect of experimental infection with *Listeria monocytogenes* on the development of pregnancy and on concentrations of progesterone, oestrone sulphate and 15-ketodihydro-PGF2α in the goat. *Anim. Reprod. Sci.* **45:**311–327.

10. **Higginbotham, J. N., T. L. Lin, and S. B. Pruett.** 1992. Effect of macrophage activation on killing of *Listeria monocytogenes*. Roles of reactive oxygen or nitrogen intermediates, rate of phagocytosis, and retention of bacteria in endosomes. *Clin. Exp. Immunol.* **88:**492–498.

11. **Iurkina, O. A., M. R. Karpova, V. V. Novitskii, and I. V. Fedorov.** 1997. The effect of *Listeria monocytogenes* on the blood system. *Zh. Mikrobiol. Epidemiol. Immunobiol.* **6:**68–70.

12. **Jakoniuk, P., W. Badmajew, W. Jablonska-Strynkowska, and J. Borowski.** 1979. Effect of *Listeria monocytogenes* lipids on the course of infections with some gram-negative bacilli in mice. *Arch. Immunol. Ther. Exp.* **27:**79–87.

13. **Jakoniuk, P., J. Borowski, and W. Jablonska-Strynkowska.** 1980a. The effect of *Listeria monocytogenes* lipids on the activity of nonspecific immune mechanisms. *Arch. Immunol. Ther. Exp.* **28:**611–618.

14. **Jakoniuk, P., W. Jablonska-Strynkowska, B. Musiatowicz, and J. Borowski.** 1980b. Effect of *Listeria monocytogenes* lipids on the immunity of mice against *Candida albicans, Cryptococcus neoformans* and *Trichomonas vaginalis*. *Arch. Immunol. Ther. Exp.* **28:**377–387.

15. **Jakoniuk, P., J. Talarczyk, and J. Borowski.** 1985. The effect of phospholipids from *Listeria monocytogenes* and *Aspergillus fumigatus* on degradation of bacterial antigens by mouse peritoneal macrophages. *Arch. Immunol. Ther. Exp.* **33:**397–404.

16. **Janoutova, J., M. Mara, and Z. Likovsky.** 1995. Accumulation of activated lymphocytes in liver of *Listeria* factor Ei treated rabbits. *Folia Microbiol.* **40:**652–654.

17. **John, C., I. Spratkova, M. Moravkova, F. Patocka, and M. Mara.** 1974. Effect of Listeria-factor Ei on spleen cells migration in rabbits hypersensitive to *Listeria monocytogenes*. *J. Hyg. Epidemiol. Microbiol. Immunol.* **18:**369–372.

18. **Johnson, J. D., W. L. Hand, N. L. King, and C. G. Hughes.** 1975. Activation of alveolar macrophages after lower respiratory tract infection. *J. Immunol.* **115:**80–84.

19. **Khalafalla, F. A.** 1993. Microbiological status of rabbit carcases in Egypt. *Z. Lebensm. Unters. Forsch.* **196:**233–235.

20. **Kral, J., M. Bastar, and B. Horyna.** 1975. Diagnosis of *Listeria monocytogenes* by immunofluorescence. *Vet. Med.* **20:**83–89.

21. **Lechner, W., F. Allerberger, A. Bergant, E. Solder, and M. P. Dierich.** 1993. Effect of *Listeria* on contractility of human uterine muscle. *Z. Geburtshilfe Perinatol.* **197:**179–183.

22. **Mazing, Yu. A., M. A. Danilova, V. N. Kokryakov, V. G. Seliverstova, V. E. Pigarevskii, S. Voros, M. Kerenyi, and B. Ralovich.** 1990. Haematological reactions of rabbits infected intravenously with *Listeria* strains of different virulence. *Acta Microbiol. Hung.* **37:**135–144.

23. **Musher, D. M., K. R. Ratzan, and L. Weinstein.** 1970. The effect of *Listeria monocytogenes* on resistance to pneumococcal infection. *Proc. Soc. Exp. Biol. Med.* **135:**557–560.

24. **Nakane, A., A. Numata, Y. Chen, and T. Minagawa.** 1991. Endogenous gamma interferon-independent host resistance against *Listeria monocytogenes* infection in CD4$^+$ T cell- and asialo GM1+ cell-depleted mice. *Infect. Immun.* **59:**3439–3445.

25. **Percy, D. H., and S. W. Barthold.** 2001. *Pathology of Laboratory Rodents and Rabbits,* 2nd ed. Iowa State University Press, Ames.

26. **Peters, M., and G. Scheele.** 1996. Listeriosis in a rabbitry. *Dtsch. Tierarztl. Wochenschr.* **103:**460–462.

27. **Siddique, I. H., and C. A. Walker.** 1967. Effects of *Listeria monocytogenes* hemolysins on the isolated ileum of rabbit. *Am. J. Vet. Res.* **28:** 1843–1849.
28. **Siddique, I. H., L. C. Ying, and B. B. Robinson.** 1969. Hematological and febrile responses of rabbits to listerial hemolysins. *Can. J. Comp. Med.* **33:**292–296.
29. **Vahidy, R., and F. Jehan.** 1996. Enhanced in vitro engulfment of Listeria monocytogenes by rabbit polymorphonuclear leukocytes in the presence of sera from immune rabbits. *FEMS Immunol. Med. Microbiol.* **14:**103–107.
30. **Vahidy, R., M. Waseem, and S. M. Khalid.** 1996. A comparative study of unpassaged and animal passaged cultures of *Listeria monocytogenes* in rabbits. *Ann. Acad. Med. Singapore* **25:**139–142.
31. **Watson, G. L., and M. G. Evans.** 1985. Listeriosis in a rabbit. *Vet. Pathol.* **22:**191–193.
32. **Williams, B. B., and I. H. Siddique.** 1972. Effects of listerial hemolysin on rabbit heart. *Am. J. Vet. Res.* **33:**591–597.
33. **Zaidman, G. W., P. Coudron, and J. Piros.** 1990. *Listeria monocytogenes* keratitis. *Am. J. Ophthalmol.* **109:**334–339.

Pasteurella multocida
1. **Al-Haddawi, M. H., S. Jasni, M. Zamri-Saad, A. R. Mutalib, and A. R. Sheikh-Omar.** 1999. Ultrastructural pathology of the upper respiratory tract of rabbits experimentally infected with *Pasteurella multocida* A:3. *Res. Vet. Sci.* **67:**163–170.
2. **Al-Haddawi, M. H., S. Jasni, M. Zamri-Saad, A. R. Mutalib, I. Zulkifli, R. Son, and A. R. Sheikh-Omar.** 2000. In vitro study of *Pasteurella multocida* adhesion to trachea, lung and aorta of rabbits. *Vet. J.* **159:**274–281.
3. **Anderson, L. C., H. G. Rush, and J. C. Glorioso.** 1984. Strain differences in the susceptibility and resistance of *Pasteurella multocida* to phagocytosis and killing by rabbit polymorphonuclear neutrophils. *Am. J. Vet. Res.* **45:**1193–1198.
4. **Bjotvedt, G., E. M. Bertke, and G. M. Hendricks.** 1979. Peritonitis due to *Pasteurella multocida* in a rabbit. *Vet. Med. Small Anim. Clin.* **74:** 215–216.
5. **Boiti, C., C. Canali, G. Brecchia, F. Zanon, and E. Facchin.** 1999. Effects of induced endometritis on the life-span of corpora lutea in pseudopregnant rabbits and incidence of spontaneous uterine infections related to fertility of breeding does. *Theriogenology* **52:**1123–1132.
6. **Bonilla-Ruz, L. F., and G. A. Garcia-Delgado.** 1993. Adherence of *Pasteurella multocida* to rabbit respiratory epithelial cells in vitro. *Rev. Latinoam. Microbiol.* **35:**361–369.
7. **Brogden, K. A.** 1980. Physiological and serological characteristics of 48 *Pasteurella multocida* cultures from rabbits. *J. Clin. Microbiol.* **11:**646–649.
8. **Cameron, C. M., L. Pienaar, and A. S. Vermeulen.** 1980. Lack of cross-immunity among *Pasteurella multocida* type A strains. *Onderstepoort J. Vet. Res.* **47:**213–219.
9. **Cary, C. J., G. K. Peter, C. E. Chrisp, and D. F. Keren.** 1984. Serological analysis of five serotypes of *Pasteurella multocida* of rabbit origin by use of an enzyme-linked immunosorbent assay with lipopolysaccharide as antigen. *J. Clin. Microbiol.* **20:**191–194.
10. **Chaffee, V. W., E. A. James, Jr., and R. J. Montali.** 1975. Suppurative mandibular osteomyelitis associated with *Pasteurella multocida* in a rabbit. *Vet. Med. Small Anim. Clin.* **70:**1411–1413.
11. **Chrisp, C. E., and N. T. Foged.** 1991. Induction of pneumonia in rabbits by use of a purified protein toxin from *Pasteurella multocida*. *Am. J. Vet. Res.* **52:**56–61.
12. **Confer, A. W., M. A. Suckow, M. Montelongo, S. M. Dabo, L. J. Miloscio, A. J. Gillespie, and G. L. Meredith.** 2001. Intranasal vaccination of rabbits with *Pasteurella multocida* A: 3 outer membranes that express iron-regulated proteins. *Am. J. Vet. Res.* **62:**697–703.
13. **Dabo, S. M., A. W. Confer, and Y. S. Lu.** 2000. Single primer polymerase chain reaction fingerprinting for *Pasteurella multocida* isolates from laboratory rabbits. *Am. J. Vet. Res.* **61:**305–309.
14. **Dabo, S. M., A. W. Confer, M. Montelongo, and Y. S. Lu.** 1999. Characterization of rabbit *Pasteurella multocida* by use of whole-cell, outer-membrane, and polymerase chain reaction typing. *Lab. Anim. Sci.* **49:**551–559.
15. **Deeb, B. J., R. F. DiGiacomo, B. L. Bernard, and S. M. Silbernagel.** 1990. *Pasteurella multocida* and *Bordetella bronchiseptica* infection in rabbits. *J. Clin. Microbiol.* **28:**70–75.
16. **Dehoux, J. P., P. Dachet, L. Gueye, A. Dieng, and A. Buldgen.** 1996. Epizootics of pasteurellosis in a semi-intensive breeding farm of indigenous rabbits in Senegal. *Rev. Elev. Med. Vet. Pays Trop.* **49:**98–101.
17. **DeLong, D., and P. J. Manning.** 1994. Bacterial diseases, p. 131–170. *In* P. J. Manning, D. H. Ringler, and C. E. Newcomer (ed.), *The Biology of the Laboratory Rabbit,* 2nd ed. Academic Press, Inc., San Diego, Calif.
18. **DeLong, D., P. J. Manning, R. Gunther, and D. L. Swanson.** 1992. Colonization of rabbits by *Pasteurella multocida*: serum IgG responses

following intranasal challenge with serologically distinct isolates. *Lab. Anim. Sci.* **42**:13–18.
19. **DiGiacomo, R. F., V. Allen, and M. H. Hinton.** 1991. Naturally acquired *Pasteurella multocida* subsp. *multocida* infection in a closed colony of rabbits: Characteristics of isolates. *Lab. Anim.* **25**:236–241.
20. **DiGiacomo, R. F., B. J. Deeb, S. J. Brodie, T. E. Zimmerman, E. R. Veltkamp, and C. E. Chrisp.** 1993. Toxin production by *Pasteurella multocida* isolated from rabbits with atrophic rhinitis. *Am. J. Vet. Res.* **54**:1280–1286.
21. **DiGiacomo, R. F., B. J. Deeb, W. E. Giddens, Jr., B. L. Bernard, and M. M. Chengappa.** 1989. Atrophic rhinitis in New Zealand white rabbits infected with *Pasteurella multocida*. *Am. J. Vet. Res.* **50**:1460–1465.
22. **DiGiacomo, R. P., L. E. Garlinghouse, Jr., and G. L. Van Hoosier, Jr.** 1983. Natural history of infection with *Pasteurella multocida* in rabbits. *J. Am. Vet. Med. Assoc.* **183**:1172–1175.
23. **DiGiacomo, R. F., C. D. Jones, and C. M. Wathes.** 1987. Transmission of *Pasteurella multocida* in rabbits. *Lab. Anim. Sci.* **37**:621–623.
24. **DiGiacomo, R. F., and C. J. Maré.** 1994. Viral Diseaes, p. 171–204. *In* P. J. Manning, D. H. Ringler, and C. E. Newcomer (ed.), *The Biology of the Laboratory Rabbit*, 2nd ed. Academic Press, Inc., San Diego, Calif.
25. **DiGiacomo, R. F., Y. M. Xu, V. Allen, M. H. Hinton, and G. R. Pearson.** 1991. Naturally acquired *Pasteurella multocida* infection in rabbits: clinicopathological aspects. *Can. J. Vet. Res.* **55**:234–238.
26. **Dillehay, D. L., K. S. Paul, R. F. DiGiacomo, and M. M. Chengappa.** 1991. Pathogenicity of *Pasteurella multocida* A:3 in Flemish giant and New Zealand white rabbits. *Lab. Anim.* **25**:337–341.
27. **Flatt, R. E., D. W. Deyoung, and R. M. Hogle.** 1977. Suppurative otitis media in the rabbit: prevalence, pathology, and microbiology. *Lab. Anim. Sci.* **27**:343–347.
28. **Glass, L. S., and J. N. Beasley.** 1989. Infection with and antibody response to *Pasteurella multocida* and *Bordetella bronchiseptica* in immature rabbits. *Lab. Anim. Sci.* **39**:406–410.
29. **Glorioso, J. C., G. W. Jones, H. G. Rush, L. J. Pentler, C. A. DaRif, and J. E. Coward.** 1982. Adhesion of type A *Pasteurella multocida* to rabbit pharyngeal cells and its possible role in rabbit respiratory tract infections. *Infect. Immun.* **35**:1103–1109.
30. **Hanan, M. S., E. M. Riad, and N. A. el-Khouly.** 2000. Antibacterial efficacy and pharmacokinetic studies of ciprofloxacin on *Pasteurella multocida* infected rabbits. *Dtsch. Tierarztl. Wochenschr.* **107**:151–155.
31. **Johnson, J. H., and A. M. Wolf.** 1993. Ovarian abscesses and pyometra in a domestic rabbit. *J. Am. Vet. Med. Assoc.* **203**:667–669.
32. **Kawamoto, E., T. Sawada, and T. Maruyama.** 1990. Prevalence and characterization of *Pasteurella multocida* in rabbits and their environment in Japan. *Nippon Juigaku Zasshi* **52**:915–921.
33. **Kluger, M. J., and B. A. Rothenburg.** 1979. Fever and reduced iron: their interaction as a host defense response to bacterial infection. *Science* **203**:374–376.
34. **Kunstyr, I., and S. Naumann.** 1985. Head tilt in rabbits caused by pasteurellosis and encephalitozoonosis. *Lab. Anim. Sci.* **19**:208–213.
35. **Lu, Y. S., D. H. Ringler, and J. S. Park.** 1978. Characterization of *Pasteurella multocida* isolates from the nares of healthy rabbits with pneumonia. *Lab. Anim. Sci.* **28**:691–697.
36. **Mahler, M., S. Stunkel, C. Ziegowski, and I. Kunstyr.** 1995. Inefficiency of enrofloxacin in the elimination of *Pasteurella multocida* in rabbits. *Lab. Anim.* **29**:192–199.
37. **McKay, S. G., D. W. Morck, J. K. Merrill, M. E. Olson, S. C. Chan, and K. M. Pap.** 1996. Use of tilmicosin for treatment of pasteurellosis in rabbits. *Am. J. Vet. Res.* **57**:1180–1184.
38. **Murray, K. A., B. A. Hobbs, and J. W. Griffith.** 1985. Acute meningoencephalomyelitis in a rabbit infected with *Pasteurella multocida*. *Lab. Anim. Sci.* **35**:169–171.
39. **Nakagawa, M., K. Nakayama, M. Saito, S. Takayama, and S. Watarai.** 1986. Bacteriological and serological studies on *Pasteurella multocida* infection in rabbits. *Jikken Dobutsu* **35**:463–469.
40. **Percy, D. H., and S. W. Barthold.** 2001. *Pathology of Laboratory Rodents and Rabbits,* 2nd ed. Iowa State University Press, Ames.
41. **Percy, D. H., J. L. Bhasin, and S. Rosendal.** 1986. Experimental pneumonia in rabbits inoculated with strains of *Pasteurella multocida*. *Can. Vet. J.* **50**:36–41.
42. **Redondo, E., A. J. Masot, A. Gazqauez, V. Roncero, E. Duran, and E. Piriz.** 1993. Experimental reproduction of acute pneumonic pasteurellosis in rabbits. *Histol. Histopathol.* **8**:97–104.
43. **Richardson, M., A. Fletch, K. Delaney, M. DeReske, L. H. Wilcox, and R. L. Kinlough-Rathbone.** 1997. Increased expression of vascular cell adhesion molecule-1 by the aortic endothelium of rabbits with *Pasteurella multocida* pneumonia. *Lab. An. Sci.* **47**:27–35.

44. Ruble, R. P., J. S. Cullor, and D. L. Brooks. 1999. The observation of reactive thrombocytosis in New Zealand white rabbits in response to experimental *Pasteurella multocida* infection. *Blood Cells Mol. Dis.* **25**:95–102.
45. Rush, H. G., J. C. Glorioso, C. A. DaRif, and L. C. Olson. 1981. Resistance of *Pasteurella multocida* to rabbit neutrophil phagocytosis and killing. *Am. J. Vet. Res.* **42**:1760–1768.
46. Scharf, R. A., S. A. Monteleone, and D. M. Stark. 1981. A modified barrier system for maintenance of *Pasteurella*-free rabbits. *Lab. Anim. Sci.* **31**:513–515.
47. Snyder, S. B., J. G. Fox, and O. A. Soave. 1973. Subclinical otitis media associated with *Pasteurella multocida* infections in New Zealand white rabbits (*Oryctolagus cuniculus*). *Lab. Anim. Sci.* **23**:270–272.
48. Suckow, M. A., C. E. Chrisp, and N. T. Foged. 1991. Heat-labile toxin-producing isolates of *Pasteurella multocida* from rabbits. *Lab. Anim. Sci.* **41**:151–156.
49. Suckow, M. A., B. J. Martin, T. L. Bowerstock, and F. A. Douglas. 1996. Derivation of *Pasteurella multocida*-free rabbit litters by enrofloxacin treatment. *Vet. Microbiol.* **51**:161–168.
50. Takashima, H., H. Sakai, T. Yanai, and T. Masegi. 2001. Detection of antibodies against *Pasteurella multocida* using immunohistochemical staining in an outbreak of rabbit pasteurellosis. *J. Vet. Med. Sci.* **63**:171–174.
51. Toth, L. A., and J. M. Krueger. 1990. Somnogenic, pyrogenic, and hematologic effects of experimental pasteurellosis in rabbits. *Am. J. Physiol.* **258**:R536–R542.
52. Zaoutis, T. E., G. R. Reinhard, C. J. Cioffe, P. B. Moore, and D. M. Stark. 1991. Screening rabbit colonies for antibodies to *Pasteurella multocida* by an ELISA. *Lab. Anim. Sci.* **41**:419–422.

Staphylococcus aureus
1. Amorena, B., J. A. Garcia de Jalon, R. Baselga, J. Ducha, M. V. Latre, L. M. Ferrer, F. Sancho, I. Mansson, K. Krovacek, and A. Faris. 1991. Infection of rabbit mammary glands with ovine mastitis bacterial strains. *J. Comp. Pathol.* **104**:289–302.
2. Bamberger, D. M., B. L. Herndon, K. M. Bettin, and D. N. Gerding. 1989. Neutrophil chemotaxis and adherence in vitro and localization in vivo in rabbits with *Staphylococcus aureus* abscesses. *J. Lab. Clin. Med.* **114**:135–141.
3. Bawdon, R. E., A. M. Fiskin, B. B. Little, L. L. Davis, and G. Vergarra. 1989. Fibronectin and postpartum infection in rabbits: an animal model. *Gynecol. Obstet. Investig.* **28**:185–190.
4. Bhambani, B. D. 1966. A case report of conjunctivitis and dermonecrosis in rabbit due to *Staphylococcus aureus*. *Indian Vet. J.* **43**:555–558.
5. Boros, I., V. Ghetie, J. Boros, G. Mota, and J. Sjoquist. 1980. *Staphylococcus aureus* and protein A as mitogens for rabbit T lymphocytes. *Immunobiology* **157**:30–40.
6. Carruth, W. A., M. P. Byron, D. D. Solomon, W. L. White, G. J. Stoddard, R. D. Marosok, and R. J. Sherertz. 1994. Subcutaneous, catheter-related inflammation in a rabbit model correlates with peripheral vein phlebitis in human volunteers. *J. Biomed. Mater. Res.* **28**:259–267.
7. Cheung, A. L., K. J. Eberhardt, E. Chung, M. R. Yeaman, P. M. Sullam, M. Ramos, and A. S. Bayer. 1994. Diminished virulence of a sar-/agr- mutant of *Staphylococcus aureus* in the rabbit model of endocarditis. *J. Clin. Investig.* **94**:1815–1822.
8. Cordero, J., L. Munuera, and M. D. Folgueira. 1996. Influence of bacterial strains on bone infection. *J. Orthop. Res.* **14**:663–667.
9. DeLong, D., and P. J. Manning. 1994. Bacterial Diseases, p. 131–170. *In* P. J. Manning, D. H. Ringler, and C. E. Newcomer (ed.), *The Biology of the Laboratory Rabbit*, 2nd ed. Academic Press, Inc., San Diego, Calif.
10. Devriese, L. A., W. Hendrickx, C. Godard, L. Okerman, and F. Haesebrouck. 1996. A new pathogenic *Staphylococcus aureus* type in commercial rabbits. *Zentbl. Vetmed.* **43**:313–315.
11. Engstrom, R. E., Jr., B. J. Mondino, B. J. Glasgow, H. Pitchekian-Halabi, and S. A. Adamu. 1991. Immune response to *Staphylococcus aureus* endophthalmitis in a rabbit model. *Investig. Ophthalmol. Vis. Sci.* **32**:1523–1533.
12. Korinteli, V. I., V. A. Akhobadze, L. S. H. Dzhidzheishvili, D. V. Gamrekeli, and D. D. Giorkhelidze. 1989. A study of the subcellular structure of the rabbit liver during the development of a bacterial infection. *Zh. Mikrobiol. Epidemiol. Immunobiol.* **4**:77–80.
13. Koupal, A., and R. H. Deibel. 1977. Rabbit intestinal fluid stimulation by an enterotoxigenic factor of *Staphylococcus aureus*. *Infect. Immun.* **18**:298–303.
14. McCollister, B. D., B. N. Kreiswirth, R. P. Novick, and P. M. Schlievert. 1990. Production of toxic shock syndrome-like illness in rabbits by *Staphylococcus aureus* D4508: association with enterotoxin A. *Infect. Immun.* **58**:2067–2070.
15. Olson, R. D., D. L. Stevens, and M. E. Melish. 1989. Direct effects of purified staphylococcal toxic shock syndrome toxin 1 on myocardial

function of isolated rabbit atria. *Rev. Infect. Dis.* **11:**S313–S315.
16. Percy, D. H., and S. W. Barthold. 2001. *Pathology of Laboratory Rodents and Rabbits,* 2nd ed. Iowa State University Press, Ames.
17. Seeger, W., R. G. Birkemeyer, L. Ermert, N. Suttorp, S. Bhakdi, and H. R. Duncker. 1990. Staphylococcal a-toxin-induced vascular leakage in isolated perfused rabbit lungs. *Lab. Investig.* **63:**341–349.
18. Siqueira, J. A., C. Speeg-Schatz, F. Freitas, J. Sahel, H. Monteil, and G. Prevost. 1997. Channel-forming leucotoxins from *Staphylococcus aureus* cause severe inflammatory reactions in a rabbit eye model. *J. Med. Microbiol.* **46:**486–494.
19. Walmrath, D., M. Scharmann, R. Konig, J. Pilch, F. Grimminger, and W. Seeger. 1993. Staphylococcal alpha-toxin induced ventilation-perfusion mismatch in isolated blood-free perfused rabbit lungs. *J. Appl. Physiol.* **74:**1972–1980.

Treponema paraluis-cuniculi
1. Baker-Zander, S. A., and S. A. Lukehart. 1992. Macrophage-mediated killing of opsonized *Treponema pallidum. J. Infect. Dis.* **165:**69–74.
2. Borenstein, L. A., T. Ganz, S. Sell, R. I. Lehrer, and J. N. Miller. 1991. Contribution of rabbit leukocyte defensins to the host response in experimental syphilis. *Infect. Immun.* **59:**1368–1377.
3. Bouis, D. A., T. G. Popova, A. Takashima, and M. V. Norgard. 2001. Dendritic cells phagocytose and are activated by *Treponema pallidum. Infect. Immun.* **69:**518–528.
4. Burgess, A. W., L. J. Paradise, D. Hilbelink, and H. Friedman. 1994. Adherence of *Treponema pallidum* subsp. *pallidum* in the rabbit placenta. *Proc. Soc. Exp. Biol. Med.* **207:**180–185.
5. Cunliffe-Beamer, T. L., and R. R. Fox. 1981. Venereal spirochetosis of rabbits: Description and diagnosis. *Lab. Anim. Sci.* **31:**366–371.
6. Cunliffe-Beamer, T. L., and R. R. Fox. 1981. Venereal spirochetosis of rabbits: Epizootiology. *Lab. Anim. Sci.* **31:**372–378.
7. Cunliffe-Beamer, T. L., and R. R. Fox. 1981. Venereal spirochetosis of rabbits: eradication. *Lab. Anim. Sci.* **31:**379–381.
8. DeLong, D., and P. J. Manning. 1994. Bacterial diseases, p. 131–170. *In* P. J. Manning, D. H. Ringler, and C. E. Newcomer (ed.), *The Biology of the Laboratory Rabbit,* 2nd ed, Academic Press, Inc., San Diego, Calif.
9. DiGiacomo, R. F., S. A. Lukehart, C. D. Talburt, S. A. Baker-Zander, J. Condon, and C. W. Brown. 1984. Clinical course and treatment of venereal spirochaetosis in New Zealand White rabbits *Br. J. Vener. Dis.* **60:**214–218.
10. DiGiacomo, R. F., S. A. Lukehart, C. D. Talburt, S. A. Baker-Zander, W. E. Giddens, Jr., J. Condon, and C. W. Brown. 1985. Chronicity of infection with *Treponema paraluis-cuniculi* in New Zealand white rabbits. *Genitourin. Med.* **61:**156–164.
11. DiGiacomo, R. F., C. D. Talburt, S. A. Lukehart, S. A. Baker-Zander, and J. Condon. 1983. *Treponema paraluis-cuniculi* infection in a commercial rabbitry: epidemiology and serodiagnosis. *Lab. Anim. Sci.* **33:**562–566.
12. Fitzgerald, T. J., and M. A. Tomai. 1991. Splenic T-lymphocyte functions during early syphilitic infection are complex. *Infect. Immun.* **59:**4180–4186.
13. Graves, S. 1980. Susceptibility of rabbits venereally infected with *Treponema paraluis-cuniculi* to superinfections with *Treponema pallidum. Br. J. Vener. Dis.* **56:**387–389.
14. Graves, S., and J. Downes. 1981. Experimental infection of man with rabbit-virulent *Treponema paraluis-cuniculi. Br. J. Vener. Dis.* **57:**7–10.
15. Graves, S. R., J. W. Edmonds, and R. C. Shepherd. 1980. Lack of serological evidence for venereal spirochaetosis in wild Victorian rabbits and the susceptibility of laboratory rabbits to *Treponema paraluis-cuniculi. Br. J. Vener. Dis.* **56:**381–386.
16. Nathan, L., D. M. Twickler, M. T. Peters, P. J. Sanchez, and G. D. Wendel, Jr. 1993. Fetal syphilis: correlation of sonographic findings and rabbit infectivity testing of amniotic fluid. *J. Ultrasound Med.* **12:**97–101.
17. Percy, D. H., and S. W. Barthold. 2001. *Pathology of Laboratory Rodents and Rabbits,* 2nd ed. Iowa State University Press, Ames.
18. Podwinska, J., and M. Chomik. 1992. Treponemicidal activity of anti-treponemal lymphotoxins and their relation to circulating immune complexes and autolymphocytotoxins. *FEMS Microbiol. Immunol.* **4:**345–351.
19. Podwinska, J., R. Zaba, M. Chomik, and J. Bowszyc. 1993. The ability of peripheral blood mononuclear cells of rabbits infected with *Treponema pallidum* to produce IL-2. *FEMS Immunol. Med. Microbiol.* **7:**257–264.
20. Sell, S., and J. Salman. 1992. Demonstration of *Treponema pallidum* in axons of cutaneous nerves in experimental chancres of rabbits. *Sex. Transm. Dis.* **19:**1–6.
21. Tight, R. R., D. Leland, and M. L. French. 1981. Incidence of positive serologic tests for treponemal infections in healthy rabbits. *Sex. Transm. Dis.* **8:**8–11.
22. Tomai, M. A., and T. J. Fitzgerald. 1991. Splenic macrophage function in early syphilitic

infection is complex. Stimulation versus down-regulation. *J. Immunol.* **146:**3171–3176.

FUNGI
Dermatomycosis
1. **Bergdall, V. K., and R. C. Dysko.** 1994. Metabolic, traumatic, mycotic, and miscellaneous diseases, p. 345–353. *In* P. J. Manning, D. H. Ringler, and C. E. Newcomer (ed.), *The Biology of the Laboratory Rabbit.* Academic Press, Inc., San Diego, Calif.
2. **Cabanes, F. J., M. L. Abarca, and M. R. Bragulat.** 1997. Dermatophytes isolated from domestic animals in Barcelona, Spain. *Mycopathologia* **137:**107–113.
3. **Connole, M. D.** 1990. Review of animal mycoses in Australia. *Mycopathologia* **111:**133–164.
4. **Morganti, L., M. P. Tampieri, R. Galuppi, and F. Menegali.** 1992. Morphological and biochemical variability of *Microsporum canis* strains. *Eur. J. Epidemiol.* **8:**340–345.
5. **Percy, D. H., and S. W. Barthold.** 2001. *Pathology of Laboratory Rodents and Rabbits,* 2nd ed. Iowa State University Press, Ames.
6. **Simaljakova, M., J. Buchvald, and B. Olexova.** 1989. *Microsporum canis*-Infektion beim Kaninchen mit Ubertragung auf den Menschen. *Mycoses* **32:**93–96.
7. **Torres-Rodriguez, J. M., M. A. Dronda, J. Rossell, and N. Madrenys.** 1992. Incidence of dermatophytoses in rabbit farms in Catalonia, Spain, and its repercussion on human health. *Eur. J. Epidemiol.* **8:**326–329.
8. **Vogtsberger, L. M., H. H. Harroff, G. E. Pierce, and G. E. Wilkinson.** 1986. Spontaneous dermatomycosis due to *Microsporum canis* in rabbits. *Lab. Anim. Sci.* **36:**294–297.

PARASITES
Cheyletiella parasitivorax
1. **Bjarke, T., L. Hellgren, and K. Orstadius.** 1973. *Cheyletiella parasitovorax* dermatitis in man. *Acta Derm. Venereol.* **53:**217–223.
2. **Clark, J. D., and H.-S. Ah.** 1976. *Cheyletiella parasitovorax* (Megnin), a parasitic mite causing mange in the domestic rabbit. *J. Parasitol.* **62:**125.
3. **Cloyd, G. G., and D. P. Moorhead.** 1976. Facial alopecia in the rabbit associated with *Cheyletiella parasitovorax. Lab. Anim. Sci.* **26:**801–803.
4. **Foxx, T. S., and S. A. Ewing.** 1969. Morphologic features, behavior and life history of *Cheyletiella yasguri. Am. J. Vet. Res.* **30:**269–285.
5. **George, J. B., S. Otobo, J. Ogunleye, and B. Adediminiyi.** 1992. Louse and mite infestation in domestic animals in northern Nigeria. *Trop. Anim. Health Prod.* **24:**121–124.
6. **Hofing, G. L., and A. L. Kraus.** 1994. Arthropod and helminth parasites, p. 231–257. *In* P. J. Manning, D. H. Ringler, and C. E. Newcomer (ed.), *The Biology of the Laboratory Rabbit,* 2nd ed. Academic Press, Inc., San Diego, Calif.
7. **Vail, E. L., and G. F. Auguston.** 1943. A new ectoparasite (Acarina: Cheyletidae) from domestic rabbits. *J. Parasitol.* **29:**419–421.

Cryptosporidium parvum
1. **Aboul-Magd, L. A., A. M. el-Ridi, and S. A. Michael.** 1989. Biological and haematological changes in experimental cryptosporidiosis. *J. Egypt. Soc. Parasitol.* **19:**49–56.
2. **Beier, T. V., N. V. Sidorenko, and N. V. Svezhova.** 1995. Cellular interactions in the intracellular parasitism of cryptosporidia. I. The effect of *Cryptosporidium parvum* on the phosphatase activity in the small intestine enterocytes of experimentally infected newborn rat pups. *Tsitologiia* **37:**829–837.
3. **Chen, X. M., G. J. Gores, C. V. Paya, and N. F. LaRusso.** 1999. *Cryptosporidium parvum* induces apoptosis in biliary epithelia by a Fas/Fas ligand-dependent mechanism. *Am. J. Physiol.* **277:**G599–G608.
4. **Cruz, J. R., G. Paraja, P. Caceres, F. Cano, and F. Chew.** 1989. Acute and persistent diarrheal disease and its nutritional consequences in Guatemalan infants. *Arch. Latinoam. Nutr.* **39:**263–277.
5. **Current, W. L., and L. S. Garcia.** 1991. Cryptosporidiosis. *Clin. Microbiol. Rev.* **4:**325–358.
6. **el-Dein, S. Z., A. M. Khalifa, H. A. Sadaka, I. H. Hegazy, and H. S. Ibrahim.** 1998. Electroencephalographic changes in rats received antigens of different parasites. *J. Egypt. Soc. Parasitol.* **28:**797–805.
7. **Guarino, A., R. B. Canani, A. Casola, E. Pozio, R. Russo, E. Bruzzese, M. Fontana, and A. Rubino.** 1995. Human intestinal cryptosporidiosis: secretory diarrhea and enterotoxic activity in Caco-2 cells. *J. Infect. Dis.* **171:**976–983.
8. **Inman, L. R., and A. Takeuchi.** 1979. Spontaneous cryptosporidiosis in an adult female rabbit. *Vet. Pathol.* **16:**89–95.
9. **Matsui, T., T. Fujino, J. Kajima, and M. Tsuji.** 2000. Infectivity to experimental rodents of *Cryptosporidium parvum* oocysts from Siberian chipmunks (*Tamias sibiricus*) originated in the People's Republic of China. *J. Vet. Med. Sci.* **62:**487–489.
10. **Mosier, D. A., K. Y. Cimon, T. L. Kuhls, R. D. Oberst, and K. R. Simons.** 1997. Experimental cryptosporidiosis in adult and neonatal rabbits. *Vet. Parasitol.* **69:**163–169.

11. **Nina, J. M. S., V. McDonald, R. M. A. Deer, S. E. Wright, D. A. Dyson, P. L. Chiodini, and K. P. W. J. McAdam.** 1992. Comparative study of the antigenic composition of oocyst isolates of *Cryptosporidium parvum* from different hosts. *Parasite Immunol.* **14:**227–232.
12. **Pakes, S. P., and L. W. Gerrity.** 1994. Protozoal Diseases, p. 205–229. *In* P. J. Manning, D. H. Ringler, and C. E. Newcomer (ed.), *The Biology of the Laboratory Rabbit,* 2nd ed. Academic Press, Inc., San Diego, Calif.
13. **Pavlasek, I., M. Lavicka, E. Tumova, and M. Skrivan.** 1996. Spontaneous *Cryptosporidium* infection in weaned rabbits. *Vet. Med. (Praha)* **41:**361–366.
14. **Rehg, J. E., G. W. Lawton, and S. P. Pakes.** 1979. *Cryptosporidium cuniculus* in the rabbit (*Oryctolagus cuniculus*). *Lab. Anim. Sci.* **29:**656–660.
15. **Reperant, J. M., M. Naciri, S. Iochmann, M. Tilley, and D. T. Bout.** 1994. Major antigens of *Cryptosporidium parvum* recognised by serum antibodies from different infected animal species and man. *Vet. Parasitol.* **55:**1–13.
16. **Rhee, J. K., H. C. Kim, S. B. Lee, and S. Y. Yook.** 1998. Immunosuppressive effect of *Cryptosporidium baileyi* infection on vaccination against Newcastle disease in chicks. *Korean J. Parasitol.* **36:**121–125.
17. **Rhee, J. K., H. J. Yang, S. Y. Yook, and H. C. Kim.** 1998. Immunosuppressive effect of *Cryptosporidium baileyi* infection on vaccination against avian infectious bronchitis in chicks. *Korean J. Parasitol.* **36:**203–206.
18. **Thulin, J. D., M. S. Kuhlenschmidt, M. D. Rolsma, W. L. Current, and H. B. Gelberg.** 1994. An intestinal xenograft model for *Cryptosporidium parvum* infection. *Infect. Immun.* **62:**329–331.

Encephalitozoon cuniculi
1. **Armstrong, J. A., Y. H. Ke, M. C. Breinig, and L. Ople.** 1973. Virus resistance in rabbit kidney cell cultures contaminated by a protozoal resembling *Encephalitozoon cuniculi*. *Proc. Soc. Exp. Biol. Med.* **142:**1205–1208.
2. **Ashton, N., C. Cook, and F. Clegg.** 1976. Encephalitozoonosis (nosematosis) causing bilateral cataract in a rabbit. *Br. J. Ophthalmol.* **60:**618–631.
3. **Boot, R., A. K. Hansen, C. K. Hansen, N. Nozari, and H. C. Thuis.** 2000. Comparison of assays for antibodies to *Encephalitozoon cuniculi* in rabbits. *Lab. Anim.* **34:**281–289.
4. **Bywater, J. E., and B. S. Kellett.** 1978. *Encephalitozoon cuniculi* antibodies in a specific-pathogen-free rabbit unit. *Infect. Immun.* **21:**360–364.
5. **Bywater, J. E., and B. S. Kellett.** 1979. Humoral immune response to natural infection with *Encephalitozoon cuniculi* in rabbits. *Lab. Anim.* **13:**293–297.
6. **Bywater, J. E., B. S. Kellett, and T. Waller.** 1980. *Encephalitozoon cuniculi* antibodies in commerciall-available rabbit antisera and serum reagents. *Lab. Anim.* **14:**87–89.
7. **Cox, J. C.** 1977. Altered immune responsiveness associated with *Encephalitozoon cuniculi* infection in rabbits. *Infect. Immun.* **15:**392–395.
8. **Cox, J. C., and H. A. Gallichio.** 1978. Serological and histological studies on adult rabbits with recent, naturally acquired encephalitozoonosis. *Res. Vet. Sci.* **24:**260–261.
9. **Cox, J. C., R. C. Hamilton, and H. D. Attwood.** 1979. An investigation of the route and progression of *Encephalitozoon cuniculi* infection in adult rabbits. *J. Protozool.* **26:**260–265.
10. **Deplazes, P., A. Mathis, R. Baumgartner, I. Tanner, and R. Weber.** 1996. Immunologic and molecular characteristics of *Encephalitozoon*-like microsporidia isolated from humans and rabbits indicate that *Encephalitozoon cuniculi* is a zoonotic parasite. *Clin. Infect. Dis.* **22:**557–559.
11. **Didier, E. S.** 1995. Reactive nitrogen intermediates implicated in the inhibition of *Encephalitozoon cuniculi* (phylum microspora) replication in murine peritoneal macrophages. *Parasite Immunol.* **17:**405–412.
12. **Flatt, R. E., and S. J. Jackson.** 1970. Renal nosematosis in young rabbits. *Pathol. Vet.* **7:**492–497.
13. **Fuentealba, I. C., N. T. Mahoney, J. A. Shadduck, J. Harvill, V. Wicher, and K. Wicher.** 1992. Hepatic lesions in rabbits infected with *Encephalitozoon cuniculi* administered per rectum. *Vet. Pathol.* **29:**536–540.
14. **Furuya, K., D. Fukui, M. Yamaguchi, Y. Nakaoka, G. Bando, and M. Kosuge.** 2001. Isolation of *Encephalitozoon cuniculi* using primary tissue culture techniques from a rabbit in a colony showing encephalitozoonosis. *J. Vet. Med. Sci.* **63:**203–206.
15. **Gannon, J.** 1080. A survey of *Encephalitozoon cuniculi* in laboratory animal colonies in the United Kingdom. *Lab. Anim.* **14:**91–94.
16. **Greenstein, G., C. K. Drozdowicz, F. G. Garcia, and L. L. Lewis.** 1991. The incidence of *Encephalitozoon cuniculi* in a commercial barrier-maintained rabbit breeding colony. *Lab Anim.* **25:**287–290.
17. **Horvath, M., L. Leng, M. Stefkovic, V. Revajova, and M. Halanova.** 1999. Lethal encephalitozoonosis in cyclophosphamide-treated rabbits. *Acta Vet. Hung.* **47:**85–93.

18. Kimman, T. G., and J. P. Addermans. 1987. *Encephalitozoon cuniculi* in a rabbit colony. *Tijdschr. Diergeneeskd.* **112**:1405–1409.
19. Koller, L. D. 1969. Spontaneous *Nosema cuniculi* infection in laboratory rabbits. *J. Am. Vet. Med. Assoc.* **155**:1108–1114.
20. Kunstyr, I., and S. Naumann. 1985. Head tilt in rabbits caused by pasteurellosis and encephalitozoonosis. *Lab. Anim. Sci.* **19**:208–213.
21. Kunstyr, I., L. Lev, and S. Naumann. 1986. Humoral antibody response of rabbits to experimental infection with *Encephalitozoon cuniculi*. *Vet. Parasitol.* **21**:223–232.
22. Levkut, M., M. Horvath, P. Balent, M. Levkutova, V. Hipikova, and V. Letkova. 1997. Catecholamines and encephalitozoonosis in rabbits. *Vet. Parasitol.* **73**:173–176.
23. Lyngset, A. 1980. A survey of serum antibodies to *Encephalitozoon cuniculi* in breeding rabbits and their young. *Lab. Anim. Sci.* **30**:558–561.
24. Mathis, A., M. Michel, H. Kuster, C. Muller, R. Weber, and P. Deplazes. 1997. Two *Encephalitozoon cuniculi* strains of human origin are infectious to rabbits. *Parasitology* **114**:29–35.
25. Nast, R., D. M. Middleton, and C. L. Wheler. 1996. Generalized encephalitozoonosis in a Jersey wooly rabbit. *Can. Vet. J.* **37**:303–305.
26. Niederkorn, J. Y., and J. A. Shadduck. 1980. Role of antibody and complement in the control of *Encephalitozoon cuniculi* infections by rabbit macrophages. *Infect. Immun.* **27**:995–1002.
27. Packham, D. K., T. D. Hewitson, J. A. Whitworth, and P. S. Kincaid-Smith. 1992. Glomerulosclerosis and hyalinosis in rabbits. *Pathology* **24**:164–169.
28. Pakes, S. P., and L. W. Gerrity. 1994. Protozoal diseases, p. 205–229. *In* P. J. Manning, D. H. Ringler, and C. E. Newcomer (ed.), *The Biology of the Laboratory Rabbit*, 2nd ed. Academic Press, Inc., San Diego, Calif.
29. Pakes, S. P., J. A. Shadduck, D. B. Feldman, and J. A. Moore. 1984. Comparison of tests for the diagnosis of spontaneous encephalitozoonosis in rabbits. *Lab. Anim. Sci.* **34**:356–359.
30. Pattison, M., F. G. Clegg, and A. L. Duncan. 1971. An outbreak of encephalomyelitis in broiler rabbits caused by *Nosema cuniculi*. *Vet. Rec.* **88**:404–405.
31. Percy, D. H., and S. W. Barthold. 2001. *Pathology of Laboratory Rodents and Rabbits*, 2nd ed. Iowa State University Press, Ames.
32. Pye, D., and J. C. Cox. 1977. Isolation of *Encephalitozoon cuniculi* from urine samples. *Lab. Anim.* **11**:223–224.
33. Rossi, P., G. La Rosa, A. Ludovisi, A. Tamburrini, M. A. Gomez Morales, and E. Pozio. 1998. Identification of a human isolate of *Encephalitozoon cuniculi* type I from Italy. *Int. J. Parasitol.* **28**:1361–1366.
34. Thomas, C., M. Finn, L. Twigg, P. Deplazes, and R. C. Thompson. 1997. Microsporida (*Encephalitozoon cuniculi*) in wild rabbits in Australia. *Aust. Vet. J.* **75**:808–810.
35. Waller, T., B. Morein, and E. Fabiansson. 1978. Humoral immune response to infection with *Encephalitozoon cuniculi* in rabbits. *Lab. Anim.* **12**:145–148.
36. Weiss, L. M., A. Cali, E. Levee, D. LaPlace, H. Tanowitz, D. Simon, and M. Wittner. 1992. Diagnosis of *Encephalitozoon cuniculi* infection by western blot and the use of cross-reactive antigens for the possible detection of microsporidiosis in humans. *Am. J. Trop. Med. Hyg.* **47**:456–462.
37. Wesonga, H. O., and M. Munda. 1992. Rabbit encephalitozoonosis in Kenya. *Lab Anim.* **26**:219–221.
38. Wicher, V., R. E. Baughn, C. Fuentealba, J. A. Shadduck, F. Abbruscato, and K. Wicher. 1991. Enteric infection with an obligate intracellular parasite, *Encephalitozoon cuniculi*, in an experimental model. *Infect. Immun.* **59**:2225–2231.
39. Wilson, J. M. 1986. Can *Encephalitozoon cuniculi* cross the placenta? *Res. Vet. Sci.* **40**:138.
40. Wolfer, J., B. Grahn, B. Wilcock, and D. Percy. 1993. Phacoclastic uveitis in the rabbit. *Prog. Vet. Comp. Ophthalmol.* **3**:92–97.

Hepatic coccidiosis
1. Abdel-Ghaffar, F., M. Marzouk, M. B. Ashour, and M. N. Mosaad. 1990. Effects of *Eimeria labbeana* and *E. stiedai* infection on the activity of some enzymes in the serum and liver of their hosts. *Parasitol. Res.* **76**:440–443.
2. Barriga, O. O., and J. V. Arnoni. 1979. *Eimeria stiedai*: weight, oocyst output, and hepatic function of rabbits with graded infections. *Exp. Parasitol.* **48**:407–414.
3. Barriga, O. O., and J. V. Arnoni. 1981. Pathophysiology of hepatic coccidiosis in rabbits. *Vet. Parasitol.* **8**:201–210.
4. Esteller, A., M. D. Torres, M. Gomez-Bautista, E. L. Marino, C. Fernandez-Lastra, and R. Jimenez. 1990. Pharmacokinetics, hepatic biotransformation and biliary and urinary excretion of bromosulfophthalein (BSP) in an experimental liver disease mimicking biliary cirrhosis. *Eur. J. Drug. Metab. Pharmacokinet.* **15**:7–14.
5. Fernandez, E., I. D. Roman, F. Cava, A. I. Galan, A. Esteller, M. E. Munoz, and R. Ji-

menez. 1996. Acid-base disturbances in the rabbit during experimental hepatic parasitosis. *Parasitol. Res.* **82**:524–528.
6. **Gomez-Bautista, M., M. V. Garcia, and F. A. Rojo-Vazquez.** 1986. The levels of total protein and protein fractions in the serum of rabbits infected with *Eimeria stiedai*. *Ann. Parasitol. Hum. Comp.* **61**:393–400.
7. **Gomez-Bautista, M., F. A. Rojo-Vazquez, and J. M. Alunda.** 1987. The effect of the host's age on the pathology of *Eimeria stiedai* infection in rabbits. *Vet. Parasitol.* **24**:47–57.
8. **Hein, B., and G. Lammler.** 1978. Alteration of enzyme activities in serum of *Eimeria stiedai* infected rabbits. *Z. Parasitenkd.* **57**:199–211.
9. **Klesius, P. H., T. T. Kramer, and J. C. Frandsen.** 1976. *Eimeria stiedai*: delayed hypersensitivity response in rabbit coccidiosis. *Exp. Parasitol.* **39**:59–68.
10. **Pakes, S. P., and L. W. Gerrity.** 1994. Protozoal diseases, p. 205–229. *In* P. J. Manning, D. H. Ringler, and C. E. Newcomer (ed.), *The Biology of the Laboratory Rabbit,* 2nd ed. Academic Press, Inc., San Diego, Calif.
11. **Percy, D. H., and S. W. Barthold.** 2001. *Pathology of Laboratory Rodents and Rabbits,* 2nd ed. Iowa State University Press, Ames.
12. **Polozowski, A.** 1993. Coccidiosis of rabbits and its control. *Wiad. Parazytol.* **39**:13–28.
13. **Revets, H., D. Dekegel, W. Deleersnijder, J. De Jonckheere, J. Peeters, E. Leysen, and R. Hamers.** 1989. Identification of virus-like particles in *Eimeria stiedai*. *Mol. Biochem. Parasitol.* **36**:209–215.
14. **Soulsby, E. J. L.** 1982. *Helminths, Arthropods and Protozoa of Domesticated Animals,* 7th ed., p. 660–661. Lea & Febiger, Philadelphia, Pa.
15. **Vanparijs, O., L. Hermans, L. van der Flaes, and R. Marsboom.** 1989. Efficacy of diclazuril in the prevention and cure of intestinal and hepatic coccidiosis in rabbits. *Vet. Parasitol.* **32**:109–117.
16. **Wang, J. S., and S. F. Tsai.** 1991. Prevalence and pathological study on rabbit hepatic coccidiosis in Taiwan. *Proc. Natl. Sci. Counc. Repub. China Part B Basic Sci.* **15**:240–243.

Intestinal coccidiosis
1. **Cere, N., J. F. Humbert, D. Licois, M. Corvione, M. Afanassieff, and N. Chanteloup.** 1996. A new approach for the identification and the diagnosis of *Eimeria media* parasite of the rabbit. *Exp. Parasitol.* **82**:132–138.
2. **Cere, N., D. Licois, and J. F. Humbert.** 1997. Comparison of the genomic fingerprints generated by the random amplicfication of polymorphic DNA between precocious lines and parental strains of *Eimeria* spp. from the rabbit. *Parasitol. Res.* **83**:300–302.
3. **Coudert, P.** 1976. Intestinal coccidiosis of the rabbit: comparison of the pathogenic power of *Eimeria intestinalis* with 3 other *Eimeria. C. R. Acad. Sci. Hebd. Seances Acad. Sci. D.* **282**:2219–2222.
4. **Coudert, P., D. Licois, F. Provot, and F. Drouet-Viard.** 1993. *Eimeria* sp. from the rabbit (*Oryctolagus cuniculus*): pathogenicity and immunogenicity of *Eimeria intestinalis*. *Parasitol. Res.* **79**:186–190.
5. **Fioramonti, J., J. M. Soraing, D. Licois, and L. Bueno.** 1982. Intestinal motor and transit disturbances associated with experimental coccidiosis (*Eimeria magna*) in the rabbit. *Ann. Rech. Vet.* **12**:413–420.
6. **Gallazzi, D.** 1977. Cyclical variations in the excretion of intestinal coccidial oocysts in the rabbit. *Folia Vet. Lat.* **7**:371–380.
7. **Hyun, C. S., C. W. Chen, N. L. Shinowara, T. Palaia, F. S. Fallick, L. A. Martello, M. Mueenuddin, V. M. Donovan, and S. Teichberg.** 1995. Morphological factors influencing transepithelial conductance in a rabbit model of ileitis. *Gastroenterology* **109**:13–23.
8. **Licois, D., P. Coudert, S. Bahagia, and G. L. Rossi.** 1992. Endogenous development of *Eimeria intestinalis* in rabbits (*Oryctolagus cuniculus*). *J. Parasitol.* **78**:1041–1048.
9. **Licois, D., and P. Mongin.** 1980. An hypothesis of the pathogenesis of diarrhoea in the rabbit based on a study of intestinal contents. *Reprod. Nutr. Dev.* **20**:1209–1216.
10. **Niilo, L.** 1967. Acquired resistance to reinfection of rabbits with *Eimeria magna*. *Can. Vet. J.* **8**:201–208.
11. **Pakandl, M., F. Drouet-Viard, and P. Coudert.** 1995. How do sporozoites of rabbit *Eimeria* species reach their target cells? *C. R. Acad. Sci. Ser. III Life Sci.* **318**:1213–1217.
12. **Pakandl, M., K. Gaca, F. Drouet-Viard, and P. Coudert.** 1996. *Eimeria coecicola* Cheissin 1947: endogenous development in gut-associated lymphoid tissue. *Parasitol. Res.* **82**:347–351.
13. **Pakes, S. P., and L. W. Gerrity.** 1994. Protozoal diseases, p. 205–229. *In* P. J. Manning, D. H. Ringler, and C. E. Newcomer (ed.), *The Biology of the Laboratory Rabbit,* 2nd ed. Academic Press, Inc., San Diego, Calif.
14. **Peeters, J. E., R. Geeroms, R. Froyman, and P. Halen.** 1981. Coccidiosis in rabbits: a field study. *Res. Vet. Sci.* **30**:328–334.
15. **Percy, D. H., and S. W. Barthold.** 2001. *Pathology of Laboratory Rodents and Rabbits,* 2nd ed. Iowa State University Press, Ames.

16. **Polozowski, A.** 1993. Coccidiosis of rabbits and its control. *Wiad. Parazytol.* **39:**13–28.
17. **Renaux, S., F. Drouet-Viard, N. K. Chanteloup, Y. Le Vern, D. Kerboieuf, M. Pakandl, and P. Coudert.** 2001. Tissues and cells involved in the invasion of the rabbit intestinal tract by sporozoites of *Eimeria coecicola*. *Parasitol. Res.* **87:**98–106.
18. **Toula, F. H., and H. H. Ramadan.** 1998. Studies on coccidia species of genus Eimeria from domestic rabbit (*Oryctolagus cuniculus* L.) in Jeddah, Saudi Arabia. *J. Egypt. Soc. Parasitol.* **28:**691–698.
19. **Vanparijs, O., L. Desplenter, and R. Marsboom.** 1989. Efficacy of diclazuril in the control of intestinal coccidiosis in rabbits. *Vet. Parasitiol.* **34:**185–190.
20. **Varga, I.** 1982. Large-scale management systems and parasite populations: Coccidia in rabbits. *Vet. Parasitol.* **11:**69–84.
21. **Vitovec, J., and M. Pakandl.** 1989. The pathogenicity of rabbit coccidium *Eimeria coecicola* Cheissin, 1947. *Folia Parasitol. (Praha)* **36:**289–293.
22. **Weisbroth, S. H., and S. Scher.** 1975. Fatal intussusception associated with intestinal coccidiosis (*Eimeria perforans*) in a rabbit. *Lab. Anim. Sci.* **25:**79–81.

Passalurus ambiguus
1. **Allan, J. C., P. S. Craig, J. Sherington, M. T. Rogan, D. M. Storey, S. Heath, and K. Iball.** 1999. Helminth parasites of the wild rabbit *Oryctolagus cuniculus* near Malham Tarn, Yorkshire, UK. *J. Helminthol.* **73:**289–294.
2. **Boag, B.** 1985. The incidence of helminth parasites from the wild rabbit *Oryctolagus cuniculus* (L.) in eastern Scotland. *J. Helminthol.* **59:**61–69.
3. **Duwel, D., and K. Brech.** 1981. Control of oxyuriasis in rabbits by fenbendazole. *Lab. Anim.* **15:**101–105.
4. **Hobbs, R. P., L. E. Twigg, A. D. Elliot, and A. G. Wheeler.** 1999. Factors influencing the fecal egg and oocyst counts of parasites of wild European rabbits *Oryctolagus cuniculus* (L.) in Southern Western Australia. *J. Parasitol.* **85:**796–802.
5. **Hofing, G. L., and A. L. Kraus.** 1994. Arthropod and Helminth Parasites, p. 231–257. *In* P. J. Manning, D. H. Ringler, and C. E. Newcomer (ed.), *The Biology of the Laboratory Rabbit*, 2nd ed. Academic Press, Inc., San Diego, Calif.
6. **Shirokova, E P., and E. A. Grishina.** 1997. Microstructural changes in the organs of the rabbit with passaluriasis. *Med. Parazitol. (Mosk.)* **April-June:**18–21.
7. **Taffs, L. F.** 1976. Pinworm infections in laboratory rodents: a review. *Lab. Anim.* **10:**1–13.

Psoroptes cuniculi
1. **Arlian, L. G., S. Kaiser, S. A. Estes, and B. Kummel.** 1981. Infestivity of *Psoroptes cuniculi* in rabbits. *Am. J. Vet. Res.* **42:**1782–1784.
2. **Bjotvedt, G., and L. W. Geib.** 1981. Otitis media associated with *Staphylococcus epidermidis* and *Psoroptes cuniculi* in a rabbit. *Vet. Med. Small Anim. Clin.* **76:**1015–1016.
3. **Cutler, S. L.** 1998. Ectopic *Psoroptes cuniculi* infestation in a pet rabbit. *J. Small Anim. Pract.* **39:**86–87.
4. **Goudie, A. C., N. A. Evans, K. A. Gration, B. F. Bishop, S. P. Gibson, K. S. Holdom, B. Kaye, S. R. Wicks, D. Lewis, A. J. Weatherley, C. I. Bruce, A. Herbert, and D. J. Seymour.** 1993. Doramectin- a potent novel endectocide. *Vet. Parasitol.* **49:**5–15.
5. **Hofing, G. L., and A. L. Kraus.** 1994. Arthropod and helminth parasites, p. 231–257. *In* P. J. Manning, D. H. Ringler, and C. E. Newcomer (ed.), *The Biology of the Laboratory Rabbit*, 2nd ed. Academic Press, Inc., San Diego, Calif.
6. **Rafferty, D. E., and J. S. Gray.** 1987. The feeding behaviour of *Psoroptes* spp. mites on rabbits and sheep. *J. Parasitol.* **73:**901–906.
7. **Ribbeck, R., and M. Steinhardt.** 1973. The effect of experimental *Psoroptes cuniculi* infection on thermoregulation in rabbits. I. Studies in the thermoneutral zone. *Angew. Parasitol.* **14:**199–207.
8. **Smith, K. E., R. Wall, E. Berriatua, and N. P. French.** 1999. The effects of temperature and humidity on the off-host survival of *Psoroptes ovis* and *Psoroptes cuniculi*. *Vet. Parasitol.* **83:**265–275.
9. **Uhlíř, J.** 1991. Humoral and cellular immune response to *Psoroptes cuniculi*, the rabbit scab mite. *Vet. Parasitol.* **40:**325–334.
10. **Uhlíř, J.** 1993. Isolation and partial characterisation of an immunogen from the mite, *Psoroptes cuniculi*. *Vet. Parasitol.* **45:**307–317.
11. **Uhlíř, J., and P. Volf.** 1992. Ivermectin: its effect on the immune system of rabbits and rats infested with ectoparasites. *Vet. Immunol. Immunopathol.* **34:**325–336.
12. **Wright, F. C., and J. R. DeLoach.** 1980. Ingestion of erythrocytes containing ^{51}Cr-labeled hemoglobin by *Psoroptes cuniculi* (Arari: Psoroptidae). *J. Med. Entomol.* **17:**186–187.
13. **Wright, F. C., and J. C. Riner.** 1985. Comparative efficacy of injection routes and doses of ivermectin against *Psoroptes* in rabbits. *Am. J. Vet. Res.* **46:**752–754.

Sarcoptes scabiei
1. **Arlian, L. G., M. Ahmed, and D. L. Vyszenski-Moher.** 1988. Effects of *S. scabiei* var.

canis (Acari: Sarcoptidae) on blood indexes of parasitized rabbits. *J. Med. Entomol.* **25**:360–369.
2. **Arlian, L. G., R. H. Bruner, R. A. Stuhlman, M. Ahmed, and D. . Vyszenski-Moher.** 1990. Histopathology in hosts parasitized by *Sarcoptes scabiei*. *J. Parasitol.* **76**:889–894.
3. **Arlian, L. G., M. S. Morgan, D. L. Vyszenski-Moher, and B. L. Stemmer.** 1994. *Sarcoptes scabiei:* the circulating antibody response and induced immunity to scabies. *Exp. Parasitol.* **78**:37–50.
4. **Arlian, L. G., C. M. Rapp, and M. S. Morgan.** 1995. Resistance and immune response in scabies-infested hosts immunized with *Dermatophagoides* mites. *Am. J. Trop. Med. Hyg.* **52**:539–545.
5. **Arlian, L. G., C. M. Rapp, D. L. Vyszenski-Moher, and M. S. Morgan.** 1994. *Sarcoptes scabiei:* histopathological changes associated with acquisition and expression of host immunity to scabies. *Exp. Parasitol.* **78**:51–63.
6. **Arlian, L. G., R. A. Runyan, and S. A. Estes.** 1984. Cross infestivity of *Sarcoptes scabiei*. *J. Am. Acad. Dermatol.* **10**:979–986.
7. **Arlian, L. G., D. L. Vyszenski-Moher, S. G. Ahmed, and S. A. Estes.** 1991. Cross-antigenicity between the scabies mite, *Sarcoptes scabiei,* and the house dust mite, *Dermatophagoides pteronyssinus*. *J. Invest. Dermatol.* **96**:349–354.
8. **Baker, D. G., J. D. Bryant, J. F. Urban, Jr., and J. K. Lunney.** 1994. Swine immunity to selected parasites. *Vet. Immunol. Immunopathol.* **43**:127–133.
9. **Cargill, C. F., and K. J. Dobson.** 1979. Experimental *Sarcoptes scabiei* infestation in pigs. 2. Effects on production. *Vet. Rec.* **104**:33–36.
10. **Hofing, G. L., and A. L. Kraus.** 1994. Arthropod and Helminth Parasites, p. 231–257. *In* P. J. Manning, D. H. Ringler, and C. E. Newcomer (ed.), *The Biology of the Laboratory Rabbit*, 2nd ed. Academic Press, Inc., San Diego, Calif.
11. **Lin, S. L., D. M. Pinson, and J. R. Lindsey.** 1984. Diagnostic exercise. Mange due to *Sarcoptes scabiei*. *Lab. Anim. Sci.* **34**:353–355.
12. **Morgan, M. S., and L. G. Arlian.** 1994. Serum antibody profiles of *Sarcoptes scabiei* infested or immunized rabbits. *Folia Parasitol. (Praha)* **41**:223–227.

PATHOGENS OF FERRETS

7

INTRODUCTION

The European ferret, *Mustela putorius furo*, has assumed a vital role as an animal model of several human conditions, including viral, parasitic, and cardiovascular diseases and in behavioral and hormonal research (1). In addition, ferrets have become extremely popular as pets in those states where ferret ownership is legal. It is hoped that all institutions utilizing ferrets in biomedical research would purchase purpose-bred animals from reputable, commercial vendors of biomedical research-quality animals. However, some institutions may on occasion purchase ferrets from sources similar to those used by pet stores. These ferrets may harbor pathogens not present in animals purchased from more tightly controlled sources, and may serve as sources of infection or infestation to the latter (2). In addition, other animal species, including humans, may transmit diseases to ferrets. Therefore, the laboratory animal veterinarian or biomedical researcher may need to consider the potential effects of particular pathogens on the biomedical usefulness of ferrets used in research.

VIRUSES

Human influenza virus

Agent

Influenza viruses are helical, enveloped, single-stranded RNA (ssRNA) viruses of the family *Orthomyxoviridae*. There are three types, A, B, and C, based on antigenic differences between nucleoproteins and matrix proteins (1). Human influenza types A and B are infectious to ferrets, with type A strains more highly pathogenic (9, 21).

Epidemiology

The prevalence of infection with influenza virus is unknown, but may be high and largely unreported. Transmission is by aerosolization of virus that may result from sneezing, and possibly by fecal shedding, and by both direct and indirect contact, the latter by contaminated husbandry articles. Infected personnel may easily transmit the infection to ferrets.

Clinical signs

Clinical signs are only observed following infection of ferrets with human influenza type

A viruses, are virus strain dependent (20), and are mild or unapparent in nursing and adult ferrets, whereas acute mortality may occur in newborns from naive (7, 8), but not from previously infected dams (11). Clinical signs in adults are usually restricted to the upper respiratory tract, and include anorexia, malaise, fever, sneezing, and serous nasal discharge; with conjunctivitis, photophobia, and otitis media seen less commonly (3, 9). Affected ferrets generally recover within 4 to 5 days (9). Immune-compromised animals may develop pneumonia (9).

Pathology
Viral replication is most often limited to the nasal mucosa, accompanied by early influx of neutrophils, and later macrophages and marked nasal congestion (5). While viral replication may also occur in intestinal (10) and pulmonary cells, these sites have a lower capacity to produce and release influenza virus than nasal mucosal cells (4). Increased susceptibility of the lower airways in neonatal ferrets accounts for the higher mortality in that age group (6). Immunity includes both cellular and humoral components (11). Experimental infection of pregnant females results in lesions in the livers and respiratory tracts of fetuses (18).

Interference with research
Influenza infection induces localized interferon, kinin, and antibody production, which can be detected in nasal secretions (2). In addition, infection induces systemic changes. For example, viral injury to airway mucosa increases adherence of bacterial pathogens, thereby facilitating bacterial infection of the respiratory tract (16, 19). Infection results in changes in hematologic profiles (9), regulation of lipid metabolism (13), and hepatic enzyme profiles (14), and increases the contractile response of airway smooth muscle to substance P (12). Also, specific viral strains cause hearing loss and alterations in brainstem auditory-evoked potentials (17). Infection does not suppress immunity (15). Natural infection of laboratory ferrets with human influenza virus may alter studies involving the enterohepatic, hematopoietic, lymphoreticular, musculoskeletal, nervous, and respiratory systems.

Diagnosis and control
A diagnosis of influenza may be suspected on the basis of clinical signs. Definitive diagnosis depends on virus isolation, serology, and more recently, PCR assay. It is important to rule out canine distemper, which, unlike human influenza virus infection, does not spontaneously resolve (9). Affected ferrets are relatively easily treated with fluids and possibly other supportive therapies. Personnel working with ferrets should themselves be free from signs of influenza. Caretakers with signs of fever, malaise, and nasal discharge should be kept away from the research ferret colony until signs abate. Annual influenza immunization of personnel will minimize human sources of infection. Caretakers and laboratory personnel should be made aware of the importance of personal hygiene in preventing the spread of infection to ferrets, as well as the zoonotic risk to their own health.

Rotavirus

Agent
Rotaviruses are double-stranded RNA (dsRNA) viruses of the family *Reoviridae*, and are responsible for causing enteritis in the young of several mammalian species, including ferrets. The interested reader is referred to chapter 2 for a more complete discussion of rotaviruses. It should be noted, however, that the rotavirus infecting ferrets is one of the "atypical" rotaviruses, probably belonging to the group C rotaviruses (2).

Epidemiology
The prevalence of infection with rotavirus is unknown but considered to be low in research colonies. However, once introduced into a breeding colony, infection may become enzootic. Morbidity and mortality can approach 100% (1). Transmission is fecal-oral, and may be spread by aerosolization of diarrheic feces, and by fomite and vector transmission.

Clinical signs and pathology
Clinical signs are generally limited to 2- to 6-week-old kits, and include variable diarrhea of acute onset, rough hair coat, and perianal erythema (2). Gross and microscopic lesions are limited to the intestinal tract. Grossly, soft, yellow-green liquid, or mucoid feces distend the terminal colon (1, 2). Histologic lesions may be noted in the small intestine and include villous atrophy and vacuolation of villar epithelium (1).

Interference with research
The author is not aware of any publications directly implicating rotavirus infection as a confounder of research data. However, the interested reader is again referred to the discussion of rotavirus infection in chapter 2 for information concerning possible physiologic changes that may alter research. Clearly, research involving the enterohepatic system, virtually any aspect of nutrition, and potentially other fields of study, could be affected.

Diagnosis and control
Diagnosis is based on clinical signs and is confirmed by electron microscopic visualization of viral particles. Currently the virus is not cultivatable (1). Ideally, infected colonies should be eliminated because, as with rotavirus infection of mice and rats, it is not known whether infection persists. Alternatively, affected kits can be provided supportive therapy, consisting of fluids, milk replacer, and antibiotics (1). Breeding should be discontinued to stop introduction of a susceptible population.

Rabies virus

Agent
Rabies virus is an ssRNA virus of the family *Rhabdoviridae*. All warm-blooded animals are susceptible (7).

Epidemiology
The occurrence of rabies in ferrets is extremely rare. It is assumed that transmission is through exposure to infectious saliva, although viral shedding in the saliva is uncommon (2, 5). At least experimentally, Ixodid ticks have been shown to transmit rabies virus to ferrets (1). This mode of infection should not be of concern in well-managed animal colonies. However, it may be a factor if animals are purchased from poorly maintained breeding operations. While some have questioned whether ferrets can transmit rabies to humans (3), and no cases of human rabies caused by ferret bites have been reported (2), virus can be shed in the saliva as noted above (5), and infected ferrets should therefore be considered a human health risk.

Clinical signs
So few cases of naturally acquired rabies virus infection have been reported that information concerning clinical signs is lacking. Experimentally, clinical signs in intramuscularly inoculated ferrets consisted of ascending paralysis, ataxia, cachexia, inactivity, anorexia, bladder atony, fever, hyperactivity, hypothermia, tremors, paresis, lethargy, constipation, paresthesia; and rarely, aggressive behavior (4). Some infected ferrets survive following experimental infection, not always with accompanying seroconversion (4, 5).

Pathology
Rabies virus infection of virtually all warm-blooded animals results in early localized intramuscular viral replication, with later uptake at motor and sensory nerve endings. Virus ascends the nerve axons to the ventral horn cells of the spinal cord, eventually arriving at the brain. The most prominent pathologic change is nonpurulent polioencephalomyelitis with perivascular cuffing. Nonspecific inflammatory lesions occur at multiple locations in the brain. Most surviving animals respond with circulating virus-neutralizing antibodies (7).

Interference with research
To the author's knowledge, there are no reports of rabies virus interfering with research involving ferrets. However, infected animals would obviously be unusable for any type of research because of the severe clinical signs, pathologic changes, and high mortality. Stud-

ies involving the enterohepatic, musculoskeletal, and nervous systems would be most affected.

Diagnosis and control
Rabies virus infection can be diagnosed by using mouse intracerebral inoculation, immunohistochemical demonstration of viral antigen, and virus isolation, and by the rapid fluorescent focus inhibition test (4). Ferrets can be vaccinated against rabies (2, 6) but that is not considered necessary. Any ferret vaccination program should be compatible with state and local rabies immunization laws. Ferrets suspected of rabies infection should be euthanized. It should be noted that the neurotropic form of canine distemper can appear similar to rabies (2). Lastly, while rabies transmission from laboratory ferrets to humans is not known to have occurred, immunization of animal care personnel may lessen any anxiety regarding that possibility.

Canine distemper virus

Agent
Canine distemper virus (CDV) is an enveloped ssRNA virus of the family *Paramyxoviridae*. Members of the family are divided into three genera, on the basis of size of nucleocapsid, presence or absence of neuraminidase, and antigenic relationships (11). Like rinderpest, measles, and phocine distemper virus of seals, CDV is one of the Morbilliviruses. Multiple strains exist, and differ in disease characteristics (2).

Epidemiology
Canine distemper is the most serious infectious disease of ferrets because of the nearly 100% mortality that accompanies infection (2). Fortunately, prevalence is very low due to improvements in husbandry and veterinary medical practices. Transmission is by aerosolization and contact. Virus is shed in conjunctival, nasal, and oral secretions; as well as in feces and urine; and in skin detritus (2). Transplacental transmission has not been demonstrated (4).

Clinical signs
The course of CDV includes two phases: the catarrhal phase, followed by the neurotropic phase. Descriptions of clinical symptoms have been reported for *M. putorius furo*, and for a closely related species, the black-footed ferret, *Mustela nigripes* (9). Observations concerning both species are included here. Clinical signs observed in the catarrhal phase may occur in about a week following infection, and include anorexia, diarrhea, pruritus, fever, photosensitivity, serous nasal discharge, erythema of the chin and inguinal area, melena, and occasionally, hyperkeratosis of the footpads (2, 9). Secondary bacterial infections, including pneumonia and dermatitis, may occur. Ferrets may die during the catarrhal phase, or enter the neurotropic phase, wherein they develop central nervous system (CNS) signs, including hyperexcitability, excessive salivation, muscular tremors, convulsions, and coma (2, 9).

Pathology
Gross lesions are limited to those associated with nasal discharge, dermatitis, footpad hyperkeratosis, and any secondary bacterial infections. One of the histologic hallmarks of CDV infection is intracytoplasmic inclusion bodies in epithelial cells of the trachea, bronchi, urinary tract, and less commonly, the skin, gastrointestinal tract, salivary and adrenal glands, spleen, lymph nodes, and brain (2, 9). Viral entry into the CNS appears to be through vascular endothelium, and may involve platelets (6).

Interference with research
There are no reports directly implicating CDV as interfering with research. However, an attenuated strain of CDV has been shown to profoundly immune suppress ferrets, and serves as a model of immune suppression (5). Any condition with nearly 100% mortality, as with CDV, clearly will render infected ferrets unusable for almost any type of research study. On the basis of the clinical signs and viral distribution, studies likely to be affected by natural infection of ferrets with CDV in-

clude the dermal, endocrine, enterohepatic, hematopoietic, lymphoreticular, musculoskeletal, nervous, respiratory, and urinary systems. Also, immunization of ferrets against CDV may itself represent an unwanted variable and should only occur after careful consideration of potential adverse effects. At least one injection-site fibrosarcoma has been reported following vaccination for CDV (7), as has the development of ataxia (1). Lastly, vaccine-derived CDV may contaminate cell cultures established from ferret tissue (3).

Diagnosis and control
Presumptive diagnosis of CDV infection is based on history and clinical signs, and confirmed by fluorescent antibody testing of blood smears or conjunctival scrapings, and finally by pathologic examination (2). More recently, PCR assays have been developed and proven reliable for detecting CDV infection (8, 10). During an outbreak, affected ferrets should be quarantined, treated with supportive therapy or euthanized, and ferrets not showing clinical signs vaccinated. The interested reader is referred to the guidance of others for discussions of the very important topic of vaccine selection (2, 10). CDV is readily inactivated by disinfectants, such as 0.2% Roccal, and by environmental factors such as exposure to light, as well as temperature and pH extremes (11). Thorough disinfection of all items having had any contact with the colony is absolutely essential. Where likelihood of infection exists, newly arriving ferrets should be vaccinated, if not so already, and quarantined for 2 weeks (2).

Parvovirus

Agent
Ferrets are susceptible to infection with parvovirus, a dsDNA virus of the family *Parvoviridae*. It is the causative agent of Aleutian disease of mustelids. Although first reported in mink with the Aleutian pelt color, it was later also reported in ferrets. Multiple strains exist, with those from mink being generally more virulent (4). The Utah I strain is among the most virulent (2).

Epidemiology
The prevalence of infection is low in laboratory ferret colonies, but is increasing in the pet-trade ferret population so that those working with ferrets in a laboratory setting should be familiar with it. In addition to mustelids, other mammals may serve as reservoir hosts, including raccoons, cats, dogs, and mice (2). Like other members of the family, the virus is highly contagious. Transmission occurs by numerous means, including aerosolization; direct contact with urine, feces, blood, or saliva; by contact with contaminated fomites; and by vertical transmission from the jill (4). The virus persists in the environment, to serve as a source of infection even 2 years after an outbreak (3). Once infected, many ferrets remain carriers for life.

Clinical signs
Clinical signs vary depending on viral strain and host age at exposure, and may be absent in persistently infected animals (4). While death with premonitory signs can occur, the most common presentation is one of chronic wasting, malaise, and melena (4, 5). Some ferrets may also develop neurologic signs, which must be distinguished from those of CDV (5, 9, 10, 11).

Pathology
Pathologic changes in parvovirus-infected ferrets are most prominent in tissues associated with the immune system, and include hepatomegaly, splenomegaly, mesenteric lymphadenopathy, membranous glomerulopathy, interstitial pneumonia, and less commonly, thymic enlargement. Histologically, there is periportal infiltration of the liver by immune cells, bile duct proliferation and fibrosis, and generalized expansion of immune cell populations in many organs (4, 5, 6, 9, 10). Virus-specific B-lymphocytes appear to be the primary target for parvovirus infection (1). The most striking, although inconsistent,

alteration in clinical chemistry is hypergammaglobulinemia (6, 10, 11). Much of the hypergammaglobulinemia represents virus-specific antibody (7). The mechanism by which this develops remains unknown. In this regard, most infected ferrets develop antiviral antibody, although it is not protective (8, 11).

Interference with research

While the author is not aware of any publications specifically reporting the effects of parvovirus on ferret research, it is clear that generalized immune stimulation would interfere with numerous areas of research involving ferrets. Likewise, hypergammaglobulinemia would confound studies evaluating serum globulin levels or, potentially, the analysis of any other protein. Also, chronic weight loss would interfere with any study in which normal growth or maintenance was expected. Acute deaths would reduce sample size. Lastly, studies involving the enterohepatic, hematopoietic, nervous, and respiratory systems could be adversely affected.

Diagnosis and control

Diagnosis is based on a history of weight loss, is supported by demonstrating hypergammaglobulinemia, and is confirmed by serologic tests for antiviral antibody (4). Seropositivity alone only indicates past infection, and does not prove that an animal is currently infected. Others have presented helpful differentials for chronic weight loss in ferrets (5). There is no effective treatment for parvovirus infection of ferrets. Infected or seropositive ferrets should be euthanized humanely to prevent additional animal infection and suffering, and because affected animals are not useful research subjects. As noted above, parvoviruses persist for long periods in the environment. Strict attention to disinfection is absolutely necessary following the occurrence of parvovirus infection in a laboratory colony. In fact, it may be necessary to assign laboratory ferrets to animal rooms not previously occupied by infected ferrets to avoid recurrence of infection.

BACTERIA

Helicobacter mustelae

Agent

Helicobacter mustelae is a gram-negative, rod-shaped, microaerophilic, gastric pathogen of ferrets. It is the cause of gastric ulcer disease in ferrets, which is analogous to a similar condition caused by *Helicobacter pylori* in humans. There appears to be little genetic heterogeneity among isolates (13, 15). For a thorough discussion on *H. mustelae,* the interested reader is referred to the writings of others (6). The most important points are summarized here.

Epidemiology

Infection with *H. mustelae,* at some time in life, appears to be nearly universal in laboratory ferrets (8), although infections may be lost later in life (10). *H. mustelae* is passed by fecal-oral transmission, and infects young ferrets shortly after weaning (6).

Clinical signs

Most infections with *H. mustelae* are asymptomatic (6). Eventually, ferrets may present with vomiting, melena, anorexia, and chronic weight loss (6).

Pathology

Initially, *H. mustelae* colonizes the gastric fundus, followed by colonization of the pyloric antrum (6). Colonization depends on urease production and flagellar induced motility (1, 6), whereas molecular mimicry of blood group antigens may facilitate immune evasion (3). Shortly after infection, *H. mustelae* causes a number of pathologic changes in the ferret stomach. These may include lymphoplasmacytic gastritis, which eventually becomes chronic and atrophic; gastric or duodenal ulcers; gastric adenocarcinoma; and mucosa-associated lymphoid tissue (MALT) lymphoma (5, 6, 7, 9). Ultrastructural and functional changes occur in the gastric mucosa, including loss of microvilli, cytoarchitectural changes in cellular junctions, and alterations in gastric mucosal hydrophobicity

(6, 11). Clinicopathologic changes include autoantibody formation, hypergastrinemia, hypochlorhydria, and lowered hematocrit (2, 6, 14). The latter is likely due to the combined effects of gastric bleeding and iron uptake by the organism (4).

Interference with research
The ferret-*H. mustelae* system is a useful model for the study of *H. pylori*-induced gastritis of humans. It is essential that ferrets intended for these studies be documented free of the pathogen. *H. mustelae* infection has been shown to induce autoantibodies; alter growth rate; weight gain; hematocrit; gastric morphology, including gastric epithelial cell proliferation rates; and gastric function (2, 6, 16). Clearly, infection with *H. mustelae* will interfere with studies in which these parameters are measured and with toxicity studies in which gastric tumor development is evaluated. Specifically, studies involving the enterohepatic, hematopoietic, and lymphoreticular systems may be altered.

Diagnosis and control
H. mustelae infection can be diagnosed serologically, and by culture of gastric necropsy or biopsy samples. Initial testing checks for urease production, which can be accomplished with a commercial kit, followed by other biochemical and morphologic tests (6). The reader is warned, however, that culture of members of the genus *Helicobacter* is difficult, and should be attempted by a laboratory with a good track record with these organisms. Clinical signs alone may suggest infection with *H. mustelae*, but are not pathognomonic. Infected ferrets can be effectively treated with antibiotics and mucosal protectants (6, 12). In cases where it is necessary to utilize *H. mustelae*-free ferrets, newly arriving ferrets should be screened and treated prior to entry into the main animal facility.

Lawsonia intracellularis

Agent
After many years of searching, the causative agent of proliferative bowel disease in ferrets has been identified as *Lawsonia intracellularis*, a gram-negative, slender, curved, obligate, intracellular rod (3). While *L. intracellularis* is morphologically similar to members of the family *Campylobacteriaceae*, significant genetic differences preclude inclusion of *L. intracellularis* in that family (3). *L. intracellularis* is genetically more closely related to the genus *Desulfovibrio*. The interested reader is referred to chapter 4 for a more detailed discussion of the biology of *L. intracellularis*.

Epidemiology
Increased awareness of this condition during nearly the past 20 years has resulted in greater case recognition. Proliferative bowel disease is now considered a common clinical condition among young ferrets (1). Fecal-oral transmission likely accounts for most infections.

Clinical signs
Clinical signs are most commonly observed in ferrets up to about 6 months of age, and include anorexia; weight loss, which may be profound; partial rectal prolapse; mucohemorrhagic, greenish, diarrheic feces; dehydration; and CNS signs, including ataxia and muscle tremors (2, 5). Some ferrets will die of the condition.

Pathology
The most prominent pathologic feature is segmentally thickened terminal colon due to marked proliferation of the apical epithelium (1), possibly under the influence of interferon γ (IFN-γ) (7). Less commonly, the ileum may also be involved. Other histopathologic changes include reduced goblet cell production, variable inflammatory cell infiltration, and changes in the glandular architecture of the affected bowel (1).

Interference with research
There is a paucity of information concerning the spectrum of physiologic effects of *L. intracellularis* on the ferret host. It is likely that future studies will reveal much about this host-pathogen interaction. At this point, it can

be concluded that infection of ferrets with *L. intracellularis* may confound studies involving the enterohepatic, hematopoietic, musculoskeletal, and nervous systems, and may affect those studies wherein growth rate is monitored. It is currently unknown what effect, if any, asymptomatic infection would have on host physiology.

Diagnosis and control
Diagnosis of *L. intracellularis* infection is complicated by the inability to grow the organism on artificial media, and is therefore based initially on clinical signs and physical examination. Careful palpation of the distal colon often reveals marked thickening. Terminal colon biopsy provides specimens that can be silver stained for identification of the organism, and routinely stained for evaluation of histopathologic changes. More specialized techniques, including immunohistochemistry, or, more recently, PCR, can also be used (4). It should be borne in mind that affected ferrets might be coinfected with other pathogens, including a *Campylobacter* sp. (1) or coccidia (6). Infected animals should either be culled, or aggressively treated with antibiotics and supportive care (1), depending on the objectives of the research project.

PARASITES

Fleas

Agent
Ferrets may be infested with fleas of the genus *Ctenocephalides* (3). Because fleas tend not to be highly host-specific, species infesting cats, dogs, and other mammals, including humans, are likely to also infest ferrets.

Epidemiology
The prevalence of flea infestation in laboratory ferrets is unknown but considered low (3). Fleas may become established in facilities where standard operating procedures for cage sanitation are not rigorously followed, where infested animals enter the colony without testing and treatment, and when feral mammals gain access to the facility. Transmission is by contact with infested animals, and by exposure to contaminated housing. Concerning the latter, while fleas spend the majority of their lives on the host, eggs will fall off and contaminate caging and animal housing areas.

Clinical signs
Infestation may be asymptomatic. More commonly, affected ferrets, like other flea-infested animals, present with pruritus, scaly skin, alopecia, and weight loss, and may develop secondary bacterial infections due to excoriation sustained while attempting to relieve the pruritus. The interscapular area, base of the tail, ventral abdomen, and thighs are the areas most often affected (2, 3).

Pathology
Pathologic changes due to flea infestation are associated with type 1 hypersensitivity reactions. Affected areas develop dermatitis, with infiltration of eosinophils, mast cells, and plasma cells. Areas secondarily infected with bacteria (usually *Staphylococcus aureus*) may become suppurative, with a neutrophilic inflammation.

Interference with research
The pruritus associated with flea infestation can markedly alter research results, by reducing food intake, leading to reduced weight gain, and weight loss; and by causing behavioral changes such as anxiety, excessive grooming, irritability, and general agitation. There is considerable evidence that ectoparasite infestation alters immune parameters, through cytokine induction (1), although this has not been evaluated in the ferret-flea model. Therefore, natural infestation of laboratory ferrets with fleas may alter research involving the dermal, enterohepatic, lymphoreticular, and nervous systems.

Diagnosis and control
Diagnosis of flea infestation is based on clinical signs and on identifying the fleas and their ex-

creta through close examination of suspect animals and bedding materials. Infested ferrets should be isolated and medicated with compounds approved for use in cats, such as pyrethrin powders or sprays, and other nontoxic compounds (2, 3). This excludes the use of organophosphates and other potentially toxic compounds. Strict attention should be paid to area and cage sanitation, including objects such as washable bedding (towels) or enrichment items. Insecticides and residual chemicals such as insect growth inhibitors can be used to treat surrounding areas, where feral rodents may live. Ideally, housing should be constructed in a manner precluding access by feral rodents. The author is personally familiar with a situation in which flea-infested feral squirrels were living underneath a portable laboratory animal housing unit. The fleas were able to gain access to the housing unit, resulting in flea infestation of the laboratory animals.

Dirofilaria immitis (heartworm)

Agent
Like many other mammals, including canids, felids, and others, ferrets are susceptible to infection with the filarial nematode parasite, *Dirofilaria immitis*. Development to the infective stage occurs in a wide range of mosquito species. In fact, about half the mosquito species in the United States are capable of hosting *D. immitis*.

Epidemiology
Ferrets housed outdoors in unscreened or poorly screened enclosures are likely to become infected with heartworms in areas where *D. immitis* is endemic. In some countries, such as in the United States, the geographic range of *D. immitis* has been expanding for several years, and is, of course, linked to the geographic ranges of host mosquitoes. Mosquitoes become infected by ingesting larval forms (microfilaria) during blood feeding. Development to the infective third larval (L_3) stage in the mosquito occurs in 2 to 3 weeks. Transmission to a susceptible ferret is through the feeding activities of infected mosquitoes. Larval worms develop in the subcutaneous connective tissues prior to migrating to the pulmonary arteries and right ventricle. Worms may be found in the heart 10 weeks after infection (7). Patent infections often do not develop, or are transient, in the ferret. The prevalence of infection in laboratory ferrets is unknown, but likely low in well-managed facilities. Wherever heartworms are found, canids serve as the primary reservoir hosts.

Clinical signs
Infection with even one adult worm can be, and with more worms is uniformly, fatal in ferrets (1, 6). Clinical signs include dyspnea, cough, lethargy, anorexia, pale mucous membranes, and in some animals, splenomegaly, dehydration, and melena (1, 4, 8). Heart sounds are muffled due to pleural effusion, and a heart murmur may be auscultated. Thoracic radiography or echocardiography reveals an enlarged right atrium, ventricle, and pulmonary artery, along with pulmonary congestion and effusion (2, 5, 6, 8). In severe cases, right-sided hypertension leads to ascites production. Death results from blockage of major vessels, with subsequent hemodynamic changes.

Pathology
Adult worms usually number less than 10 (6), but can exceed 20 in naturally infected ferrets (3). Pathologic changes occur in the pulmonary arteries and smaller vessels, and consist of intimal damage, thickening of the arterial walls, and endarteritis. Thromboembolic disease occurs as vessels become occluded with worms and worm fragments. The resulting pulmonary hypertension causes compensatory right ventricular hypertrophy; congestive heart failure; and chronic passive congestion, leading to chylous effusion, pulmonary edema, and ascites (6, 8).

Interference with research
The author is not aware of any publications concerning studies compromised by *D. immi-*

tis. It can be safely anticipated that infection would render ferrets unusable for many kinds of research studies, most prominently those involving the cardiovascular, enterohepatic, and respiratory systems. In addition, studies where weight gain, food consumption, and activity levels are to be measured would certainly be compromised by infection.

Diagnosis and control

Clinical signs, radiographic and echocardiographic findings, and a history of possible or likely exposure to mosquitoes in a heartworm-endemic area strongly suggest dirofilariasis. Diagnosis is complicated by the inconsistent finding of microfilaria in blood smears. Antigen detection kits offer the best opportunity for detection. As with infected dogs and cats, treatment is often unsuccessful and risky, and too often it results in the death of the animal. However, inclusion of antithrombotic therapy greatly increases survival rate (6). Given the uniform mortality of this disease in ferrets, prevention is extremely important. Ferrets should be obtained from reputable breeders that either house ferrets indoors, or in mosquito-proof enclosures, or that prophylactically medicate ferrets with larvacidal anthelmintics. Ferrets should be housed indoors after arrival at the animal facility.

REFERENCES

INTRODUCTION

1. **Fox, J. G.** 1998. *Biology and Diseases of the Ferret*, 2nd ed. Lippincott Williams & Wilkins, Baltimore, Md.
2. **Williams, E. S., and E. T. Thorne.** 1994. Infectious and parasitic diseases of captive carnivores, with special emphasis on the black-footed ferret (*Mustela nigripes*). *Rev. Sci. Tech.* **15:**91–114.

VIRUSES

Human influenza virus

1. **Ardans, A. A.** 1999. *Orthomyxoviridae*, p. 396–402. *In:* D. C. Hirsh and Y. C. Zee (ed.), *Veterinary Microbiology*. Blackwell Science, Inc., Malden, Mass.
2. **Barnett, J. K., L. W. Cruse, and D. Proud.** 1990. Kinins are generated in nasal secretions

TABLE 7-1. Body systems known or likely to be affected by pathogen indicated.

Pathogen	Cardio-vascular	Dermal	Endocrine	Entero-hepatic	Hema-topoietic	Lympho-reticular	Musculo-skeletal	Nervous	Reproductive	Respiratory	Urinary
Human influenza virus				X		X	X	X		X	
Rotavirus				X							
Rabies virus				X				X			
Canine distemper virus		X	X	X	X	X	X	X		X	X
Parvovirus				X	X		X	X			
Helicobacter mustelae				X	X	X					
Lawsonia intracellularis				X			X	X			
Fleas		X				X					
Dirofilaria immitis (heartworm)	X									X	

during influenza A infections in ferrets. *Am. Rev. Respir. Dis.* **142**:162–166.
3. Buchman, C. A., J. D. Swarts, J. T. Seroky, N. Panagiotou, F. Hayden, and W. J. Doyle. 1995. Otologic and systemic manifestations of experimental influenza A virus infection in the ferret. *Otolaryngol. Head Neck Surg.* **112**:572–578.
4. Cavanagh, D., F. Mitkis, C. Sweet, M. H. Collie, and H. Smith. 1979. The localization of influenza virus in the respiratory tract of ferrets: susceptible nasal mucosa cells produce and release more virus than susceptible lung cells. *J. Gen. Virol.* **44**:505–514.
5. Chen, K. S., S. S. Bharaj, and E. C. King. 1995. Induction and relief of nasal congestion in ferrets infected with influenza virus. *Int. J. Exp. Pathol.* **76**:55–64.
6. Coates, D. M., R. H. Husseini, M. H. Collie, C. Sweet, and H. Smith. 1984. The role of cellular susceptibility in the declining severity of respiratory influenza of ferrets with age. *Br. J. Exp. Pathol.* **65**:29–39.
7. Coates, D. M., R. H. Husseini, D. I. Rushton, C. Sweet, and H. Smith. 1984. The role of lung development in the age-related susceptibility of ferrets to influenza virus. *Br. J. Exp. Pathol.* **65**:543–547.
8. Collie, M. H., D. L. Rushton, C. Sweet, and H. Smith. 1980. Studies of influenza virus infection in newborn ferrets. *J. Med. Microbiol.* **13**:561–571.
9. Fox, J. G. 1998. *Biology and Diseases of the Ferret*, 2nd ed. Lippincott Williams & Wilkins, Baltimore, Md.
10. Glathe, H., M. Hilgenfeld, A. Lebhardt, H. U. Strittmatter, P. Schulze, and B. Brandt. 1984. The intestine of ferret—a possible site of virus replication. *Acta. Virol.* **28**:287–293.
11. Husseini, R. H., C. Sweet, H. Overton, and H. Smith. 1984. Role of maternal immunity in the protection of newborn ferrets against infection with a virulent influenza virus. *Immunology* **52**:389–394.
12. Jacoby, D. B., J. Tamaoki, D. B Borson, and J. A. Nadel. 1988. Influenza infection causes airway hyperresponsiveness by decreasing enkephalinase. *J. Appl. Physiol.* **64**:2653–2658.
13. Kang, E. S., M. S. Galloway, W. Bean, G. A. Cook, and G. Olson. 1991. Acute alterations in the regulation of lipid metabolism after intravascular reesposure to a single bolus of homologous virus during influenza B infection in ferrets: possible model of epiphenomena associated with influenza. *Int. J. Exp. Pathol.* **72**:319–327.
14. Kang, E. S., H. J. Lee, J. Boulet, L. K. Myers, G. A. Cook, and W. Bean. 1992. Potential for hepatic and renal dysfunction during influenza B infection, convalescence, and after induction of secondary viremia. *J. Exp. Pathol.* **6**:133–144.
15. Kauffman, C. A., G. M. Schiff, and J. P. Phair. 1978. Influenza in ferrets and guinea pigs: effect on cell-mediated immunity. *Infect. Immun.* **19**:547–552.
16. Ramphal, R., P. M. Small, J. W. Shands, Jr., W. Fishchlschweiger, and P. A. Small, Jr. 1980. Adherence of *Pseudomonas aeruginosa* to tracheal cells injured by influenza infection or by endotracheal intubation. *Infect. Immun.* **27**:614–619.
17. Rarey, K. E., M. A. DeLacure, S. A. Sandridge, and P. A. Small, Jr. 1987. Effect of upper respiratory infection on hearing in the ferret model. *Am. J. Otolaryngol.* **8**:161–170.
18. Rushton, D. I., M. H. Collie, C. Sweet, R. H. Husseini, and H. Smith. 1983. The effects of maternal viraemia in late gestation on the conceptus of the pregnant ferret. *J. Pathol.* **140**:181–191.
19. Sanford, B. A., and M. A. Ramsay. 1989. In vivo localization of Staphylococcus aureus in nasal tissues of healthy and influenza A virus-infected ferrets. *Proc. Soc. Exp. Biol. Med.* **191**:163–169.
20. Sweet, C., J. C. Macartney, R. A. Bird, D. Cavanagh, M. H. Collie, R. H. Husseini, and H. Smith. 1981. Differential distribution of virus and histological damage in the lower respiratory tract of ferrets infected with influenza viruses of differing virulence. *J. Gen. Virol.* **54**:103–114.
21. Zitzow, L. A., T. Rowe, T. Morken, W. J. Shieh, S. Zaki, and J. M. Katz. 2002. Pathogenesis of avian influenza A (H5N1) viruses in ferrets. *J. Virol.* **76**:4420–4429.

Rotavirus
1. Fox, J. G. 1998. *Biology and Diseases of the Ferret*, 2nd ed. Lippincott Williams & Wilkins, Baltimore, Md.
2. Torres-Medina, A. 1987. Isolation of an atypical Rotavirus causing diarrhea in neonatal ferrets. *Lab. Anim. Sci.* **37**:167–171.

Rabies virus
1. Aubert, M. F. 1982. Experimental transmission of rabies to the ferret by an Ixodidate: *Pholeoixodes rugicollis* (Schultze and Schlottke, 1929). *Acarologia* **23**:125–132.
2. Fox, J. G. 1998. *Biology and Diseases of the Ferret*, 2nd ed. Lippincott Williams & Wilkins, Baltimore, Md.
3. Gunby, P. 1981. Can you catch rabies from your ferret? Probably not. *JAMA* **245**:1628.

4. **Niezgoda, M., D. J. Briggs, J. Shaddock, D. W. Dreesen, and C. E. Rupprecht.** 1997. Pathogenesis of experimentally induced rabies in domestic ferrets. *Am. J. Vet. Res.* **58:**1327–1331.
5. **Niezgoda, M., D. J. Briggs, J. Shaddock, and C. E. Rupprecht.** 1998. Viral excretion in domestic ferrets (*Mustela putorius furo*) inoculated with a raccoon rabies isolate. *Am. J. Vet. Res.* **59:**1629–1632.
6. **Rupprecht, C. E., J. Gilbert, R. Pitts, K. R. Marshall, and H. Koprowski.** 1990. Evaluation of an inactivated rabies virus vaccine in domestic ferrets. *J. Am. Vet. Med. Assoc.* **196:**1614–616.
7. **Zee, Y. C.** 1999. *Rhabdoviridae*, p. 412–417. In D. C. Hirsh and Y.C. Zee (ed.), *Veterinary Microbiology*. Blackwell Science, Inc., Malden, Mass.

Canine distemper virus
1. **Donnelly, T. M., and C. J. Orcutt.** 2001. Acute ataxia in a young ferret following canine distemper vaccination. Renal failure after epinepherine overdose. *Lab. Anim.* **30:**25–27.
2. **Fox, J. G.** 1998. *Biology and Diseases of the Ferret*, 2nd ed. Lippincott Williams & Wilkins, Baltimore, Md.
3. **Groelke, J. W., L. W. Dixon, C. Cummings, and J. B. Baseman.** 1986. Virus contamination and cytopathology of ferret tracheal epithelial cells in culture caused by vaccination with distemper virus. *Lab. Anim. Sci.* **36:**527–529.
4. **Hagen, K. W., H. Goto, and J. R. Gorham.** 1970. Distemper vaccine in pregnant ferrets and mink. *Res. Vet. Sci.* **11:**458–460.
5. **Kauffman, C. A., A. G. Bergman, and R. P. O'Connor.** 1982. Distemper virus infection in ferrets: an animal model of measles-induced immunosuppression. *Clin. Exp. Immunol.* **47:**617–625.
6. **Krakowka, S., M. K. Axthelm, and J. R. Gorham.** 1987. Effects of induced thrombocytopenia on viral invasion of the central nervous system in canine distemper virus infection. *J. Comp. Pathol.* **97:**441–450.
7. **Murray, J.** 1998. Vaccine injection-site sarcoma in a ferret. *J. Am. Vet. Med. Assoc.* **213:**955.
8. **Rzezutka, A., and B. Mizak.** 2002. Application of N-PCR for diagnosis of distemper in dogs and fur animals. *Vet. Microbiol.* **88:**95–103.
9. **Williams, E. S., E. T. Thorne, M. J. Appel, and D. W. Belitsky.** 1988. Canine distemper in black-footed ferrets (*Mustela nigripes*) from Wyoming. *J. Wildl. Dis.* **24:**385–398.
10. **Wimsatt, J., M. T. Jay, K. E. Innes, M. Jensen, and J. K. Collins.** 2001. Serologic evaluation, efficacy, and safety of a commercial modified-live canine distemper vaccine in domestic ferrets. *Am. J. Vet. Res.* **62:**736–740.
11. **Zee, Y. C.** 1999. *Paramyxoviridae*, p. 403–411. In D. C. Hirsh and Y. C. Zee (ed.), *Veterinary Microbiology*. Blackwell Science, Inc., Malden, Mass.

Parvovirus
1. **Aasted, B., and R. G. Leslie.** 1991. Virus-specific B-lymphocytes are probably the primary targets for Aleutian disease virus. *Vet. Immunol. Immunopathol.* **28:**127–141.
2. **Alexandersen, S., A. U. Jensen, M. Hansen, and B. Aasted.** 1985. Experimental transmission of Aleutian disease virus (ADV) to different animal species. *Acta Pathol. Microbiol. Immunol. Scand.* **93:**195–200.
3. **Daoust, P. Y., and D. B. Hunter.** 1978. Spontaneous Aleutian disease in ferrets. *Can. Vet. J.* **19:**133–135.
4. **Fox, J. G.** 1998. *Biology and Diseases of the Ferret*, 2nd ed. Lippincott Williams & Wilkins, Baltimore, Md.
5. **Palley, L. S., B. F. Corning, J. G. Fox, J. C. Murphy, and D. H. Gould.** 1992. Parvovirus associated syndrome (Aleutian disease) in two ferrets. *J. Am. Vet. Med. Assoc.* **201:**100–106.
6. **Porter, H. G., D. D. Porter, and A. E. Larsen.** 1982. Aleutian disease in ferrets. *Infect. Immun.* **36:**379–386.
7. **Porter, H. G., D. D. Porter, and A. E. Larsen.** 1984. Much of the increased IgG in Aleutian disease of mink is viral antibody. *J. Exp. Pathol.* **1:**79–88.
8. **Porter, H. G., D. D. Porter, and A. E. Larsen.** 1990. Aleutian disease parvovirus infection of mink and ferrets elicits an antibody response to a second nonstructural viral protein. *J. Virol.* **64:**1859–1860.
9. **Rozengurt, N., D. Stewart, and S. Sanchez.** 1995. Diagnostic exercise: ataxia and incoordination in ferrets. *Lab. Anim. Sci.* **45:**432–434.
10. **Une, Y., Y. Wakimoto, Y. Nakano, M. Konishi, and Y. Nomura.** 2000. Spontaneous Aleutian disease in a ferret. *J. Vet. Med. Sci.* **62:**553–555.
11. **Welchman, D. D., M. Oxenham, and S. H. Done.** 1993. Aleutian disease in domestic ferrets: diagnostic findings and survey results. *Vet. Rec.* **132:**479–484.

BACTERIA

Helicobacter mustelae
1. **Andrutis, K. A., J. G. Fox, D. B. Schauer, R. P. Marini, J. C. Murphy, L. Yan, and J. V. Solnick.** 1995. Inability of an isogenic urease-negative mutant strain of *Helicobacter mustelae* to colonize the ferret stomach. *Infect. Immun.* **63:**3722–3725.

2. **Croinin, T. O., M. Clyne, B. J. Appelmelk, and B. Drumm.** 2001. Antigastric autoantibodies in ferrets naturally infected with *Helicobacter mustelae*. *Infect. Immun.* **69:**2708–2713.
3. **Croinin, T. O, M. Clyne, and B. Drumm.** 1998. Molecular mimicry of ferret gastric epithelial blood group antigen A by *Helicobacter mustelae*. *Gastroenterology* **114:**690–696.
4. **Dhaenens, L., F. Szczebara, S. Van Nieuwenhuyse, and M. O. Husson.** 1999. Comparison of iron uptake in different *Helicobacter* species. *Res. Microbiol.* **150:**475–481.
5. **Erdman, S. E., P. Correa, L. A. Coleman, M. D. Schrenzel, X. Li, and J. G. Fox.** 1997. *Helicobacter mustelae*-associated gastric MALT lymphoma in ferrets. *Am. J. Pathol.* **151:**273–380.
6. **Fox, J. G.** 1998. *Biology and Diseases of the Ferret*, 2nd ed. Lippincott Williams & Wilkins, Baltimore, Md.
7. **Fox, J. G., C. A. Dangler, W. Sager, R. Borkowski, and J. M. Gliatto.** 1997. *Helicobacter mustelae*-associated gastric adenocarcinoma in ferrets (*Mustela putorius furo*). *Vet. Pathol.* **34:**225–229.
8. **Fox, J. G., G. Otto, J. C. Murphy, N. S. Taylor, and A. Lee.** 1991. Gastric colonization of the ferret with *Helicobacter* species: natural and experimental infections. *Rev. Infect. Dis.* **13:**S671–S680.
9. **Fox, J. G., G. Otto, N. S. Taylor, W. Rosenblad, and J. C. Murphy.** 1991. *Helicobacter mustelae*-induced gastritis and elevated gastric pH in the ferret (*Mustela putorius furo*). *Infect. Immun.* **59:**1875–1880.
10. **Fox, J. G., B. J. Paster, F. E. Dewhirst, N. S. Taylor, L. L. Yan, P. J. Macuch, and L. M. Chmura.** 1992. *Helicobacter mustelae* insolation from feces of ferrets: evidence to support fecal-oral transmission of a gastric *Helicobacter*. *Infect. Immun.* **60:**606–611.
11. **Gold, B. D., P. Islur, Z. Policova, S. Czinn, A. W. Neumann, and P. M. Sherman.** 1996. Surface properties of *Helicobacter mustelae* and ferret gastrointestinal mucosa. *Clin. Investig. Med.* **19:**92–100.
12. **Marini, R. P., J. G. Fox, N. S. Taylor, L. Yan, A. A. McColm, and R. Williamson.** 1999. Ranitidine bismuth citrate and clarithromycin, alone or in combination, for eradication of *Helicobacter mustelae* infection in ferrets. *Am. J. Vet. Res.* **60:**1280–1286.
13. **Morgan, D. D., and R. J. Owen.** 1990. Use of DNA restriction endonuclease digest and ribosomal RNA gene probe patterns to fingerprint *Helicobacter pylori* and *Helicobacter mustelae* isolated from human and animal hosts. *Mol. Cell. Probes* **4:**321–334.
14. **Perkins, S. E., J. G. Fox, and J. H. Walsh.** 1996. *Helicobacter mustelae*-associated hypergastrinemia in ferrets (*Mustela putorius furo*). *Am. J. Vet. Res.* **57:**147–150.
15. **Taylor, D. E., N. Chang, N. S. Taylor, and J. G. Fox.** 1994. Genome conservation in *Helicobacter mustelae* as determined by pulsed-field gel electrophoresis. *FEMS Microbiol. Lett.* **118:**31–36.
16. **Yu, J., R. M. Russell, R. N. Salomon, J. C. Murphy, L. S. Palley, and J. G. Fox.** 1995. Effect of *Helicobacter mustelae* infection on ferret gastric epithelial cell proliferation. *Carcinogenesis* **16:**1927–1931.

Lawsonia intracellularis

1. **Fox, J. G.** 1998. *Biology and Diseases of the Ferret*, 2nd ed. Lippincott Williams & Wilkins, Baltimore, Md.
2. **Fox, J. G., J. C. Murphy, J. I. Ackerman, K. S. Prostak, C. A. Gallagher, and V. J. Rambow.** 1982. Proliferative colitis in ferrets. *Am. J. Vet. Res.* **43:**858–864.
3. **Hirsh, D. C.** 1999. Spiral organisms I: Campylobacter—arcobacter—lawsonia (digestive tract), p. 89–92. *In* D. C. Hirsh and Y. C. Zee (ed.), *Veterinary Microbiology*. Blackwell Science, Inc., Malden, Mass.
4. **Kim, J., C. Choi, W. S. Cho, and C. Chae.** 2000. Immunohistochemistry and polymerase chain reaction for the detection of *Lawsonia intracellularis* in porcine intestinal tissues with proliferative enteropathy. *J. Vet. Med. Sci.* **62:**771–773.
5. **Krueger, K. L., J. C. Murphy, and J. G. Fox.** 1989. Treatment of proliferative colitis in ferrets. *J. Am. Vet. Med. Assoc.* **194:**1435–1436.
6. **Li, X., J. Pang, and J. G. Fox.** 1996. Coinfection with intracellular *Desulfovibrio* species and coccidia in ferrets with proliferative bowel disease. *Lab. Anim. Sci.* **46:**569–571.
7. **Smith, D. G., S. C. Mitchell, T. Nash, and S. Rhind.** 2000. Gamma interferon influences intestinal epithelial hyperplasia caused by *Lawsonia intracellularis* infection in mice. *Infect. Immun.* **68:**6737–6743.

PARASITES

Fleas

1. **Baker, D. G., J. D. Bryant, J. F. Urban, Jr., and J. K. Lunney.** 1994. Swine immunity to selected parasites. *Vet. Immunol. Immunopathol.* **43:**127–133.
2. **Fox, J. G.** 1998. *Biology and Diseases of the Ferret*, 2nd ed. Lippincott Williams & Wilkins, Baltimore, Md.
3. **Orcutt, C.** 1997. Dermatologic diseases, p. 115–125. *In* E. V. Hillyer and K. E. Quesenberry (ed.), *Ferrets, Rabbits, and Rodents: Clinical Medicine and Surgery*. W.B. Saunders Co., Philadelphia, Pa.

Dirofilaria immitis **(heartworm)**
1. **Fox, J. G.** 1998. *Biology and Diseases of the Ferret,* 2nd ed. Lippincott Williams & Wilkins, Baltimore, Md.
2. **McCall, J. W.** 1998. Dirofilariasis in the domestic ferret. *Clin. Tech. Small Anim. Pract.* **13:**109–112.
3. **Moreland, A. F., A. H. Battles, and J. H. Nease.** 1986. Dirofilariasis in a ferret. *J. Am. Vet. Med. Assoc.* **188:**864.
4. **Parrott, T. Y., E. C. Greiner, and J. D. Parrott.** 1984. *Dirofilaria immitis* infection in three ferrets. *J. Am. Vet. Med. Assoc.* **184:**582–583.
5. **Sasai, H., K. Kato, T. Sasaki, S. Koyama, T. Kotani, and T. Fukata.** 2000. Echocardiographic diagnosis of dirofilariasis in a ferret. *J. Small Anim. Pract.* **41:**172–174.
6. **Stamoulis, M. E., M. S. Miller, and E. V. Hillyer.** 1997. Cardiovascular diseases, p. 63–76. *In* E. V. Hillyer and K. E. Quesenberry (ed.), *Ferrets, Rabbits, and Rodents: Clinical Medicine and Surgery.* W.B. Saunders Co., Philadelphia, Pa.
7. **Supakorndej, P., J. W. McCall, and J. J. Jun.** 1994. Early migration and development of *Dirofilaria immitis* in the ferret, *Mustela putorius furo. J. Parasitol.* **80:**237–244.
8. **Williams, J., and M. A. Mitchell.** 2000. What is your diagnosis? Severe pleural effusion and pulmonary atelectasis. *J. Am. Vet. Med. Assoc.* **217:**1625–1626.

PATHOGENS OF CATS

8

INTRODUCTION

The domestic cat (*Felis sylvestris catus*) is commonly used as a model for research into a variety of physiologic systems and several human diseases, including vision, trauma, neurophysiology, myocardial injury, vestibular disease, viral pathophysiology, pharmacokinetics, pulmonary conditions, dental caries, and renal ischemia research. In addition, veterinary research on feline diseases has increased markedly, as the cat has replaced the dog as the most commonly owned pet animal. Therefore, the number of cats in research animal facilities remains high. Most cats used in research are purpose bred, of very high quality, and of low pathogen status, and are purchased from reputable dealers. However, on occasion, a research facility may purchase cats from other sources, in particular, if the cats are only to be used for teaching laboratories. These cats may bring pathogens into an animal facility. Similarly, caretakers may unknowingly transmit pathogens from their own pet cats to those in the animal facility. For these reasons, it is imperative that the laboratory animal veterinarian and biomedical researcher be aware of the natural pathogens of cats, and their documented or potential effects on research.

For many pathogens, no studies have been conducted that specifically sought to examine the role of feline pathogens as confounding variables through their physiologic effects on the host. In these cases, the literature covering natural case reports and experimental infections has been reviewed to allow a reasonable synthesis of the known and potential physiologic effects these pathogens may have on the feline research subject.

VIRUSES

Feline calicivirus

Agent
Caliciviruses are nonenveloped single-stranded RNA (ssRNA) viruses of the family *Caliciviridae* (36). There appears to be considerable serologic cross protection among isolates, suggesting that while strains differ in pathogenicity, they retain considerable antigenic similarity (3, 9, 15, 21, 23). More recently, sequence-based methods have been used for typing feline calicivirus (CV) (12, 24).

Epidemiology
CV is extremely common throughout the world (17, 36). Risk factors for infection include young age (4 to 11 months of age), multiple cat households, and contact with dogs with or without respiratory tract disease (2).

Transmission is primarily through inhalation or ingestion of infectious aerosols of oral and nasal secretions, but can also occur in utero (8). Recovered cats carry virus in oropharyngeal tissues, principally the tonsils, for up to 2 years, and thereby serve as reservoirs of infection for other cats (6, 36). In these cats, reactivation of CV excretion occurs but does not appear to be triggered by stress (34). These asymptomatic cats differ in the amount of virus shed, and can be divided into high-, medium-, or low-level excretors (34).

Clinical signs
Clinical signs of infection are strain dependent, develop within 2 to 3 days of exposure, and are primarily associated with the upper respiratory tract and oral cavity. Traditionally, two biotypes of CV have been recognized. One biotype causes primarily acute oral and respiratory disease, while the other causes primarily chronic gingivitis and stomatitis (22). Taken together, clinical signs may include oculonasal discharge, rhinitis, conjunctivitis, sneezing, mild fever, oral ulcerations, inappetance, and depression (11, 23, 26, 28, 36). In addition, immune complex-induced joint pain (1, 4) and abortions (8, 33) have been linked to calicivirus infection. Clinical signs usually resolve within 7 to 10 days in the absence of secondary bacterial infections (36). More recently, a highly virulent strain causing hemorrhagic-like fever, systemic illness, and high mortality was reported (21). Coinfection with immunosuppressive viruses may increase the severity of calicivirus infection (27, 31).

Pathology
Following infection, virus replication occurs in epithelial cells of the oral cavity, conjunctiva, and respiratory tract (35). Like clinical signs, pathogenicity is strain dependent (20). Lesions most often occur in and around the oral cavity, and consist of vesicles that later ulcerate, on the tongue, hard palate, and external nares. Without secondary bacterial infections, ulcers heal within a few weeks. Severe cases may also involve interstitial pneumonia, with replacement of type I with type II epithelial cells, fibroblasts, and inflammatory cells (14). Naturally infected or vaccinated cats develop serum-neutralizing antibodies, which are passed to kittens in colostrum, and decline after weaning (36).

Interference with research
Few reports have been published describing physiologic effects of feline calicivirus, which might be useful in predicting interference of the pathogen with research studies. Feline calicivirus has been shown to elevate blood levels of α_1-acid glycoprotein (32), while in vitro studies have demonstrated release of neutrophil chemotactic factors from infected alveolar cells (14). Clearly, studies involving the dermal, enterohepatic, musculoskeletal, reproductive, and respiratory systems would be at least temporarily compromised by natural infection with feline calicivirus.

Diagnosis and control
Traditional methods of diagnosis have included virus isolation and demonstration by indirect immunofluorescence assay (IFA), similar to that described for feline herpesvirus 1 (see below). More recently, reverse transcriptase (RT)-PCR assays have been developed which should improve the speed and reliability of diagnosis (18, 30). As for most other viral infections, treatment is primarily supportive, and includes administration of broad-spectrum antibiotics, fluid therapy in cases of dehydration, and nasal antihistamine drops (36). Unless cats are to be held under strict barrier conditions, early and annual vaccination with inactivated or modified live vaccines is recommended (5). Concerning the modified live vaccines, considerable evidence exists that vaccine strains may mutate and cause clinical disease (25). This problem may be overcome by use of recombinant vaccines such as the recombinant myxoma virus vaccine, which expresses CV capsid protein (16). Feline calicivirus is resistant to inactivation by ultraviolet light (20), as well as by many common disinfectants, including some quaternary

ammonium compounds, but is inactivated by dilute sodium hypochlorite (1:128 or less), chlorine dioxide, and potassium peroxymonosulfate (7, 10, 29).

Feline coronavirus

Agent
Feline coronavirus (FCV) is an ssRNA virus antigenically related to other coronaviruses, including feline enteric coronavirus (FECV), a nearly ubiquitous, persistent, mildly pathogenic, small intestinal virus. In fact, it has been proposed that FCV originates, through mutation, from intestinal FECV (2, 12).

Epidemiology
Arising by mutation from FECV, FCV has a nearly global distribution, and is common in domestic cat populations. Exotic cats are also susceptible to infection. As one would expect of viruses arising by mutation, multiple strains have been isolated, and can be grouped by virulence (3). Additionally, virus may undergo genetic alteration under selective pressures inherent in different organs within a host, resulting in the presence of different "quasi species" within a given cat (10). Persistently infected cats serve as reservoirs and shed virus intermittently in the feces for several months, and in some cases, for life (1, 4, 7). It has been proposed that pregnancy-induced immune suppression facilitates reactivation of latent FCV infections, followed by transplacental transmission to unborn kittens (15), although data generated by others do not support this (4). Kittens nursing infected queens may shed virus as early as 3 weeks. In all cases, transmission is primarily by ingestion. Virus gains entry into, and remains in, a laboratory animal colony if cats are not purchased specific pathogen free (SPF) from reputable suppliers, and if protocols are not followed to prevent or detect infection.

Clinical signs
Most infections with feline coronaviruses are asymptomatic, or are mild, and occur in 4- to 12-week-old kittens. Clinical signs include ocular or nasal discharge, and in some cases, mild, transient vomiting and diarrhea (11). This is the typical presentation for what has historically been referred to as FECV infection. In few cases, FECV mutates to FCV and gains the ability to replicate in macrophages. When these occur, and initial immune responses are subsequently avoided (2), cats may develop feline infectious peritonitis (FIP), a severe disease in young (6 months to 5 years old) and old (>14 years old) cats. Two distinct forms of FIP may be seen. The effusive or "wet" form is more common, and is characterized by pleuritis and peritonitis, resulting in fluid accumulation in the thorax and peritoneum. Clinical signs include fever, weight loss, dyspnea, and abdominal distension (15). In contrast, the noneffusive or "dry" form is a disease of the internal organs, central nervous system (CNS), and eyes. In that form, clinical signs vary, and are dependent on the organs or tissues affected. In both forms, mortality may be high, and is related to, among other things, overall environmental levels of coronavirus, notably and interestingly, FECV (5). Lastly, in utero infection may result in stillbirths, or birth of kittens that quickly develop clinical disease.

Pathology
Considering only pathogenic FCV infections, the pathogenesis of FIP is complex, and largely depends on the host immune response and viral strain virulence (14). Following ingestion, infected intestinal macrophages disseminate virus throughout the body. A humoral immune response, without a cellular response, facilitates phagocytosis, and results in the effusive form of FIP, which is characterized by pyogranulomatous vasculitis around small venules in the visceral peritoneum, pleura, omentum, and solid organs (8, 13). It is thought that the pathogenesis is associated with specific antibody and immune complex formation (8, 15). In contrast, if a cellular immune response occurs, a more localized granulomatous response occurs in the lymph

nodes, kidneys, meninges, and ependyma of the brain and spinal cord, without fluid accumulation (15). While less common, clinical FECV enteritis is characterized by histologic changes in the small intestinal villus epithelium (9). Immunity to FCV is primarily cellular, while immunity to FECV is primarily humoral (5).

Interference with research

To the best of this author's knowledge, there is no literature directly reporting interference of feline coronaviruses with research. However, given the multiple sites of viral replication, differences in strain virulence, and the range of pathologic presentations and organ involvement, one can assume that infection with FCV or FECV could alter research involving the cardiovascular, enterohepatic, hematopoietic, lymphoreticular, nervous, reproductive, respiratory, and urinary systems. In addition, alterations may be noted in growth parameters and animal behavior. It is unknown what level of infection is required before organ systems are affected. It is likely that asymptomatic cats would be less affected physiologically, although it cannot be stated with certainty that there would be no physiologic effects whatsoever.

Diagnosis and control

Diagnosis of FCV infection is based on clinical signs, histopathology, and serologic findings. The "wet" form has a more characteristic presentation and is therefore more easily diagnosed clinically. Also, antibodies are routinely produced and are detectable. The noneffusive form presents a greater diagnostic challenge. It should be noted that some cats may have antibodies cross-reactive with antigenically related non-FIP coronaviruses. More recently, PCR assays have been developed, and are highly reliable for detecting virus shedding (1) or viremia (6). There are no effective treatments for FCV infection. Treatment of cats with effusive disease is mostly palliative, including thoracocentesis and abdominocentesis. Unless contraindicated by the needs of the research project, cats should be vaccinated. If eradication of the virus is necessary, the premises should be thoroughly disinfected with quaternary ammonium compounds. Infected cats should be isolated or euthanized, depending on programmatic needs. Reportedly, the keys to controlling FCV infections in catteries include reduction of FECV-shedding rates and selection for genetically resistant cats (5).

Feline herpesvirus type 1

Agent

The family *Herpesviridae* contains a diverse group of double-stranded DNA (dsDNA) viruses, representatives of which have been found in nearly every host species investigated. Feline herpesvirus type 1 (FHV-1) is a member of the subfamily Alphaherpesvirinae. Members of this subfamily grow rapidly; are highly cytopathic in cell culture; and establish latent infections, primarily in sensory ganglia (2, 16). FHV-1 is the cause of feline viral rhinotracheitis (FVR). While mostly similar serologically, FHV-1 strains differ in pathogenicity and can be distinguished by restriction enzyme digestion pattern (2, 8). For an excellent review of the biology and clinical aspects of infection, the interested reader is referred elsewhere (24).

Epidemiology

Infection of cats with FHV-1 is common throughout the world (3, 15, 24, 26). Latently infected, frequently asymptomatic cats serve as reservoirs of infection. Within a few to several weeks following some physiologic stress such as parturition, dietary changes, or housing alterations, virus is shed for up to about 10 days (5, 30). Shed virus serves as a source of infection for other cats. Transmission is by direct contact with infectious discharges, and is facilitated by overcrowding and close housing. Fomites and human vectors, including animal facility personnel, may also facilitate transmission (2, 24). It is thought that all cats infected with FHV-1 become life-long carriers (30).

Clinical signs

Clinical signs are most severe in very young and very old cats, and most often include signs related to upper respiratory disease, such as nasal discharge, sneezing, and coughing (1, 24, 26). Additional clinical signs may include ulcerative keratitis, keratoconjunctivitis sicca, uveitis, blepharospasm, symblepharon, corneal sequestration, ulcerative stomatitis, dermatitis, abortions, fever, lethargy, inappetence, and pneumonia (1, 2, 6, 13, 17, 23, 24). Antibody responses are largely ineffectual for controlling the infection, although titers remain elevated for up to a year (2).

Pathology

The pathogenesis of FHV-1 infection depends on the route of infection. Experimental inoculations of the nasal passages, thought to be analogous to natural infection, cause rapid and severe cytolytic infections of the local epithelium (2). Intranuclear inclusion body conjunctivitis, uveitis, hyperemia, chemosis, and keratitis, may accompany upper respiratory tract disease. Virus persists in the upper respiratory tract for approximately 2 weeks. Pathologic changes also develop in the lungs, and consist of interstitial pneumonitis with focal necrotic lesions and inflammatory cell accumulation found from the level of the bronchi to the alveoli (2). Clinicopathologic changes include neutrophilia, followed later by mild lymphocytosis (27). Eventually, the infection becomes latent in the trigeminal ganglia and other tissues, such as the cornea, until the next stressful event (18, 20, 24).

Interference with research

Latent infection could compromise studies in which the architecture of neural ganglia is under study. Clinically affected cats clearly are unsuitable for studies involving the dermal, enterohepatic, hematopoietic, lymphoreticular, nervous, reproductive, and respiratory systems. Studies in which growth rates are measured would also be affected. In addition, FHV-1 has been shown to cause transient immune suppression (21), stimulate gene expression of feline immunodeficiency virus (9), bind heparin (12), and induce tracheal hyperresponsiveness to vagal stimulation (11).

Diagnosis and control

FHV-1 infection, particularly in acute cases, is suggested by clinical, primarily ophthalmic signs. Visual diagnosis is more complicated in recurrent or chronic disease but may be assisted by the clinical history (24). A diagnosis of FVR has traditionally been confirmed by immunofluorescence staining of nasal and conjunctival tissues or impressions made from swabs. More recently, an enzyme-linked immunosorbent assay (ELISA) has been developed (22). Virus isolation, following inoculation using swabs from the same sites, may also be accomplished, and in some reports (3, 19), though not in all (14), is more sensitive than IFA. Also, paired serology can be used to evaluate infection status. Lastly, quantitative (28) and nonquantitative (25, 29) PCR assays have been developed for both active and latent infections, and will likely become the diagnostic test of choice. Treatment of affected cats is mostly supportive, although newer, nontoxic, topically applied antiviral drugs such as vidarabine or trifluridine may ameliorate ophthalmic signs (17, 24). Supportive therapy should include systemic and ophthalmic broad-spectrum antibiotics, and frequent cleansing of the eyes and nose (24). Where virus eradication is desired, viral culturing after corticosteroid-induced reactivation of excretion, followed by culling of all positive animals, was largely successful in eliminating the pathogen from a large laboratory cat colony (7). FHV-1 is readily inactivated in the animal facility environment by commonly used disinfectants, including bleach, iodinated and quaternary ammonium compounds, and chlorhexidine (10, 31). Therefore, disinfection following a clinical case should greatly reduce the pathogen load in the environment. Prevention of severe infection involves stress reduction and annual or semiannual vaccination (2, 4), although it should be noted that vaccination does not completely protect against infection with field strains (30).

Feline immunodeficiency virus

Agent
Feline immunodeficiency virus (FIV) is the most thoroughly investigated pathogen infecting cats. This is because FIV is an excellent animal model of human immunodeficiency virus (HIV) infection and AIDS. FIV is an enveloped ssRNA virus of the family *Retroviridae* and genus *Lentivirus*. Isolates are grouped on the basis of envelope protein fusogenic properties (37, 65), and in addition, may differ in pathogenicity, T lymphotropism, and in vitro cytopathic effect (58, 68).

Epidemiology
FIV infection is globally prevalent. Seroprevalence may be high in multiple cat households, and among cohorts of sick cats. Risk factors for FIV infection include aggression; roaming, and therefore gender, with males at greater risk for infection; mixed breed (versus purebred); and advancing age (males only) (15, 16, 87). It has been reported that male orange cats gain weight faster and are heavier than nonorange cats, and have a higher incidence of FIV infection (73). These data support studies reporting that transmission is primarily by exposure to infectious saliva. However, transmission has also been demonstrated to occur pre- and postnatally (63, 79, 82), and by semen (45), although sexual contact is not considered a major route of transmission. Lastly, anecdotal evidence suggests that FIV may also be transmitted by reused suture material (23). Casual, nonaggressive contact between cats does not efficiently facilitate transmission. Dual infection with feline leukemia virus is not uncommon. Interspecies transmission of FIV occurs between domestic and exotic felids (60). In this regard, antibodies to FIV have been found in many species of exotic cats (59, 62).

Clinical signs
Clinical disease due to FIV infection develops through three stages (59). An acute stage is characterized by lymphadenopathy, malaise, and recurrent fever of undetermined origin. During this time the popliteal lymph node is a good indicator node for the assessment of lymphoreticular status in FIV infection (21). Severity of clinical disease is inversely correlated with age at infection, with cats infected as neonates developing the most severe signs (28). Next comes a long, largely asymptomatic, subclinical stage. Finally, several months to years after infection, a minority of cats enter a terminal stage characterized by tumor formation, degenerative disease, and opportunistic infections (47, 59). Plasma viral load has been shown to correlate with clinical stage, survival time, and disease progression in naturally infected cats, and may therefore be a useful prognostic marker (30). Opportunistic pathogens shown to be associated with FIV include viral (feline poxvirus, feline calicivirus), bacterial (*Chlamydophila felis*, *Listeria monocytogenes*), mycotic (*Microsporum canis*, *Malassezia* spp., *Candida albicans*, *Cryptococcus neoformans*), and parasitic (*Toxoplasma gondii*) agents (19, 20, 53, 77, 84). Credible anecdotal reports suggest others as well (3, 4, 13, 29). Late-stage clinical signs are nonspecific, and may include wasting, lethargy, inappetence, lymphadenopathy, oculonasal discharge, diarrhea, fever, chronic oral infections, respiratory distress, and neurologic disorders such as psychomotor disturbances, dementia, and convulsions (22, 59, 90). For an excellent comparison of clinical indicators of FELV versus FIV infection, the interested reader is referred elsewhere (76).

Pathology
Following infection, virus gains access to cells via chemokine receptors (26). Macrophages represent the primary target of FIV infection (6). Viral replication also occurs in salivary ductal epithelium and local lymph nodes, then disseminates to essentially all lymphoid tissue, resulting in generalized lymphadenopathy (5,

21, 61, 67, 81). Infection results in both humoral and cellular immune responses, which temporarily expands lymphocyte populations and limits progression of disease (2, 14, 17, 38, 39, 40, 75, 89). Both cytolytic and noncytolytic T cells are involved in the control of FIV in asymptomatic cats (25). The humoral response is directed against a variety of T-cell-dependent and independent antigens, including FIV reverse transcriptase (24). FIV also infects $CD4^+$ and $CD8^+$ T lymphocytes. The primary pathophysiologic event in FIV infection is eventual, profound loss of $CD4^+$ T lymphocytes, resulting in an inversion of the CD4/CD8 ratio and loss of immune competence (2). In addition, infected macrophages release neurotoxins, resulting in CNS pathology (44). Prenatal infection results in the most profound thymic lymphocyte depletion (8, 42, 80). Cell death is induced by tumor necrosis factor α (TNFα) and appears to be mediated by activation of the caspase cascade (57). This results in thymic involution (35) and lymphoid atrophy (9). In addition, B-cell lymphomas and myeloproliferative disorders have been associated with FIV infection (27, 69). Associated clinicopathologic changes include lymphopenia, thrombocytopenia, neutropenia, hyperglobulinemia, increased cellularity of bronchoalveolar lavage (BAL) preparations, alterations in coagulation times, and circulating immune complexes (54), resulting in a variety of pathologic effects (32, 34, 83). Additional pathologic changes are most commonly noted in the intestine, brain, lung, gingivae, kidney, skeletal muscle, and eyes; and are most often inflammatory in nature (1, 9, 36, 51, 55, 56, 71, 72). Later, as opportunistic infections begin, the spectrum of pathologic changes broadens considerably, and may involve virtually any organ system. FIV infection persists for the life of the cat (59).

Interference with research

Many body systems are either directly or indirectly affected as a result of FIV or opportunistic infections, respectively. These include the enterohepatic, hematopoietic, lymphoreticular, musculoskeletal, nervous, respiratory, and urinary systems. In addition, opportunistic infections may occur in many of these same organ systems, in addition to the dermal system. Reported direct effects of FIV infection on host physiology include anemia (83), altered hematopoietic function (88), hemostatic disorders (32), induction of apoptosis (64, 91), alteration of cytokine profiles (48, 50, 52, 78), modulation of host cell activation (7, 85, 93), increased cellularity of BAL preparations (34), increased susceptibility and/or altered immune responsiveness to other infectious diseases (47, 76), suppressed blastogenic responsiveness (49), diminution of innate immunity (loss of neutrophil and natural killer cell function) (31, 92), neuronal cytoskeletal changes (41), decreased expression of microtubule-associated protein 2 (MAP-2) and glutamic acid decarboxylase (GAD) in neurons (46), altered glutathione metabolism (66), reduced cell-cell communication (18), central nervous system electrophysiologic alterations (70, 75), and altered behavior (86).

Diagnosis and control

FIV infection may be readily diagnosed by serology, including ELISA, IFA, and Western immunoblotting (11, 33); and recently, by PCR amplification of proviral DNA in peripheral blood mononuclear cells (12). For many years, ELISA has been used as a screening test, and immunoblotting as a confirmatory test (22). However, with the increased use of RT-PCR, that paradigm will likely change. Indeed, PCR is already in use experimentally (79). Caution should be exercised when interpreting serologic titers of kittens, since passively transferred antibody may give false positive results. Lastly, FIV infection may be identified through viral isolation, although this is not routine. A variety of FIV vaccines have been developed. However, this author questions the appropriateness of vaccinating against a pathogen whose presence in a research animal warrants euthanasia. While antiviral therapy is available and, combined with supportive therapies, can relieve the clinical condition, infected cats should be removed from the colony, because FIV represents a significant confounder of research. Research colonies can be maintained FIV free by only purchasing cats from reputable, commercial vendors, and by preventing contact with cats of unknown viral status. FIV is readily inactivated by a variety of common disinfectants, including chlorine bleach, quaternary ammonium compounds, phenolic compounds, and alcohol (22). Interestingly, while FIV is not considered zoonotic (10), cynomolgus macaques (*Macaca fasicularis*) can be infected and develop clinical signs (43). Therefore, it would seem prudent that persons with immune deficiencies utilize personal protective clothing, and adhere to strict standards of personal hygiene when handling FIV-infected cats.

Feline leukemia virus

Agent
Feline leukemia virus (FELV) is a mammalian type C, enveloped, ssRNA, exogenous replication-competent virus of the family *Retroviridae* and genus *Gammaretrovirus*. There are three antigenic types: A, B, and C. These designations are based on differences in envelope antigens (22). In addition, isolates differ in pathogenicity, due to differences in envelope and/or nucleocapsid proteins (25, 29).

Epidemiology
On a worldwide basis, FELV is the most common cause of neoplastic and nonneoplastic disease, and therefore the most common cause of nonaccidental death of cats. Mortality due to FELV has been estimated at 250 per 100,000 cats per year (22). Seroprevalence may be as high as 50% in urban and colony populations (22). Transmission is by contact with virus shed in body secretions, most notably saliva. In utero transmission also occurs (9). Dual infection with FIV is not uncommon. Of further epidemiologic interest is the association between FELV and Feline Sarcoma Virus (FSV), another retrovirus, which causes fibrosarcomas in cats. All strains of FSV lack genes encoding envelope proteins. Therefore, FSV utilizes exclusively envelope proteins encoded by FELV (22).

Clinical signs
Most infections with FELV are self-limiting, since the majority of cats infected with FELV rapidly develop antibodies against feline oncovirus membrane-associated antigen (FOCMA). These cats do not shed virus, or do so only transiently, and do not exhibit clinical signs (18). Experimental corticosteroid administration impairs this early viral containment and therefore enhances susceptibility (31). For similar mechanistic reasons, young cats are more susceptible to infection than are adults (16). Other naturally infected cats either do not develop anti-FOCMA antibodies, or do so only transiently. These cats become persistently viremic, and may eventually develop a variety of disease syndromes, including neoplastic and nonneoplastic conditions (6, 18, 28). Neoplastic conditions include lymphosarcoma and myeloproliferative disease, while nonneoplastic conditions include anemia and immunopathologic disease (22). As a consequence of these conditions, other conditions may develop, most notably opportunistic infections. Given the latter, it would be impossible to delineate the full range of clinical signs one might encounter in cats infected with FELV. Clinical signs directly associated with FELV also vary depending on tissue involvement, and can include poor reproductive performance, including infertility, fetal deaths, and abortion (22), icterus, depression, lethargy, weakness, pallor, weight loss, vomiting, decreased appetite, diarrhea or constipation, fecal blood, ocular opacity, lymph-node enlargement, respiratory distress, exercise intolerance, excessive drinking and urination, geophagia, and neurologic signs (9). Secondary or opportunistic infections with viral, bacterial, mycotic, and parasitic agents add variety to the clinical signs indirectly attributable to FELV infection. Recurrent, unusual, or unresponsive infectious diseases suggest immune suppression, and justify evaluation of

the FELV status of the feline host (28). In those cats destined to develop clinical disease, the induction period, the time from the onset of viremia to the appearance of clinical disease, ranges from 2 to 52 months, with an average of about 2 years (9). Most persistently viremic cats die within 3.5 years (9). For an excellent comparison of clinical indicators of FELV versus FIV infection, the interested reader is referred elsewhere (27).

Pathology

Lymphosarcoma is one of the most important infectious disease of cats, and accounts for roughly a third of all tumors in cats. FELV can be demonstrated in about 65% of those tumors (22). Lymphosarcoma occurs in four forms, including multicentric lymphosarcoma, in which tumors occur in lymphoid and nonlymphoid tissues; thymic lymphosarcoma, usually occurring in kittens; alimentary B-cell lymphosarcoma in intestinal or mesenteric lymphoid tissue of older cats; and unclassified lymphosarcoma, which occurs in a variety of nonlymphoid tissues (22). Other than the alimentary form, lymphosarcomas caused by FELV are of T-cell origin, with virus infecting both $CD4^+$ and $CD8^+$ T cells, in addition to myeloid cells (22). Myeloproliferative disease results from FELV-induced transformation of bone marrow cells. Cell types affected include erythroid (erythromyelosis), granulocytic myeloid (granulocytic leukemia), erythroid and granulocytic myeloid (erythroleukemia), and lastly, fibroblast and cancellous bone cells (myelofibrosis) (15, 22). Resulting myeloproliferation may lead to nonregenerative (aplastic) anemia, pancytopenia, lymphopenia, neutropenia, thrombocytopenia, and immunosuppression (5, 9, 15, 22). FELV-associated myelopathy rarely occurs in cats with neither neoplastic nor hematologic disease (3). Early appearance of virus-specific antibodies and cytotoxic T lymphocytes is associated with immunologic control of infection (12, 14). Cellular immune responses are augmented by involvement of interleukin 12 (IL-12) and IL-18 (13). In contrast, persistent viremia and subsequent immune pathology occur when there is a silencing of virus-specific humoral and cell-mediated host immune effector mechanisms (12). Immunopathologic diseases caused by FELV include both immune complex and immunodeficiency conditions (22). Release of FELV antigens results in immune complex glomerulonephritis. Alternatively, lymphoid depletion occurs due to antibody-mediated destruction of $FOCMA^+$ cells. Loss of immune cells facilitates secondary infection with a variety of microbial pathogens (22).

Interference with research

Natural infection of laboratory cats with FELV may profoundly alter a variety of research efforts. These include studies involving the endocrine, enterohepatic, hematopoietic, lymphoreticular, musculoskeletal, nervous, reproductive, respiratory, and urinary systems. Reported effects on host physiology include anemia and other hematologic abnormalities (2, 5, 15, 30, 33), liver degradation and enteritis (17, 28), neuroendocrine dysfunction (35), suppressed blastogenic responses (4, 23, 36), reduced T-cell cytolytic activity (23), impaired cytokine secretion (11, 24), loss of short-term suppressor cell function (34), neutrophil dysfunction (7, 18), prolonged allograft rejection times (26), reduced complement and antibody levels (22), thymic atrophy (32), lymphocyte depletion (8, 25, 32), and profoundly altered cytokine expression (19, 34). Lastly, in vitro studies also reveal effects of FELV, including increased release of hematopoietic growth factors in fibroblast cultures (1), cytolysis of early erythroid progenitor cells (10), envelope protein-induced neurotoxicity (21), altered cell metabolism, and reduction of growth-inhibitory activity by bone marrow stromal cells (20).

Diagnosis and control

FELV is rarely isolated from tumors, although its presence can be demonstrated by using antigen or genomic detection methods. Antigen detection methods include ELISA and IFA. Molecular techniques include RT-PCR. Vaccination with inactivated whole virus or subunit vaccines will considerably reduce the incidence of clinical disease. This strategy may be used to prevent the development of clinical disease. However, in a laboratory setting, it will likely be more desirable to test and eliminate infected cats from the colony. Multiple tests may be required to correctly determine the infection status of an individual cat. The interested reader is referred elsewhere for an excellent discussion of test and cull strategies (27). All cats purchased from questionable sources should be tested prior to and after arrival. Cats obtained from animal shelters should not be mixed with virus-free cats in the research colony, since the likelihood of infection is high. While FELV is not considered zoonotic, persons with immune deficiencies would be wise to utilize personal protective clothing, and adhere to strict standards of personal hygiene when handling FELV-infected cats.

Feline parvovirus

Agent
Feline parvovirus was the first feline virus associated with disease, and is the causative agent of feline panleukopenia, a highly contagious, acute viral infection of domestic and exotic cats (22). Mink, raccoon, and coatimundi are also susceptible (10). The virus is a small, nonenveloped ssDNA virus. Cats are also susceptible to a closely related canine strain, and transmission of this infection from dogs is possible (21)

Epidemiology
Feline parvovirus occurs globally, with the majority of cats seropositive in some populations (7). Most epidemics occur in the summer months, as maternally transferred immunity wains in large numbers of kittens born in the spring (16). Infected cats, whether symptomatic or not, serve as reservoirs and sources of infection for others. Transmission is primarily from cat to cat, by the oral and respiratory routes, although intrauterine transmission also occurs. Contaminated fomites such as cleaning utensils, fleas, and humans may serve as mechanical vectors (2, 14). Virus is excreted in saliva, vomitus, urine, and feces for variable periods of time depending on many factors, including age at infection, with those infected in utero shedding virus for up to a year (17, 21).

Clinical signs
Clinical signs of infection can be observed in cats of any age, with mortality highest among kittens without maternally transmitted antibodies. Clinical signs appear within 2 to 4 days of infection, and include high fever; anorexia; dehydration; diarrhea that may be watery or hemorrhagic; depression; vomiting; rapid loss of body condition; and frequently, death due to overwhelming bacterial infection and septicemic shock resulting from leukopenia of less than 1,000 leukocytes (WBC)/ml of blood (9, 14, 21). Peracute cases may have subnormal temperatures without diarrhea (21). Subclinical cases also occur, and are the rule rather than the exception in cats infected as adults. Depending on age at infection, intrauterine infection leads to neonatal death, with or without fetal resorption, or CNS signs such as cerebellar ataxia, wide gait, and intention tremor, which become evident at 2 to 3 weeks of age.

Pathology
Following infection, the virus gains entry to cells through binding to the feline transferrin receptor (15). Thereafter, replication occurs in pharyngeal or intestinal lymphoid tissue. Viremia, lasting up to a week, disseminates the virus throughout the body. Viral replication is most evident in highly mitotic cells. Virus may be recovered from the thymus, spleen, mesenteric lymph nodes, cerebellum, and cerebrospinal fluid within 48 h of infection, and thereafter for up to about 2 weeks, after which it is cleared from most tissues. Notable exceptions to viral clearing include persistence of the virus in the kidneys (21), myocardium (12, 21), and possibly peripheral blood mononuclear cells (13) and the CNS (23), although those isolations may have been due to pre-

clinical viremia. In some animals, virus can be shed from the kidneys for several months (21). Gross pathologic findings are most evident in the thymus and intestinal tract, and include thymic atrophy in young cats, and dilated intestinal loops in all cats. Microscopically, one finds lymphocyte depletion and neutrophil infiltration in tissues of the immune system, including thymus, lymph nodes, spleen, Peyer's patches, and bone marrow. These findings are due to preferential replication in highly mitotic cells (14, 21), accelerated rates of apoptosis (1), and possibly direct inhibition of hematopoietic colony formation by myeloid progenitor cells in bone marrow (11). Also, one observes small intestinal epithelial crypt necrosis, with subsequent shortening and denuding of villi, as villus tip cells continue to turn over but are not replaced. Few if any small intestinal lesions are seen in axenic cats, likely due to reduced epithelial cell turnover (10). Inflammatory lesions may also be found in the myocardium (12, 21). Lastly, kittens infected early in life may develop cerebellar hypoplasia, hydrocephalus, and syringomyelia (14, 20). The clinicopathologic hallmarks of infection are leukopenia and thrombocytopenia, although anemia may also develop secondary to intestinal epithelial necrosis. Neutrophilia with a left shift is indicative of recovery (21). Leukopenia can render young cats immune compromised and susceptible to systemic opportunistic infections with enteric bacteria. Cats infected in utero may be born with cerebellar hypoplasia, and have perivascular cuffing, neuronal degeneration, and loss of the granule cell layer in the cerebellum, again due to preferential replication of virus in rapidly dividing cells (14). Immunity involves both cellular and humoral components.

Interference with research

Because of widespread distribution within the body, and preferential replication in highly mitotic cells, feline parvovirus may affect a wide range of scientific studies, including those involving the cardiovascular, enterohepatic, hematopoietic, lymphoreticular, nervous, reproductive, respiratory, and urinary systems. In addition, secondary bacterial infections will render cats at least temporarily unsuitable as research subjects, and of course may kill them outright.

Diagnosis and control

Feline panleukopenia is suggested by clinical signs, and clinicopathologic and histopathologic findings, and is confirmed by virus isolation, immunodiagnosis, or molecular methods, including PCR (8). Suspected cases should be isolated. There are no published reports regarding effective antiviral treatment. Medical care is therefore limited to supportive therapy, which may include prophylactic antibiotics, fluid therapy, "forced" feeding, and leukocyte transfusions. Vaccination of at-risk cats in the face of an outbreak will prevent development of clinical signs (3). Unless precluded by research project needs, all cats should be vaccinated annually, including those housed in barrier facilities, with modified live-virus vaccines. However, care must be taken not to use modified live-virus vaccines in cats infected with feline immunodeficiency virus (4). Also, recent reports suggest that the use of high-titer modified live triple-virus vaccine may predispose kittens to other opportunistic infections (6), or to in utero infection when pregnant queens are vaccinated (19). Disease prevention should include minimizing animal stress. Feline parvovirus is highly resistant to environmental factors. Therefore, many common disinfectants are ineffective for eliminating feline parvovirus from the animal room environment (18), especially when large amounts of organic material are present. However, sodium hypochlorite (1:30 dilution), chlorine dioxide, and potassium peroxymonosulfate are effective after removal of organic material (5).

BACTERIA

Chlamydophila felis

Agent

Chlamydophila felis, formerly known as *Chlamydia psittaci* var. *felis* (11, 16), is an obligate, intracellular, gram-negative coccobacillus. The life cycle alternates between noninfectious proliferative stages and infectious nonproliferative stages (1, 23). Infectious elementary bodies enter cells, where they transform into reticulate bodies that divide, generating more elementary bodies. This cycle requires 30 to 40 h in vitro (1).

Epidemiology
C. felis has a worldwide distribution, and may be common in some cat colonies, since commensal intestinal or latent infections are common. *C. felis* is primarily transmitted by inhalation or ingestion of elementary bodies. Infection may occur in kittens at birth during vaginal passage (5). For this reason, the prevalence of infection is highest in recently weaned cats up to about 9 months of age (5). Infection rates decline somewhat thereafter. Transmission by arthropod vectors has been reported for *Chlamydia trachomatis* (6). It remains to be demonstrated whether this mode may also be used by *C. felis*. At least one anecdotal report suggests that although they have their own strain of organism, cats can also be infected with *Chlamydophila psittaci* from birds (13, 14).

Clinical signs
While *C. felis* may localize to a number of body systems, the respiratory system seems to be the preferred site, resulting in a condition termed feline pneumonitis. Clinical infection is usually asymptomatic. In general, conjunctivitis may be noted within 3 to 10 days of infection, is initially unilateral, then spreads to the other eye and may last for up to about 45 days (5, 9, 11, 24, 29). Kittens may fail to open their eyes normally at 10 to 17 days, and the closed eyes may bulge, with exudate noted at the lid margins (5). Conjunctivitis may be accompanied by transient fever, serous nasal discharge, sneezing, blepharospasm, conjunctival hyperemia, and chemosis, and may become more severe with the involvement of secondary pathogens such as feline calicivirus, feline herpesvirus, streptococci, staphylococci, mycoplasma, *Pasteurella* spp., and *Pseudomonas* spp. (5, 9, 20, 24, 28). These signs are common to a syndrome known as "cat flu," which can be caused by a variety of infectious agents including some of those noted above. Therefore, correct diagnosis of the causative agent(s) is critical. For guidance on differentiating the various infectious causes of cat flu, the interested reader is referred elsewhere (28). Rarely, *C. felis* causes enteritis, which presents as intermittent vomiting and diarrhea; peritonitis (4); or abortion (28, 29).

Pathology
Following attachment, elementary bodies are endocytosed by epithelial cells, where they multiply as reticulate bodies, and survive lysosomal destruction of the host cell, which results in their release (27). Elementary, but not reticulate bodies produce cytotoxic factors, including a soluble hemagglutinin and a cell-bound heat-labile toxin (23). Pathologic changes depend somewhat on location within the host, but have as a common feature a granulomatous reaction. In pulmonary infections, a mild bronchopneumonia may develop and result in consolidation, although in many cases, pathologic lesions are either not found, or are minimal (9). Other pathologic findings may include hepatitis, splenic enlargement, lymph-node hyperplasia, peritonitis, and renal disease (4).

Interference with research
Reports of the influence of *C. felis* on research involving cats are scarce. However, one can glean and judiciously transpose information from reports on the effects of *C. psittaci* in vitro and in other hosts, although even this information is relatively scant. *C. psittaci* has been shown to transiently depress lymphocyte blastogenic responses (12); regulate peritoneal macrophage lysosomal enzyme activities (17); slow, and at high multiplicities of infection, halt host cell division (10); locally elevate immunoglobulin and albumin levels (25); modulate host cell apoptosis at several levels simultaneously (3, 19), alter host cell mor-

phology and metabolism (23), and induce enzymatic and cytokine activities (2), as well as major histocompatibility complex (MHC) molecule expression (18). On the basis of these reports, one can conclude that infection with *C. felis* would interfere with studies involving the enterohepatic, lymphoreticular, reproductive, respiratory, and urinary systems, as well as those where metabolic parameters are measured.

Diagnosis and control
C. felis can not be grown on cell-free media, but can be grown on embryonated chicken eggs and in tissue culture (24). Diagnosis has traditionally been accomplished by recovery of *C. felis* from ocular swabs, or by identification of intracellular inclusions following immunofluorescent or Giemsa staining. Intracytoplasmic inclusions are seen most often in the first 4 to 7 days of clinical signs (5). Molecular techniques such as PCR are becoming incorporated into the diagnostic armamentarium, and because they are quicker and more sensitive, they are to some extent replacing traditional culture and identification methods (8, 15, 26). Serology is not commonly used for definitive diagnosis, since many healthy cats are antibody positive. Infected cats can be treated with broad-spectrum antibiotics, and are particularly responsive to either topical or systemic tetracyclines. However, systemic treatment with doxycycline (5 mg/kg orally [p.o.] twice a day [b.i.d.] for 21 days) is more likely to eliminate the organism (26, 28), and hypersensitivity to ophthalmic preparations has been reported (5). Supportive care, including regular cleaning of nasal and ocular discharges, should be incorporated to improve the comfort of the animal. Some cats remain persistently infected and serve as a source of infection for others. Control of clinical disease is through vaccination and good husbandry practices. However, vaccination will not protect against infection. Without disinfection, elementary bodies may persist in the environment for long periods, although a variety of disinfectants effectively inactivate the organism. Because *C. felis* has zoonotic potential (7, 21, 22, 30), personnel caring for infected cats should protect themselves against infection by practicing good hygiene, and by protecting against inhalation of aerosolized, infectious material.

FUNGI

Dermatomycosis

Agents
More than 40 species of dermatophytes have been reported from humans and animals. Dermatophytes may be considered phylogenetically by genus, including the genera *Epidermophyton, Microsporum,* and *Trichophyton;* or can be grouped by reservoir, whether soil (geophilic), humans (anthropophilic), or animals (zoophilic) (8). Among the dermatophytes infecting cats, *M. canis* is by far the most common, often accounting for more than 90% of cases in surveys. Less common species include *Trichophyton mentagrophytes, Microsporum persicolor,* and others (3, 8, 14).

Epidemiology
Cats are the natural reservoir of *M. canis*. Most of the remaining species of dermatophytes found on cats have other animals such as rodents, as reservoir hosts; or are geophilic. Dermatomycosis is common among the general cat population, and so occurs with some regularity among the laboratory cat population as well. Infection rates are highest in warm, humid areas. These same conditions may promote infection in laboratory colonies when temperature and humidity are poorly controlled. Cats less than one year of age, those with concurrent FIV infection, and those with long hair, are predisposed to infection (7, 8, 14). Most dermatophytes infect the stratum corneum and the hairs, where they produce a sheath of arthrospores around the latter. These arthrospores represent the infectious stage, and are transmitted to a susceptible host through direct contact or by fomites, such as brushes, cat toys, and other husbandry items. In addi-

tion, animal care staff may serve as a source of infection for cats (13, 17). Because the arthrospores may survive up to 18 months in the environment, infected skin detritus may also transmit infection (8).

Clinical signs
Many cats harboring dermatophytes never develop clinical signs, and so are asymptomatic carriers (12, 13). When present, signs of dermatomycosis may vary depending on fungal species and immunologic state of the host. In general, signs develop within 3 weeks of infection, and most often consist of discrete, often round areas of hair loss.

Pathology
Hair infected with dermatophytes is quite fragile, and so is easily pulled out, exposing an area of crusty, scaly, thickened, erythematous skin. New hair growth begins in the center of the alopecic area. Some infections clear spontaneously, while others become chronic, lasting for months or even years. Infection rarely becomes generalized, and involves large portions of the skin and pelage. In one report, a Persian cat developed mycetoma-like granulomas at the site of dermatomycosis (18). Immunity involves both innate and acquired components, including neutrophils, macrophages, lymphocytes, and fungal species-specific immunoglobulin G (IgG) antibodies (4, 6, 15, 16).

Interference with research
Few reports exist of dermatophyte infection interfering with research involving cats. In humans, dermatophyte infection increases the number but not the kinds of microbial flora isolated from lesioned areas (2). A peptide extract from *T. mentagrophytes* inhibits guinea pig macrophage migration in vitro (1). Similarly, an antigen preparation of *T. rubrum* has been shown to inhibit human lymphocyte proliferation (9). Clearly, clinical dermatomycosis could interfere with research involving the dermal and lymphoreticular systems, and may interfere with other studies in which normal skin flora is essential.

Diagnosis and control
Signs of dermatomycosis are nonspecific, and so must be differentiated from signs caused by other pathogens or conditions. Diagnosis is by direct microscopic examination of plucked hairs; fungal culture on dermatophyte test media; or examination under ultraviolet light, although only some isolates of *M. canis,* and none of the other species of dermatophytes, fluoresce. Ideally, all three methods should be used. Among them, culture is the least reliable when used alone (14). While many infections are self-limiting, infected cats should be separated from uninfected cats and treated to speed resolution of the infection, reduce environmental contamination, and minimize the risk of zoonotic transmission. A number of products are available for treating feline dermatomycosis. These include topical and systemic treatments. Topical treatments may speed resolution but are unable to penetrate to the infected hair, and so should be combined with systemic treatment. One commonly used systemic treatment is griseofulvin. However, this compound can be toxic in pregnant cats and humans, and is slightly less effective than itraconazole or terbinafine at eliminating the infection (5, 8, 11). In one study, complete resolution of infection required 56 days with itraconazole but 70 days with griseofulvin (11). Cats, especially those with long hair, should be clipped 2 to 4 weeks after beginning systemic therapy to remove infectious hair that may otherwise serve as a lingering source of infection for other cats (8). Uninfected cats should ideally be treated prophylactically with systemic therapy, or at the least, with antifungal shampoos or dips. Two negative brush cultures, 4 weeks apart, should be obtained prior to discontinuing therapy (8, 10). Cats with generalized disease should be culled from the colony. The animal facility should be thoroughly cleaned with dilute (0.5 to 5%) bleach to reduce the fungal load in the environment (8, 10). Persons working with

infected cats should know that many dermatophytes are zoonotic. Therefore, appropriate personal protective equipment should be used. At a minimum this should include gloves and a laboratory coat.

PARASITES

Fleas

Agents
The flea most commonly found infesting cats is the cat flea, *Ctenocephalides felis*. Rarely, fleas of other hosts, such as the "Sticktight" flea of poultry, *Echidnophaga gallinacea,* may infest cats, since fleas tend not to be nearly as host specific as many other parasites. However, these more unusual flea species are unlikely to be encountered in the laboratory animal environment.

Epidemiology
Flea infestation may be common in animal facilities when caretakers own cats, when unconditioned cats are brought into the facility, or when structural deficiencies allow entry of vermin such as wild rodents. Adult female fleas deposit eggs on the host. Eggs drop into the primary enclosure and hatch as larvae. Larvae feed on adult flea feces, and molt twice before pupating. An adult flea emerges from the cocoon upon perception of temperature and humidity cues given off by nearby hosts. Cocoons may remain viable in the environment for several months under conditions of low temperature (5). Adult fleas suck blood from the host. Most of this blood passes through the flea digestive tract and is deposited as feces or "flea dirt". The entire life cycle may be completed in about 2 weeks under ideal conditions (2, 5). In addition to directly causing disease, *C. felis* serves as an intermediate host for *Dipylidium caninum*, a tapeworm capable of infecting cats, and may vector blood-borne pathogens such as *Haemobartonella felis, Bartonella henselae, Rickettsia felis,* and others (9, 10, 15).

Clinical signs
Flea infestation is often more severe in immunologically compromised cats, such as aged cats, or in otherwise debilitated animals. Clinical signs consist of those associated with pruritus, and those associated with blood-loss anemia. Infested cats are restless, and scratch and groom excessively. This may result in loss of condition, reduced feed intake, weight and hair loss, trichobezoars ("hairballs"), and skin irritation to the point of self-excoriation (1, 10). Alopecia is usually symmetrical, and is more often noted in the dorsal, more distal regions of the trunk (12). Anemic cats may become lethargic and pale, and may show signs of congestive heart failure (10, 16).

Pathology
Dermatitis due to scratching may result in secondary bacterial infections. In addition, immediate, and later delayed hypersensitivity reactions occur at the site of entry of various biologically active salivary substances, such as diphosphohydrolases (3, 4), esterases (4), and antigens (8, 11). The latter bind to collagen in the skin. These hypersensitivity reactions result in local release of vasoactive substances from mast cells, and numerous small papules ("miliary dermatitis") consisting of localized tissue eosinophilia, epidermal spongiosis, crusting, and ulceration (6, 14). The severity of immune responsiveness and hypersensitivity are genetically based and therefore vary among animals. Other pathologic findings occasionally associated with flea infestation may include cardiomegaly (16) and trichobezoars (1).

Interference with research
This author is aware of no reports concerning alterations in host physiology that directly affected research. However, because flea infestation has been documented to directly or indirectly alter cytoarchitecture and/or function of the cardiovascular, dermal, hematopoietic, and lymphoreticular systems, studies involving these organ systems would likely be affected in research using flea-infested cats. In addition, studies in which behavioral or met-

abolic parameters are measured would also be affected. For these reasons, fleas should be excluded or eradicated from the research colony. Lastly, flea control is an important component of the institution's occupational health and safety program. Not only is the *C. felis* zoonotic and a nuisance, but some humans with asthma react to flea allergens.

Diagnosis and control

Flea infestation is suspected when cats are seen scratching and grooming excessively. Suspected flea dirt may be placed on a piece of white paper and a small amount of water applied. Flea feces will run red, since it consists mainly of host blood. Finding adult fleas on a cat may require diligence, since few fleas are required to elicit considerable scratching. It may be useful to determine the species of fleas infesting the colony cats, as a means of identifying the source. Many standard veterinary texts contain keys to the common flea species. Of course a diagnosis of *D. caninum* infection indicates flea infestation. Serologic or immunologically based skin tests may be useful adjuncts in establishing a diagnosis, but they are rarely definitive (10, 13). A number of newer and safer ectoparasiticides are available for eliminating fleas from the colony (2). It is essential to treat all cats simultaneously, whether symptomatic or not, and to disinfect the environment at the same time. Apparent treatment failures are common, and are often due to the failure to adequately treat all places, on and off all hosts present, where flea life-cycle stages may be found (5). It is especially important to clean cracks and crevices in the environment, and to clean or destroy bedding. Severely affected cats may require supportive therapy such as blood transfusions, supplemental iron therapy, and dietary supplementation including essential fatty acids, in addition to elimination of the fleas (7, 10). Prevention of flea infestation involves testing or treatment of all cats prior to entry into the facility, purchase of cats from reputable vendors, and education of caretaker and scientific staff concerning the risks of transmitting fleas from pet cats to research colony cats.

Intestinal nematodes

Agents

Laboratory cats may be infected with a number of intestinal nematodes. Most commonly, these include the "hookworms" *Ancylostoma braziliense, Ancylostoma tubaeforme,* and *Uncinaria stenocephala;* and the ascarids, or "roundworms" *Toxocara cati* and *Toxascaris leonina.* Cats may also be infected with the dog ascarid, *Toxocara canis,* although that aberrant infection will not be discussed further. For this discussion these parasites will be considered as a group, although important features particular to specific worms will be mentioned. Adult worms are readily identified using morphologic features described in standard veterinary parasitology reference texts (2). All hookworms have a large buccal cavity bearing "teeth" or cutting plates, while ascarids have three "lips," and lateral alae, or wing-like structures near their anterior end. Eggs from most are also readily identifiable, although for the hookworms, an ocular micrometer is of great value because, although the hookworm eggs appear somewhat similar, they differ in size. It is important to properly speciate these nematodes because of differences in pathogenicity and transmission strategies.

Epidemiology

Infection with hookworms occurs by ingestion or skin penetration of infective larvae. Larvae migrate extensively during development until arriving at the small intestine where they mature to the adult stage. Transmission may also occur by consumption of paratenic hosts; and during nursing of kittens, when inhibited larvae mobilize from mammary tissue and are passed in the milk. However, the latter has only been demonstrated for *Ancylostoma* spp., and is of questionable clinical significance. Developing larvae undergo a pulmonary migration before developing to adulthood in the small intestine. Infection with ascarids occurs by ingestion of infectious, embryonated eggs; by ingestion of paratenic hosts, including cockroaches, or their feces; and for *T. cati,* by transmammary transmission (2, 4, 8). *T. cati,* but not *T. leonina,* migrates through the liver and lungs, and eventually matures to adulthood in the small intestine. The intestinal nematodes discussed here are all prolific egg layers. Therefore, large numbers of infective stages can build up in the animal facility if appropriate sanitation is not practiced. In addition, ascarid eggs remain viable for up to several years. Kittens are more commonly found infected with intestinal nematodes. Intact animals of both sexes are more often parasitized than are their neutered counterparts (9).

Clinical signs

Clinical signs are seen when large numbers of parasites are present, although some species may cause clinical disease with fewer worms. Among the hookworms, *U. stenocephala* is least significant since it causes less pathology and consumes less blood; whereas among the ascarids, *T. leonina* is less pathogenic than *T. cati,* primarily because of the lack of extraintestinal migration. Clinical signs may include poor growth, weight loss, diarrhea, dehydration, vomiting, rough hair coat, a "pot-bellied" appearance, and pale mucous membranes.

Pathology

Pathologic changes are due to either direct intestinal damage, including focal enteritis and blood consumption by the adult worms; or to tissue damage during larval migration. Extraintestinal visceral lesions may include peritonitis, hepatic necrosis (*T. cati*), glomerular shrinking and periglomerular fibrosis due to glomerular ischemia (*T. cati*), and pulmonary arterial hypertrophy (*T. cati*) (2, 5, 6). Immunity is primarily humoral and reagenic, and once attained, may result in peracute expulsion of a large percentage of infecting worms. This is particularly the case for ascarid infections, where immunity is attained by about 6 months of age. Hookworm infections are more often retained into adulthood.

Interference with research

There is an enormous volume of literature on the physiologic effects of intestinal nematode infections in various host species, most prominently, swine, rodents, and humans. Considerably less information is available that deals specifically with feline nematodiases. Depending on the specific parasite involved, feline nematode infection may result in anemia, enteritis, eosinophilia, alterations in serum chemistries, pneumonitis, pulmonary vascular changes, histamine release, and dermatitis (2, 5, 7, 10). Effects reported in other intestinal host-parasite systems should be applied to the cat with caution. Considering the documented effects of intestinal nematode infections on the physiology of the laboratory cat, it is not necessary to describe the full range of physiologic effects reported from other host-nematode systems, although the interested reader is referred elsewhere for that information (1, 3). Clearly, infection with the intestinal nematodes discussed could alter research involving the cardiovascular, dermal, enterohepatic, hematopoietic, respiratory, and urinary systems; and influence studies measuring behavior, weight gain, and other aspects of host metabolic activity.

Diagnosis and control

Diagnosis is suspected on the basis of clinical and clinicopathologic indicators. Definitive diagnosis is based on identification of eggs in fecal examinations, or on recovery of adult worms at necropsy. Hookworm infections can be treated with a number of compounds, including dichlorvos (11.1 mg/kg), febantel (10 to 15 mg/kg), and others (2). *Uncinaria* spp. are more refractory to treatment than are *Ancylostoma* spp. (2). These treatments and others are also effective at removing adult ascarid infections (2). Few data are available on preventing transmammary transmission by

TABLE 8-1. Body systems known or likely to be affected by pathogen indicated

Pathogen	Cardio-vascular	Dermal	Endocrine	Entero-hepatic	Hema-topoietic	Lympho-reticular	Musculo-skeletal	Nervous	Reproductive	Respiratory	Urinary
Feline calicivirus		X					X			X X	X
Feline coronavirus	X			X	X X	X X		X X	X X	X	X
Feline herpesvirus type 1		X		X	X		X	X	X	X	
Feline immunodeficiency virus			X	X		X		X	X		
Feline leukemia virus	X			X	X	X	X	X	X	X	X
Feline parvovirus	X			X X		X X X X	X	X	X X	X	X X
Chlamydophila felis		X X								X	
Dermatomycosis		X									
Fleas	X X	X			X X						
Intestinal nematodes	X			X						X	X

carefully scheduled anthelmintic administration. Control is based on screening and/or treatment of cats prior to admission into the animal facility. Once the animal facility is contaminated with eggs, especially ascarid eggs, they can be extremely difficult to eliminate. Cleaning protocols should also prevent the entry of potentially infected paratenic hosts such as cockroaches. Because most of these nematodes will infect humans, at least long enough to allow for some somatic migration of larvae, personnel working with infected cats should be careful to protect themselves from accidental infection, through the wearing of proper personal protective clothing, and the washing of hands following work in the animal facility.

REFERENCES

VIRUSES

Feline calicivirus

1. Bennett, D., R. M. Gaskell, A. Mills, J. Knowles, S. Carter, and F. McArdle. 1989. Detection of feline calicivirus antigens in the joints of infected cats. *Vet. Rec.* **124**:329–332.
2. Binns, S. H., S. Dawson, A. J. Speakman, L. E. Cuevas, C. A. Hart, C. J. Gaskell, K. L. Morgan, and R. M. Gaskell. 2000. A study of feline upper respiratory tract disease with reference to prevalence and risk factors for infection with feline calicivirus and feline herpesvirus. *J. Feline Med. Surg.* **2**:123–133.
3. Burki, F., B. Starustka, and O. Ruttner. 1976. Attempts to serologically classify feline caliciviruses on a national and an international basis. *Infect. Immun.* **14**:876–881.
4. Dawson, S., D. Bennett, S. D. Carter, M. Bennett, J. Meanger, P. C. Turner, M. J. Carter, I. Milton, and R. M. Gaskell. 1994. Acute arthritis of cats associated with feline calicivirus infection. *Res. Vet. Sci.* **56**:133–143.
5. Dawson, S., K. Willoughby, R. M. Gaskell, G. Wood, and W. S. Chalmers. 2001. A field trial to assess the effect of vaccination against feline herpesvirus, feline calicivirus and feline panleucopenia virus in 6-week-old kittens. *J. Feline Med. Surg.* **3**:17–22.
6. Dick, C. P., R. P. Johnson, and S. Yamashiro. 1989. Sites of persistence of feline calicivirus. *Res. Vet. Sci.* **47**:367–373.
7. Eleraky, N. Z., L. N. Potgeiter, and M. A. Kennedy. 2002. Virucidal efficacy of four new

disinfectants. *J. Am. Anim. Hosp. Assoc.* **38**:231–234.
8. Ellis, T. M. 1981. Jaundice in a Siamese cat with in utero feline calicivirus infection. *Aust. Vet. J.* **57**:383–385.
9. Geissler, K., K. Schneider, G. Platzer, B. Truyen, O. R. Kaaden, and U. Truyen. 1997. Genetic and antigenic heterogeneity among feline calicivirus isolates from distinct disease manifestations. *Virus Res.* **48**:193–206.
10. Kennedy, M. A., V. S. Mellon, G. Caldwell, and L. N. Potgieter. 1995. Virucidal efficacy of the newer quaternary ammonium compounds. *J. Am. Anim. Hosp. Assoc.* **31**:254–258.
11. Knowles, J. O., F. McArdle, S. Dawson, S. D. Carter, C. J. Gaskell, and R. M. Gaskell. 1991. Studies on the role of feline calicivirus in chronic stomatitis in cats. *Vet. Microbiol.* **27**:205–219.
12. Kreutz, L. C., R. P. Johnson, and B. S. Seal. 1998. Phenotypic and genotypic variation of feline calicivirus during persistent infection of cats. *Vet. Microbiol.* **59**:229–236.
13. Langloss, J. M., E. A. Hoover, and D. E. Kahn. 1978. Ultrastructural morphogenesis of acute viral pneumonia produced by feline calicivirus. *Am. J. Vet. Res.* **39**:1577–1583.
14. Langloss, J. M., E. A. Hoover, D. E. Kahn, and A. J. Kniazeff. 1979. Elaboration of chemotactic substances by alveolar cells: possible mechanism for the initial neutrophilic response in feline caliciviral pneumonia. *Am. J. Vet. Res.* **40**:186–189.
15. Lauritzen, A., O. Jarrett, and M. Sabara. 1997. Serological analysis of feline calicivirus isolates from the United States and United Kingdom. *Vet. Microbiol.* **56**:55–63.
16. McCabe, V. J., I. Tarpey, and N. Spibey. 2002. Vaccination of cats with an attenuated recombinant myxoma virus expressing feline calicivirus capsid protein. *Vaccine* **20**:2454–2462.
17. Mochizuki, M., K. Kawakami, M. Hashimoto, and T. Ishida. 2000. Recent epidemiological status of feline upper respiratory infections in Japan. *J. Vet. Med. Sci.* **62**:801–803.
18. Nuanualsuwan, S., and D. O. Cliver. 2002. Pretreatment to avoid positive RT-PCR results with inactivated viruses. *J. Virol. Methods* **104**:217–225.
19. Nuanualsuwan, S., T. Mariam, S. Himathongkham, and D.-O. Cliver. 2002. Ultraviolet inactivation of feline calicivirus, human enteric viruses and coliphages. *Photochem. Photobiol.* **76**:406–410.
20. Ormerod, E., I.-A. McCandlish, and O. Jarrett. 1979. Diseases produced by feline caliciviruses when administered to cats by aerosol or intranasal instillation. *Vet. Rec.* **104**:65–69.
21. Pedersen, N. C., J. B. Elliot, A. Glasgow, A. Poland, and K. Keel. 2000. An isolated epizootic of hemorrhagic-like fever in cats caused by a novel and highly virulent strain of feline calicivirus. *Vet. Microbiol.* **73**:281–300.
22. Poulet, H., S. Brunet, M. Soulier, V. Leroy, S. Goutebroze, and G. Chappuis. 2000. Comparison between acute oral/respiratory and chronic stomatitis/gingivitis isolates of feline calicivirus: pathogenicity, antigenic profile and cross-neutralisation studies. *Arch. Virol.* **145**:243–261.
23. Povey, C., and J. Ingersoll. 1975. Cross-protection among feline caliciviruses. *Infect. Immun.* **11**:877–885.
24. Radford, A. D., S. Dawson, C. Wharmby, R. Ryvar, and R. M. Gaskell. 2000. Comparison of serological and sequence-based methods for typing feline calicivirus isolates from vaccine failures. *Vet. Rec.* **146**:117–123.
25. Radford, A. D., L. Sommerville, R. Ryvar, M. B. Cox, D. R. Johnson, S. Dawson, and R. M. Gaskell. 2001. Endemic infection of a cat colony with a feline calicivirus closely related to an isolate used in live attenuated vaccines. *Vaccine* **19**:4358–4362.
26. Ramsey, C. T. 2000. Feline chlamydia and calicivirus infections. *Vet. Clin. North Am. Small Anim. Pract.* **30**:1015–1028.
27. Reubel, G. H., J. W. George, J. Higgins, and N. C. Pedersen. 1994. Effect of chronic feline immunodeficiency virus infection on experimental feline calicivirus-induced disease. *Vet. Microbiol.* **39**:335–351.
28. Reubel, G. H., D. E. Hoffman, and N. C. Pedersen. 1992. Acute and chronic faucitis of domestic cats. A feline calicivirus-induced disease. *Vet. Clin. North Am. Small Anim. Pract.* **22**:1347–1360.
29. Scott, F. W. 1980. Virucidal disinfectants and feline viruses. *Am. J. Vet. Res.* **41**:410–414.
30. Sykes, J. E., J.–E. Allen, V.–P. Studdert, and G.–F. Browning. 2001. Detection of feline calicivirus, feline herpesvirus 1 and *Chlamydia psittaci* mucosal swabs by multiplex RT-PCR/PCR. *Vet. Microbiol.* **81**:95–108.
31. Tenorio, A. P., C. E. Franti, B. R. Madewell, and N. C. Pedersen. 1991. Chronic oral infections of cats and their relationship to persistent oral carriage of feline calici-, immunodeficiency, or leukemia viruses. *Vet. Immunol. Immunopathol.* **29**:1–14.
32. TerWee, J., A. Y. Lauritzen, M. Sabara, K. J. Dreier, and K. Kokjohn. 1997. Comparison of the primary signs induced by experi-

mental exposure to either a pneumotrophic or a 'limping' strain of feline calicivirus. *Vet. Microbiol.* **56:**33–45.

33. **van Vuuren, M., K. Geissler, D. Gerber, J. O. Nothling, and U. Truyen.** 1999. Characterization of a potentially abortigenic strain of feline calicivirus isolated from a domestic cat. *Vet. Rec.* **144:**636–638.
34. **Wardley, R. C.** 1976. Feline calicivirus carrier state. A study of the host/virus relationship. *Arch. Virol.* **52:**243–249.
35. **Wardley, R. C., and R. C. Povey.** 1977. The pathology and sites of persistance with three different strains of feline calicivirus. *Res. Vet. Sci.* **23:**15–19.
36. **Zee, Y. C.** 1999. Caliciviridae, p. 379–384. *In* D. C. Hirsh and Y. C. Zee (ed.), *Veterinary Microbiology.* Blackwell Science, Inc., Malden, Mass.

Feline coronavirus

1. **Addie, D. D., and O. Jarrett.** 2001. Use of a reverse-transcriptase polymerase chain reaction for monitoring the shedding of feline coronavirus by healthy cats. *Vet. Rec.* **148:**649–653.
2. **Evermann, J. F., A. J. McKeirnan, and R. L. Ott.** 1991. Perspectives on the epizootiology of feline enteric coronavirus and the pathogenesis of feline infectious peritonitis. *Vet. Microbiol.* **28:**243–255.
3. **Fiscus, S. A., and Y. A. Teramoto.** 1987. Antigenic comparison of feline coronavirus isolates: evidence for markedly different peplomer glycoproteins. *J. Virol.* **61:**2607–2613.
4. **Foley, J. E., A. Poland, J. Carlson, and N. C. Pedersen.** 1997. Patterns of feline coronavirus and fecal shedding from cats in multiple-cat environments. *J. Am. Vet. Med. Assoc.* **210:**1307–1312.
5. **Foley, J. E., A. Poland, J. Carlson, and N. C. Pedersen.** 1997. Risk factors for feline infectious peritonitis among cats in multiple-cat environments with endemic feline enteric coronavirus. *J. Am. Vet. Med. Assoc.* **210:**1313–1318.
6. **Gunn-Moore, D. A., T. J. Gruffydd-Jones, and D. A. Harbour.** 1998. Detection of feline coronaviruses by culture and reverse transcriptase-polymerase chain reaction of blood samples from healthy cats and cats with clinical feline infectious peritonitis. *Vet. Microbiol.* **62:**193–205.
7. **Harpold, L. M., A. M. Legendre, M. A. Kennedy, P. J. Plummer, K. Millsaps, and B. Rohrbach.** 1999. Fecal shedding of feline coronavirus in adult cats and kittens in an Abyssinian cattery. *J. Am. Vet. Med. Assoc.* **215:**948–951.
8. **Kipar, A., S. Bellmann, J. Kremendahl, K. Kohler, and M. Reinacher.** 1998. Cellular composition, coronavirus antigen expression and production of specific antibodies in lesions in feline infectious peritonitis. *Vet. Immunol. Immunopathol.* **65:**243–257.
9. **Kipar, A., J. Kremendahl, D. D. Addie, W. Leukert, C. K. Grant, and M. Reinacher.** 1998. Fatal enteritis associated with coronavirus infection in cats. *J. Comp. Pathol.* **119:**1–14.
10. **Kiss, I., S. Kecskemeti, J. Tanyi, B. Klingeborn, and S. Belak.** 2000. Preliminary studies on feline coronavirus distribution in naturally and experimentally infected cats. *Res. Vet. Sci.* **68:**237–242.
11. **Mochizuki, M., N. Osawa, and T. Ishida.** 1999. Feline coronavirus participation in diarrhea of cats. *J. Vet. Med. Sci.* **61:**1071–1073.
12. **Pedersen, N. C., J. F. Boyle, K. Floyd, A. Fudge, and J. Barker.** 1981. An enteric coronavirus infection in cats and relationship to feline infectious peritonitis. *Am. J. Vet. Res.* **42:**368–377.
13. **Savary, K. C., R. K. Sellon, and J. M. Law.** 2001. Chylous abdominal effusion in a cat with feline infectious peritonitis. *J. Am. Anim. Hosp. Assoc.* **37:**35–40.
14. **Stoddart, C. A., and F. W. Scott.** 1989. Intrinsic resistance of feline peritoneal macrophages to coronavirus infection correlates with in vivo virulence. *J. Virol.* **63:**436–440.
15. **Stott, J. L.** 1999. Coronaviridae, p. 418–429. *In* D. C. Hirsh and Y. C. Zee (ed.), *Veterinary Microbiology.* Blackwell Science, Inc., Malden, Mass.

Feline herpesvirus type 1

1. **Andrews, S. E.** 2001. Ocular manifestations of feline herpesvirus. *J. Feline Med. Surg.* **3:**9–16.
2. **Ardans, A. A.** 1999. Herpesviridae, p. 350–364. *In* D. C. Hirsh and Y. C. Zee (ed.), *Veterinary Microbiology.* Blackwell Science, Inc., Malden, Mass.
3. **Burgesser, K. M., S. Hotaling, A. Schiebel, S. E. Ashbaugh, S. M. Roberts, and J. K. Collins.** 1999. Comparison of PCR, virus isolation, and indirect fluorescent antibody staining in the detection of naturally occurring feline herpesvirus infections. *J. Vet. Diagn. Investig.* **11:**122–126.
4. **Dawson, S., K. Willoughby, R. M. Gaskell, G. Wood, and W. S. Chalmers.** 2001. A field trial to assess the effect of vaccination against feline herpesvirus, feline calicivirus and feline panleucopenia virus in 6-week-old kittens. *J. Feline Med. Surg.* **3:**17–22.
5. **Gaskell, R. M., and R. C. Povey.** 1977. Experimental induction of feline viral rhinotracheitis virus re-excretion in FVR-recovered cats. *Vet. Rec.* **100:**128–133.

6. **Hargis, A. M., and P. E. Ginn.** 1999. Feline herpesvirus 1-associated facial and nasal dermatitis and stomatitis in domestic cats. *Vet. Clin. North Am. Small Anim. Pract.* **29:**1281–1290.

7. **Hickman, M. A., G. H. Reubel, D. E. Hoffman, J. G. Morris, Q. R. Rogers, and N. C. Pedersen.** 1994. An epizootic of feline herpesvirus, type 1 in a large specific pathogen-free cat colony and attempts to eradicate the infection by identification and culling of carriers. *Lab. Anim.* **28:**320–329.

8. **Horimoto, T., J. A. Limcumpao, X. Xuan, M. Ono, K. Maeda, Y. Kawaguchi, C. Kai, E. Takahashi, and T. Mikami.** 1992. Heterogeneity of feline herpesvirus type 1 strains. *Arch. Virol.* **126:**283–292.

9. **Kawaguchi, Y., and T. Mikami.** 1995. Molecular interactions between retroviruses and herpesviruses. *J. Vet. Med. Sci.* **57:**801–811.

10. **Kennedy, M. A., V. S. Mellon, G. Caldwell, and L. N. Potgieter.** 1995. Virucidal efficacy of the newer quaternary ammonium compounds. *J. Am. Anim. Hosp. Assoc.* **31:**254–258.

11. **Killingsworth, C. R., N. E. Robinson, T. Adams, R. K. Maes, C. Berney, and E. Rozanski.** 1990. Cholinergic reactivity of tracheal smooth muscle after infection with feline herpesvirus 1. *J. Appl. Physiol.* **69:**1953–1960.

12. **Maeda, K., N. Yokoyama, K. Fujita, M. Maejima, and T. Mikami.** 1997. Heparin-binding activity of feline herpesvirus type 1 glycoprotein. *Virus Res.* **52:**169–176.

13. **Maggs, D. J., M. R. Lappin, and M. P. Nasisse.** 1999. Detection of feline herpesvirus-specific antibodies and DNA in aqueous humor from cats with or without uveitis. *Am. J. Vet. Res.* **60:**932–936.

14. **Maggs, D. L., M. R. Lappin, J. S. Reif, J. K. Collins, J. Carman, D. A. Dawson, and C. Bruns.** 1999. Evaluation of serologic and viral detection methods for diagnosing feline herpesvirus.1. Infection in cats with acute respiratory tract or chronic ocular disease. *J. Am. Vet. Med. Assoc.* **214:**502–507.

15. **Mochizuki, M., K. Kawakami, M. Hashimoto, and T. Ishida.** 2000. Recent epidemiological status of feline upper respiratory infections in Japan. *J. Vet. Med. Sci.* **62:**801–803.

16. **Murphy, F. A., E. P. J. Gibbs, M. C. Horzinek, and M. J. Studdert.** 1999. *Veterinary Virology,* 3rd ed. Academic Press, Inc., San Diego, Calif.

17. **Nasisse, M. P.** 1990. Feline herpesvirus ocular disease. *Vet. Clin. North Am. Small Anim. Pract.* **20:**667–680.

18. **Nasisse, M. P., B. J. Davis, J. S. Guy, M. G. Davidson, and W. Sussman.** 1992. Isolation of feline herpesvirus 1 from the trigeminal ganglia of acutely and chronically infected cats. *J. Vet. Intern. Med.* **6:**102–103.

19. **Nasisse, M. P., J. S. Guy, J. B. Stevens, R. V. English, and M. G. Davidson.** 1993. Clinical and laboratory findings in chronic conjunctivitis in cats: 91 cases (1983–1991). *J. Am. Vet. Med. Assoc.* **203:**834–837.

20. **Ohmura, Y., E. Ono, T. Matsuura, H. Kida, and Y. Shimizu.** 1993. Detection of feline herpesvirus 1 transcripts in trigeminal ganglia of latently infected cats. *Arch. Virol.* **129:**341–347.

21. **Reubel, G. H., J. W. George, J. E. Barlough, J. Higgins, C. K. Grant, and N. C. Pedersen.** 1992. Interaction of acute feline herpesvirus-1 and chronic feline immunodeficiency virus infections in experimentally infected specific pathogen free cats. *Vet. Immunol. Immunopathol.* **35:**95–119.

22. **Satoh, Y., K. Iizuka, M. Fukuyama, S. Kishikawa, Y. Nishino, T. Ikeda, A. Kiuchi, M. Hara, and K. Tabuchi.** 1999. An enzyme-linked immunosorbent assay using nuclear antigen for detection of feline herpesvirus 1 antibody. *J. Vet. Diagn. Investig.* **11:**334–340.

23. **Smith, K. C.** 1997. Herpesviral abortion in domestic animals. *Vet. J.* **153:**253–268.

24. **Stiles, J.** 2000. Feline herpesvirus. *Vet. Clin. North Am. Small Anim. Pract.* **30(5):**1001–1014.

25. **Stiles, J., M. McDermott, D. Bigsby, M. Willis, C. Martin, W. Roberts, and C. Greene.** 1997. Use of nested polymerase chain reaction to identify feline herpesvirus in ocular tissue from clinically normal cats and cats with corneal sequestra or conjunctivitis. *Am. J. Vet. Res.* **58:**338–342.

26. **Sykes, J. E., G. A. Anderson, V. P. Studdert, and G. F. Browning.** 1999. Prevalence of feline *Chlamydia psittaci* and feline herpesvirus 1 in cats with upper respiratory tract disease. *J. Vet. Intern. Med.* **13:**153–162.

27. **Tham, K. M., and M. J. Studdert.** 1987. Clinical and immunological responses of cats to feline herpesvirus type 1 infection. *Vet. Rec.* **120:**321–326.

28. **Vogtlin, A., C. Fraefel, S. Albini, C. M. Leutenegger, E. Schraner, B. Spiess, H. Lutz, and M. Ackerman.** 2002. Quantification of feline herpesvirus 1 DNA in ocular fluid samples of clinically diseased cats by real-time TaqMan PCR. *J. Clin. Microbiol.* **40:**519–523.

29. **Weigler, B. J., C. A. Babineau, B. Sherry, and M. P. Nasisse.** 1997. High sensitivity polymerase chain reaction assay for active and latent feline herpesvirus. 1. Infections in domestic cats. *Vet. Rec.* **140:**335–338.

30. **Willoughby, K., and S. Dawson.** 2001. The respiratory tract, p. 89–115. *In* I. Ramsey and B.

Tennant (ed.), *Manual of Canine and Feline Infectious Diseases*. British Small Animal Veterinary Association, Gloucester, England.
31. Yagami, K., S. Ando, Y. Omata, T. Furukawa, and M. Fukui. 1982. Studies on viral respiratory disease in laboratory cats. I. Isolation of feline herpesvirus and choice of proper disinfectant. *Jikken Dobutsu* **31:**27–35.

Feline immunodeficiency virus
1. Abramo, F., S. Bo, M. G. Canese, and A. Poli. 1995. Regional distribution of lesions in the central nervous system of cats infected with feline immunodeficiency virus. *AIDS Res. Hum. Retrovir.* **11:**1247–1253.
2. Ackley, C. D., J. K. Yamamoto, N. Levy, N. C. Pedersen, and M. D. Cooper. 1990. Immunologic abnormalities in pathogen-free cats experimentally infected with feline immunodeficiency virus. *J. Virol.* **64:**5652–5655.
3. Baneth, G., I. Aroch, N. Tal, and S. Harrus. 1998. *Hepatozoon* species infection in domestic cats: a retrospective study. *Vet. Parasitol.* **79:**123–133.
4. Barrs, V. R., P. Martin, R. G. Nicoll, J. A. Beatty, and R. Malik. 2000. Pulmonary cryptococcosis and *Capillaria aerophila* infection in an FIV-positive cat. *Aust. Vet. J.* **78:**154–158.
5. Beebe, A. M., N. Dua, T. G. Faith, P. F. Moore, N. Pedersen, and S. Dandekar. 1994. Primary stage of feline immunodeficiency virus infection: viral dissemination and cellular targets. *J. Virol.* **68:**3080–3091.
6. Bingen, A., H. Nonnenmcher, M. Bastien-Valle, and J. P. Martin. 2002. Tissues rich in macrophagic cells are the major sites of feline immunodeficiency virus uptake after intravenous inoculation into cats. *Microb. Infect.* **4:**795–803.
7. Bishop, S. A., N. A. Williams, T. J. Gruffydd-Jones, D. A. Harbour, and C. R. Stokes. 1992. An early defect in primary and secondary T cell responses in asymptomatic cats during acute feline immunodeficiency virus (FIV) infection. *Clin. Exp. Immunol.* **90:**491–496.
8. Bragg, D. C., L. C. Hudson, Y. H. Liang, M. B. Tompkins, A. Fernandes, and R. B. Meeker. 2002. Choroid plexus macrophages proliferate and release toxic factors in response to feline immunodeficiency virus. *J. Neurovirol.* **8:**225–239.
9. Brown, P. J., C. D. Hopper, and D. A. Harbour. 1991. Pathological features of lymphoid tissues in cats with natural feline immunodeficiency virus infection. *J. Comp. Pathol.* **104:**345–355.
10. Butera, S. T., J. Brown, M. E. Callahan, S. M. Owen, A. L. Matthews, D. D. Weigner, L. E. Chapman, and P. A. Sandstrom. 2000. Survey of veterinary conference attendees for evidence of zoonotic infection by feline retroviruses. *J. Am. Vet. Med. Assoc.* **217:**1475–1479.
11. Calandrella, M., D. Matteucci, P. Mazzetti, and A. Poli. 2001. Densitometric analysis of Western blot assays for feline immunodeficiency virus antibodies. *Vet. Immunol. Immunopathol.* **79:**261–271.
12. Celer, V., Jr., H. Kulhankova, and V. Celer. 2000. Detection of feline immunodeficiency provirus by seminested polymerase chain reaction. *Folia Microbiol. (Praha)* **45:**161–165.
13. Chalmers, S., R. O. Schick, and J. Jeffers. 1989. Demodicosis in two cats seropositive for feline immunodeficiency virus. *J. Am. Vet. Med. Assoc.* **194:**256–257.
14. Choi, I. S., R. Hokanson, and E. W. Collisson. 2000. Anti-feline immunodeficiency virus (FIV) soluble factor(s) produced from antigen-stimulated feline CD8(+) T lymphocytes suppresses FIV replication. *J. Virol.* **74:**676–683.
15. Courchamp, F., and D. Pontier. 1994. Feline immunodeficiency virus: an epidemiological review. *C. R. Acad. Sci. Ser. III Life Sci.* **317:**1123–1134.
16. Courchamp, F., N. G. Yoccoz, M. Artois, and D. Pontier. 1998. At-risk individuals in Feline Immunodeficiency Virus epidemiology: evidence from a multivariate approach in a natural population of domestic cats (*Felis catus*). *Epidemiol. Infect.* **121:**227–236.
17. Crawford, P. C., G. P. Papadi, J. K. Levy, N. A. Benson, A. Mergia, and C. M. Johnson. 2001. Tissue dynamics of CD8 lymphocytes that suppress viral replication in cats infected neonatally with feline immunodeficiency virus. *J. Infect. Dis.* **184:**671–681.
18. Danave, I. R., E. Tiffany-Castiglioni, E. Zenger, R. Barhoumi, R. C. Burghardt, and E. W. Collisson. 1994. Feline immunodeficiency virus decreases cell-cell communication and mitochondrial membrane potential. *J. Virol.* **68:**6745–6750.
19. Davidson, M. G., J. R. Rottman, R. V. English, M. R. Lappin, and M. B. Tompkins. 1993. Feline immunodeficiency virus predisposes cats to acute generalized toxoplasmosis. *Am. J. Pathol.* **143:**1486–1497.
20. Dean, G. A., J. A. Bernales, and N. C. Pedersen. 1998. Effect of feline immunodeficiency virus on cytokine response to *Listeria monocytogenes* in vivo. *Vet. Immunol. Immunopathol.* **65:**125–138.
21. del Fierro, G. M., J. Meers, J. Thomas, B. Chadwick, H. S. Park, and W. F. Robinson.

1995. Quantification of lymphadenopathy in experimentally induced feline immunodeficiency virus infection in domestic cats. *Vet. Immunol. Immunopathol.* **46**:3–12.
22. **Donovan, R. M.** 1999. Retroviridae, p. 442–460. *In* D. C. Hirsh and Y. C. Zee (ed.), *Veterinary Microbiology*. Blackwell Science, Inc., Malden, Mass.
23. **Druce, J. D., W. F. Robinson, S. A. Locarnini, M. T. Kyaw-Tanner, S. F. Sommerlad, and C. J. Birch.** 1997. Transmission of human and feline immunodeficiency viruses via reused suture material. *J. Med. Virol.* **53**:13–18.
24. **Fevereiro, M., C. Roneker, and F. de Noronha.** 1991. Antibody response to reverse transcriptase in cats infected with feline immunodeficiency virus. *Viral Immunol.* **4**:225–235.
25. **Flynn, J. N., S. Dunham, A. Mueller, C. Cannon, and O. Jarrett.** 2002. Involvement of cytolytic and non-cytolytic T cells in the control of feline immunodeficiency virus infection. *Vet. Immunol. Immunopathol.* **85**:159–170.
26. **Frey, S. C., E. A. Hoover, and J. I. Mullins.** 2001. Feline immunodeficiency virus cell entry. *J. Virol.* **75**:5433–5440.
27. **Gabor, L. J., D. N. Love, R. Malik, and P. J. Canfield.** 2001. Feline immunodeficiency virus status of Australian cats with lymphosarcoma. *Aust. Vet. J.* **79**:540–545.
28. **George, J. W., N. C. Pedersen, and J. Higgins.** 1993. The effect of age on the course of experimental feline immunodeficiency virus infection in cats. *AIDS Res. Hum. Retrovir.* **9**:897–905.
29. **Gothe, R., P. Beelitz, H. Schol, and B. Beer.** 1992. Trichomonad infections of the oral cavity in cats in south Germany. *Tieraerztl. Prax.* **20**:195–198.
30. **Goto, Y., Y. Nishimura, K. Baba, T. Mizuno, Y. Endo, K. Masuda, K. Ohno, and H. Tsujimoto.** 2002. Association of plasma viral RNA load with prognosis in cats naturally infected with feline immunodeficiency virus. *J. Virol.* **76**:10079–10083.
31. **Hanlon, M. A., J. M. Marr, K. A. Hayes, L. E. Mathes, P. C. Stromberg, S. Ringler, S. Krakowka, and L. J. Lafrado.** 1993. Loss of neutrophil and natural killer cell function following feline immunodeficiency virus infection. *Viral Immunol.* **6**:119–124.
32. **Hart, S. W., and I. Nolte.** 1994. Hemostatic disorders in feline immunodeficiency virus-seropositive cats. *J. Vet. Intern. Med.* **8**:355–362.
33. **Hartmann, K., R. M. Werner, H. Egberink, and O. Jarrett.** 2001. Comparison of six in-house tests for the rapid diagnosis of feline immunodeficiency and feline leukaemia virus infection. *Vet. Rec.* **149**:317–320.
34. **Hawkins, E. C., S. Kennedy-Stoskopf, J. K. Levy, D. J. Meuten, L. Cullins, W. A. Tompkins, and M. B. Tompkins.** 1996. Effect of FIV infection on lung inflammatory cell populations recovered by bronchoalveolar lavage. *Vet. Immunol. Immunopathol.* **51**:21–28.
35. **Hayes, K. A., A. J. Phipps, S. Francke, and L. E. Mathes.** 2000. Antiviral therapy reduces viral burden but does not prevent thymic involution in young cats infected with feline immunodeficiency virus. *Antimicrob. Agents Chemother.* **44**:2399–2405.
36. **Hofman-Lehmann, R., M. Berger, B. Sigrist, P. Schawalder, and H. Lutz.** 1998. Feline immunodeficiency virus (FIV) infection leads to increased incidence of feline odontoclastic resorptive lesions (FORL). *Vet. Immunol. Immunopathol.* **65**:299–308.
37. **Hohdatsu, T., H. Hirabayashi, K. Motokawa, and H. Koyama.** 1996. Comparative study of the cell tropism of feline immunodeficiency virus isolates of subtypes A, B and D classified on the basis of the *env* gene V3-V5 sequence. *J. Gen. Virol.* **77**:93–100.
38. **Hohdatsu, T., N. Miyagawa, M. Ohkubo, K. Kida, and H. Koyama.** 2000. Studies on feline CD8$^+$ T cell non-cytolytic anti-feline immunodeficiency virus (FIV) activity. *Arch. Virol.* **145**:2525–2538.
39. **Hohdatsu, T., M. Okubo, and H. Koyama.** 1998. Feline CD8$^+$ cell non-cytolytic anti-feline immunodeficiency virus activity mediated by a soluble factor(s). *J. Gen. Virol.* **79**:2729–2735.
40. **Hohdatsu, T., T. Sasagawa, A. Yamazaki, K. Motokawa, H. Kusuhara, T. Kaneshima, and H. Koyama.** 2002. CD8$^+$ T cells from feline immunodeficiency virus (FIV) infected cats suppress exogenous FIV replication of their peripheral blood mononuclear cells in vitro. *Arch. Virol.* **147**:1517–1529.
41. **Jacobson, S., S. J. Henriksen, O. Prospero-Garcia, T. R. Phillips, J. H. Elder, W. G. Young, F. E. Bloom, and H. S. Fox.** 1997. Cortical neuronal cytoskeletal changes associated with FIV infection. *J. Neurovirol.* **3**:283–289.
42. **Johnson, C. M., S. J. Bortnick, P. C. Crawford, and G. P. Papadi.** 2001. Unique susceptibility of the fetal thymus to feline immunodeficiency virus infection: an animal model for HIV infection in utero. *Am. J. Reprod. Immunol.* **45**:273–288.
43. **Johnston, J. B., M. E. Olson, E. W. Rud, and C. Power.** 2001. Xenoinfection of nonhuman primates by feline immunodeficiency virus. *Curr. Biol.* **11**:1109–1113.

44. Johnston, J. B., C. Silva, and C. Power. 2002. Envelope gene-mediated neurovirulence in feline immunodeficiency virus infection: induction of matrix metalloproteinases and neuronal injury. *J. Virol.* **76:**2622–2633.
45. Jordan, H. L., J. G. Howard, J. G. Bucci, J. L. Butterworth, R. English, S. Kennedy-Stoskopf, M. B. Tompkins, and W. A. Tompkins. 1998. Horizontal transmission of feline immunodeficiency virus with semen from seropositive cats. *J. Reprod. Immunol.* **41:**341–357.
46. Koirala, T. R., K. Nakagaki, T. Ishida, S. Nonaka, S. Morikawa, and T. Tabira. 2001. Decreased expression of MAP-2 and GAD in the brain of cats infected with feline immunodeficiency virus. *Tohoku J. Exp. Med.* **195:**141–151.
47. Lappin, M. R., A. Marks, C. E. Greene, B. J. Rose, P. W. Gasper, C. C. Powell, and J. S. Reif. 1993. Effect of feline immunodeficiency virus infection on *Toxoplasma gondii*-specific humoral and cell-mediated immune responses of cats with serologic evidence of toxoplasmosis. *J. Vet. Intern. Med.* **7:**95–100.
48. Liang, Y., L. C. Hudson, J. K. Levy, J. W. Ritchey, W. A. Tompkins, and M. B. Tompkins. 2000. T cells overexpressing interferon-γ and interleukin-10 are found in both the thymus and secondary lymphoid tissues of feline immunodeficiency virus-infected cats. *J. Infect. Dis.* **181:**564–575.
49. Lin, D. S., D. D. Bowman, R. H. Jacobson, M. C. Barr, M. Fevereiro, J. R. Williams, F. M. Noronha, F. W. Scott, and R. J. Avery. 1990. Suppression of lymphocyte blastogenesis to mitogens in cats experimentally infected with feline immunodeficiency virus. *Vet. Immunol. Immunopathol.* **26:**183–189.
50. Linenberger, M. L., and T. Deng. 1999. The effects of feline retroviruses on cytokine expression. *Vet. Immunol. Immunopathol.* **72:**343–368.
51. Loesenbeck, G., W. Drommer, and H. J. Heider. 1995. Findings in the eyes of serologically FIV (feline immunodeficiency virus) positive cats. *Dtsch. Tieraerztl. Wochenschr.* **102:**348–351.
52. Ma, J., S. Kennedy-Stoskopf, R. Sellon, S. Tonkonogy, E. C. Hawkins, M. B. Tompkins, and W. A. Tompkins. 1995. Tumor necrosis factor-α responses are depressed and interleukin-6 responses unaltered in feline immunodeficiency virus infected cats. *Vet. Immunol. Immunopathol.* **46:**35–50.
53. Mancianti, F., C. Giannelli, M. Bendinelli, and A. Poli. 1992. Mycological findings in feline immunodeficiency virus-infected cats. *J. Med. Mycol.* **30:**257–259.
54. Matsumoto, H., N. Takemura, T. Sako, H. Koyama, S. Motoyoshi, and Y. Inada. 1997. Serum concentration of circulating immune complexes in cats infected with feline immunodeficiency virus detected by immune adherence hemagglutination method. *J. Vet. Med. Sci.* **59:**395–396.
55. Mitchell, T. W., P. S. Buckmaster, E. A. Hoover, L. R. Whalen, and F. E. Dudek. 1998. Axonal sprouting in hippocampus of cats infected with feline immunodeficiency virus (FIV). *J. Acquir. Immune Defic. Syndr. Hum. Retrovirol.* **17:**1–8.
56. Mitchell, T. W., P. S. Buckmaster, E. A. Hoover, L. R. Whalen, and F. E. Dudek. 1999. Neuron loss and axon reorganization in the dentate gyrus of cats infected with the feline immunodeficiency virus. *J. Comp. Neurol.* **411:**563–577.
57. Mizuno, T., Y. Goto, K. Baba, K. Masuda, K. Ohno, and H. Tsujimoto. 2001. TNF-α-induced cell death in feline immunodeficiency virus-infected cells is mediated by the caspase cascade. *Virology* **287:**446–455.
58. Moraillon, A., F. Barre-Sinoussi, A. Parodi, R. Moraillon, and C. Dauguet. 1992. In vitro properties and experimental pathogenic effect of three strains of feline immunodeficiency virus (FIV) isolated from cats with terminal disease. *Vet. Microbiol.* **31:**41–54.
59. Murphy, F. A., E. P. J. Gibbs, M. C. Horzinek, and M. J. Studdert. 1999. *Veterinary Virology*, 3rd ed. Academic Press, Inc., San Diego, Calif.
60. Nishimura, Y., Y. Goto, K. Yoneda, Y. Endo, T. Mizuno, M. Hamachi, H. Maruyama, H. Kinoshita, S. Koga, M. Komori, S. Fushuku, K. Ushinohama, M. Akuzawa, T. Watari, A. Hasegawa, and H. Tsujimoto. 1999. Interspecies transmission of feline immunodeficiency virus from the domestic cat to the Tsushima cat (*Felis bengalensis euptilura*) in the wild. *J. Virol.* **73:**7916–7921.
61. Obert, L. A., and E. A. Hoover. 2002. Early pathogenesis of transmucosal feline immunodeficiency virus infection. *J. Virol.* **76:**6311–6322.
62. Olmstead, R. A., R. Langley, M. E. Roelke, R. M. Goeken, D. Adger-Johnson, J. P. Goff, J. P. Albert, C. Packer, M. K. Laurenson, T. M. Caro, L. Scheepers, D. E. Wildt, M. Bush, J. S. Martenson, and S. J. O'Brien. 1992. Worldwide prevalence of lentivirus infection in wild feline species: epidemiologic and phylogenetic aspects. *J. Virol.* **66:**6008–6018.
63. O'Neil, L. L., M. J. Burkhard, and E. A. Hoover. 1996. Frequent perinatal transmission

of feline immunodeficiency virus by chronically infected cats. *J. Virol.* **70:**2894–2901.
64. Ohno, K., T. Nakano, Y. Matsumoto, T. Watari, R. Goitsuka, H. Nakayama, H. Tsujimoto, and A. Hasegawa. 1999. Apoptosis induced by tumor necrosis factor in cells chronically infected with feline immunodeficiency virus. *J. Virol.* **67:**2429–2433.
65. Pancino, G., S. Castelot, and P. Sonigo. 1995. Differences in feline immunodeficiency virus host cell range correlates with envelope fusogenic properties. *Virology* **206:**796–806.
66. Paolicchi, A., P. Tonarelli, S. Silva, P. Bandecchi, and G. Malvaldi. 1996. Changes of glutathione metabolism during feline immunodeficiency virus infection. *J. Acquir. Immune Defic. Syndr. Hum. Retrovirol.* **13:**94–96.
67. Park, H. S., M. Kyaw-Tanner, J. Thomas, and W. F. Robinson. 1995. Feline immunodeficiency virus replicates in salivary gland ductular epithelium during the initial phase of infection. *Vet. Microbiol.* **46(1–3):**257–267.
68. Pedersen, N. C., C. M. Leutenegger, J. Woo, and J. Higgins. 2001. Virulence differences between two field isolates of feline immunodeficiency virus (FIV-APetaluma and FIV-CPGammar) in young adult specific pathogen free cats. *Vet. Immunol. Immunopathol.* **79:**53–67.
69. Pedersen, N. C., J. K. Yamamoto, T. Ishida, and H. Hansen. 1989. Feline immunodeficiency virus infection. *Vet. Immunol. Immunopathol.* **21:**111–129.
70. Phipps, A. J., K. A. Hayes, W. R. Buck, M. Podell, and L. E. Mathes. 2000. Neurophysiologic and immunologic abnormalities associated with feline immunodeficiency virus molecular clone FIV-PPR DNA inoculation. *J. Acquir. Immune Defic. Syndr.* **23:**8–16.
71. Podell, M., E. Chen, and G. D. Shelton. 1998. Feline immunodeficiency virus associated myopathy in the adult cat. *Muscle Nerve* **21:**1680–1685.
72. Poli, A., F. Abramo, E. Taccini, G. Guidi, P. Barsotti, M. Bendinelli, and G. Malvaldi. 1993. Renal involvement in feline immunodeficiency virus infection: a clinicopathological study. *Nephron* **64:**282–288.
73. Pontier, D., E. Fromont, F. Courchamp, M. Artois, and N. G. Yoccoz. 1998. Retroviruses and sexual size dimorphism in domestic cats (*Felis catus* L.). *Proc. R. Soc. Lond. B Biol. Sci.* **265:**167–173.
74. Pontzer, C. H., J. K. Yamamoto, F. W. Bazer, T. L. Ott, and H. M. Johnson. 1997. Potent anti-feline immunodeficiency virus and anti-human immunodeficiency virus effect of IFN-γ. *J. Immunol.* **158:**4351–4357.
75. Prospero-Garcia, O., S. Huitron-Resendiz, S. C. Casalman, M. Sanchez-Alavez, O. Diaz-Ruiz, L. Navarro, D. L. Lerner, T. R. Phillips, J. H. Elder, and S. J. Henriksen. 1999. Feline immunodeficiency virus envelope protein (FIVgp120) causes electrophysiological alterations in rats. *Brain Res.* **836:**201–209.
76. Ramsey, I., D. Gunn-Moore, and S. Shaw. 2001. The haematopoietic and lymphoreticular systems, p. 65–88. *In* I. Ramsey and B. Tennant, *Manual of Canine and Feline Infectious Diseases.* British Small Animal Veterinary Association, Gloucester, England.
77. Reubel, G. H., G. A. Dean, J. W. George, J. E. Barlough, and N. C. Pedersen. 1994. Effects of incidental infections and immune activation on disease progression in experimentally feline immunodeficiency virus-infected cats. *J. Acquir. Immune Defic. Syndr.* **7:**1003–1015.
78. Ritchey, J. W., J. K. Levy, S. K. Bliss, W. A. Tompkins, and M. B. Tompkins. 2001. Constitutive expression of types 1 and 2 cytokines by alveolar macrophages from feline immunodeficiency virus-infected cats. *Vet. Immunol. Immunopathol.* **79:**83–100.
79. Rogers, A. B., and E. A. Hoover. 1998. Maternal-fetal feline immunodeficiency virus transmission: timing and tissue tropisms. *J. Infect. Dis.* **178:**960–967.
80. Rogers, A. B., and E. A. Hoover. 2002. Fetal feline immunodeficiency virus is prevalent and occult. *J. Infect. Dis.* **186:**895–904.
81. Sandy, J. R. W. F. Robinson, B. Bredhauer, M. Kyaw-Tanner, and C. R. Howlett. 2002. Productive infection of the bone marrow in feline immunodeficiency virus infected cats. *Arch. Virol.* **147:**1053–1059.
82. Sellon, R. K., H. L. Jordan, S. Kennedy-Stoskopf, M. B. Tompkins, and W. A. Tompkins. 1994. Feline immunodeficiency virus can be experimentally transmitted via milk during acute maternal infection. *J. Virol.* **68:**3380-3385.
83. Shelton, G. H., and M. L. Linenberger. 1995. Hematologic abnormalities associated with retroviral infections in the cat. *Semin. Vet. Med. Surg. (Small Anim.)* **10:**220–233.
84. Sierra, P., J. Guillot, H. Jacob, S. Bussieras, and R. Chermette. 2000. Fungal flora on cutaneous and mucosal surfaces of cats infected with feline immunodeficiency virus or feline leukemia virus. *Am. J. Vet. Res.* **61:**158–161.
85. Silvotti, L., L. Kramer, A. Corradi, L. Busani, F. Tedeschi, G. Brandi, M. Bendinelli, and G. Piedimonte. 1997. Modulation of host

cell activation during feline immunodeficiency virus (FIV) infection. *J. Comp. Pathol.* **116:**263–271.
86. **Steigerwald, E. S., M. Sarter, P. March, and M. Podell.** 1999. Effects of feline immunodeficiency virus on cognition and behavioral function in cats. *J. Acquir. Immune Defic. Syndr. Hum. Retrovirol.* **20:**411–419.
87. **Sukura, A., Y. T. Grohn, J. Junttila, and T. Palolahti.** 1992. Association between feline immunodeficiency virus antibodies and host characteristics in Finnish cats. *Acta Vet. Scand.* **33:**325–334.
88. **Tanabe, T., and J. K. Yamamoto.** 2001. Phenotypic and functional characteristics of FIV infection in the bone marrow stroma. *Virology* **282:**113–122.
89. **Taniguchi, A., T. Ishida, T. Washizu, and I. Tomoda.** 1991. Humoral immune response to T cell dependent and independent antigens in cats infected with feline immunodeficiency virus. *J. Vet. Med. Sci.* **53:**333–335.
90. **Tenorio, A. P., C. E. Franti, B. R. Madewell, and N. C. Pedersen.** 1991. Chronic oral infections of cats and their relationship to persistent oral carriage of feline calici-, immunodeficiency, or leukemia viruses. *Vet. Immunol. Immunopathol.* **29:**1–14.
91. **Tompkins, M. B., M. E. Bull, J. L. Dow, J. M. Ball, E. W. Collisson, B. J. Winslow, A. P. Phadke, T. W. Vahlenkamp, and W. A. Tompkins.** 2002. Feline immunodeficiency virus infection is characterized by B7$^+$DTLA4$^+$ T cell apoptosis. *J. Infect. Dis.* **185:**1077–1093.
92. **Zaccaro, L., M. L. Falcone, S. Silva, L. Bigalli, A. Cecchettini, F. Giorgi, G. Malvaldi, and M. Bendinelli.** 1995. Defective natural killer cell cytotoxic activity in feline immunodeficiency virus-infected cats. *AIDS Res. Hum. Retrovir.* **11:**747–752.
93. **Zhao, Y., D. Gebhard, R. English, R. Sellon, M. Tompkins, and W. Tompkins.** 1995. Enhanced expression of novel CD57$^+$CD8$^+$ LAK cells from cats infected with feline immunodeficiency virus. *J. Leukoc. Biol.* **58:**423–431.

Feline leukemia virus
1. **Abkowitz, J. L., R. D. Holly, G. M. Segal, and J. W. Adamson.** 1986. Multilineage, nonspecies specific hematopoietic growth factor(s) elaborated by a feline fibroblast cell line: enhancement by virus infection. *J. Cell. Physiol.* **127:**189–196.
2. **Abkowitz, J. L., R. L. Ott, R. D. Holly, and J. W. Adamson.** 1987. Lymphocytes and antibody in retrovirus-induced feline pure red cell aplasia. *J. Natl. Cancer Inst.* **78:**135–139.
3. **Carmichael, K. P., D. Bienzle, and J. J. McDonnell.** 2002. Feline leukemia virus-associated myelopathy in cats. *Vet. Pathol.* **39:**536–545.
4. **Cockerell, G. L., and E. A. Hoover.** 1977. Inhibition of normal lymphocyte mitogenic reactivity by serum from feline leukemia virus-infected cats. *Cancer Res.* **37:**3985–3989.
5. **Cotter, S. M.** 1979. Anemia associated with feline leukemia virus infection. *J. Am. Vet. Med. Assoc.* **175:**1191–194.
6. **Cotter, S. M., W. D. Hardy, Jr., and M. Essex.** 1975. Association of feline leukemia virus with lymphosarcoma and other disorders in the cat. *J. Am. Vet. Med. Assoc.* **166:**449–454.
7. **Dezzutti, C. S., K. A. Wright, M. G. Lewis, L. J. Lafrado, and R. G. Olsen.** 1989. FeLV-induced immunosuppression through alterations in signal transduction: down regulation of protein kinase C. *Vet. Immunol. Immunopathol.* **21:**55–67.
8. **Donahue, P. R., S. L. Quackenbush, M. V. Gallo, C. M. deNoronha, J. Overbaugh, E. A. Hoover, and J. Mullins.** 1991. Viral genetic determinants of T-cell killing and immunodeficiency disease induction by the feline leukemia virus FeLV-FAIDS. *J. Virol.* **65:**4461–4469.
9. **Donovan, R. M.** 1999. Retroviridae, p. 442–460. *In* D. C. Hirsh and Y. C. Zee (ed.), *Veterinary Microbiology*. Blackwell Science, Inc., Malden, Mass.
10. **Dornsife, R. E., P. W. Gasper, J. I. Mullins, and E. A. Hoover.** 1989. In vitro erythrocytopathic activity of an aplastic anemia-inducing feline retrovirus. *Exp. Hematol.* **17:**138–144.
11. **Engleman, R. W., R. W. Fulton, R. A. Good, and N. K. Day.** 1985. Suppression of gamma interferon production by inactivated feline leukemia virus. *Science* **227:**1368–1370.
12. **Flynn, J. N., S. P. Dunham, V. Watson, and O. Jarrett.** 2002. Longitudinal analysis of feline leukemia virus-specific cytotoxic T lymphocytes: correlation with recovery from infection. *J. Virol.* **76:**2306–2315.
13. **Hanlon, L., D. Argyle, D. Bain, L. Nicolson, S. Dunham, M. C. Golder, M. McDonald, C. McGillivray, O. Jarrett, J. C. Neil, and D. E. Onions.** 2001. Feline leukemia virus DNA vaccine efficacy is enhanced by co-administration with interleukin-12 (IL-12) and IL-18 expression vectors. *J. Virol.* **75:**8424–8433.
14. **Harbour, D. A., D. A. Gunn-Moore, T. J. Gruffydd-Jones, S. M. Caney, J. Bradshaw, O. Jarrett, and A. Wiseman.** 2002. Protection against oronasal challenge with virulent feline leukaemia virus lasts for at least 12 months fol-

lowing a primary course of immunisation with Leukocell 2 vaccine. *Vaccine* **20**:2866–2872.
15. **Hisasue, M., H. Okayama, T. Okayama, T. Suzuki, T. Mizuno, Y. Fujino, K. Naganobu, A. Hasegawa, T. Watari, N. Matsuki, K. Masuda, K. Ohno, and H. Tsujimoto.** 2001. Hematologic abnormalities and outcome of 16 cats with myelodysplastic syndromes. *J. Vet. Intern. Med.* **15**:471–477.
16. **Hoover, E. A., J. L. Rojko, P. L. Wilson, and R. G. Olsen.** 1981. Determinants of susceptibility and resistance to feline leukemia virus infection. I. Role of macrophages. *J. Natl. Cancer Inst.* **67**:889-898.
17. **Kipar, A., J. Kremendahl, M. L. Jackson, and M. Reinacher.** 2001. Comparative examination of cats with feline leukemia virus-associated enteritis and other relevant forms of feline enteritis. *Vet. Pathol.* **38**:359–371.
18. **Lafrado, L. J., C. S. Dezzutti, M. G. Lewis, and R. G. Olsen.** 1989. Immunodeficiency in latent feline leukemia virus infections. *Vet. Immunol. Immunopathol.* **21**:39–46.
19. **Linenberger, M. L., and T. Deng.** 1999. The effects of feline retroviruses on cytokine expression. *Vet. Immunol. Immunopathol.* **72**:343–368.
20. **Linenberger, M. L., S. W. Dow, and J. L. Abkowitz.** 1995. Feline leukemia virus infection downmodulates the production of growth-inhibitory activity by marrow stromal cells. *Exp. Hematol.* **23**:1069–1079.
21. **Mitchell, T. W., J. L. Rojko, J. R. Hartke, A. R. Mihajlov, G. A. Kasemeyer, P. W. Gasper, and L. R. Whalen.** 1997. FeLV envelope protein (gp70) variable region 5 causes alterations in calcium homeostasis and toxicity of neurons. *J. Acquir. Immune Defic. Syndr. Hum. Retrovirol.* **14**:307–320.
22. **Murphy, F. A., E. P. J. Gibbs, M. C. Horzinek, and M. J. Studdert.** 1999. *Veterinary Virology*, 3rd ed. Academic Press, Inc., San Diego, Calif.
23. **Orosz, C. G., N. E. Zinn, R. G. Olsen, and L. E. Mathes.** 1985. Retrovirus-mediated immunosuppression. I. FeLV-UV and specific FeLV proteins alter T lymphocyte behavior by inducing hyporesponsiveness to lymphokines. *J. Immunol.* **134**:3396–3403.
24. **Orosz, C. G., N. E. Zinn, R. G. Olsen, and L. E. Mathes.** 1985. Retrovirus-mediated immunosuppression. II. FeLV-UV alters in vitro murine T lymphocyte behavior by reversibly impairing lymphokine secretion. *J. Immunol.* **135**:583–590.
25. **Overbaugh, J., E. A. Hoover, J. I. Mullins, D. P. Burns, L. Rudensey, S. L. Quackenbush, V. Stallard, and P. R. Donahue.** 1992. Structure and pathogenicity of individual variants within an immunodeficiency disease-inducing isolate of FeLV. *Virology* **188**:558–569.
26. **Perryman, L. E., E. A. Hoover, and D. S. Yohn.** 1972. Immunologic reactivity of the cat: Immunosuppression in experimental feline leukemia. *J. Natl. Cancer Inst.* **49**:1357–1365.
27. **Ramsey, I., D. Gunn-Moore, and S. Shaw.** 2001. The Haematopoietic and Lymphoreticular Systems, p. 65–88. *In* I. Ramsey and B. Tennant (ed.), *Manual of Canine and Feline Infectious Diseases*. British Small Animal Veterinary Association, Gloucester, England.
28. **Reinacher, M.** 1989. Diseases associated with spontaneous feline leukemia virus (FeLV) infection in cats. *Vet. Immunol. Immunopathol.* **21**:85–95.
29. **Rohn, J. L., M. S. Moser, S. R. Gwynn, D. N. Baldwin, and J. Overbaugh.** 1998. In vivo evolution of a novel, syncytium-inducing and cytopathic feline leukemia virus variant. *J. Virol.* **72**:2686–2896.
30. **Rojko, J. L., C. M. Cheney, P. W. Gasper, K. L. Hamilton, E. A. Hoover, L. E. Mathes, and G. J. Kociba.** 1986. Infectious feline leukaemia virus is erythrosuppressive in vitro. *Leukoc. Res.* **10**:1193–1199.
31. **Rojko, J. L., E. A. Hoover, L. E. Mathes, S. Krakowka, and R. G. Olsen.** 1979. Influence of adrenal corticosteroids on the susceptibility of cats to feline leukemia virus infection. *Cancer Res.* **39**:3789–3791.
32. **Rojko, J. L., J. R. Hartke, C. M. Cheney, A. J. Phipps, and J. C. Neil.** 1996. Cytopathic feline leukemia viruses cause apoptosis in hemolymphatic cells. *Prog. Mol. Subcell. Biol.* **16**:13-43.
33. **Shelton, G. H., and M. L. Linenberger.** 1995. Hematologic abnormalities associated with retroviral infections in the cat. *Semin. Vet. Med. Surg.* (*Small Anim.*) **10**:220–233.
34. **Stiff, M. I., and R. G. Olsen** 1982. Loss of the short-lived suppressive function of peripheral leukocytes in feline retrovirus-infected cats. *J. Clin. Lab. Immunol.* **7(2)**:133–138.
35. **Wang, S. W., and C. S. Teng.** 1995. Induction of feline acquired immune deficiency syndrome by feline leukemia virus: alteration in response to hormones in the hypothalamic-pituitary-gonadal system. *Proc. Soc. Exp. Biol. Med.* **208**:404–412.
36. **Yasuda, M., R. A. Good, and N. K. Day.** 1987. Influence of inactivated feline retrovirus on feline alpha interferon and immunoglobulin production. *Clin. Exp. Immunol.* **69**:240–245.

Feline parvovirus
1. **Bauder, B., A. Suchy, C. Gabler, and H. Weissenbock.** 2000. Apoptosis in feline panleu-

kopenia and canine parvovirus enteritis. *J. Vet. Med. Ser. B* **47:**775–784.
2. **Berthier, K., M. Langlais, P. Auger, and D. Pontier.** 2000. Dynamics of a feline virus with two transmission modes within exponentially growing host populations. *Proc. R. Soc. Lond. B Biol. Sci.* **267:**2049–2056.
3. **Brun, A., G. Chappuis, P. Precausta, and J. Terre.** 1979. Immunisation against panleukopenia: early development of immunity. *Comp. Immunol. Microbiol. Infect. Dis.* **1:**335–339.
4. **Buonavoglia, C., F. Marsilio, M. Tempesta, D. Buonavoglia, P. G. Tiscar, A. Cavalli, and M. Campagnucci.** 1993. Use of a feline panleukopenia modified live virus vaccine in cats in the primary-stage of feline immunodeficiency virus infection. *Zentbl. Vetmed. Reihe B* **40:**343–346.
5. **Eleraky, N. Z., L. N. Potgeiter, and M. A. Kennedy.** 2002. Virucidal efficacy of four new disinfectants. *J. Am. Anim. Hosp. Assoc.* **38:**231–234.
6. **Foley, J. E., U. Orgad, D. C. Hirsh, A. Poland, and N. C. Pedersen.** 1999. Outbreak of fatal salmonellosis in cats following use of a high-titer modified-live panleukopenia virus vaccine. *J. Am. Vet. Med. Assoc.* **214:**67–70.
7. **Goto, H., M. Horimoto, K. Shimizu, T. Hiraga, T. Matsuoka, T. Nakano, Y. Morohoshi, K. Maejima, and T. Urano.** 1981. *Jikken Dobutsu* **30:**283–290.
8. **Horiuchi, M., K. Yuri, T. Soma, H. Katae, H. Nagasawa, and M. Shinagawa.** 1996. Differentiation of vaccine virus from field isolates of feline panleukopenia virus by polymerase chain reaction and restriction fragment length polymorphism analysis. *Vet. Microbiol.* **53:**283–293.
9. **Ikegami, T., K. Shirota, K. Goto, A. Takakura, T. Itoh, S. Kawamura, Y. Une, Y. Nomura, and K. Fujiwara.** 1999. Enterocolitis associated with dual infection by *Clostridium piliforme* and feline panleukopenia virus in three kittens. *Vet. Pathol.* **36:**613–615.
10. **Kahn, D. E.** 1978. Pathogenesis of feline panleukopenia. *J. Am. Vet. Med. Assoc.* **173:**628–630.
11. **Kurtzman, G. J., L. Plantanias, L. Lustig, N. Frickhofen, and N. S. Young.** 1989. Feline parvovirus propagates in cat bone marrow cultures and inhibits hematopoietic colony formation in vitro. *Blood* **74:**71–81.
12. **Meurs, K. M., P. R. Fox, A. L. Magnon, S. Liu, and J. A. Towbin.** 2000. Molecular screening by polymerase chain reaction detects panleukopenia virus DNA in formalin-fixed hearts from cats with idiopathic cardiomyopathy and myocarditis. *Cardiovasc. Pathol.* **9:**119–126.
13. **Miyazawa, T., Y. Ikeda, K. Nakamura, R. Naito, M. Mochizuki, Y. Tohya, D. Vu, T. Mikami, and E. Takahashi.** 1999. Isolation of feline parvovirus from peripheral blood mononuclear cells of cats in northern Vietnam. *Microbiol. Immunol.* **43:**609–612.
14. **Murphy, F. A., E. P. J. Gibbs, M. C. Horzinek, and M. J. Studdert.** 1999. *Veterinary Virology,* 3rd ed. Academic Press, Inc., San Diego, Calif.
15. **Parker, J. S., W. J. Murphy, D. Wang, S. J. O'Brien, and C. R. Parrish.** 2001. Canine and feline parvoviruses can use human or feline transferrin receptors to bind, enter, and infect cells. *J. Virol.* **75:**3896–3902.
16. **Reif, J. S.** 1976. Seasonality, natality and herd immunity in feline panleukopenia. *Am. J. Epidemiol.* **103:**81–87.
17. **Rusbridge, C.** 2001. The nervous system, p. 231–249. *In* I. Ramsey and B. Tennant (ed.), *Manual of Canine and Feline Infectious Diseases.* British Small Animal Veterinary Association, Gloucester, England.
18. **Scott, F. W.** 1980. Virucidal disinfectants and feline viruses. *Am. J. Vet. Res.* **41:**410–414.
19. **Sharp, N. J., B. J. Davis, J. S. Guy, J. M. Cullen, S. F. Steingold, and J. N. Kornegay.** 1999. Hydranencephaly and cerebellar hypoplasia in two kittens attributed to intrauterine parvovirus infection. *J. Comp. Pathol.* **121:**39–53.
20. **Tani, K., A. Taga, K. Itamoto, T. Iwanaga, S. Une, M. Nakaichi, and Y. Taura.** 2001. Hydrocephalus and syringomyelia in a cat. *J. Vet. Med. Sci.* **63:**1331–1334.
21. **Tennant, B.** 2001. The alimentary tract, p. 129–150. *In* I. Ramsey and B. Tennant (ed.), *Manual of Canine and Feline Infectious Diseases.* British Small Animal Veterinary Association, Gloucester, England.
22. **van Vuuren, M., A. Steinel, T. Goosen, E. Lane, J. van der Lugt, J. Pearson, and U. Truyen.** 2000. Feline panleukopenia virus revisited: molecular characteristics and pathological lesions associated with three recent isolates. *J. S. Afr. Vet. Assoc.* **71:**140–143.
23. **Wilcox, G. E., R. L. Flower, and R. D. Cook.** 1984. Recovery of viral agents from the central nervous system of cats. *Vet. Microbiol.* **9:**355–366.

BACTERIA

Chlamydophila felis

1. **Biberstein, E. L., and D. C. Hirsh.** 1999. Chlamydiae, p. 173–177. *In* D. C. Hirsh and Y. C. Zee (ed.), *Veterinary Microbiology.* Blackwell Science, Inc., Malden, Mass.

2. **Carlin, J. M., and J. B. Weller.** 1995. Potentiation of interferon-mediated inhibition of Chlamydia infection by interleukin-1 in human macrophage cultures. *Infect. Immun.* **63:**1870–1875.
3. **Coutinho-Silva, R., J. L. Perfettini, P. M. Persechini, A. Dautry-Varsat, and D. M. Ojcius.** 2001. Modulation of P2Z/P2X$_7$ receptor activity in macrophages infected with *Chlamydia psittaci*. *Am. J. Physiol.* **280:**C81–C89.
4. **Dickie, C. W., and E. S. Sniff.** 1980. Chlamydia infection associated with peritonitis in a cat. *J. Am. Vet. Med. Assoc.* **176:**1256–1259.
5. **Dorin, S. E., W. W. Miller, and J. K. Goodwin.** 1993. Diagnosing and treating chlamydial conjunctivitis in cats. *Vet. Med.* **88:**322–330.
6. **Forsey, T., and S. Darougar.** 1981. Transmission of chlamydiae by the housefly. *Br. J. Ophthalmol.* **65:**147–150.
7. **Hartley, J. C., S. Stevenson, A. J. Robinson, J. D. Littlewood, C. Carder, J. Cartledge, C. Clark, and G. L. Ridgway.** 2001. Conjunctivitis due to *Chlamydophila felis* (*Chlamydia psittaci* Feline Pneumonitis Agent) acquired from a cat: Case report with molecular characterization of isolates from the patient and cat. *J. Infect.* **43:**7–11.
8. **Helps, C., N. Reeves, S. Tasker, and D. Harbour.** 2001. Use of real-time quantitative PCR to detect *Chlamydophila felis* infection. *J. Clin. Microbiol.* **39:**2675–2676.
9. **Hoover, E. A., D. E. Kahn, and J. M. Langloss.** 1978. Experimentally induced feline chlamydial infection (feline pneumonitis). *Am. J. Vet. Res.* **39:**541–547.
10. **Horoschak, K. D., and J. W. Moulder.** 1978. Division of single host cells after infection with chlamydiae. *Infect. Immun.* **19:**281–286.
11. **Johnson, F. W.** 1984. Isolation of *Chlamydia psittaci* from nasal and conjunctival exudate of a domestic cat. *Vet. Rec.* **114:**342–344.
12. **Lammert, J. K., and P. B. Wyrick.** 1982. Modulation of the host immune response as a result of *Chlamydia psittaci* infection. *Infect. Immun.* **35:**537–545.
13. **Lipman, N. S., L. L. Yan, and J. C. Murphy.** 1994. Probable transmission of *Chlamydia psittaci* from a macaw to a cat. *J. Am. Vet. Med. Assoc.* **204:**1479–1480.
14. **McClenaghan, M., N. F. Inglis, and A. J. Herring.** 1991. Comparison of isolates of *Chlamydia psittaci* of ovine, avian and feline origin by analysis of polypeptide profiles from purified elementary bodies. *Vet. Microbiol.* **26:**269–278.
15. **McDonald, M., B. J. Willett, O. Jarrett, and D. D. Addie.** 1998. A comparison of DNA amplification, isolation and serology for the detection of *Chlamydia psittaci* infection in cats. *Vet. Rec.* **143:**97–101.
16. **Meijer, A., S. A. Morre, A. J. van den Brule, P. H. Savelkoul, and J. M. Ossewaarde.** 1999. Genomic relatedness of Chlamydia isolates determined by amplified fragment length polymorphism analysis. *J. Bacteriol.* **181:**4469–4475.
17. **Morland, B., G. I. Byrne, and T. C. Jones.** 1987. The effect of intracellular *Chlamydia psittaci* on lysosomal enzyme activities in mouse peritoneal macrophages. *Acta Pathol. Microbiol. Immunol. Scand. Sect. C Immunol.* **95:**291–193.
18. **Ojcius, D. M., R. Hellio, and A. Dautry-Varsat.** 1997. Distribution of endosomal, lysosomal, and major histocompatibility complex markers in a monocytic cell line infected with *Chlamydia psittaci*. *Infect. Immun.* **65:**2437–2442.
19. **Ojcius, D. M., P. Souque, J. L. Perfettini, and A. Dautry-Varsat.** 1998. Apoptosis of epithelial cells and macrophages due to infection with the obligate intracellular pathogen *Chlamydia psittaci*. *J. Immunol.* **161:**4220–4226.
20. **Ramsey, C. T.** 2000. Feline chlamydia and calicivirus infections. *Vet. Clin. North Am. Small Anim. Pract.* **30:**1015–1028.
21. **Regan, R. J., J. R. Dathan, and J. D. Treharne.** 1979. Infective endocarditis with glomerulonephritis associated with cat chlamydia (*C. psittaci*) infection. *Br. Heart J.* **42:**349–352.
22. **Schmeer, N., G. J. Jahn, A. A. Bialasiewicz, and A. Weber.** 1987. The cat as a possible infection source for *Chlamydia psittaci* keratoconjunctivitis in humans. *Tieraerztl. Prax.* **15:**201–204.
23. **Storz, J., and P. Spears.** 1977. Chlamydiales: properties, cycle of development and effect on eukaryotic host cells. *Curr. Top. Microbiol. Immunol.* **76:**167–214.
24. **Studdert, M. J., V. P. Studdert, and H. J. Wirth.** 1981. Isolation of *Chlamydia psittaci* from cats with conjunctivitis. *Aust. Vet. J.* **57:**515–517.
25. **Suri, A. K., B. Guerin, P. Humblot, and M. Thibier.** 1986. Effect of infection of the genital tract on the concentration of IgG and albumin in bull serum and semen. *Vet. Immunol. Immunopathol.* **13:**273–278.
26. **Sykes, J. E., V. P. Studdert, and G. F. Browning.** 1999. Comparison of the polymerase chain reaction and culture for the detection of feline *Chlamydia psittaci* in untreated and doxycycline-treated experimentally infected cats. *J. Vet. Intern. Med.* **13:**146–152.
27. **Todd, W. J., and J. Storz.** 1975. Ultrastructural cytochemical evidence for the activation of lysosomes in the cytocidal effect of *Chlamydia psittaci*. *Infect. Immun.* **12:**638–646.

28. **Willoughby, K., and S. Dawson.** 2001. The respiratory tract, p. 89-115. *In* I. Ramsey and B. Tennant (ed.), *Manual of Canine and Feline Infectious Diseases.* British Small Animal Veterinary Association, Gloucester, England.
29. **Wills, J., T. J. Gruffydd-Jones, S. Richmond, and I. D. Paul.** 1984. Isolation of *Chlamydia psittaci* from cases of conjunctivitis in a colony of cats. *Vet. Rec.* **114:**344–346.
30. **Yan, C., H. Fukushi, H. Matsudate, K. Ishihara, K. Yasuda, H. Kitagawa, T. Yamaguchi, and K. Hirai.** 2000. Seroepidemiological investigation of feline chlamydiosis in cats and humans in Japan. *Microbiol. Immunol.* **44:**155–160.

FUNGI
Dermatomycosis
1. **Asahi, M., S. Ueda, M. Kurakazu, and H. Urabe.** 1982. Purification and characterization of a new peptide antigen extracted from dermatophyte mycelia. *J. Investig. Dermatol.* **78:**38–43.
2. **Bibel, D. J., and J. R. LeBrun.** 1975. Effect of experimental dermatophyte infection on cutaneous flora. *J. Investig. Dermatol.* **64:**119–123.
3. **Cabanes, F. J., M. L. Abarca, and M. R. Bragulat.** 1997. Dermatophytes isolated from domestic animals in Barcelona, Spain. *Mycopathologia* **137:**107–113.
4. **Calderon, R. A., and R. J. Hay.** 1987. Fungicidal activity of human neutrophils and monocytes on dermatophyte fungi, *Trichophyton quinckeanum* and *Trichophyton rubrum*. *Immunology* **61:**289–295.
5. **Castanon-Olivares, L. R., P. Manzano-Gayosso, R. Lopez-Martinez, I. A. De la Rosa-Velazquez, and E. Soto-Reyes-Solis.** 2001. Effectiveness of terbinafine in the eradication of *Microsporum canis* from laboratory cats. *Mycoses* **44:**95–97.
6. **DeBoer, D. J., and K. A. Moriello.** 1993. Humoral and cellular immune responses to *Microsporum canis* in naturally occurring feline dermatophytosis. *J. Med. Vet. Mycol.* **31:**121–132.
7. **Mancianti, F., C. Giannelli, M. Bendinelli, and A. Poli.** 1992. Mycological findings in feline immunodeficiency virus-infected cats. *J. Med. Mycol.* **30:**257–259.
8. **Mason, I., R. Bond, D. A. Gunn-Moore, and A. Sparks.** 2001. The skin, p.197–218. *In* I. Ramsey and B. Tennant (ed.), *Manual of Canine and Feline Infectious Diseases.* British Small Animal Veterinary Association, Gloucester, England.
9. **McGregor, J. M., A. J. Hamilton, and R. J. Hay.** 1992. Possible mechanisms of immune modulation in chronic dermatophytes: an in vitro study. *Br. J. Dermatol.* **127:**233–238.
10. **Moriello, K. A.** 1990. Mangement of dermatophyte infections ni catteries and multiple-cat households. *Vet. Clin. North Am. Small Anim. Pract.* **20:**1457–1474.
11. **Moriello, K. A., and D. J. DeBoer.** 1995. Efficacy of griseofulvin and itraconazole in the treatment of experimentally induced dermatophytosis in cats. *J. Am. Vet. Med. Assoc.* **207:**439–444.
12. **Pier, A. C., and K. A. Moriello.** 1998. Parasitic relationship between *Micrsporum canis* and the cat. *Med. Mycol.* **36:**271–275.
13. **Romano, C.** 1999. Tinea capitis in Siena, Italy. An 18-year study. *Mycoses* **42:**559–562.
14. **Sparkes, A. H., T. J. Gruffydd-Jones, S. E. Shaw, A. I. Wright, and C. R. Stokes.** 1993. Epidemiological and diagnostic features of canine and feline dermatophytosis in the United Kingdom from 1956 to 1991. *Vet. Rec.* **133:**57–61.
15. **Sparkes, A. H., T. J. Gruffydd-Jones, and C. R. Stokes.** 1996. Acquired immunity in experimental feline *Microsporum canis* infection. *Res. Vet. Sci.* **61:**165–168.
16. **Sparkes, A. H., C. R. Stokes, and T. J. Gruffydd-Jones.** 1993. Humoral immune responses in cats with dermatophytosis. *Am. J. Vet. Res.* **54:**1869–1873.
17. **Tan, J. S.** 1997. Human zoonotic infections transmitted by dogs and cats. *Arch. Intern. Med.* **157:**1933–1943.
18. **Yager, J. A., B. P. Wilcock, J. A. Lynch, and A. R. Thompson.** 1986. Mycetoma-like granuloma in a cat caused by *Microsporum canis*. *J. Comp. Pathol.* **96:**171–176.

PARASITES
Fleas
1. **Barrs, V. R., J. A. Beatty, P. L. Tisdall, G. B. Hunt, M. Gunew, R. G. Nicoll, and R. Malik.** 1999. Intestinal obstruction by trichobezoars in five cats. *J. Feline Med. Surg.* **1:**199–207.
2. **Bowman, D., C. M. Hendrix, D. S. Lindsay, and S. C. Barr.** 2002. *Feline Clinical Parasitology*, 1st ed. Iowa State University Press, Ames.
3. **Cheeseman, M. T.** 1998. Characterization of apyrase activity from the salivary glands of the cat flea *Ctenocephalides felis*. *Insect Biochem. Mol. Biol.* **28:**1025–1030.
4. **Cheeseman, M. T., P. A. Bates, and J. M. Crampton.** 2001. Preliminary characterization of esterase and platelet-activating factor (PAF)-acetylhydrolase activities from cat flea (*Ctenocephalides felis*) salivary glands. *Insect Biochem. Mol. Biol.* **31:**157–164.

5. **Dryden, M. W., and M. K. Rust.** 1994. The cat flea: biology, ecology and control. *Vet. Parasitol.* **52:**1–19.
6. **Gross, T. L., K. W. Kwochka, and G. A. Kunkle.** 1986. Correlation of histologic and immunologic findings in cats with miliary dermatitis. *J. Am. Vet. Med. Assoc.* **189:**1322–1325.
7. **Harvey, R. G.** 1991. Management of feline miliary dermatitis by supplementing the diet with essential fatty acids. *Vet. Rec.* **128:**326–329.
8. **Lee, S. E., I. P. Johnstone, R. P. Lee, and J. P. Opdebeeck.** 1999. Putative salivary allergens of the cat flea, *Ctenocephalides felis felis*. *Vet. Immunol. Immunopathol.* **69:**229–237.
9. **Marquez, F. J., M. A. Muniain, J. M. Perez, and J. Pachon.** 2002. Presence of *Rickettsia felis* in the cat flea from Southwestern Europe. *Emerg. Infect. Dis.* **8:**89–91.
10. **Mason, I., R. Bond, D. A. Gunn-Moore, and A. Sparks.** 2001. The skin, p. 197–218. *In* I. Ramsey and B. Tennant (ed.), *Manual of Canine and Feline Infectious Diseases*. British Small Animal Veterinary Association, Gloucester, England.
11. **McDermott, M. J., E. Weber, S. Hunter, K. E. Stedman, E. Best, G. R. Frank, R. Wang, J. Escudero, J. Kuner, and C. McCall.** 2000. Identification, cloning, and characterization of a major cat flea salivary allergen (Cte f 1). *Mol. Immunol.* **37:**361–375.
12. **O'Dair, H. A., and A. P. Foster.** 1995. Focal and generalized alopecia. *Vet. Clin. North Am. Small Anim. Pract.* **25:**851–870.
13. **Slacek, B., and J. P. Opdebeeck.** 1993. Reactivity of dogs and cats to feeding fleas and to flea antigens injected intradermally. *Aust. Vet. J.* **70:** 313–314.
14. **Thoday, K. L.** 1979. Skin diseases of dogs and cats transmissible to man. *In Pract.* **1:**5–15.
15. **Windsor, J. J.** 2001. Cat-scratch disease: epidemiology, aetiology and treatment. *Br. J. Biomed. Sci.* **58:**101 *In Pract.* **1110**.
16. **Yaphe, W., S. Giovengo, and N. S. Moise.** 1993. Severe cardiomegaly secondary to anemia in a kitten. *J. Am. Vet. Med. Assoc.* **202:**961 *In Pract.* **1964**.

Intestinal nematodes
1. **Bowman, D.** 1999. *Georgis' Parasitology for Veterinarians,* 7th ed. W.B. Saunders Co., Philadelphia, Pa.
2. **Bowman, D., C. M. Hendrix, D. S. Lindsay, and S. C. Barr.** 2002. *Feline Clinical Parasitology,* 1st ed. Iowa State University Press, Ames.
3. **Despommier, D. D., R. W. Gwadz, P. J. Hotez, and C. A. Knirsch.** 2000. *Parasitic Diseases,* 4th ed. Apple Tree Productions, New York, N.Y.
4. **Dubinsky, P., K. Havasiova-Reiterova, B. Petko, I. Hovorka, and O. Tomasovicova.** 1995. Role of small mammals in the epidemiology of toxocariasis. *Parasitology* **110:**187 *In Pract.* **1193**.
5. **Hamilton, J. M., J. Naylor, and A. Weatherley.** 1982. Glomerular lesions associated with infestation with *Toxocara cati*. *Vet. Rec.* **111:**583 *In Pract.* **1584**.
6. **Jonas, A. M., T. W. Swerczek, and S. E. Downing.** 1972. Vaso-occlusive pulmonary artery disease in the cat. A preliminary report. *Acta Radiol. Suppl.* **319:**237–244.
7. **Onwuliri, C. O., A. B. Nwosu, and A. O. Anya.** 1981. Experimental *Ancylostoma tubaeforme* infection of cats: changes in blood values and worm burdens in relation to single infections of varying size. *Z. Parasitenkd.* **64:**149–155.
8. **Swerczek, T. W., S. W. Nielsen, and C. F. Helmboldt.** 1971. Transmammary passage of *Toxocara cati* in the cat. *Am. J. Vet. Res.* **32:**89–92.
9. **Visco, R. J., R. M. Corwin, and L. A. Selby.** 1978. Effect of age and sex on the prevalence of intestinal parasitism in cats. *J. Am. Vet. Med. Assoc.* **172:**797–800.
10. **Weatherley, A. J., and J. M. Hamilton.** 1984. Possible role of histamine in the genesis of pulmonary arterial disease in cats infected with *Toxocara cati*. *Vet. Rec.* **114:**347–349.

PATHOGENS OF DOGS

9

INTRODUCTION

The domestic dog (*Canis familiaris*) is a commonly used animal model for many types of research. The dog serves as a model for research involving the cardiopulmonary, gastrointestinal, renal, orthopedic, reproductive, and other systems. Because of the similarities between many aspects of canine and human physiology, much of what is learned utilizing dogs is considered directly applicable to human physiology and medicine. In addition, veterinary research on dogs has increased over the past years, and has contributed significantly to the overall improvements made in the field of canine health and well-being.

Most dogs used in research are purpose bred, of very high quality and with low pathogen status, and are purchased from reputable dealers. However, some research facilities continue to purchase conditioned dogs from "Class B" dog dealers. These are dealers who purchase and/or resell dogs. Less commonly, dogs are obtained from local animal control facilities, although this source of dogs is dwindling as a result of pressure brought on municipalities by animal activists. Clearly, dogs from the latter two sources are still appropriate for certain types of research and/or teaching activities. However, because they are from generally less well controlled environments, they are more likely to be infected with various pathogens. In this author's experience, nearly all dogs from animal control centers harbor some pathogen(s). These pathogens have a way of gaining entry into the purpose-bred research colony, and can thereby disrupt research at many levels. In addition, even purpose-bred dogs from reputable vendors may occasionally be found harboring pathogens. Lastly, animal caretakers may unknowingly transmit pathogens from their personal pets to the animal facility population. For these reasons, it is imperative that the laboratory animal veterinarian and biomedical researchers be aware of the natural pathogens of dogs and their documented or potential effects on research.

As for the pathogens of cats, and the reader will note for most of the other larger research animals discussed in this text, there are very few reports directly describing the research-altering effects of pathogens on their canine hosts. This is surprising considering the high cost of dogs, the practice of directly relating research findings to human physiology and medicine, and the elevated position dogs occupy in society in general. It would seem that greater effort should be made to ensure that infectious agents do not confound research involving dogs, yet this does not seem to be the case. Apparently, there is a level of acceptance of "background" infections in research dogs that would not be tolerated in laboratory rodents. Once again, the literature covering natural case reports and experimental infections has been reviewed to allow a reasonable synthesis of the known and potential physiologic effects these pathogens may have on the canine research subject.

VIRUSES

Canine adenoviruses

Agent
Canine adenoviruses (CAV) are nonenveloped, double-stranded DNA (dsDNA) viruses of the family *Adenoviridae*. CAV-1 causes infectious canine hepatitis, while both CAV-1 and CAV-2 are two of many causes of infectious tracheobronchitis or "kennel cough." The two virus strains are antigenically related but distinct in a variety of ways (1, 9). Likewise, strain differences exist between viral isolates (21).

Epidemiology
Both strains of CAV are highly contagious. Prevalence is difficult to establish due to maternal or vaccination-induced antibodies, but is likely quite low (14). Transmission of CAV-1 is through exposure to infectious urine in the environment, and to a lesser extent, exposure to other body fluids (23). CAV-2 is transmitted through exposure to infectious respiratory secretions.

Clinical signs
Clinical signs associated with CAV-1 are either systemic or respiratory, change during the course of infection, and are in large part dependent on the route of infection (27). In many cases, the earliest sign of CAV-1 infection is a high but short-lived fever. Other signs of systemic infection include photophobia, hemorrhagic diarrhea, lethargy, anorexia, weight loss, thirst, and petechiation and ecchymosis of the abdominal skin. The abdomen becomes tender as hepatitis develops and the liver swells. This is most prominent in the xyphoid region. Development of hepatic enlargement may be followed by subcutaneous edema in the region of the head and neck. In most cases clinical signs abate within a week (18, 22, 25, 31). One to three weeks later, dogs develop painful but usually transient, iridocyclitis, anterior uveitis, corneal edema, and opacity ("blue eye"). The latter is due to immune complex deposition in the cornea, resulting from a type III hypersensitivity reaction (4, 27). Corneal opacity may not reverse (D. Baker, unpublished observation). Affected dogs may die peracutely within a few hours of onset of clinical signs (31). Infection during pregnancy results in fetal death, or birth of weak puppies that soon die. Clinical disease may be more serious when accompanied by infection with other pathogens (11, 15). On occasion, CAV-1 infection will present with signs of kennel cough in addition to those signs previously described for infectious hepatitis and systemic infection (18). In these cases one observes conjunctivitis, oculonasal discharge, tachypnea, and a harsh cough (30; D. Baker, unpublished observation). Susceptibility to infection appears to be greater in the Afghan breed versus others (6). Clinical signs of CAV-2 infection are those of kennel cough, and include a harsh cough, oculonasal discharge, and fever. CAV-2 has also rarely been associated with diarrheal disease, although a causal relationship has yet to be conclusively demonstrated (8, 12).

Pathology
Following exposure to CAV-1, virus localizes in the tonsils, spreads to regional lymph nodes, and then disseminates hematogenously to virtually all organs, including the liver. Hepatic parenchymal and vascular endothelial cells are primary targets for viral replication and injury (31). The wide tissue distribution and cytolytic propensity leads to pathologic changes in several organs. In this regard, pathologic findings of systemic CAV-1 infection include tonsilitis; leukopenia, encephalitis, enteritis,

anterior uveitis, widespread mucosal congestion and hemorrhages; and an enlarged, thickened gall bladder and spleen. In addition, hepatitis, nephritis, and iridocyclitis occur, and represent the most deleterious changes (2, 28, 31). Renal lesions are due to a type IV hypersensitivity reaction (27). Loss of clotting factors and thrombocytopenia result in increased clotting times and hemorrhages. Cowdry type A bodies can be identified in many hepatic and endothelial cells (31). Unfortunately, glomerular immune complex deposition is a common sequela to antibody response (4, 29). Dogs dying acutely have edematous and hemorrhagic lymph nodes, serosal hemorrhages, abdominal fibrin deposition, and serosanguinous or hemorrhagic ascites. Pathologic findings in respiratory infections include necrotizing bronchiolitis, followed by bronchiolar epithelial hyperplasia (30). Antibody response is rapid, results in viral clearing within about a week after infection, and lasts several years (31). Unlike infection with CAV-1, viremia is not a prominent feature of CAV-2 infection. Generalized disease therefore does not develop and the range of pathologic involvement is far less extensive. Lesions associated with CAV-2 infection are usually limited to the upper respiratory tract, and include pharyngitis, tonsillitis, and tracheobronchitis (31). CAV-2 may also be isolated from the intestinal tract, without lesion development. Virus persists in the respiratory tract for up to a month. Acquired immunity is once again humoral, but may not be as long lasting.

Interference with research
Little information is available describing interference with research by CAV-1 or CAV-2. In hamsters, both strains are oncogenic. This has not been demonstrated in dogs (31). CAV-1 infection can cause immune suppression with induction of leukopenia, thrombocytopenia, coagulation disorders, and elevated liver enzymes (23, 31). Given the widespread tissue distribution of CAV-1, natural infection could compromise studies involving virtually any organ system in the body. However, the cardiovascular, dermal, enterohepatic, hematopoietic, lymphoreticular, nervous, reproductive, respiratory, and urinary systems appear most severely affected. CAV-2 infection has been shown to alter the cellular architecture and mechanics of the lung, and increase histamine airway reactivity (16, 17, 26). Natural infection with CAV-2 would compromise studies involving the respiratory, and possibly the enterohepatic systems. In vitro studies may also be compromised if cell cultures are contaminated with adenovirus (19, 24).

Diagnosis and control
Infection with CAV-1 should be strongly suspected when fever, leukopenia, pain on palpation of the liver, prolonged clotting times, and ocular opacity occur, in that order. However, other infectious and noninfectious conditions may mimic some of these signs. Diagnosis is confirmed by virus isolation or rising serum titers. More recently, PCR assays have been developed for rapid diagnosis of virus in tissue culture, paraffin-embedded tissues, and clinical specimens (9, 10, 13). Treatment of CAV-1 infection is primarily supportive. For a description of treatment and vaccination strategies, the interested reader is referred elsewhere (23, 31). Because CAV-1 may be shed in the urine for up to a year, infected dogs continue to be a source of environmental contamination long after the resolution of signs (31). Given the wide range of agents associated with kennel cough, a definitive diagnosis of CAV-2 requires virus isolation or serologic confirmation. Modified live (7), but not killed (5), CAV-1 and CAV-2 vaccines are cross protective. However, CAV-2 vaccines are now regularly used to immunize dogs against both strains of virus (3). This strategy confers protection, while preventing postvaccinal ocular lesions. CAV are modestly resistant to mild environmental stresses. However, common disinfectants such as iodine, phenol, bleach, or lysol, readily inactivate them, as does steam (23, 31). Serologic studies indicate that humans can become infected

with CAV-1, although clinical signs do not develop (20).

Canine coronavirus

Agent
Canine coronavirus (CCV) is a single-stranded RNA (ssRNA) virus in the family *Coronaviridae,* genus *Coronavirus.* Multiple antigenic variants have been reported (1, 9). Coronaviruses are uniquely shaped, somewhat resembling a crown bearing "club-shaped" projections.

Epidemiology
On the basis of seroprevalence studies, infection with CCV is common and worldwide, with seroprevalence of up to 100% in some kennels (2, 3, 4, 7, 12). Transmission is fecal-oral. Viral shedding by asymptomatic carriers facilitates transmission within a colony setting. Incidence of infection is higher during the winter months, possibly due to cold tolerance of the virus, and closer contact of animals.

Clinical signs
Clinical signs of CCV infection are uncommon. When present, they occur in pups 6 to 12 weeks of age, are usually mild, and are limited to watery diarrhea (10, 13). Mortality is rare in uncomplicated infections. In cases where clinical signs are severe, it is likely that CCV is acting as a copathogen rather than as a primary pathogen (10).

Pathology
CCV infects primarily intestinal epithelium, but may also be found incidentally in pulmonary alveoli, tonsils, liver, lung, spleen, and mesenteric lymph nodes (9, 10, 13). Colonization begins in the duodenum, and extends to the rest of the small intestine. Viral shedding occurs within a week of infection, and persists for about 2 weeks (4, 10). Gross pathologic changes are often absent (13), or may include distended, fluid-filled bowel loops; serosal congestion; and enlarged mesenteric lymph nodes (9). Histopathologic lesions include loss of epithelial cells, villous atrophy, and villous fusion (9, 10). These changes result in diarrhea through loss of enzymatic activity and absorptive capability (9). Intestinal cytoarchitectural recovery occurs rapidly, although diarrhea may persist for up to about 2 weeks (10). Intestinal immunoglobulin A (IgA) is responsible for recovery, and protects against reinfection. Systemic antibody responses following parenteral immunization are detectable, but not protective (5, 7, 10,13).

Interference with research
There are no reports of CCV interfering with research studies. However, inclusion of pups in studies involving the gastrointestinal tract could be compromised by natural infection with CCV. Relatedly, CCV has been shown to increase severity of disease caused by canine parvovirus and canine adenovirus type 1 (8, 10). This is likely because the loss of intestinal epithelial cells by CCV leads to epithelial regeneration, and, as noted in the discussion of canine parvovirus (CPV), below, rapidly dividing cells are prime targets for CPV infection (10). CCV may therefore interfere with experimental infections using other enteric pathogens, particularly parvoviruses.

Diagnosis and control
Because of the innocuous nature of CCV, definitive diagnosis is rarely attempted. Fecal virus isolation is definitive, but false negatives occur due to loss of fragile virus particles during sample handling (11). Fluorescent staining of fecal or necropsy samples, and paired serology, seeking demonstration of a fourfold rise in titer, are also diagnostic, but are not usually performed. Newer methods, including reverse transcriptase (RT)-PCR, have been developed and are more reliable than virus isolation or electron microscopy (4, 6). Affected animals should be treated symptomatically, with fluids and electrolytes. Due to the low significance of this pathogen, vaccination is generally not warranted but should be determined by program requirements. Coronaviruses are easily inactivated by a variety of

disinfectants that function as lipid solvents and heat. CCV is acid stable (pH of 3.0) and cold resistant (9).

Canine distemper virus

Agent
Canine distemper virus (CDV) is an enveloped, ssRNA virus in the family *Paramyxoviridae*. Members of the family are grouped as morbilliviruses, paramyxoviruses, and pneumoviruses, on the basis of nucleocapsid size, presence or absence of neuraminidase, and antigenic relationships (39). CDV belong to the morbillivirus group, along with rinderpest and others. Other than rabies virus, which is zoonotic, CDV is the most serious viral disease of dogs. Multiple virus strains have been identified (4, 6, 24, 28).

Epidemiology
In most parts of the world, infection with CDV is common in the feral dog population. In contrast, CDV is rarely seen in laboratory dog colonies. Entrance into the colony is gained through the purchase of dogs from animal control facilities. Transmission is by inhalation or contact exposure to nasal and ocular secretions, urine, and feces from infected dogs. Transplacental transmission also occurs (18). Contaminated fomites, such as kennel-cleaning items, may carry the virus between and among dog colonies. Likewise, contaminated animal caretakers moving between colonies may transmit the infection. In the wild, CDV may infect other animal species, including many carnivores and omnivores (25). This concern may affect husbandry practices, for example, when ferrets or raccoons, both susceptible species, are also housed in the animal facility.

Clinical signs
Clinical signs of CDV infection are dependent on many host and viral factors. For example, dogs have an age-related immunity, seemingly dependent on the physiological maturity of the immune system (19). Also, CDV disseminates widely in the host; resulting in lesions in many different organ systems. Essentially any organ system may be involved. Lastly, viral hemagglutins differ, which determines cellular tropisms and cytopathogenicity (36). Therefore, clinical signs are variable, with up to 50% of cases subclinical (38). When present, signs range from unapparent to fatal. Most commonly, clinical signs appear 3 to 5 days postinfection, and include diphasic fever, ocular and nasal discharges, dry cough, anorexia, depression, vomiting, diarrhea, dehydration, respiratory distress, reduced litter sizes, dental discoloration, skin rash, hardening of the foot pads and nasal planum, muscle spasms, seizures and other central nervous system (CNS) signs, and death (38, 39). Nervous system, dental, and dermal signs generally occur weeks later in the course of the disease (26). Mortality ranges from 30 to 80%, and is highest among nonvaccinated animals, in unprotected puppies, and in cases complicated by pneumonia or encephalitis (26, 39).

Pathology
Following infection, CDV gains entry into target cells by binding to CD9, a cell-surface protein (20). CDV multiplies within T lymphocytes and macrophages in the bronchial lymph nodes and tonsils. Sequential waves of viremia and lymphatic invasion quickly spread virus throughout the body, where infection of mononuclear cells within virtually all body systems occurs. Dogs with adequate serum-neutralizing antibodies eliminate the virus and recover. Those lacking adequate antibody titers develop severe, even fatal infection (39). The lymphoreticular, enterohepatic, respiratory, nervous, and dermal systems are most affected. Secondary bacterial infections may follow infection, especially within the gastrointestinal system. Infection of, and damage to, mononuclear cells results in widespread tissue damage. Pathologic findings may therefore include bronchointerstitial pneumonia (23), encephalitis (14), metaphyseal osteopathy (3), dental enamel hypoplasia (5), cardiomyopathy (15), parathyroid degeneration (37), rhinitis,

pleuritis, optic neuritis, conjunctivitis, gastroenteritis, hyperkeratosis, and others (38). Infection of the CNS results in a progressive, demyelinating disease caused by down-regulation of myelin gene transcription (30). Brain cell tropisms differ among viral strains, and influence CNS effects (28). In utero or neonatal infection may result in fetal death or permanent immunodeficiency in surviving pups (18, 29). Immunity is both humoral and cellular, and is usually strong and long lasting (27), although some dogs develop chronic neurologic disease (31, 33, 34).

Interference with research
Infection of laboratory dogs with CDV would render dogs at least temporarily unusable for essentially all research purposes. Dogs recovering from infection may be utilized for some research applications, but the principal investigator should be warned that cytoarchitectural changes, including lymphoid hyperplasia, resulting from infection, may remain for several weeks. Host physiologic changes documented in CDV infection include depletion of lymphocytes (17), immune depression (33), leukopenia and thrombocytopenia (2), induction of cytokines (7, 12, 33), up-regulation of major histocompatibility complex (MHC) class II antigen expression (1), thymic hypoplasia (17), anemia (15), parathyroid dysfunction and hypocalcemia (37), increased arachidonic acid metabolism (9), hypogammaglobulinemia, and increased susceptibility to other pathogens (29, 39). However, as noted previously, virtually all body systems could be affected by CDV infection, rendering infected dogs unsuitable for research. In vitro cellular effects of CDV infection include induction of apoptosis (13), vacuolar degeneration (11), necrosis (40), syncytial cell formation (22), reorganization of cytoskeletal structures (16), and interference with the growth of other pathogens (10).

Diagnosis and control
CDV infection may be suspected on the basis of clinical signs, especially when "hard-pad disease" is noted. However, because of the variability of clinical symptoms, laboratory tests should be used to confirm the diagnosis. Confirmatory tests include virus isolation in cell culture, demonstration of viral antigen in conjunctival scrapings, and rising IgG titers (32). Newer methodologies, including RT-PCR will surely supplant older, less reliable, and more time-consuming methods of diagnosis (8, 21). Confirmed or suspected cases should be isolated immediately and treated symptomatically (38), or euthanized. Because virus may remain in protected sites following recovery (38), and thereby serve as a potential source of infection for other dogs, this author recommends euthanasia of all cases. Canine distemper is preventable by routine vaccination (39). Unless precluded by study needs, all incoming dogs should be immunized prior to arrival at the research facility, or should be isolated and immunized on arrival. Regular booster vaccinations should be a routine part of the colony management. CDV is relatively unstable in the environment, and is inactivated by temperature or pH extremes, light, and a variety of disinfectants including quaternary ammonium compounds, phenols, and bleach (39).

Parainfluenza virus type 2

Agent
Parainfluenza virus is an enveloped, ssRNA virus in the family *Paramyxoviridae*. Members of the family are grouped as morbilliviruses, paramyxoviruses, and pneumoviruses, on the basis of nucleocapsid size, presence or absence of neuraminidase, and antigenic relationships (27). Parainfluenza viruses belong to the paramyxovirus group, along with Newcastle disease virus. There are five serotypes of parainfluenza viruses causing upper respiratory disease in humans and animals. Canine parainfluenza virus is one member of the type 2 serotype group. While some consider that parainfluenza virus type 2 (PV2) may be identical to simian virus 5 (SV5) (14), others have conducted virus neutralization and other antigen-binding studies, and consider them

different (19, 21). Adding to the controversy, some consider human and canine isolates of SV5 to be nearly identical (3), while others report that they are antigenically distinct (20).

Epidemiology
PV2 is highly contagious (2, 5), and is transmitted by aerosol exposure or contact with contaminated fomites. In those cases where colony dogs are not vaccinated, such as when dogs are obtained from animal control facilities, it is typical for a large percentage of dogs to break with clinical signs within a week of the appearance of the first case.

Clinical signs
PV2 is one of several causes of acute tracheobronchitis ("kennel cough") in dogs (1). Clinical signs are generally not observed in vaccinated dogs. While clinical disease can be induced with PV2 alone, clinical signs are more severe when other pathogens, such as *Bordetella bronchiseptica,* are also present (2). Onset of clinical signs is acute, and generally includes fever, reduced appetite, variable lethargy, purulent nasal discharge, tonsillitis, and a harsh, nonproductive cough. The condition is self-limiting, and will resolve within 2 weeks if untreated. However, with treatment, most clinical signs resolve within about 3 to 4 days, leaving only a mild cough, which resolves within a week. In this author's experience, if clinical signs do not resolve, or broaden to include corneal changes, increases in clotting times, and/or a cyclic, nonresponsive fever, one should consider adenovirus or distemper virus infection in the differential diagnosis.

Pathology
Following infection, virus replicates in the epithelial cells of the upper respiratory tract, causing cellular necrosis and loss of ciliary clearing of the upper airways (27). Histopathologic changes can occur without the onset of clinical signs (24). Cellular damage and loss of ciliary function facilitate establishment of secondary invaders, such as *B. bronchiseptica,* resulting in the development of exudative pneumonia (7, 13). In at least one case, PV2 was isolated from the prostatic fluid of a dog (23). In another case, PV2 was isolated from the cerebrospinal fluid of a dog with neurologic signs. This isolate also induced encephalitis in experimentally infected pups (4, 8, 9). Typically, virus can be isolated from nasal secretions from 1 to 8 days after infection (27). Immunity is primarily cellular (26), although infected dogs develop pronounced antibody responses (22).

Interference with research
Canine PV2 has been shown to alter host physiology in a number of ways. These include altering olfactory function (15), compromising and/or altering pulmonary function (16, 18, 24, 25), increasing histamine responsiveness (11, 18), and inducing thromboxane production and release into brochoalveolar lavage fluid when coinfecting with *B. bronchiseptica* (17). Airway dysfunction appears to be associated with neutrophil infiltration (7). Clearly, infection of laboratory dogs with PV2 can alter studies involving the enterohepatic, nervous, and respiratory systems. Additional information is needed to determine whether infection with PV2 also interferes with studies involving the lymphoreticular system.

Diagnosis and control
Because there are several causes of kennel cough in dogs, a definitive diagnosis of PV2 cannot be made on clinical signs alone. Definitive diagnosis requires virus isolation or evaluation of rising serum antibody titers (6). These diagnostic steps are generally not necessary, as most of the causes of kennel cough respond similarly to antibiotics. As noted earlier, those not responding to routine treatments are likely due to other, more serious causes. Antibiotics such as chloramphenicol (still a great drug), sulfonamides, tetracycline, fluroquinolones, or cephalosporins tend to alleviate signs rapidly. Dogs with kennel cough should be immediately isolated to minimize the potential for spread within the research colony. However, given the highly contagious

nature of this disease, by the time clinical signs appear in the first case, other dogs within the colony may have already been exposed (5). Unless contraindicated by the research protocol, all dogs in the colony should be vaccinated annually against PV2 infection. PV2 is relatively unstable in the environment, and is therefore easily killed with a variety of common disinfectants. To the best of this author's knowledge, clinical signs associated with PV2 have not been reported in humans. However, on the basis of serologic surveys, humans may become infected with SV5 (10). Immune-compromised persons would be wise to exercise caution when working with infected dogs because it has not yet been determined with certainty that PV2 and SV5 are different viruses (12).

Parvovirus

Agent

Canine parvovirus (CPV) is a nonenveloped, ssDNA virus of the family *Parvoviridae* (29). Many features of the biology of this virus are similar to those of other parvoviruses, including Kilham rat virus and minute virus of mice, and some clinical features are shared with feline panleukopenia. Regarding the latter, it is widely accepted that the CPV initially associated with disease in dogs, CPV type 2, was actually a variant of feline panleukopenia virus (24). CPV type 2 has essentially disappeared from the dog population, and has been replaced with newer variants, designated CPV type-2a, type-2b, and type-2c (14, 25). Currently CPV type-2b predominates in the canine population (23, 24, 29). All of these variants replicate in cats (12, 14, 23).

Epidemiology

Canine parvoviral disease was first recognized in the United States in 1978, and in most other regions of the world soon thereafter (15, 29). Parvoviral disease is common in animal facilities. Outbreaks are especially high in breeding facilities containing large numbers of young, immunologically naive puppies. CPV is highly infectious, and is transported from one location to another with remarkable speed and ease. Transmission is fecal-oral, with infected dogs shedding virus in the feces for up to 10 days after the onset of clinical signs (29). Transmission is facilitated by direct contact, contaminated fomites, and biological vectors such as animal caretakers and, possibly, tissue culture (6).

Clinical signs

Severity of infection with CPV is strongly influenced by many factors, including age at exposure, level of maternal or actively acquired immunity, immune competence, concurrent infection, diet changes, stress level, and dog breed (23). Concerning the dog breed, clinical disease is more severe in the Doberman and rottweiler breeds. While these breeds are not traditionally used as purpose-bred research dogs, they may be obtained from animal control centers or class B dog dealers, and used for terminal experiments or teaching laboratories. When present, clinical signs are those of acute, severe enteritis, and include bloody diarrhea, dehydration, depression, anorexia, vomiting, and fever (10). The character and odor of the diarrhea is quite distinct, and often readily recognizable after experience with even a few cases. Dogs less than one year of age are more severely affected than adult dogs (23). Maternal immunity protects puppies from infection or lessens disease severity until about 8 to 12 weeks of age (23). Puppies less than about 4 weeks of age may develop myocarditis and accompanying pulmonary involvement, without enteric signs. In this case, puppies are lethargic, and death may occur secondary to ventricular fibrillation and pulmonary complications (13).

Pathology

Following an initial viremia, CPV replicates in the thymus, tonsils, retropharyngeal, mesenteric lymph nodes, spleen, bone marrow, and other tissues (13, 27, 29). Within a week of infection there is widespread colonization of intestinal mucosa. Colonization occurs most in the jejunum and ileum. Cellular entry is by endocytosis (26). The tissue distribution is typical of parvoviruses, and reflects a preference for tissues comprising rapidly dividing cells, such as cells in the hematopoietic, lymphoreticular, and enterohepatic systems. In this regard, CPV, like other parvoviruses, requires cells in the S phase of the cell division cycle for its replication (13). This is most pronounced in the young, where multiple tissues are growing, and in part explains why infections are more severe in puppies versus adult dogs. Virus is generally detected in the feces from days 3 to 12, with peak viral shedding occurring between days 4 and 7. However, virus has been detected in the feces as long as 22 days postinfection (13, 29). Grossly, affected bowel loops are thickened and hemorrhagic (10), while acute enteritis may also predispose dogs to intestinal intussusception (19). Local enteric lymph nodes are edematous and enlarged. In acute cases of myocarditis, white streaks occur in the myocardium, often accompanied by pulmonary edema (29). In just one report, CPV was considered the cause of canine erythema multiforme (5). Histopathologic lesions of enteritis include severe intestinal crypt necrosis and villus atrophy (10, 15). Epithelial regeneration occurs in those dogs that survive the acute phase (10). There is widespread lymphocyte destruction in the thymus and other lymphoid tissues. This may result in profound leukopenia consisting primarily of a relative lymphopenia, a diagnostic hallmark of CPV infection (10). Neutropenia is also frequently present (3). Secondary bacterial infections may result in septicemia and endotoxemia. Myocarditis is characterized by myocardial necrosis, mononuclear cell infiltration, and intranuclear inclusion bodies (1). Development of humoral immunity is rapid, pronounced, and persists for at least 24 months (13, 16, 29). Local secretory immunity appears to be more important than systemic immunity, and serves as the first line of defense against reinfection.

Interference with research
Little information is available which directly describes the effects of CPV on research involving dogs. It has been reported that CPV modulates immune responses to immunization against other pathogens (9). CPV also may induce a pronounced leukopenia (3, 10), tumor regression in experimental studies (28), leukoencephalomalacia secondary to myocardial lesions (1), cytokine production and release (4), hypercoagulability (17), and increased rates of apoptosis (2). CPV may also increase susceptibility to other pathogens, particularly those for which neutrophils are protective (20). Clearly, studies involving the cardiovascular, enterohepatic, hematopoietic, lymphoreticular, nervous, and respiratory systems will be profoundly affected by natural infection with CPV. Less commonly affected is the dermal system. Other organ systems may also be affected depending on age at infection. Lastly, studies wherein nutritional parameters are measured, outside of direct involvement of the enterohepatic system, will also be affected.

Diagnosis and control
With experience, a presumptive diagnosis can often be made on the basis of the history and clinical signs. However, laboratory confirmation is necessary to rule out other causes of bloody diarrhea, including infection with *Campylobacter jejuni* and other enteric pathogens. Antigen detection kits are useful for confirming the diagnosis early in the course of illness (22). Rapid confirmation is essential if appropriate control measures are to be instituted. Virus isolation, serology, histopathology, and immunochemistry are also useful but require more time. Newer methods such as PCR will likely become important diagnostic tools as well (11, 21). If at all possible, infected dogs should be immediately removed from the research colony and either euthanized, or nursed back to health. Where treatment is attempted, it should include, at a minimum, fluid and electrolyte replacement and broad-spectrum antibiotic coverage. The interested reader is referred elsewhere for treatment and vaccination recommendations (23). The non-enveloped nature of CPV renders it highly resistant to environmental stresses, including heat, pH extremes, dessication, and chemicals whose virucidal action involves destruction of

the envelope (7). CPV is inactivated by bleach (1:30) but not by quaternary ammonium compounds (8, 29). In this author's opinion, once a facility is contaminated with CPV, sporadic infections due to lingering environmental contamination may render the facility permanently unsuitable for housing dogs. Protective clothing worn while working with infected dogs or in contaminated areas should be thoroughly disinfected, or disposed of, along with all other contaminated material. To prevent entry of CPV into the facility, dogs should be obtained only from reputable vendors, and should be adequately immunized. Unfortunately, vaccines incorporating CPV type 2 may not induce adequate protection against the heterologous and more common strain CPV type-2b (18). In facilities that breed dogs for research use, infected pups should be isolated from other dogs to minimize opportunities for exposure. This is especially true during their most vulnerable period, from the waning of maternal antibody, until a protective immune response develops (13). Because CVP types 2a to 2c have been isolated from cats (12, 14), feral cats should be excluded from the animal facility.

BACTERIA

Bordetella bronchiseptica

Agent
First isolated in 1911, *Bordetella bronchiseptica* is an aerobic, motile, gram-negative rod commonly found inhabiting the ciliated respiratory epithelium of dogs and other animals (8). Isolates from several host species have been compared and grouped using a variety of parameters, including antigenic polymorphism (14), restriction enzyme analysis and ribotyping schemes (9, 13, 16), and pathogenicity (6, 11). It appears that little host specificity exists, although additional research is needed in this area (9). The interested reader is referred to chapters 6 and 10 for additional information concerning *B. bronchiseptica*.

Epidemiology
Subclinical infection with *B. bronchiseptica* is common in dogs, which therefore represent a significant reservoir of the pathogen. In addition, humans, as well as laboratory animals including rats, rabbits, cats, guinea pigs, primates, and swine, may serve as reservoirs for infection. Transmission is by aerosol, fomites, and contact.

Clinical signs
Most infections with *B. bronchiseptica* are subclinical. However, *B. bronchiseptica* is recognized as a primary pathogen, and is one of the more common causes of canine infectious tracheobronchitis ("kennel cough") in dogs (1, 15). In those cases, clinical signs include mucoid to mucopurulent nasal discharge, moist to hacking cough, occasional dyspnea in cases of pneumonia, and rarely, death (8). Clinical disease is more common in young pups (2, 3, 4). Infection may be complicated by concurrent infection with *Mycoplasma* spp., canine parainfluenza virus type 2, canine adenoviruses, and canine herpesvirus (8). Uncomplicated cases of bordetellosis recover without intervention in 1 to 2 weeks, although bacteria may be shed for up to 3 months (3, 4). Clinical cases respond rapidly to antibiotic therapy.

Pathology
Following infection, *B. bronchiseptica* colonizes the ciliated epithelium of the respiratory tract. Bacterial proliferation results in ciliary paralysis and inflammation. It should be noted that ciliostasis is dependent on the presence of bacterial somatic pili (6). Alterations to normal ciliary function facilitate infection with co-pathogens. *B. bronchiseptica* is capable of surviving inside phagolysosomes, and can escape into an endosomal compartment that does not fuse with a lysosome (8). Several virulence factors have been identified, including a dermonecrotic toxin, hemolysin, proteases, adenylate cyclase, hemagglutinins, a tracheal cytotoxin, somatic pili, and others (6, 8). The collective actions of these products in large

part explain the pathology induced by *B. bronchiseptica*. When present, typical pathologic changes of the lower respiratory tract are those of bronchitis, suppurative bronchopneumonia, and interstitial pneumonitis (2). Microscopically, there may be prominent peribronchial lymphocyte cuffing. Local humoral immunity develops by the fourth day postinfection, and is important for recovery (4, 7).

Interference with research
B. bronchiseptica is primarily a respiratory tract pathogen. Effects on host physiology include depression of respiratory clearance mechanisms through ciliostasis (5, 6), and alteration of alveolar macrophage and dendritic cell function (8, 18). Clearly, clinical bordetellosis would compromise the usefulness of laboratory dogs in respiratory studies, and may also influence studies involving the lymphoreticular system.

Diagnosis and control
Diagnosis of infection is based on clinical signs and recovery of the organism from transtracheal washes, nasal swabs, and oropharyngeal swabs cultured on blood or MacConkey agar (10). All *Bordetella* spp. are strict aerobes and are relatively easily grown. Affected dogs should be administered antibiotics such as tetracycline, chloramphenicol, clavulanate-potentiated amoxycillin, potentiated sulfonamides, or any of the fluoroquinolones; and kept well hydrated (17). A number of vaccines are available commercially. However, in this author's opinion, their routine use is unwarranted. *B. bronchiseptica* is easily killed by heat and commonly used disinfectants such as diluted bleach. Because humans are common carriers of *B. bronchiseptica* (12), and given the high prevalence of infection in dog colonies, it would be difficult and costly to develop and maintain a *Bordetella*-free dog colony, with little benefit in return.

Brucella canis

Agent
Brucella canis is one of six species of *Brucella*. *B. canis* is an obligate, slow-growing, gram-negative bacterial pathogen causing chronic disease in dogs and humans. All *Brucella* spp. are coccobacilli that can easily be mistaken for cocci. They most often appear singly but can also be found in pairs and clusters (22).

Epidemiology
Historically, *B. canis* infection has been considered common in the Americas, less so in Europe, and not present in the United Kingdom (6). The current prevalence of infection is unknown, but may still be regionally high. Therefore, this agent may occasionally gain access to research colonies if dogs are obtained from animal control facilities or from sources other than purpose-bred dog dealers. Transmission may be direct or indirect. Direct transmission occurs by ingestion, inhalation, congenital, or mucous membrane exposure to bodily fluids such as semen, urine, and other secretions (1, 19). Dogs most often become infected during breeding, or by contact with infectious tissues and fluids associated with abortions (22). Indirect transmission occurs when caretakers serve as vectors. Clearly, kennel environments facilitate the spread of infection. Canine body fluids can serve as primary sources of infection for humans (18).

Clinical signs
Most infections are subclinical, or are limited to signs of reproductive failure (2, 3). In this regard, clinical signs are often limited to the reproductive system. Male dogs present with scrotal swelling and reduced fertility (20). Also, scrotal pain induces frequent scrotal licking, which leads to local dermatitis. In one report, infection with *B. canis* reduced successful matings from 90% to 28.8%, and the number of pups produced per bitch per year decreased from 6 to 1.51 (15). Infected bitches may abort at 45 to 55 days of gestation. Less commonly, fetal resorptions, stillbirths, or the birth of weak pups may result (3). Some dogs recover spontaneously while others do not (14). In some cases, extragenital infection may be the first signs noticed, such as anterior uveitis.

Pathology

Following exposure, *B. canis* penetrates intact mucosal surfaces, such as the epithelium covering ileal Peyer's patches. Phagocytosis by macrophages and neutrophils quickly follows. Pathogen survival within these cells is facilitated by a variety of mechanisms, including inhibition of phagolysosome fusion, suppression of oxygen radicals, and production of stress proteins (22). Porins are protein components of the outer membrane that are thought to stimulate delayed-type hypersensitivity reactions (22). Infection localizes and amplifies in the regional lymph nodes. Thereafter, the agent disseminates by the blood to tissues of the lymphoid and reproductive systems (3). In this regard, both bacteremia (19) and tissue colonization (2) may be prolonged. Hematogenous dissemination has led to a number of unusual case reports (4, 5, 17). There is a generalized lymphoreticular response, leading to genitourinary tract infiltration (13). Lesions of the reproductive tract include placentitis, orchitis, and prostatitis. The pathogenesis of abortion is uncertain, but may involve circulatory changes, endotoxin, or fetal compromise. Aborted pups have bronchitis and bronchopneumonia (22). Extragenital infection may result in osteomyelitis (21), discospondylitis (9, 11), splenitis (2), nephritis and cystitis (14), meningoencephalitis (8), endocarditis (24), lymphocytic endophthalmitis, and anterior uveitis (6, 22). Effective immunity is primarily cellular, through cytokine-induced macrophage activation. Antibodies are also produced, but may be more detrimental than helpful. For example, production of IgG, IgM, and IgA autoantibody may facilitate infertility (7, 20).

Interference with research

Surprisingly little information is available on the effects of *B. canis* on host physiology. It has been reported that *B. canis* causes induction of IgA autoantibody (22), spermatozoal abnormalities (6), and altered lymphocyte responses (10). However, as noted previously, hematogenous dissemination may allow establishment of infection, lymphoreticular responses, and cytoarchitectural changes in a variety of tissues. At a minimum, natural infection of dogs with *B. canis* would interfere with studies involving the lymphoreticular and reproductive systems. In other cases, the cardiovascular, dermal, hematopoietic, musculoskeletal, nervous, reproductive, respiratory, and urinary systems may be affected. Concerning the reproductive system, for example, dogs continue to be a prime model for research involving the prostate. Such studies would clearly be altered as a result of infection with *B. canis*. It is also likely that *Brucella*-infected dogs may experience physiologic alterations in association with systemic infection. These changes would render affected animals unsuitable for use in research.

Diagnosis and control

B. canis infection may be diagnosed by culture, serology, animal inoculation, histopathology, and immunohistochemistry of target adult and fetal tissues (22). No one test has proven definitive, including serology (23). More recently, PCR assays have been developed for rapid identification (12). Special laboratory practices are required to culture and identify *B. canis,* and a *Brucella* reference laboratory should be consulted prior to sample collection. Historically, eradication of the pathogen has involved test and cull strategies (15, 16). When deciding on a course of action for affected dogs, economic and research value should be carefully weighed against zoonotic potential and difficulty of pathogen clearance. If infected dogs are to be retained, they should be neutered, if intact. Treatment is prolonged, and consists of antibiotic administration for up to 4 weeks. Even with such long treatment regimens, treatment failures are common (22). Prevention of disease consists of limiting dog purchases to those made from reputable vendors, serologic screening prior to inclusion in a breeding program, and physical examination of males (22). *B. canis* is relatively environmentally resistant, surviving particularly well in cold temperatures. Most disinfectants in use in animal facilities are effective against *B. canis*.

Campylobacter jejuni

Agent
Dogs may be infected with several members of the genus *Campylobacter*, including *C. jejuni*, *C. coli*, *C. helveticus*, *C. lari*, and *C. upsaliensis* (13, 20, 27). They are microaerophilic, gram-negative, motile, slender, curved rods. These bacteria are considered commensals of the oral cavity and genital and intestinal tracts. As such, they are viewed as opportunistic pathogens, causing disease only under certain conditions that upset the normal balance of intestinal flora (28). *C. jejuni* is the most important species, and is most commonly associated with disease in dogs. Multiple strains have been identified.

Epidemiology
C. jejuni infects a wide range of vertebrate hosts, including poultry, cats, cattle, and humans. This pathogen is found in human and animal populations worldwide. Prevalence of infection may be quite high in dog kennels (8, 28, 29) and in the stray dog population (6). Feces from symptomatic and asymptomatic dogs appear to be the primary source of infection for naive dogs. Transmission is fecal-oral, and may be direct or indirect. Direct transmission occurs when dogs consume contaminated feces. Indirect transmission occurs when dogs consume contaminated animal products, or are exposed to contaminated fomites or vectors.

Clinical signs
Most dogs infected with *C. jejuni* are asymptomatic. Stressors, such as overcrowding, unsanitary conditions, nutritional stress, and concurrent disease, may result in changes in the intestinal flora which facilitate overgrowth of *C. jejuni*. When this occurs, clinical signs are likely to follow. These may include a watery to mucoid, occasionally hemorrhagic or bile-streaked diarrhea; vomiting; depression; tenesmus; fever; inappetance; and an unkempt appearance (9, 10, 23, 25). Animals less than 6 months of age are most commonly affected (21). Affected dogs tend to recover within 5 to 15 days (10). Occasionally, the infection may become systemic (16). Clinical signs associated with systemic infection may vary, and can include abortion (3, 16, 22), or be absent altogether.

Pathology
Following infection, *C. jejuni* adheres to intestinal epithelial cells, multiplies locally, and then invades target cells. Toxins liberated by the bacteria facilitate invasion and disrupt cellular processes (31). Toxins and other virulence factors known or suspected of facilitating disease include cholera-like toxins, "heat-labile" toxins, cytotoxins, hemolysins, lipopolysaccharides, and adhesin molecules. The relationships of these virulence factors to disease continue to be explored (11, 15, 17, 26). There is a marked inflammatory response to the organism and its toxins, resulting in further mucosal epithelial disruption, cellular necrosis, and localized fluid imbalance. These pathogenic mechanisms result in diarrhea. At necropsy, gross lesions consist of congestion of colonic mucosa, fluid distension of the cecum, and mesenteric lymph node enlargement (16). Microscopic lesions are not always evident. When present, they consist of typhlitis and colitis, loss of goblet cells, attenuation and exfoliation of surface epithelium, glandular hypertrophy, and neutrophilic infiltration of the lamina propria (25). Immunity is primarily humoral, with all immunoglobulin classes induced. IgA is primarily involved in eliminating organisms within the intestine, while other immunoglobulin classes prevent or limit bacteremia (30, 31). Infection with *Campylobacter* spp. has been associated with the acute motor axonal neuropathy pattern of Guillain-Barré syndrome in people (14). Similar postinfection sequelae have not been reported in animals.

Interference with research
Few reports have described effects of *C. jejuni* on research involving dogs. When reports

from other host systems are also considered, it is found that *C. jejuni* causes leukocytosis (9), lymphocyte apoptosis (32), impaired fetal development (24), elevated eicosanoid and cAMP levels (5), and disruption of cell cultures (1, 2, 7, 11). Clearly, natural infection of research dogs with *C. jejuni* could interfere with studies involving the enterohepatic and hematopoietic, and under some conditions, the lymphoreticular and reproductive systems. In addition, studies in which growth or nutritional parameters are measured would also be affected.

Diagnosis and control
A diagnosis of campylobacteriosis may be suspected following direct examination or special staining of fecal smears. However, definitive diagnosis requires enzyme immunoassay or fecal culture (12). *Campylobacter* spp. require special conditions for growth and isolation (13). It is advisable to discuss sample processing with the diagnostic laboratory prior to collection of samples to ensure correct sample handling (19). More recently, fecal PCR assays have been developed (4). These provide a rapid means of diagnosis, without the problems of sample handling. Infected dogs with diarrhea should receive supportive treatment and antibiotic therapy. The interested reader is referred elsewhere for effective antibiotic regimens (18, 28). Recovered dogs may continue to shed the organism for long periods. The decision to cull affected dogs, or treat with antibiotics to more rapidly ameliorate clinical signs and possibly clear the infection (18), should be made with the research goals and risks of infection to humans and other animals in mind. It is unlikely that all dogs in the colony could be cleared with antibiotics, that *C. jejuni* could be completely eradicated from the facility, or that a *C. jejuni*-free colony could be maintained. In this author's opinion, the goal of antibiotic therapy should be limited to the amelioration of clinical signs and removal of a significant zoonotic hazard. Contaminated material should be disposed of in a manner that prevents exposure of personnel or other research animals. Caretakers should be instructed to follow strict personal hygiene and disinfection protocols when working around *C. jejuni* (28). *Campylobacter* spp. tolerate water and cold temperatures, but are sensitive to drying, direct sunlight, and many disinfectants (13).

FUNGI

Dermatomycosis

Agents
Dermatophytes are filamentous fungi capable of parasitizing keratinized structures such as the superficial skin, hair, and nails. Important structures of the parasitic stages include hyphae and arthroconidia, an asexual reproductive unit. Dermatophytes also exist in nonparasitic stages, for example, in culture. Important structures of the nonparasitic stage include septate, branching hyphae, collectively called mycelium; and asexual reproductive structures called conidia. The particular features of the conidia are diagnostic for individual species. Several species of dermatophytes have been isolated. Dogs may be infected with at least three species of dermatophytes. These include *Microsporum canis, M. gypseum,* and *Trichophyton mentagrophytes*. Of these, *M. canis* is the most common (8, 10).

Epidemiology
Globally, dermatophytes are extremely common. Warm, humid environments offer ideal conditions for survival (5). *M. canis* and *T. mentagrophytes* are zoophilic. That is, they have other animals as natural reservoirs. The natural reservoirs of *M. canis* and *T. mentagrophytes* are cats and rodents, respectively. *M. gypseum* is geophilic, with soil being the natural reservoir (3). It is unlikely that these reservoirs constitute significant sources of infection in the research colony. It is more likely that transmission is by exposure to other infected dogs. This may occur directly, as when dogs are turned out to exercise, or indirectly, through the common use of contaminated utensils (fo-

mites) such as brushes and combs (3). Humans can become infected with all three species affecting dogs, and may serve as an additional source of infection in the laboratory colony environment (12).

Clinical signs

Some dogs may be asymptomatic when infected with dermatophytes (5, 7). Clinical signs of infection are most common in dogs less than one year of age. Signs develop within about 3 weeks of infection, and include roughly circular areas of hair loss and scurfy, flaking skin. *T. mentagrophytes-* and *M. gypseum*-induced lesions may be more severe, spreading, and extensive, and include suppurative to crusty or erosive areas over large portions of the face or other regions. In these cases, inflammation may be pronounced. The common name designation "ringworm" arose out of the roughly circular shape of the lesion. Lesions are usually nonpruritic. Signs may abate spontaneously within a few weeks or months, though the organism persists in the tissues (3, 8). Failure of an infection to resolve may indicate a more serious condition, such as generalized immune suppression.

Pathology

Infectious spores enter through a defect in the skin. Following colonization and germination, hyphal strands grow out and invade adjacent hair follicles and the outer portions of associated hair shafts. Eventually, proteolytic enzymes are produced by the parasitic stages. These break down keratinized structures, facilitate invasion of adjacent skin, and incite inflammation. There are few lesions initially. Alopecia occurs due to increased fragility of the hairs. Later, there is hypertrophy of the stratum corneum, variable erythema, accelerated keratinization, and exfoliation (3). More severe reactions occur with *T. mentagrophytes,* and include vesiculopustular reactions, suppuration, and occasionally, granuloma formation (1). In uncomplicated cases of dermatomycosis, lesions generally regress as immunity develops. Immunity to dermatophytes is primarily cellular. Although antidermatophyte antibodies are detectable, they are not thought to play a functional role (3). Resistance to reinfection is variable.

Interference with research

Infection of laboratory dogs with dermatophytes would interfere with studies involving the skin. Besides causing dermal lesions, dermatophytes have been shown to affect total populations of skin flora (2). *T. rubrum,* another species of *Trichophyton* infecting humans, produces a mannan cell wall component that may locally inhibit lymphoproliferative responses (4). It is unknown whether similar, localized immune suppression occurs in dogs infected with other dermatophytes. In addition, a number of fungi have been shown to produce message molecules that have sequence homology with mammalian hormones (11). It is also unknown whether dermatophytes infecting dogs produce message molecules that interfere with host endocrine functions. Both of these questions warrant examination. Lastly, antifungal agents may also alter host physiology and interfere with research (6).

Diagnosis and control

Dermatomycosis may be suspected on the basis of clinical signs. Infection may be confirmed using a number of diagnostic tests (9). One method involves plucking a few hairs from lesion margins, and inoculating them into and onto special media, such as Sabouraud's agar, or Dermatophyte Test Medium (DTM). An alkaline reaction on a DTM plate suggests the presence of a dermatophyte. However, up to 3 weeks are required for growth of some isolates, so a definitive diagnosis by culture methods may be slow in coming. Also, culture methods are not highly reliable when serving as the sole diagnostic test, due to the occurrence of false positives and false negatives (10). Diagnosis may be more rapidly and reliably accomplished by microscopic examination of plucked hair shafts for hyphae and arthroconidia, following partial digestion with KOH on a heated glass slide (9). Lastly, diagnosis of *M. canis* infection may be facilitated by shining a Wood's light on a lesion and observing for green fluorescence. Most isolates of *M. canis* produce a tryptophan metabolite in vivo that fluoresces green under these conditions. Like direct microscopy, this method has high predictive value (10). Most dermatophytes respond well to combinations of systemic and topical antifungal agents. The interested reader is referred elsewhere for specific treatment recommendations (8). Affected dogs should be treated to reduce environmental contamination and zoonotic risk (12). Dermatophytes are susceptible to common disinfectants, including iodinated compounds and dilute bleach. Without chemical disinfection, dermatophytes may live several years in the environment (3). It is therefore recommended that contaminated items be disposed of or disinfected, and that contaminated facilities be thoroughly disinfected.

Malassezia pachydermatis

Agent
Malasezia pachydermatis, formerly referred to as *Pityrosporum canis* or *P. pachydermatis*, is a yeast commonly found on the skin and mucous membranes of dogs and many other animals. Humans may also become infected (7). *M. pachydermatis* is most commonly found in the external ear canal, interdigital skin, the haired skin of the lip region, and the anal mucosa (6). Multiple strains of *M. pachydermatis* have been described (1, 12).

Epidemiology
Because *M. pachydermatis* is considered a commensal organism, dog-to-dog transmission is not considered important or necessary for development of disease. However, the author is familiar with at least one case in which a dog that had never developed *M. pachydermatis* otitis externa, did so only after being housed in a particular kennel. It was thought that the dog may have encountered a more virulent strain of yeast, been unusually stressed, or was exposed to numbers of yeast that were sufficient to overcome resistance. Lastly, *M. pachydermatis* has been demonstrated on the exoskeleton of *Sarcoptes scabiei*, indicating that mites may serve as mechanical vectors for the yeast (21). However, this route of transmission should not be of concern in a well-managed animal facility.

Clinical signs
M. pachydermatis is considered a commensal under normal conditions. As such, clinical signs are not observed. Factors that trigger clinical episodes are poorly understood, but likely include host, pathogen, and environmental factors. Some host factors might include underlying immunologic or endocrine disorders, stress, concurrent infectious or noninfectious skin disease, recent antibiotic therapy, breed, anatomical conformation, and lipid production in the external ear canal (2, 4, 14, 19). Some of these factors have a genetic basis. Dogs with allergic skin disease are especially prone to *M. pachydermatis* dermatitis (18), while dogs with poorly draining ears are especially prone to otitis externa (14). Environmental factors include temperature and humidity, with warm, humid environments favoring expansion of yeast populations. Clinical disease most commonly presents as otitis externa, and less commonly as generalized dermatitis of the face, ventral neck, axillae, groin, interdigital skin, and other skin locations that remain warm and moist (2).

Pathology
As noted above, *M. pachydermatis* is normally considered a commensal organism. The factors promoting transition to opportunistic infection are poorly understood. When clinical disease occurs, affected external ear canals are pruritic, malodorous, and exudative. Canine cerumen seems to promote the growth of *M. pachydermatis* (9). This is relevant because adherence of *M. pachydermatis* to cornified epithelial cells of the skin is mediated by lipid (15). Other affected body parts are characterized by erythema, alopecia, scaly or greasy ex-

udation, mild to severe pruritus, and a foul odor. If the condition persists, hyperpigmentation and thickening of the skin occur. Rarely, *M. pachydermatis* may cause obstruction of the lacrimal canaliculus (20). Affected dogs frequently have concurrently increased populations of *Staphyloccus* spp. and *Pseudomonas aeruginosa* (10). The presence of these pathogens complicates the establishment of a cause relative to dermatitis. *M. pachydermatis* produces numerous enzymes, including esterase, proteinase, phospholipase, hyaluronidase, and chondroitin sulfatase (8, 13). It is not known what roles, if any, these enzymes play in pathogenesis. Immunity to *M. pachydermatis* is primarily cellular, although anti-*M. pachydermatis* antibodies are detectable (3). In predisposed dogs, these reactivities may contribute to immune-related dermatitis, including atopy (17).

Interference with research

There is virtually no information directly implicating *M. pachydermatis* as an unwanted research variable. However, it is known that *M. pachydermatis* alters normal microbial flora (10), activates macrophages and prolongs survival of mice implanted with tumors (22, 23), and accentuates type-1 hypersensitivity reactions (18). Therefore, the presence of clinical mycosis caused by *M. pachydermatis* could alter research involving the lymphoreticular system, and would certainly alter dermatologic studies in general, and studies of skin microflora in particular. Also, behavioral changes induced by pruritus could invalidate studies in which behavioral parameters are important. Lastly, secondary bacterial infections could interfere with research in a variety of areas, including those involving local immunity. The interested reader is referred to chapter 2 for information on potential effects of bacterial pathogens commonly associated with dermatitis.

Diagnosis and control

M. pachydermatis may be diagnosed by cytological examination of stained swab material or tape preparations (11, 16). The stained sample should be examined for organisms with the characteristic "shoe print" or "peanut" shape, typical of budding yeasts. When evaluating numbers of organisms recovered one must consider the body location from which the sample was obtained. For example, lip folds and interdigital skin normally harbor larger yeast populations than do the axillae and groin (5, 6, 11). These population differences highlight the need to evaluate yeast numbers before and after treatment. This approach will aid in case management. Treatment is aimed at reducing yeast populations, and addressing any underlying conditions that may have allowed for the transition from commensal to opportunistic pathogen (16). Poorly draining ears may need to be corrected surgically. Cases of otitis externa not requiring surgery may be successfully treated with topical combinations of antifungal, antibiotic, and anti-inflammatory compounds (10). For more generalized dermatitis, products that cleanse, degrease, and dry the skin are likely to be effective therapies for dermatitis. One of these includes 2% miconazole plus 2% chlorhexidine shampoo applied every 3 days. However, it is unlikely that even the best treatments will eradicate *M. pachydermatis* from a colony.

PARASITES

Demodex canis

Agent

Demodex canis is a member of the family Demodicidae. These mites live in the hair follicles and sebaceous glands of various mammals. Parasites that occur in different hosts are generally considered different species. *Demodex* spp. are elongate, and have a head, thorax which bears four pairs of short legs, and an elongate abdomen that is transversely striated. Life-cycle stages consist of egg, larva, protonymph, deutonymph, and adult. The entire life cycle is spent on the host, and is completed in 18 to 24 days. Parasite stages develop deep in the hair follicles or sebaceous glands, depending somewhat on species. Males are generally found at the skin surface, while the females are often found in the hair follicle. Adults feed on epithelial cells and skin detritus. Larvae and nymphs move along with the sebaceous flow to the mouth of the follicle, where they mature (1).

Epidemiology
D. *canis* is considered a commensal organism, and is globally distributed in the canine population. Infestation occurs within a few hours of birth (10). As a result, dog-to-dog transmission later in life is not considered important, since the majority of dogs carry the organism. The occurrence of disease caused by D. *canis* is regionally distributed within the United States, and is highest in southern regions (21). More recently, a shorter form of *Demodex* mite (D. *cornei*) (20, 22), and an unnamed long-bodied species (20) have also been recovered from dogs on several continents. However, patterns of clinical disease and response to treatment appear to be similar to those of D. *canis* (20).

Clinical signs
D. *canis* preferentially infests the skin of the muzzle, the skin around the eyes, and the extremities (1). Considering that most, if not all, dogs carry D. *canis,* clinical disease is uncommon. Factors predisposing for disease include young age (<1 year), poor condition, short hair, concurrent infection with other pathogens, hyperadrenocorticism, excessive use of drying shampoos, and genetic predisposition to immune suppressive conditions (1, 7, 9, 16, 24, 25). Immune dysfunction reflects an inability to mount an effective cell-mediated immune response. The majority of cases of canine demodicosis are classified as localized or generalized, with the localized form roughly twice as common as the generalized form (16). The localized form most often occurs in puppies, and presents as erythema and alopecia around the eyes and mouth, and over bony projections on the extremities (20). Lesions are nonpruritic. The prognosis for localized demodicosis is good. Spontaneous recovery generally occurs around the time of sexual maturity. In some cases, infestation becomes generalized. In these cases, secondary bacterial infection occurs, resulting in abscess or pustule formation. Generalized demodicosis occurs in both young (<1 year old) and older (>5 years old) dogs (7). Affected dogs develop widespread alopecia; and the skin becomes coarse, dry, and erythematous (20). Pustules break open and ooze. Dogs so affected are malodorous. Prognosis for generalized demodicosis is guarded for all ages of dog affected. On occasion, dogs develop other forms of demodicosis, including pododermatitis (7) and otitis externa (4). Extremely severe cases of mite infestation rarely result in death due to toxicosis or emaciation.

Pathology
There is no association between the different clinical forms of demodicosis and the histopathologic character of associated lesions (7). Differences lie mainly in degree of skin involvement. In the localized form, the hair follicles are distended with mites and cellular debris. Histologically, there is follicular epithelial atrophy, nodular dermatitis, hyperkeratosis, perifolliculitis, and exfoliation. The hair becomes fragile and so is split or shed. Sebaceous glands may atrophy or hypertrophy (7). The generalized form is essentially the localized form but widespread, and with pyoderma. The secondary bacterial component is frequently *Staphylococcus* spp., *Pseudomonas aeruginosa,* gram-positive cocci, *Malassezia pachydermatis,* and others (7). Bacterial infection is followed by infiltration of neutrophils, cytotoxic T lymphocytes, and plasma cells, resulting in suppurative dermatitis, perifolliculitis, and furunculosis (6, 7). The number of mites in the skin is proportional to the severity of lesion development. Immunity is cellular, and involves $CD3^+$ $CD8^+$ (cytotoxic) T lymphocytes (6).

Interference with research
Dogs with generalized demodicosis have been shown to have increased concentrations of circulating immune complexes (8), reduction of

circulating $CD4^+$:$CD8^+$ cell ratio (6), stimulation of cytokine production (15), activation of epidermal Langerhans cells expressing MHC class II antigens (7), suppressed neutrophil chemotaxis (14), and suppressed in vitro reactivity of peripheral lymphocytes to mitogen (2, 11, 13, 17). It is not completely known which of these are due to the bacterial component of the infection, versus *D. canis*. In this regard, suppression of in vitro reactivity of lymphocytes to mitogens and other indicators of immune dysfunction have been shown to be due to the accompanying pyoderma (3, 23). Interestingly, similar immune suppression has on occasion been reported with localized demodicosis (18), where one would not expect bacteria-induced suppression. Lastly, acaracidal preparations used for the treatment of demodicosis may themselves alter host physiology. For example, amitraz has been shown to induce hyperglycemia in part by inhibiting insulin release (12). Studies involving the dermal and lymphoreticular systems would be profoundly affected by generalized, and possibly to a lesser extent, by localized demodicosis.

Diagnosis and control

Diagnosis is by direct examination of deep skin scrapings and sebaceous or pustule material for large numbers of mites. Scrapings should be deep enough to include the hair follicle, and so should cause some capillary oozing (20). Consistent recovery of only low numbers of mites should make one cautious in ascribing the clinical symptoms to *D. canis*. While resolution of advanced cases may be difficult, effective treatment regimens have been reported. These include amitraz solutions, high-dose ivermectin, and high-dose milbemycin (19, 20). Apparent treatment failure is often due to improper use of acaricidal compounds, or concurrent underlying disease (5).

Dirofilaria immitis (heartworm)

Agent

Dirofilaria immitis is a filarial nematode parasite causing potentially severe disease in dogs. *D. immitis* infects a range of mammalian hosts, including dogs, ferrets, cats, and humans. Disease severity is greatest in ferrets and cats, while humans are a "dead-end" host. Lesions of *D. immitis* infection in humans are often misdiagnosed as neoplasia (25, 26).

Epidemiology

D. immitis is endemic to most warm regions of the world. In the United States, the range of *D. immitis* has been steadily expanding over the past decades, and now includes most regions of the country where there is appreciable rainfall. The life cycle is somewhat complex, and requires about 6 months for completion. Embryonic forms, termed microfilaria, are ingested with the blood meal of a mosquito feeding on an infected dog. Development to the third-stage larva (L_3) occurs in the Malpighian tubules of the mosquito. The L_3 migrate to the salivary glands of the mosquito where they await the taking of another blood meal. On feeding by the mosquito, the L_3 gain entry into the next dog. Larvae develop through to the L_5 (young-adult) stage in the skin and connective tissues. Young-adult worms then migrate to the pulmonary arteries, presumably through the venous circulation. After a prepatent period of 6 to 7 months, sexually mature adults mate and microfilaria are once again released into the blood. Adult worms may live 5 years or more (2), and microfilaremia has been documented to extend up to 7.5 years from a single infection (20). Several species of mosquitoes are suitable intermediate hosts, although the number that actually play a significant role in the epidemiology of the disease is rather small. However, this mosquito host tolerance contributes to the wide geographic range of the parasite. While transmission of *D. immitis* occurs primarily through the bite of an infected mosquito, transplacental transmission has occasionally been reported (29). The transplacental route, however, is not considered clinically relevant.

Clinical signs

Clinical signs are absent during the prepatent period, and in dogs infected with only about

25 worms. As the worm burden increases to about 50, evidence of infection becomes apparent. The first clinical sign noted is exercise intolerance and cough, brought on by physical occlusion of pulmonary arteries. Greater worm burdens result in respiratory distress. Affected dogs appear lethargic and unthrifty. Overwhelming infections may result in signs compatible with liver failure, such as abdominal distension, weight loss, and icterus (12). Postcaval occlusion causes acute collapse and death (8). A number of case reports exists describing unusual presentations of dirofilariasis, including formation of skin nodules (23), posterior paralysis or paresis (4, 27), muscular weakness (30), depression (4), mucocoele (14), pneumothorax (3), hindlimb lameness (10), CNS dysfunction (7, 21), and possibly a cutaneous syndrome (24).

Pathology
Pathologic changes are most evident in the heart, alveoli, and pulmonary vasculature, and consist of pulmonary endarteritis, intimal proliferation, alveolar septal thickening, eosinophilic pneumonia, and obstructive fibrosis (5, 18, 28). These lead to pulmonary hypertension, tricuspid regurgitation, right heart enlargement and eventual failure. Vascular damage and inflammation are exacerbated by dead worm emboli (28). In addition, microfilaria may obstruct virtually any capillary bed. Chronically elevated pulmonary hypertension leads not only to right heart failure, but also to back pressure on the liver and kidneys, with hepatomegaly, centrilobular necrosis, ascites, renal hemosiderosis, hemoglobinuric casts, and death (8, 18). Immune complex formation or immune-mediated destruction of microfilaria may result in pulmonary immune complex deposition, glomerulonephritis, and anemia (9, 13, 28, 30). On occasion, larval or adult heartworms are found in aberrant locations, including cerebral, femoral, iliac, popliteal, and testicular arteries (4, 16, 21, 27), skin (23), salivary duct (14), hindlimb peripheral vasculature (10), abdominal aorta and liver (12), peritoneal cavity (1), lateral ventricle and brain (4, 7, 18), renal tubules (6), and eye (15, 16). The capacity for the worm to migrate to or develop in these aberrant locations allows for the potential development of pathologic changes in a wide range of organs. Immunity to *D. immitis* is primarily humoral, and is relatively slow in developing (11).

Interference with research
Alterations in host physiology brought about by *D. immitis* include pulmonary hypertension and an accelerated pulmonary hypertensive response to hypoxia (22), generation of circulating immune complexes (19), and alteration of hepatic enzyme levels, leukocytosis, and anemia (12, 16). Infection with *D. immitis* clearly would interfere with research involving the cardiovascular, hematopoietic, hepatobiliary, lymphoreticular, respiratory, and urinary systems. Less commonly affected systems include the dermal, musculoskeletal, nervous, and reproductive. Immune-mediated destruction of microfilaria, as well as worm development in aberrant locations, may occur in many organs, widening the potential scope of organ involvement and further compromising the usefulness of the dog as a research subject. Lastly, studies in which exercise or activity levels are to be measured would likely be altered.

Diagnosis and control
Diagnosis may be approached using several methods, depending on the clinical condition of the dogs involved. The interested reader is referred to other sources for extensive discussions of heartworm diagnosis (2). In brief, examination of the blood for microfilaria provides direct evidence of infection. This can be done by examining the buffy coat of a spun microhematocrit sample, or by performing a "Knott's" test. Care must be taken to differentiate *D. immitis* from *Dipetalonema reconditum,* a nonpathogenic filarial nematode. False-negative tests are common. These may result from prepatency, mild or single-sex infections, or immune clearance of microfilaria. Commercially available antigen detec-

tion kits are generally reliable and technically simple, although they suffer from some of the same limitations as direct methods. Thoracic radiography is useful for evaluating the clinical severity of infection, since pathognomonic radiographic lesions are often discernable. Elimination of infection presents considerable risk to the dog, as dying microfilaria and adult worms may result in hypersensitivity reactions and/or embolic events. The interested reader is referred to other sources for discussions of treatment approaches and risks (2). Infection with *D. immitis* can be avoided by incorporating chemoprophylaxis into the facility's standard operating procedures. Several highly effective chemoprophylactic compounds are available, including the avermectins. These are generally given once per month. More recently, moxidectin, given as a sustained-release formulation at 0.17 mg/kg has been effective at preventing establishment of infection for up to 180 days (17). Heartworm infection is easily prevented, and yet can render valuable dogs unsuitable for research. Therefore, all research dogs with outside access should be on a heartworm-prevention regimen.

Fleas

Agent

Fleas belong to the order *Siphonaptera*. They are ectoparasites of dogs and other animals, including humans. Fleas are wingless, laterally flattened, blood-feeding insects. Body segments include a head, thorax, and abdomen. Species are differentiated by such morphologic characteristics as the shape of the head, and the presence and features of genal and pronotal "combs," found on the head. Life-cycle stages consist of egg, three larval stages, pupa, and adult. The life cycle is completed in as little as 14 days under optimal conditions. Larval fleas feed on skin detritus, and on the feces of adult fleas, which consist primarily of digested host blood. Adult fleas can survive for several weeks without a blood meal. The flea most commonly found infesting dogs is the cat flea, *Ctenocephalides felis*. Less commonly, *C. canis* is found on dogs. Fleas of other hosts, such as the "Sticktight" flea of poultry, *Echidnophaga gallinacea,* rarely may infest dogs, but this and other less common flea species are unlikely to be encountered in the laboratory animal environment.

Epidemiology

Flea infestation can be a common problem in many laboratory animal facilities housing dogs. Fleas exhibit little host specificity, allowing for infestation to become established from a variety of sources. Fleas gain access to the colony when unconditioned dogs are brought into the facility, on the clothing of caretakers that own infested dogs, or rarely, on other host species. Fleas serve as intermediate hosts of the dog tapeworm, *Dipylidium caninum,* and the filarial nematode, *Dipetalonema reconditium*. In addition to these, fleas serve as biologic vectors of a number of more rare, but important diseases. (1).

Clinical signs

Even large populations of fleas may be well tolerated by some dogs. In contrast, dogs that are prone to hypersensitivity reactions to flea saliva react strongly to the bites of even a few fleas. In these animals, clinical signs include intense pruritus with associated frequent scratching, general agitation, loss of condition, reduced feed intake, weight loss, and a characteristic pattern of hair loss over the tail head and dorsum. Secondary bacterial infections may occur as a result of self-excoriation. Young pups may show signs of blood-loss anemia, including pale mucous membranes, poor condition, failure to thrive, and occasionally, death.

Pathology

Dermatitis is associated with hypersensitivity reactions, excessive scratching, and secondary bacterial infections. Immediate, delayed, and cutaneous basophil hypersensitivity reactions occur at bite sites (7). Fleas produce a number of biologically active salivary substances, such as diphosphohydrolases, esterases, and antigens (3, 4, 6, 8, 10). Additional pathologic findings include hyperpigmentation, scale formation, and pyoderma (9).

Interference with research
There are no reports, of which this author is aware, concerning alterations in host physiology that directly affected research. However, because flea infestation has been documented to directly or indirectly alter cytoarchitecture and/or function of the dermal and lymphoreticular systems, studies involving these organ systems would certainly be affected. In addition, studies in which behavioral or metabolic parameters are measured would also be affected. Also, studies involving the enterohepatic system might be affected because of pruritus-induced decreases in food intake. Lastly, transmission of *D. caninum* or *D. reconditum* would further compromise dogs as research subjects. For these reasons, fleas should be excluded from the research colony. Also, flea control is an important component of an institution's Occupational Health and Safety Program. Not only is *C. felis* zoonotic and a nuisance, but some humans with asthma experience severe reactions to flea allergens.

Diagnosis and control
Flea infestation is suspected when characteristic clinical signs are observed. The reader is directed to chapter 8 for a complete discussion of diagnostic methods. In brief, diagnosis is accomplished by finding flea dirt or fleas on dogs or in the immediate environment. In addition, a diagnosis of *D. caninum* or *D. reconditum* infection indicates a history of recent flea infestation. A number of newer and safer ectoparasiticides are available for eliminating fleas from a dog colony (2, 11). Unfortunately, these do not include most avermectin derivatives (12). Also, fleas must still feed to be affected by insecticides. The advent of "once-a-month" treatments has markedly reduced the prevalence of fleas in many areas. The interested reader is directed elsewhere for a complete discussion of flea-control strategies (1). The reader is reminded that it is essential to treat all dogs simultaneously, whether symptomatic or not, and to disinfect the environment at the same time. Apparent treatment failures are common, and are often due to the failure to adequately treat all host and environmental locations where flea life-cycle stages may be found (5). It is especially important to clean cracks and crevices in the environment, and to clean or destroy bedding. Severely affected pups may require supportive therapy such as blood transfusions, supplemental iron therapy, and dietary supplementation. Prevention of flea infestation involves testing or treatment of all dogs prior to entry into the facility, purchase of dogs from reputable vendors, and education of caretaker and scientific staff concerning the risks of transmitting fleas from pet dogs to research colony dogs.

Intestinal nematodes

Agents
Dogs housed in laboratory environments are susceptible to a plethora of gastrointestinal nematodes. However, husbandry practices in a modern research facility preclude completion of multiple host life cycles, thereby eliminating a large number of potential pathogens. The interested reader is referred to any standard veterinary parasitology text for a more complete presentation of parasites infecting dogs. This discussion is limited to intestinal nematodes most likely to be found in the research colony. Most commonly, these include the "hookworms," *Ancylostoma caninum, Ancylostoma braziliense,* and *Uncinaria stenocephala;* the ascarids, or "roundworms," *Toxocara canis* and *Toxascaris leonina;* and the "whipworm," *Trichuris vulpis.* For this discussion these parasites will be considered as a group, although important features particular to specific worms will be mentioned. Adult worms are readily identified using morphologic features described in standard veterinary parasitology reference texts (2). All hookworms infecting dogs have a large buccal cavity bearing

"teeth" or cutting plates, depending on the species. Ascarids have three "lips" and lateral alae or wing-like structures near their anterior end. Whipworms have a long, slender anterior end and a stouter, shorter, posterior region. Eggs from these nematodes are also readily identifiable, although an ocular micrometer is of great value for hookworm egg identification, because the various species exhibit similar appearances but differ in size. It is important to properly assign these parasites to species because of significant differences in pathogenicity and transmission strategies. This is especially true for the ascarids.

Epidemiology
Infection with hookworms occurs by ingestion or skin penetration of infective larvae. Larvae migrate extensively during development until arriving at the small intestine where they mature to the adult stage. Transmission may also occur during nursing of pups, after inhibited larvae in the bitch are mobilized from skeletal muscle and migrate to the intestine, where they develop to adults, or to the mammary glands where they are passed in the milk. The latter is especially significant in the last 2 weeks of pregnancy. Lastly, transmission may occur through consumption of paratenic hosts. Developing larvae undergo a pulmonary migration before developing to adulthood in the small intestine. Infection with ascarids occurs by ingestion of infectious, embryonated eggs, by ingestion of paratenic hosts, and for *T. canis*, by transmammary and transplacental transmission (3, 6). *T. canis*, but not *T. leonina*, migrates through somatic tissues, including the lungs, liver, and others, where they may encyst. Encysted larvae appear to be impervious to host immunity, possibly because of local immune suppression by *T. canis* excretory/secretory products (5). The migratory fate of *T. canis* larvae is profoundly affected by the age and exposure history of the host. Both species eventually mature to adulthood in the small intestine. Infection with *T. vulpis* occurs by consumption of embryonated eggs. Larvae develop within the wall of the large intestine, and emerge as adult worms. Other than *T. vulpis*, the intestinal nematodes discussed here are all very prolific egg layers. Therefore, large numbers of infective stages can build up in the animal facility if suitable substrates are available, such as loose, sandy soil, and if appropriate sanitation is not practiced. Ascarid and trichurid eggs remain viable for several years under optimal conditions. Coprologic surveys indicate that ascarid infections are more common in intact versus neutered dogs, and in young dogs up to about 6 months of age. In contrast, coprologic evidence of hookworm and whipworm infections peak around one year of age and decline thereafter (1, 8).

Clinical signs
For each of these intestinal nematodes, clinical signs are seen when large numbers of parasites are present, although some species may cause clinical disease with relatively fewer worms. Among the hookworms, *A. caninum* is most pathogenic, causing severe blood loss, especially in pups. In fact, transmammary inoculations of even 50 to 100 larvae represent overwhelming infections in newborn pups (2). In these cases, pups appear healthy for about a week, then decline rapidly to death. Pups are very pale and have soft, dark feces. The latter is due to intestinal blood loss. Older dogs exposed to high numbers of infective larvae develop an acute condition characterized by signs of anemia, poor hair coat, decreased weight gain or weight loss, lethargy, and occasionally, death. Chronic infections may present with few if any clinical signs other than anemia, unless the dog decompensates under the added stress of another, concurrent medical condition (2). In contrast, *U. stenocephala* is least significant, causing less pathology and consuming less blood. Among the ascarids, *T. canis* is much more pathogenic than *T. leonina*, primarily because *T. canis* undergoes extraintestinal migration during development. Clinical signs may include poor growth, weight loss, diarrhea, dehydration, vomiting, rough hair coat, a "pot-bellied" appearance, gastrointestinal discomfort, and pale

mucous membranes (6). Infection with *T. vulpis* is usually asymptomatic. However, heavy infections may cause intermittent mucoid to bloody diarrhea and weight loss.

Pathology
Pathologic changes associated with intestinal nematode infection are due to either direct intestinal damage, including focal enteritis and blood consumption by the adult worms, or to tissue damage during larval migration for those species that migrate. Extraintestinal visceral lesions may occur in virtually any organ, but are most common in the lungs and liver of dogs with ascariasis. Associations between hookworm infection and biliary carcinoma, and between *T. canis* infection and biliary angiocholitis have been suggested (4, 7). Immunity to all of these nematode infections is primarily humoral. Induction of IgE and immediate hypersensitivity reactions are reflected in white blood cell profiles, and may result in peracute expulsion of a large percentage of infecting worms. Again, this is particularly the case for ascarid infections, where immunity is attained by about 6 months of age. Hookworm and whipworm infections are more often retained into adulthood.

Interference with research
There is an enormous volume of literature on the physiologic effects of intestinal nematode infections in various host species, most prominently, swine, rodents, and humans. Somewhat surprisingly, a paucity of information exists describing the physiologic effects of canine intestinal nematodiases. Depending on the specific parasite involved, canine nematode infection may result in anemia, enteritis, eosinophilia, alterations in serum chemistries, pneumonitis, pulmonary vascular changes, histamine release, and dermatitis (2). Effects reported in other intestinal host-parasite systems should be applied to the dog with caution. Infection with the intestinal nematodes discussed could clearly alter research involving the cardiovascular, dermal, enterohepatic, hematopoietic, lymphoreticular, reproductive, and respiratory systems; and influence studies measuring behavior, weight gain, and other aspects of host metabolic activity.

Diagnosis and control
Infection may be suspected based on clinical and clinicopathologic indicators. Definitive diagnosis is based on identification of eggs in fecal examinations, or on recovery of adult worms at necropsy. Intestinal nematode infections can be treated with a number of anthelmintic compounds. The interested reader is referred to any current veterinary parasitology text or formulary for specific drugs and dosages. Special efforts must be expended to address the problem of contaminated environments, especially outdoor environments contaminated with ascarid or whipworm eggs. Control is based on screening and/or treatment of dogs prior to admission into the animal facility. Prior to purchase of dogs from a vendor, medical histories should be requested and examined to gain a sense of whether the dogs are likely harboring encysted larvae. Strongyles and ascarids will infect humans but will not reach patency. Regardless, zoonotic infection can cause serious disease in humans. Therefore, personnel working with infected dogs should protect themselves from accidental infection through the wearing of proper personal protective clothing, and the washing of hands following handling of infected dogs or their waste. Ascarid eggs are particularly "sticky," and are thus easily moved about a facility on clothing, cleaning utensils, etc.

Intestinal protozoa

Agents
Dogs may be found infected with a number of intestinal protozoa, including *Isospora canis, Isospora ohioensis, Neospora caninum, Giardia duodenalis,* and others (3). Except for *G. duodenalis,* a mucosoflagellate, all of these belong to the Subphylum Apicomplexa, and share many biological similarities. Apicomplexan parasites infect the intestinal mucosal epithelium, where they undergo multiple rounds of

asexual cell division, destroying infected cells with the release of each round of progeny. This is followed by sexual multiplication. Oocysts are released in the feces, and after sporulation, are infective to another host. *G. duodenalis* is morphologically similar to a number of *Giardia* isolates, each recoverable from a different mammalian host. It is questionable that they all represent separate species. It appears more likely that there are fewer species, with wider host ranges. For the purposes of this discussion, the name *G. duodenalis* is used to describe the morphologic type found in dogs, cats, ruminants, humans, and other mammals. Extracellular trophozoites inhabit the surfaces of intestinal mucosal epithelial cells. Trophozoites usually form infectious, environmentally resistant cysts prior to being passed with the feces.

Epidemiology
Among the many protozoa of dogs, laboratory colonies most commonly harbor *Isospora* spp. and *G. duodenalis*. Pups are infected within the first weeks of life. Transmission is fecal-oral. Considering the environmental resistance of infectious forms, even mildly contaminated kennels facilitate maintenance of infection within the colony. In the case of *G. duodenalis*, other mammalian hosts may serve as sources of infection for dogs. However, contact among different host species should not occur in laboratory animal settings, and so this source of infection should not play a significant role. Transmission patterns of *N. caninum* appear to be more complex and not completely understood. The primary route of transmission appears to be transmammary (5). However, additional research is needed to elucidate the significance of this and other potential routes.

Clinical signs
Most protozoan infections are asymptomatic. Clinical effects appear to be directly correlated with parasite burden. However, not all of the parasites named are equally pathogenic, and so the number of parasites needed to induce clinical signs differs with species. When present, clinical signs are generally confined to the intestinal tract, or are related to intestinal dysfunction. Affected dogs lose weight or fail to gain weight, have poor hair coats, and exhibit diarrhea of various character (6). Diarrhea caused by Apicomplexa is often watery, and may include blood, while diarrhea induced by *G. duodenalis* is often malodorous, fatty and of a "cow pie" consistency. Clinical signs of giardiasis may begin as early as 5 days postinfection, while onset of signs compatible with coccidiosis appear shortly thereafter. It should be remembered that diagnostic stages may not appear in feces for a week or more after signs begin, since intestinal damage may occur as a result of early life-cycle stages, well before the point of fecal shedding. Diarrhea caused by coccidia may be acute or persist for several weeks, while that caused by *G. duodenalis* is very often chronic. Severe cases may experience signs associated with secondary bacterial infection, including sepsis. Anemia may accompany infection; either from blood loss (coccidiosis) or nutrient deprivation (*G. duodenalis*). Instead of intestinal signs, dogs infected with *N. caninum* more often show signs related to neurologic and muscular dysfunction, including limb paralysis and muscle atrophy (19).

Pathology
Pathologic changes induced by intestinal protozoal infection are commonly restricted to the intestinal tract. Exact location along the tract depends on parasite species. Lesions often include enteritis, and histiocytic proliferation of the lamina propria (6). As noted above, *N. caninum* infection is associated with neuropathy, myopathy, and encephalitis, but *N. caninum* can also cause pneumonia, nodular dermatitis, hepatitis, ophthalmitis, and myocarditis (5, 12, 13, 17). *N. caninum* stages have been found in a wide range of tissues, including brain, spinal cord, retina, muscles, thymus, heart, liver, kidney, stomach, adrenal gland, and skin (14). *G. duodenalis* attaches to the intestinal epithelium by a sucking disc. There-

TABLE 9-1. Body systems known or likely to be affected by pathogen indicated

Pathogen	Cardio-vascular	Dermal	Endocrine	Entero-hepatic	Hema-topoietic	Lympho-reticular	Musculo-skeletal	Nervous	Reproductive	Respiratory	Urinary
Canine coronavirus				×		×					
Canine adenovirus	×	×		×	×	×		×	×	×	×
Canine distemper virus	×	×	×	×	×	×	×	×		×	×
Parainfluenza virus type 2				×				×		×	
Parvovirus	×	×		×	×	×		×		×	
Bordetella bronchiseptica						×				×	
Brucella canis	×	×			×	×	×		×	×	×
Campylobacter jejuni				×	×	×			×		
Dermatomycosis		×				×					
Malassezia pachydermatis		×				×					
Demodex canis		×									
Fleas		×		×		×					
Dirofilaria immitis (heartworm)	×	×		×	×	×	×	×	×	×	×
Intestinal nematodes	×	×		×	×	×			×	×	
Intestinal protozoa	×		×	×	×		×	×		×	×

fore, infection with *G. duodenalis* causes pathologic changes compatible with loss of nutrient absorptive capacity and physical denuding of microvilli. Immunity to intestinal protozoa involves both cellular and humoral components, but is primarily cellular (8). While infections with the Apicomplexa are generally "self-limiting," immune protection is highly species specific. Subsequent infection with a previously "unseen" parasite species is not ameliorated by prior experience with other species.

Interference with research
There is a surprising paucity of information directly describing physiologic effects of intestinal coccidial infections of dogs. Light infections with intestinal protozoa are probably inconsequential. However, heavy infections early in life may slow body weight gain, while later infections may result in weight loss. Information reported from other host species infected with intestinal coccidia can suggest potential pathophysiologic changes, which may occur in dogs, but which have not yet been investigated or reported. Coccidial infections alter feed digestibility and nitrogen balance, lower serum glucose, albumin concentrations, and packed cell volume, and shift gut microfloral populations from gram-positive to gram-negative in goats (2, 11); slow reproductive maturation (18), alter bacterial population dynamics following coinfection (15, 16), induce nitric oxide compound and cytokine production, decrease circulating carotenoid levels, and elevate alkaline phosphatase activity in poultry (1, 4, 9); and alter electrolyte transport and electrical conductance in rabbits (7, 10). *G. duodenalis* is known to cause alterations in intestinal disaccharidases, in addition to cytoarchitectural changes associated with malabsorption. Clearly, enteric protozoal infections of dogs may result in a wide range of physiologic alterations. Studies involving the intestinal tract would be altered most consistently. However, interference with research involving the cardiovascular, dermal, endocrine, hematopoietic, musculoskeletal, nervous, respiratory, and urinary systems may also be affected, depending on the parasite species involved.

Diagnosis and control
Intestinal protozoal infections are relatively easily diagnosed by routine fecal examinations for diagnostic or infectious stages. The interested reader is referred to standard veterinary parasitology texts for diagnostic methods and therapeutic regimens (3). Diagnosis of *N. caninum* is more difficult than for other intestinal protozoa, but is also less likely to be present in the laboratory animal environment. Given the environmental resistance of infectious stages, it is impractical to attempt complete eradication of intestinal protozoa from the laboratory environment. Effort should be directed toward facility cleanliness, avoidance of severe physiologic stress on the dogs, and rapid diagnosis, isolation, and treatment of clinical cases. These measures will markedly reduce the environmental parasite burden, thereby avoiding or ameliorating most clinical episodes. While treatment may not always be necessary to get dogs past a clinical episode, the marked reduction in environmental contamination justifies treatment in all cases. Dogs with coccidiosis respond more slowly to treatment than dogs with giardiasis because anticoccidial drugs have therapeutic action only at specific points in what are rather complicated life cycles. Considerable damage to the intestinal epithelium may be done before individual organisms reach a point of vulnerability. In contrast, the life cycle of *G. duodenalis* is much simpler. The final verdict is still out concerning the zoonotic potential of *G. duodenalis*. It is this author's opinion that there is little host specificity among mammalian isolates. Therefore, personnel should practice good personal hygiene when working with potentially infected dogs.

REFERENCES

VIRUSES

Canine adenoviruses
1. **Adair, B. M.** 1979. Differences in cytopathology between canine adenovirus serotypes. *Br. Vet. J.* **135:**328–330.

2. **Aguirre, G., L. Carmichael, and S. Bistner.** 1975. Corneal endothelium in viral induced anterior uveitis. Ultrastructural changes following canine adenovirus type 1 infection. *Arch. Ophthalmol.* **93:**219–224.
3. **Appel, M., S. L. Bistner, M. Menegus, D. A. Albert, and L. E. Carmichael.** 1973. Pathogenicity of low-virulence strains of two canine adenovirus types. *Am. J. Vet. Res.* **34:**543–550.
4. **Carmichael, L. E., B. L. Medic, S. L. Bistner, and G. D. Aguirre.** 1975. Viral-antibody complexes in canine adenovirus type 1 (CAV-1) ocular lesions: leukocyte chemotaxis and enzyme release. *Cornell Vet.* **65:**331–351.
5. **Cornwell, H. J., S. D. Paterson, I. A. McCandlish, H. Thompson, and N. G. Wright.** 1983. Immunity to canine adenovirus respiratory disease: effect of vaccination with an inactivated vaccine. *Vet. Rec.* **113:**509–512.
6. **Curtis, R., and K. C. Barnett.** 1981. Canine adenovirus-induced ocular lesions in the Afghan hound. *Cornell Vet.* **71:**85–95.
7. **Emery, J. B., J. A. House, and W. R. Brown.** 1978. Cross-protective immunity to canine adenovirus type 2 by canine adenovirus type 1 vaccination. *Am. J. Vet. Res.* **39:**1778–1783.
8. **Hamelin, C., P. Jouvenne, and R. Assaf.** 1985. Association of a type-2 canine adenovirus with an outbreak of diarrhoeal disease among a large dog congregation. *J. Diarrhoeal Dis. Res.* **3:**84–87.
9. **Hu, R. L., G. Huang, W. Qiu, Z. H. Zhong, X. Z. Xia, and Z. Yin.** 2001. Detection and differentiation of CAV-1 and CAV-2 by polymerase chain reaction. *Vet. Res. Commun.* **25:**77–84.
10. **Kiss, I., K. Matiz, E. Bajmoci, M. Rusvai, and B. Harrach.** 1996. Infectious canine hepatitis: detection of canine adenovirus type 1 by polymerase chain reaction. *Acta Vet. Hung.* **44:**253–258.
11. **Kobayashi, Y., K. Ochiai, and C. Itakura.** 1993. Dual infection with canine distemper virus and infectious canine hepatitis virus (canine adenovirus type 1) in a dog. *J. Vet. Med. Sci.* **55:**699–701.
12. **Macartney, L., H. M. Cavanagh, and N. Spibey.** 1988. Isolation of canine adenovirus-2 from the faeces of dogs with enteric disease and its unambiguous typing by restriction endonuclease mapping. *Res. Vet. Sci.* **44:**9–14.
13. **Maxson, T. R., K. M. Meurs, L. B. Lehmkuhl, A. L. Magnon, S. E. Weisbrode, and C. E. Atkins.** 2001. Polymerase chain reaction analysis for viruses in paraffin-embedded myocardium from dogs with dilated cardiomyopathy or myocarditis. *Am. J. Vet. Res.* **62:**130–135.
14. **Olson, P., B. Klingeborn, and A. Hedhammar.** 1988. Serum antibody response to canine parvovirus, canine adenovirus-1, and canine distemper virus in dogs with known status of immunization: study of dogs in Sweden. *Am. J. Vet. Res.* **49:**1460–1466.
15. **Pratelli, A., V. Martella, G. Elia, M. Tempesta, F. Guarda, M. T. Capucchio, L. E. Carmichael, and C. Buonavoglia.** 2001. Severe enteric disease in an animal shelter associated with dual infections by canine adenovirus type 1 and canine coronavirus. *J. Vet. Med. B* **48:**385–392.
16. **Quan, S. F., M. L. Witten, R. Grad, C. G. Ray, and R. J. Lemen.** 1991. Changes in lung mechanics and histamine responsiveness after sequential canine adenovirus 2 and canine parainfluenza 2 virus infection in beagle puppies. *Pediatr. Pulmonol.* **10:**236–243.
17. **Quan, S. F., M. L. Witten, R. Grad, R. E. Sobonya, C. G. Ray, N. N. Dambro, and R. J. Lemen.** 1990. Acute canine adenovirus 2 infection increases histamine airway reactivity in beagle puppies. *Am. Rev. Respir. Dis.* **141:**414–420.
18. **Ramsey, I., D. Gunn-Moore, and S. Shaw.** 2001. The haemopoietic and lymphoreticular systems, p. 65–88. *In* I. Ramsey and B. Tennant (ed.), *Manual of Canine and Feline Infectious Diseases.* British Small Animal Veterinary Association, Gloucester, England.
19. **Shahrabadi, M. S., and T. Yamamoto.** 1975. Cytoplasmic inclusions in canine cells infected with infectious canine laryngotracheitis (ICL) adenovirus. *Can. J. Microbiol.* **21:**1421–1427.
20. **Smith, K. O., W. D. Gehle, and W. T. Kniker.** 1970. Serologic evidence that infectious canine hepatitis virus commonly infects humans and is related to human adenovirus type 8. *J. Immunol.* **105:**1036–1039.
21. **Spibey, N., and H. M. Cavanagh.** 1989. Molecular cloning and restriction endonuclease mapping of two strains of canine adenovirus type 2. *J. Gen. Virol.* **70:**165–172.
22. **Tennant, B.** 2001. The alimentary tract, p. 129–150. *In* I. Ramsey and B. Tennant (ed.), *Manual of Canine and Feline Infectious Diseases.* British Small Animal Veterinary Association, Gloucester, England.
23. **Tennant, B.** 2001. The liver, pancreas and spleen, p. 175–184. *In* I. Ramsey and B. Tennant (ed.), *Manual of Canine and Feline Infectious Diseases.* British Small Animal Veterinary Association, Gloucester, England.
24. **Thompson, H., H. J. Cornwell, N. G. Wright, and R. S. Campbell.** 1972. Canine

adenovirus in organ cultures. *Res. Vet. Sci.* **13**: 191–193.
25. **Willoughby, K., and S. Dawson.** 2001. The respiratory tract, p. 89–115. *In* I. Ramsey and B. Tennant (ed.), *Manual of Canine and Feline Infectious Diseases.* British Small Animal Veterinary Association, Gloucester, England.
26. **Witten, M. L., J. L. McKee, R. C. Lantz, A. M. Hays, S. F. Quan, R. E. Sobonya, and R. J. Lemen.** 1993. Fractal and morphometric analysis of lung structures after canine adenovirus-induced bronchiolitis in beagle puppies. *Pediatr. Pulmonol.* **16:**62–68.
27. **Wright, N. G.** 1976. Canine adenovirus: its role in renal and ocular disease: a review. *J. Small Anim. Pract.* **17:**25–33.
28. **Wright, N. G., and H. J. Cornwell.** 1983. Experimental canine adenovirus glomerulonephritis: histological, immunofluorescence and ultrastructural features of the early glomerular changes. *Br. J. Exp. Pathol.* **64:**312–319.
29. **Wright, N. G., A. S. Nash, and H. J. Cornwell.** 1981. experimental canine adenovirus glomerulonephritis: persistence of glomerular lesions after oral challenge. *Br. J. Exp. Pathol.* **62:**183–189.
30. **Wright, N. G., H. Thompson, and H. J. Cornwell.** 1971. Canine adenovirus pneumonia. *Res. Vet. Sci.* **12:**162–167.
31. **Zee, Y. C.** 1999. Adenoviridae, p. 346–349. *In* D. C. Hirsh and Y. C. Zee (ed.), *Veterinary Microbiology.* Blackwell Science, Inc., Malden, Mass.

Canine coronavirus
1. **Horsburgh, B. C., and T. D. Brown.** 1995. Cloning, sequencing and expression of the S protein gene from two geographically distinct strains of canine coronavirus. *Virus Res.* **39:**63–74.
2. **Mainka, S. A., X. Qiu, T. He, and M. J. Appel.** 1994. Serologic survey of giant pandas (*Ailuropoda melanoleuca*), and domestic dogs and cats in the Wolong Reserve, China. *J. Wildl. Dis.* **30:**86–89.
3. **Mochizuki, M., M. Hashimoto, and T. Ishida.** 2001. Recent epidemiological status of canine viral enteric infections and *Giardia* infection in Japan. *J. Vet. Med. Sci.* **63:**573–575.
4. **Naylor, M. J., G. A. Harrison, R. P. Monckton, S. McOrist, P. R. Lehrbach, and E. M. Deane.** 2001. Identification of canine coronavirus strains from feces by S gene nested PCR and molecular characterization of a new Australian isolate. *J. Clin. Microbiol.* **39:**1036–1041.
5. **Naylor, M. J., R. P. Monckton, P. R. Lehrbach, and E. M. Deane.** 2001. Canine coronavirus in Australian dogs. *Aust. Vet. J.* **79:**116–119.
6. **Pratelli, A., D. Buonavoglia, V. Martella, M. Tempesta, A. Lavazza, and C. Buonavoglia.** 2000. Diagnosis of canine coronavirus infection using nested-PCR. *J. Virol. Methods* **84:** 91–94.
7. **Pratelli, A., G. Elia, V. Martella, A. Palmieri, F. Cirone, A. Tinelli, M. Corrente, and C. Buonavoglia.** 2002. Prevalence of canine coronavirus antibodies by an enzyme-linked immunosorbent assay in dogs in the south of Italy. *J. Virol. Methods* **102:**67–71.
8. **Pratelli, A., V. Martella, G. Elia, M. Tempesta, F. Guarda, M. T. Capucchio, L. E. Carmichael, and C. Buonavoglia.** 2001. Severe enteric disease in an animal shelter associated with dual infections by canine adenovirus type 1 and canine coronavirus. *J. Vet. Med. Ser. B* **48:** 385–392.
9. **Stott, J. L.** 1999. Coronaviridae, p. 418–429. *In* D. C. Hirsh and Y. C. Zee (ed.), *Veterinary Microbiology.* Blackwell Science, Inc., Malden, Mass.
10. **Tennant, B.** 2001. The alimentary tract, p. 129–150. *In* I. Ramsey and B. Tennant (ed.), *Manual of Canine and Feline Infectious Diseases.* British Small Animal Veterinary Association, Gloucester, England.
11. **Tennant, B. J., R. M. Gaskell, and C. J. Gaskell.** 1994. Studies on the survival of canine coronavirus under different environmental conditions. *Vet. Microbiol.* **42:**255–259.
12. **Tennant, B. J., R. M. Gaskell, R. C. Jones, and C. J. Gaskell.** 1993. Studies on the epizootiology of canine coronavirus. *Vet. Rec.* **132:**7–11.
13. **Tennant, B. J., R. M. Gaskell, D. F. Kelly, S. D. Carter, and C. J. Gaskell.** 1991. Canine coronavirus infection in the dog following oronasal inoculation. *Res. Vet. Sci.* **51:**11–18.

Canine distemper virus
1. **Alldinger, S., A. Wunschmann, W. Baumgartner, C. Voss, and E. Kremmer.** 1996. Up-regulation of major histocompatibility complex class II antigen expression in the central nervous system of dogs with spontaneous canine distemper virus encephalitis. *Acta Neuropathol.* (Berl.) **92:**273–280.
2. **Axthelm, M. K., and S. Krakowka.** 1987. Canine distemper virus-induced thrombocytopenia. *Am. J. Vet. Res.* **48:**1269–1275.
3. **Baumgartner, W., R. W. Boyce, S. Alldinger, M. K. Axthelm, S. E. Weisbrode, S. Krakowka, and K. Gaedke.** 1995. Metaphyseal bone lesions in young dogs with systemic canine distemper virus infection. *Vet. Microbiol.* **44:**201–209.
4. **Bolt, G., T. D. Jensen, E. Gottschalck, P. Arctander, M. J. Appel, R. Buckland, and

M. Blixenkron-Moller. 1997. Genetic diversity of the attachment (H) protein gene of current field isolates of canine distemper virus. *J. Gen. Virol.* **78:**367–372.

5. Dubielzig, R. R., R. J. Higgins, and S. Krakowka. 1981. Lesions of the enamel organ of developing dog teeth following experimental inoculation of gnotobiotic puppies with canine distemper virus. *Vet. Pathol.* **18:**684–689.

6. Evans, M. B., T. O. Bunn, H. T. Hill, and K. B. Platt. 1991. Comparison of *in vitro* replication and cytopathology caused by strains of canine distemper virus of vaccine and field origin. *J. Vet. Diagn. Investig.* **3:**127–132.

7. Frisk, A. L., W. Baumgartner, and A. Grone. 1999. Dominating interleukin-10 mRNA expression induction in cerebrospinal fluid cells of dogs with natural canine distemper virus induced demyelinating and non-demyelinating CNS lesions. *J. Neuroimmunol.* **97:**102–109.

8. Frisk, A. L., M. Konig, A. Moritz, and W. Baumgartner. 1999. Detection of canine distemper virus nucleoprotein RNA by reverse transcription-PCR using serum, whole blood, and cerebrospinal fluid from dogs with distemper. *J. Clin. Microbiol.* **37:**3634–3643.

9. Fu, S. C., R. Mozzi, S. Krakowka, R. J. Higgins, and L. A. Horrocks. 1980. Plasmalogenase and phospholipase A1, A2, and L1 activities in white matter in canine distemper virus-associated demyelinating encephalomyelitis. *Acta Neuropathol. (Berl.)* **49:**13–18.

10. Gemma, T., C. Kai, and T. Mikami. 1995. Suppression of canine parvovirus growth in CRFK cells by canine distemper virus. *J. Vet. Med. Sci.* **57:**535–537.

11. Glaus, T., C. Griot, A. Richard, U. Althaus, N. Herschkowitz, and M. Vendevelde. 1990. Ultrastructural and biochemical findings in brain cell cultures infected with canine distemper virus. *Acta Neuropathol. (Berl.)* **80:**59–67.

12. Grone, A., S. Alldinger, and W. Baumgartner. 2000. Interleukin-1β, -6, -12 and tumor necrosis factor-a expression in brains of dogs with canine distemper virus infection. *J. Neuroimmunol.* **110:**20–30.

13. Guo, A., and C. Lu. 2000. Canine distemper virus causes apoptosis of Vero cells. *J. Vet. Med. Ser. B* **47:**183–190.

14. Higgins, R. J., G. Child, and M. Vendevelde. 1989. Chronic relapsing demyelinating encephalomyelitis associated with persistent spontaneous canine distemper virus infection. *Acta Neuropathol. (Berl.)* **77:**441–444.

15. Higgins, R. J., S. Krakowka, A. E. Metzler, and A. Koestner. 1981. Canine distemper virus-associated cardiac necrosis in the dog. *Vet. Pathol.* **18:**472–486.

16. Howard, J. M., B. S. Eckert, and L. Y. Bourguignon. 1983. Comparison of cytoskeletal organization in canine distemper virus-infected and uninfected cells. *J. Gen. Virol.* **64:**2379–2385.

17. Iwatsuki, K., M. Okita, F. Ochikubo, T. Gemma, Y. S. Shin, N. Miyashita, T. Mikami, and C. Kai. 1995. Immunohistochemical analysis of the lymphoid organs of dogs naturally infected with canine distemper virus. *J. Comp. Pathol.* **113:**185–190.

18. Krakowka, S., E. A. Hoover, A. Koestner, and K. Ketring. 1977. Experimental and naturally occurring transplacental transmission of canine distemper virus. *Am. J. Vet. Res.* **38:**919–922.

19. Krakowka, S., and A. Koestner. 1976. Age-related susceptibility to infection with canine distemper virus in gnotobiotic dogs. *J. Infect. Dis.* **134:**629–632.

20. Loffler, S., F. Lottspeich, F. Lanza, D. O. Azorsa, V. ter Meulen, and J. Schneider-Schaulies. 1997. CD9, a tetraspan transmembrane protein, renders cells susceptible to canine distemper virus. *J. Virol.* **71:**42–49.

21. Mee, A. P., J. A. Dixon, J. A. Hoyland, M. Davies, P. L. Selby, and E. B. Mawer. 1998. Detection of canine distemper virus in 100% of Paget's disease samples by in situ-reverse transcriptase-polymerase chain reaction. *Bone* **23:**171–175.

22. Mee, A. P., C. May, D. Bennett, and P. T. Sharpe. 1995. Generation of multinucleated osteoclast-like cells from canine bone marrow: effects of canine distemper virus. *Bone* **17:**47–55.

23. Miry, C., R. Ducatelle, H. Thoonen, and J. Hoorens. 1983. Immunoperoxidase study of canine distemper virus pneumonia. *Res. Vet. Sci.* **34:**145–148.

24. Mori, T., Y. S. Shin, M. Okita, N. Hirayama, N. Miyashita, T. Gemma, C. Kai, and T. Mikami. 1994. The biological characterization of field isolates of canine distemper virus from Japan. *J. Gen. Virol.* **75:**2403–2408.

25. Morrell, V. 1994. Canine distemper virus. Serengeti's big cats going to the dogs. *Science* **264:**1664.

26. Murphy, F. A., E. P. J. Gibbs, M. C. Horzinek, and M. J. Studdert. 1999. *Veterinary Virology*, 3rd ed. Academic Press, Inc., San Diego, Calif.

27. Olson, P., H. Finnsdóttir, B. Klingeborn, and Å. Hedhammar. 1997. Duration of antibodies elicited by canine distemper virus vaccinations in dogs. *Vet. Rec.* **141:**654–655.

28. **Pearce-Kelling, S., W. J. Mitchell, B. A. Summers, and M. J. Appel.** 1991. Virulent and attenuated canine distemper virus infects multiple dog brain cell types in vitro. *Glia* **4**:408–416.
29. **Ramsey, I., D. Gunn-Moore, and S. Shaw.** 2001. The haemopoietic and lymphoreticular systems, p. 65–88. *In* I. Ramsey and B. Tennant (ed.), *Manual of Canine and Feline Infectious Diseases*. British Small Animal Veterinary Association, Gloucester, England.
30. **Schobesberger, M., A. Zurbriggen, M. G. Doherr, H. Weissenbock, M. Vandevelde, H. Lassmann, and C. Griot.** 2002. Demyelination precedes oligodendrocyte loss in canine distemper virus-induced encephalitis. *Acta Neuropathol. (Berl.)* **103**:11–19.
31. **Shapshak, P., M. C. Graves, and D. T. Imagawa.** 1987. Autologous and allogenic antibody responses to canine distemper virus isolates from dogs with chronic neurologic diseases. *Viral Immunol.* **1**:45–54.
32. **Soma, T., H. Ishii, M. Hara, S. Yamamoto, T. Yoshida, T. Kinoshita, and K. Nomura.** 2001. Comparison of immunoperoxidase plaque staining and neutralizing tests for canine distemper virus. *Vet. Res. Commun.* **25**:311–325.
33. **Tipold, A., P. Moore, A. Zurbriggen, I. Burgener, G. Barben, and M. Vandevelde.** 1999. Early T cell response in the central nervous system in canine distemper virus infection. *Acta Neuropathol.* **97**:45–56.
34. **Tipold, A., M. Vandevelde, R. Wittek, P. Moore, A. Summerfield, and A. Zurbriggen.** 2001. Partial protection and intrathecal invasion of CD8$^+$ T cells in acute canine distemper virus infection. *Vet. Microbiol.* **83**:189–203.
35. **Vandevelde, M., B. Kristensen, K. G. Braund, C. E. Greene, L. J. Swango, and B. F. Hoerlein.** 1980. Chronic canine distemper virus encephalitis in mature dogs. *Vet. Pathol.* **17**:17–28.
36. **von Messling, V., G. Zimmer, G. Herrler, L. Haas, and R. Cattaneo.** 2001. The hemagglutinin of canine distemper virus determines tropism and cytopathogenicity. *J. Virol.* **75**:6418–6427.
37. **Weisbrode, S. E., and S. Krakowka.** 1979. Canine distemper virus-associated hypocalcemia. *Am. J. Vet. Res.* **40**:147–149.
38. **Willoughby, K., and S. Dawson.** 2001. The respiratory tract, p. 89–115. *In* I. Ramsey and B. Tennant (ed.), *Manual of Canine and Feline Infectious Diseases*. British Small Animal Veterinary Association, Gloucester, England.
39. **Zee, Y. C.** 1999. Paramyxoviridae, p. 403–411. *In* D. C. Hirsh and Y. C. Zee (ed.), *Veterinary Microbiology*. Blackwell Science, Inc., Malden, Mass.
40. **Zurbriggen, A., and M. Vandevelde.** 1983. Canine distemper virus-induced glial cell changes in vitro. *Acta Neuropathol. (Berl.)* **62**:51–58.

Parainfluenza virus type 2
1. **Appel, M., and D. A. Bemis.** 1978. The canine contagious respiratory disease complex (kennel cough). *Cornell Vet.* **68**:70–75.
2. **Appel, M. J., and D. H. Percy.** 1970. SV-5-like parainfluenza virus in dogs. *J. Am. Vet. Med. Assoc.* **156**:1778–1781.
3. **Baty, D. U., J. A. Southern, and R. E. Randall.** 1991. Sequence comparison between the haemagglutinin-neuraminidase genes of simian, canine and human isolates of simian virus 5. *J. Gen. Virol.* **72**:3103–3107.
4. **Baumgartner, W. K., S. Krakowka, A. Koestner, and J. Evermann.** 1982. Acute encephalitis and hyrdocephalus in dogs caused by canine parainfluenza virus. *Vet. Pathol.* **19**:79–92.
5. **Binn, L. N., and E. C. Lazar.** 1970. Comments on epizootiology of parainfluenza SV-5 in dogs. *J. Am. Vet. Med. Assoc.* **156**:1774–1777.
6. **Crandell, R. A., W. B. Brumlow, and V. E. Davison.** 1968. Isolation of a parainfluenza virus from sentry dogs with upper respiratory disease. *Am. J. Vet. Res.* **29**:2141–2147.
7. **Dambro, N. N., R. Grad, M. L. Witten, S. F. Quan, R. E. Sobonya, C. G. Ray, L. Devine, and R. J. Lemen.** 1992. Bronchoalveolar lavage fluid cytology reflects airway inflammation in beagle puppies with acute bronchiolitis. *Pediatr. Pulmonol.* **12**:213–220.
8. **Evermann, J. F., S. Krakowka, A. J. McKeirnan, and W. Baumgartner.** 1981. Properties of an encephalitogenic canine parainfluenza virus. *Arch. Virol.* **68**:165–172.
9. **Evermann, J. F., J. D. Lincoln, and A. J. McKeirnan.** 1980. Isolation of a paramyxovirus from the cerebrospinal fluid of a dog with posterior paresis. *J. Am. Vet. Med. Assoc.* **177**:1132–1134.
10. **Goswami, K. K., L. S. Lange, D. N. Mitchell, K. R. Cameron, and W. C. Russell.** 1984. Does simian virus 5 infect humans? *J. Gen. Virol.* **65**:1295–1303.
11. **Lemen, R. J., S. F. Quan, M. L. Witten, R. E. Sobonya, C. G. Ray, and R. Grad.** 1990. Canine parainfluenza type 2 bronchiolitis increases histamine responsiveness in beagle puppies. *Am. Rev. Respir. Dis.* **141**:199–207.
12. **Mayr, A.** 1989. Infections which humans in the household transmit to dogs and cats. *Zentbl. Bakteriol. Mikrobiol. Hyg. Abt B* **187**:508–526.
13. **McCandlish, I. A., H. Thompson, H. J. Cornwell, and N. G. Wright.** 1978. A study

of dogs with kennel cough. *Vet. Rec.* **102:**293–301.
14. **Murphy, F. A., E. P. J. Gibbs, M. C. Horzinek, and M. J. Studdert.** 1999. *Veterinary Virology,* 3rd ed. Academic Press, Inc., San Diego, Calif.
15. **Myers, L. J., K. E. Nusbaum, L. J. Swango, L. N. Hanrahan, and E. Sartin.** 1988. Dysfunction of sense of smell caused by canine parainfluenza virus infection in dogs. *Am. J. Vet. Res.* **49:**188–190.
16. **Quan, S. F., R. J. Lemen, M. L. Witten, D. L. Sherrill, R. Grad, R. E. Sobonya, and C. G. Ray.** 1990. Changes in lung mechanics and reactivity with age after viral bronchiolitis in beagle puppies. *J. Appl. Physiol.* **69:**2034–2042.
17. **Quan, S. F., M. L. Witten, N. N. Dambro, and R. J. Lemen.** 1991. Canine parainfluenza type 2 and *Bordetella bronchiseptica* infection produces increased bronchoalveolar lavage thromboxane concentrations in beagle puppies. *Prostaglandins Leukot. Essent. Fatty Acids* **44:**171–175.
18. **Quan, S. F., M. L. Witten, R. Grad, C. G. Ray, and R. J. Lemen.** 1991. Changes in lung mechanics and histamine responsiveness after sequential canine adenovirus 2 and canine parainfluenza 2 virus infection in beagle puppies. *Pediatr. Pulmonol.* **10:**236–243.
19. **Randall, R. E., and D. F. Young.** 1988. Comparison between parainfluenza virus type 2 and simian virus 5: monoclonal antibodies reveal major antigenic differences. *J. Gen. Virol.* **69:**2051–2060.
20. **Randall, R. E., D. F. Young, K. K. Goswami, and W. C. Russell.** 1987. Isolation and characterization of monoclonal antibodies to simian virus 5 and their use in revealing antigenic differences between human, canine and simian isolates. *J. Gen. Virol.* **68:**2769–2780.
21. **Tsurudome, M., M. Nishio, H. Komada, H. Bando, and Y. Ito.** 1989. Extensive antigenic diversity among human parainfluenza type 2 virus isolates and immunological relationships among paramyxoviruses revealed by monoclonal antibodies. *Virology* **171:**38–48.
22. **Ueland, K.** 1990. Serological, bacteriological and clinical observations on an outbreak of canine infectious tracheobronchitis in Norway. *Vet. Rec.* **126:**481–483.
23. **Vieler, E., W. Herbst, W. Baumgartner, and S. Breuker.** 1994. Isolation of a parainfluenza virus type 2 from the prostatic fluid of a dog. *Vet. Rec.* **135:**384–385.
24. **Wagener, J. S., L. Minnich, R. Sobonya, L. M. Taussig, C. G. Ray, and V. Fulginiti.** 1983. Parainfluenza type II infection in dogs. A model for viral lower respiratory tract infection in humans. *Am. Rev. Respir. Dis.* **127:**771–775.
25. **Wagener, J. S., R. Sobonya, L. Minnich, and L. M. Taussig.** 1984. Role of canine parainfluenza virus and *Bordetella bronchiseptica* in kennel cough. *Am. J. Vet. Res.* **45:**1862–1866.
26. **Young, D. F., R. E. Randall, J. A. Hoyle, and B. E. Souberbielle.** 1990. Clearance of a persistent paramyxovirus infection is mediated by cellular immune responses but not by serum-neutralizing antibody. *J. Virol.* **64:**5403–5411.
27. **Zee, Y. C.** 1999. Paramyxoviridae, p. 403–411. *In* D. C. Hirsh and Y. C. Zee (ed.), *Veterinary Microbiology.* Blackwell Science, Inc., Malden, Mass.

Parvovirus
1. **Agungpriyono, D. R., K. Uchida, H. Tabaru, R. Yamaguchi, and S. Tateyama.** 1999. Subacute massive necrotizing myocarditis by canine parvovirus type 2 infection with diffuse leukoencephalomalacia in a puppy. *Vet. Pathol.* **36:**77–80.
2. **Bauder, B., A. Suchy, C. Gabler, and H. Weissenbock.** 2000. Apoptosis in feline panleukopenia and canine parvovirus enteritis. *J. Vet. Med. Ser. B* **47:**775–784.
3. **Brown, M. R., and K. S. Rogers.** 2001. Neutropenia in dogs and cats: a retrospective study of 261 cases. *J. Am. Anim. Hosp. Assoc.* **37:**131–139.
4. **Cohn, L. A., J. M. Rewerts, D. McCaw, G. D. Boon, C. Wagner-Mann, and C. D. Lothrop, Jr.** 1999. Plasma granulocyte colony-stimulating factor concentrates in neutropenic, parvoviral enteritis-infected puppies. *J. Vet. Intern. Med.* **13:**581–586.
5. **Favrot, C., T. Olivry, S. M. Dunston, F. Degorce-Rubiales, and J. S. Guy.** 2000. Parvovirus infection of keratinocytes as a cause of canine erythema multiforme. *Vet. Pathol.* **37:**647–649.
6. **Gemma, T., C. Kai, and T. Mikami.** 1995. Suppression of canine parvovirus growth in CRFK cells by canine distemper virus. *J. Vet. Med. Sci.* **57:**535–537.
7. **Gordon, J. C., and E. J. Angrick.** 1986. Canine parvoviruses: environmental effects on infectivity. *Am. J. Vet. Res.* **47:**1464–1467.
8. **Kennedy, M. A., V. S. Mellon, G. Caldwell, and L. N. Potgieter.** 1995. Virucidal efficacy of the newer quaternary ammonium compounds. *J. Am. Anim. Hosp. Assoc.* **31:**254–258.
9. **Krakowka, S., R. G. Olsen, M. K. Axthelm, J. Rice, and K. Winters.** 1982. Canine parvovirus infection potentiates canine distemper encephalitis attributable to modified live-virus vaccine. *J. Am. Vet. Med. Assoc.* **180:**137–139.

10. Macartney, L., I. A. McCandlish, H. Thompson, and H. J. Cornwell. 1984. Canine parvovirus enteritis I: Clinical, haematological and pathological features of experimental infection. *Vet. Rec.* **115:**201–210.
11. Maxson, T. R., K. M. Meurs, L. B. Lehmkuhl, A. L. Magnon, S. E. Weisbrode, and C. E. Atkins. 2001. Polymerase chain reaction analysis for viruses in paraffin-embedded myocardium from dogs with dilated cardiomyopathy or myocarditis. *Am. J. Vet. Res.* **62:**130–135.
12. Mochizuki, M., M. Horiuchi, H. Hiragi, M. C. San Gabriel, N. Yasuda, and T. Uno. 1996. Isolation of canine parvovirus from a cat manifesting clinical signs of feline panleukopenia. *J. Clin. Microbiol.* **34:**2101–2105.
13. Murphy, F. A., E. P. J. Gibbs, M. C. Horzinek, and M. J. Studdert. 1999. *Veterinary Virology*, 3rd ed. Academic Press, Inc., San Diego, Calif.
14. Nakamura, K., M. Sakamoto, Y. Ikeda, E. Sato, K. Kawakami, T. Miyazawa, Y. Tohya, E. Takahashi, T. Mikami, and M. Mochizuki. 2001. Pathogenic potential of canine parvovirus types 2a and 2c in domestic cats. *Clin. Diagn. Lab. Immunol.* **8:**663–668.
15. Nelson, D. T., S. L. Eustis, J. P. McAdaragh, and I. Stotz. 1979. Lesions of spontaneous canine viral enteritis. *Vet. Pathol.* **16:**680–686.
16. Olson, P., B. Klingeborn, and Å. Hedhammar. 1988. Serum antibody response to canine parvovirus, canine adenovirus-1, and canine distemper virus in dogs with known status of immunization: study of dogs in Sweden. *Am. J. Vet. Res.* **49:**1460–1466.
17. Otto, C. M., T. M. Rieser, M. B. Brooks, and M. W. Russell. 2000. Evidence of hypercoagulability in dogs with parvoviral enteritis. *J. Am. Vet. Med. Assoc.* **217:**1500–1504.
18. Pratelli, A., A. Cavalli, V. Martella, M. Tempesta, N. Decaro, L. E. Carmichael, and C. Buonavoglia. 2001. Canine parvovirus (CPV) vaccination: comparison of neutralizing antibody responses in pups after inoculation with CPV2 or CPV2b modified live virus vaccine. *Clin. Diagn. Lab. Immunol.* **8:**612–615.
19. Rallis, T. S., L. G. Papazoglou, K. K. Adamama-Moraitou, and N. N. Prassinos. 2000. Acute enteritis or gastroenteritis in young dogs as a predisposing factor for intestinal intussusception: a retrospective study. *J. Vet. Med. Ser. A* **47:**507–511.
20. Rodriguez, F., A. Fernandez, A. Espinosa de los Monteros, P. Wohlsein, and H. E. Jensen. 1998. Acute disseminated candidiasis in a puppy associated with parvoviral infection. *Vet. Rec.* **142:**434–436.
21. Schunck, B., W. Kraft, and D. Truyen. 1995. A simple touch-down polymerase chain reaction for the detection of canine parvovirus and feline panleukopenia virus in feces. *J. Virol. Methods* **55:**427–433.
22. Singh, B. R., R. C. Yadav, S. P. Singh, and V. D. Sharma. 1998. Coagglutination test: a simple and rapid immunodiagnostic test for parvovirus infection in dogs. *Indian J. Exp. Biol.* **36:**622–624.
23. Tennant, B. 2001. The alimentary tract, p. 129–150. *In* I. Ramsey and B. Tennant (ed.), *Manual of Canine and Feline Infectious Diseases*. British Small Animal Veterinary Association, Gloucester, England.
24. Truyen, U. 1999. Emergence and recent evolution of canine parvovirus. *Vet. Microbiol.* **69:**47–50.
25. Truyen, U., G. Platzer, and C. R. Parrish. 1996. Antigenic type distribution among canine parvoviruses in dogs and cats in Germany. *Vet. Rec.* **138:**365–366.
26. Vihinen-Ranta, M., A. Kalela, P. Makinen, L. Kakkola, V. Marjomaki, and M. Vuento. 1998. Intracellular route of canine parvovirus entry. *J. Virol.* **72:**802–806.
27. Vlemmas, I., P. Wohlsein, G. Trautwein, G. Kanakudis, and T. Tsangaris. 1990. Experimental parvovirus infection of puppies: immunohistochemical findings. *Berl. Muench. Tieraerztl. Wochenschr.* **103:**422–425.
28. Yang, T. J. 1987. Parvovirus-induced regression of canine transmissible venereal sarcoma. *Am. J. Vet. Res.* **48:**799–800.
29. Zee, Y. C. 1999. Parvoviridae, p. 333–339. *In* D. C. Hirsh and Y. C. Zee (ed.), *Veterinary Microbiology*. Blackwell Science, Inc., Malden, Mass.

BACTERIA

Bordetella bronchiseptica

1. Appel, M., and D. A. Bemis. 1978. The canine contagious respiratory disease complex (kennel cough). *Cornell Vet.* **68:**70–75.
2. Batey, R. G., and A. F. Smits. 1976. The isolation of *Bordetella bronchiseptica* from an outbreak of canine pneumonia. *Aust. Vet. J.* **52:**184–186.
3. Bemis, D. A., L. E. Carmichael, and M. J. Appel. 1977. Naturally occurring respiratory disease in a kennel caused by *Bordetella bronchiseptica*. *Cornell Vet.* **67:**282–293.
4. Bemis, D. A., H. A. Greisen, and M. J. Appel. 1977. Pathogenesis of canine bordetellosis. *J. Infect. Dis.* **135:**753–762.
5. Bemis, D. A., and J. R. Kennedy. 1981. An improved system for studying the effect of *Bor-*

detella bronchiseptica on the ciliary activity of canine tracheal epithelial cells. *J. Infect. Dis.* **144:**349–357.
6. **Bemis, D. A., and S. A. Wilson.** 1985. Influence of potential virulence determinants on *Bordetella bronchiseptica*-induced ciliostasis. *Infect. Immunol.* **50:**35–42.
7. **Bey, R. F., F. J. Shade, R. A. Goodnow, and R. C. Johnson.** 1981. Intranasal vaccination of dogs with liver avirulent *Bordetella bronchiseptica*: correlation of serum agglutination titer and the formation of secretory IgA with protection against experimentally induced infectious tracheobronchitis. *Am. J. Vet. Res.* **42:**1130–1132.
8. **Biberstein, E. L., and D. C. Hirsh.** 1999. Bordetella, p. 148–150. *In* D. C. Hirsh and Y. C. Zee (ed.), *Veterinary Microbiology*. Blackwell Science, Inc., Malden, Mass.
9. **Binns, S. H., A. J. Speakman, S. Dawson, M. Bennett, R. M. Gaskell, and C. A. Hart.** 1998. The use of pulsed-field gel electrophoresis to examine the epidemiology of *Bordetella bronchiseptica* isolated from cats and other species. *Epidemiol. Infect.* **120:**201–208.
10. **Garlinghouse, L. E., Jr., R. F. DiGiacomo, G. L. Van Hoosier, Jr., and J. Condon.** 1981. Selective media for *Pasteurella multocida* and *Bordetella bronchiseptica*. *Lab. Anim. Sci.* **31:**39–42.
11. **Goodnow, R. A., S. C. Causey, S. J. Geary, and W. S. Wren.** 1983. Comparison of an infective avirulent and canine virulent *Bordetella bronchiseptica*. *Am. J. Vet. Res.* **44:**207–211.
12. **Gueirard, P., C. Weber, A. Le Coustumier, and N. Guiso.** 1995. Human *Bordetella bronchiseptica* infection related to contact with infected animals: persistence of bacteria in host. *J. Clin. Microbiol.* **33:**2002–2006.
13. **Keil, D. J., and B. Fenwick.** 1999. Evaluation of canine *Bordetella bronchiseptica* isolates using randomly amplified polymorphic DNA fingerprinting and ribotyping. *Vet. Microbiol.* **66:**41–51.
14. **Le Blay, K., P. Gueirard, N. Guiso, and R. Chaby.** 1997. Antigenic polymorphism of the lipopolysaccharides from human and animal isolates of *Bordetella bronchiseptica*. *Microbiology* **143:**1433–1441.
15. **McCandlish, I. A., H. Thompson, H. J. Cornwell, and N. G. Wright.** 1978. A study of dogs with kennel cough. *Vet. Rec.* **102:**293–301.
16. **Sacco, R. E., K. B. Register, and G. E. Nordholm.** 2000. Restriction endonuclease analysis discriminates *Bordetella bronchiseptica* isolates. *J. Clin. Microbiol.* **38:**4387–4393.
17. **Willoughby, K., and S. Dawson.** 2001. The respiratory tract, p. 89–115. *In* I. Ramsey and B. Tennant (ed.), *Manual of Canine and Feline Infectious Diseases*. British Small Animal Veterinary Association, Gloucester, England.
18. **Zeligs, B. J., J. D. Zeligs, and J. A. Bellanti.** 1986. Functional and ultrastructural changes in alveolar macrophages from rabbits colonized with *Bordetella bronchiseptica*. *Infect. Immun.* **53:**702–706.

Brucella canis
1. **Carmichael, L. E., and J. C. Joubert.** 1988. Transmission of *Brucella canis* by contact exposure. *Cornell Vet.* **78:**63–73.
2. **Carmichael, L. E., and R. M. Kenney.** 1968. Canine abortion caused by *Brucella canis*. *J. Am. Vet. Med. Assoc.* **152:**605–616.
3. **Carmichael, L. E., and R. M. Kenney.** 1970. Canine brucellosis: the clinical disease, pathogenesis, and immune response. *J. Am. Vet. Med. Assoc.* **156:**1726–1734.
4. **Dawkins, B. G., S. V. Machotka, D. Suchmann, and R. M. McLaughlin.** 1982. Pyogranulomatous dermatitis associated with *Brucella canis* infection in a dog. *J. Am. Vet. Med. Assoc.* **181:**1432–1433.
5. **Dillon, A. R., and R. A. Henderson.** 1981. *Brucella canis* in a uterine stump abscess in a bitch. *J. Am. Vet. Med. Assoc.* **178:**987–988.
6. **England, G.** 2001. The reproductive tract and neonate, p. 185–195. *In* I. Ramsey and B. Tennant (ed.), *Manual of Canine and Feline Infectious Diseases*. British Small Animal Veterinary Association, Gloucester, England.
7. **George, L., and L. Carmichael.** 1984. Antisperm response in male dogs with chronic *Brucella canis* infections. *Am. J. Vet. Res.* **45:**274–281.
8. **Harris, A. M., M. L. Horton, R. M. Letscher, E. E. McConnell, and A. E. New.** 1974. Enzootic *Brucella canis*: an occult disease in a research canine colony. *Lab. Anim. Sci.* **24:**796–799.
9. **Henderson, R. A., B. F. Hoerlein, T. T. Kramer, and M. E. Meyer.** 1974. Discospondylitis in three dogs infected with *Brucella canis*. *J. Am. Vet. Med. Assoc.* **165:**451–455.
10. **Johnson, C. A., R. W. Bull, and R. G. Schirmer.** 1983. Peripheral lymphocyte function in dogs with *Brucella canis* infection. *Vet. Immunol. Immunopathol.* **4:**425–431.
11. **Kerwin, S. C., D. D. Lewis, T. N. Hribernik, B. Partington, G. Hosgood, and B. E. Eilts.** 1992. Diskospondylitis associated with *Brucella canis* infection in dogs: 14 cases (1980–1991). *J. Am. Vet. Med. Assoc.* **201:**1253–1257.
12. **Kulakov, I. K., M. M. Zheludkov, T. A. Tolmacheva, N. V. Alekseeva, I. N. Kovalev, A. G. Skavronskaia, A. L. Gintsburg, I. P. Mikhailova, V. V. Kalmykov, and

K. V. Shumilov. 2000. Use of molecular-biological methods for identifying *Brucella* in a comparative analysis of strains, isolated from sick dogs. *Mol. Genet. Mikrobiol. Virusol.* **4:**7–12.
13. Moore, J. A., and B. N. Gupta. 1970. Epizootiology, diagnosis, and control of *Brucella canis*. *J. Am. Vet. Med. Assoc.* **156:**1737–1740.
14. Moore, J. A., and T. J. Kakuk. 1967. Male dogs naturally infected with *Brucella canis*. *J. Am. Vet. Med. Assoc.* **155:**1352–1358.
15. Pickerill, P. A., and L. E. Carmichael. 1972. Canine brucellosis: control programs in commercial kennels and effect on reproduction. *J. Am. Vet. Med. Assoc.* **160:**1607–1615.
16. Rhoades, H. E., and G. M. Mesfin. 1980. *Brucella canis* infection in a kennel. *Vet. Med. Small Anim. Clin.* **75:**595–599.
17. Riecke, J. A., and H. E. Rhoades. 1975. *Brucella canis* isolated from the eye of a dog. *J. Am. Vet. Med. Assoc.* **166:**583–384.
18. Rumley, R. L., and S. W. Chapman. 1986. *Brucella canis:* an infectious cause of prolonged fever of undetermined origin. *South. Med. J.* **79:**626–628.
19. Serikawa, T., T. Muraguchi, J. Yamada, and H. Takada. 1981. Long-term observation of canine brucellosis: excretion of *Brucella canis* into urine of infected male dogs. *Jikken Dobutsu* **30:**7–14.
20. Serikawa, T., H. Takada, Y. Kondo, T. Muraguchi, and J. Yamada. 1984. Multiplication of *Brucella canis* in male reproductive organs and detection of autoantibody to spermatozoa in canine brucellosis. *Dev. Biol. Stand.* **56:**295–305.
21. Smeak, D. D., M. L. Olmstead, and R. B. Hohn. 1987. *Brucella canis* osteomyelitis in two dogs with total hip replacement. *J. Am. Vet. Med. Assoc.* **191:**986–990.
22. Walker, R. L. 1999. *Brucella,* p. 198–203. *In* D. C. Hirsh and Y. C. Zee (ed.), *Veterinary Microbiology.* Blackwell Science, Inc., Malden, Mass.
23. Wooley, R. E., P. L. Hitchcock, J. L. Blue, M. A. Neuman, J. Brown, and E. B. Shotts, Jr. 1978. Isolation of *Brucella canis* from a dog seronegative for brucellosis. *J. Am. Vet. Med. Assoc.* **173:**387–388.
24. Ying, W., M. Q. Nguyen, and J. A. Jahre. 1999. *Brucella canis* endocarditis: case report. *Clin. Infect. Dis.* **29:**1593–1594.

Campylobacter jejuni
1. Akhtar, S. Q., and F. Huq. 1989. Effect of *Campylobacter jejuni* extracts and culture supernatants on cell culture. *J. Trop. Med. Hyg.* **92:**80–85.
2. Aragon, V., K. Chao, and L. A. Dreyfus. 1997. Effect of cytolethal distending toxin on F-actin assembly and cell division in Chinese hamster ovary cells. *Infect. Immun.* **65:**3774–3780.
3. Bulgin, M. S., A. C. Ward, N. Sriranganathan, and P. Saras. 1984. Abortion in the dog due to *Campylobacter* species. *Am. J. Vet. Res.* **45:**555–556.
4. Denis, M., C. Soumet, K. Rivoal, G. Ermel, D. Blivet, G. Salvat, and P. Colin. 1999. Development of a m-PCR assay for simultaneous identification of *Campylobacter jejuni* and *C. coli. Lett. Appl. Microbiol.* **29:**406–410.
5. Everest, P. H., A. T. Cole, C. J. Hawkey, S. Knutton, H. Goossens, J. P. Butzler, J. M. Ketley, and P. H. Williams. 1993. Roles of leukotriene B_4, prostaglandin E_2, and cyclic AMP in *Campylobacter jejuni*-induced intestinal fluid secretion. *Infect. Immun.* **61:**4885–4887.
6. Fernandez, H., and R. Martin. 1991. *Campylobacter* intestinal carriage among stray and pet dogs. *Rev. Saude Publica* **25:**473–475.
7. Florin, I., and F. Antillon. 1992. Production of enterotoxin and cytotoxin in *Campylobacter jejuni* strains isolated in Costa Rica. *J. Med. Microbiol.* **37:**22–29.
8. Fox, J. G., M. C. Claps, N. S. Taylor, K. O. Maxwell, J. I. Ackerman, and S. B. Hoffman. 1988. *Campylobacter jejuni/coli* in commercially reared beagles: prevalence and serotypes. *Lab. Anim. Sci.* **38:**262–265.
9. Fox, J. G., K. O. Maxwell, and J. I. Ackerman. 1984. *Campylobacter jejuni* associated diarrhea in commercially reared beagles. *Lab. Anim. Sci.* **34:**151–155.
10. Fox, J. G., R. Moore, and J. I. Ackerman. 1983. *Campylobacter jejuni*-associated diarrhea in dogs. *J. Am. Vet. Med. Assoc.* **183:**1430–1433.
11. Hanel, I., F. Schulze, H. Hotzel, and E. Schubert. 1998. Detection and characterization of two cytotoxins produced by *Campylobacter jejuni* strains. *Zentbl. Bakteriol.* **288:**131–143.
12. Hindiyeh, M., S. Jense, S. Hohmann, H. Benett, C. Edwards, W. Aldeen, A. Croft, J. Daly, S. Mottice, and K. C. Carroll. 2000. Rapid detection of *Campylobacter jejuni* in stool specimens by an enzyme immunoassay and surveillance for *Campylobacter upsaliensis* in the greater Salt Lake City area. *J. Clin. Microbiol.* **38:**3076–3079.
13. Hirsh, D. C. 1999. Spiral organisms I: *Campylobacter-Arcobacter-Lawsonia* (Digestive tract), p. 89–92. *In* D. C. Hirsh and Y. C. Zee (ed.), *Veterinary Microbiology.* Blackwell Science, Inc., Malden, Mass.
14. Ho, T. W., S. T. Hsieh, I. Nachamkin, H. J. Willison, K. Sheikh, J. Kiehlbauch, K. Flanigan, J. C. McArthur, D. R. Cornblath, G. M. McKhann, and J. W. Griffin. 1997.

Motor nerve terminal degeneration provides a potential mechanism for rapid recovery in acute motor axonal neuropathy after *Campylobacter* infection. *Neurology* **48:**717–724.
15. Konkel, M. E., M. R. Monteville, V. Rivera-Amill, and L. A. Jones. 2001. The pathogenesis of *Campylobacter jejuni*-mediated enteritis. *Curr. Issues Intest. Microbiol.* **2:**55–71.
16. Macartney, L., R. R. Al-Mashat, D. J. Taylor, and I. A. McCandlish. 1988. Experimental infection of dogs with *Campylobacter jejuni*. *Vet. Rec.* **122:**245–249.
17. Misawa, N., K. Hirayama, K. Itoh, and E. Takahashi. 1995. Detection of alpha- and beta-hemolytic-like activity from *Campylobacter jejuni*. *J. Clin. Microbiol.* **33:**729–731.
18. Monfort, J. D., J. P. Donahoe, H. F. Stills, Jr., and S. Bech-Nielsen. 1990. Efficacies of erythromycin and chloramphenicol in extinguishing fecal shedding of *Campylobacter jejuni* in dogs. *J. Am. Vet. Med. Assoc.* **196:**1069–1072.
19. Monfort, J. D., H. F. Stills, Jr., and S. Bech-Nielsen. 1989. Effects of sample holding time, temperature, and atmosphere on the isolation of *Campylobacter jejuni* from dogs. *J. Clin. Microbiol.* **27:**1419–1420.
20. Moreno, G. S., P. L. Griffiths, I. F. Connerton, and R. W. Park. 1993. Occurrence of campylobacters in small domestic and laboratory animals. *J. Appl. Bacteriol.* **75:**49–54.
21. Nair, G. B., R. K. Sarkar, S. Chowdhury, and S. C. Pal. 1985. *Campylobacter* infection in domestic dogs. *Vet. Rec.* **116:**237–238.
22. Odendaal, M. W., K. G. de Cramer, M. L. van der Walt, A. D. Botha, and P. M. Pieterson. 1994. First isolation of *Campylobacter jejuni* from the vaginal discharge of three bitches after abortion in South Africa. *Onderstepoort J. Vet. Res.* **61:**193–195.
23. Olson, P., and K. Sandstedt. 1987. *Campylobacter* in the dog: a clinical and experimental study. *Vet. Rec.* **121:**99–101.
24. O'Sullivan, A. M., C. J. Dore, S. Boyle, C. R. Coid, and A. P. Johnson. 1988. The effect of campylobacter lipopolysaccharide on fetal development in the mouse. *J. Med. Microbiol.* **26:**101–105.
25. Prescott, J. F., I. K. Barker, K. I. Manninen, and O. P. Miniats. 1981. *Campylobacter jejuni* colitis in gnotobiotic dogs. *Can. J. Comp. Med.* **45:**377–383.
26. Rivera-Amill, V., B. J. Kim, J. Seshu, and M. E. Konkel. 2001. Secretion of the virulence-associated *Campylobacter* invasion antigens from *Campylobacter jejuni* requires a stimulatory signal. *J. Infect. Dis.* **183:**1607–1616.
27. Steinhauserova, I., K. Fojtikova, and J. Klimes. 2000. The incidence and PCR detection of *Campylobacter upsaliensis* in dogs and cats. *Lett. Appl. Microbiol.* **31:**209–212.
28. Tennant, B. 2001. The alimentary tract, p. 129–150. *In* I. Ramsey and B. Tennant (ed.), *Manual of Canine and Feline Infectious Diseases*. British Small Animal Veterinary Association, Gloucester, England.
29. Torre, E., and M. Tello. 1993. Factors influencing fecal shedding of *Campylobacter jejuni* in dogs without diarrhea. *Am. J. Vet. Res.* **54:**260–262.
30. Torres, O., and J. R. Cruz. 1993. Protection against *Campylobacter* diarrhea: role of milk IgA antibodies against bacterial surface antigens. *Acta Paediatr.* **82:**835–838.
31. Wallis, M. R. 1994. The pathogenesis of *Campylobacter jejuni*. *Br. J. Biomed. Sci.* **51:**57–64.
32. Zhu, J., R. J. Meinersmann, K. L. Hiett, and D. L. Evans. 1999. Apoptotic effect of outer-membrane proteins from *Campylobacter jejuni* on chicken lymphocytes. *Curr. Microbiol.* **38:**244–249.

FUNGI

Dermatomycosis

1. Bergman, R. L., L. Medleau, K. Hnilica, and E. Howerth. 2002. Dermatophyte granulomas caused by *Trichophyton mentagrophytes* in a dog. *Vet. Dermatol.* **13:**51–54.
2. Bibel, D. J., and J. R. LeBrun. 1975. Effect of experimental dermatophyte infection on cutaneous flora. *J. Investig. Dermatol.* **64:**119–123.
3. Biberstein, E. L. 1999. Dermatophytes, p. 214–219. *In* D. C. Hirsh and Y. C. Zee (ed.), *Veterinary Microbiology*. Blackwell Science, Inc., Malden, Mass.
4. Blake, J. S., M. V. Dahl, M. J. Herron, and R. D. Nelson. 1991. An immunoinhibitory cell wall glycoprotein (mannon) from *Trichophyton rubrum*. *J. Investig. Dermatol.* **96:**657–661.
5. Cabanes, F. J., M. L. Abarca, M. R. Bragulat, and G. Castella. 1996. Seasonal study of the fungal biota of the fur of dogs. *Mycopathologia* **133:**1–7.
6. Das, M., H. Mukhtar, B. J. Del Tito, Jr., D. L. Marcelo, and D. R. Bickers. 1986. Clotrimazole, an inhibitor of benzo(a)pyrene metabolism and its subsequent glucuronidation, sulfation, and macromolecular binding in BALB/c mouse cultured keratinocytes. *J. Investig. Dermatol.* **87:**4–10.
7. Komarek, J., and Z. Wurst. 1989. Dermatophytes in clinically healthy dogs and cats. *Vet. Med. (Praha)* **34:**59–63.

8. **Mason, I., R. Bond, D. A. Gunn-Moore, and A. Sparkes.** 2001. The skin, p. 197–218. *In* I. Ramsey and B. Tennant (ed.), *Manual of Canine and Feline Infectious Diseases*. British Small Animal Veterinary Association, Gloucester, England.
9. **Moriello, K. A.** 2001. Diagnostic techniques for dermatophytosis. *Clin. Tech. Small Anim. Pract.* **16:**219–224.
10. **Sparkes, A. H., T. J. Gruffydd-Jones, S. E. Shaw, A. I. Wright, and C. R. Stokes.** 1993. Epidemiological and diagnostic features of canine and feline dermatophytosis in the United Kingdom from 1956 to 1991. *Vet. Rec.* **133:**57–61.
11. **Stevens, D. A.** 1989. The interface of mycology and endocrinology. *J. Med. Vet. Mycol.* **27:**133–140.
12. **Tan, J. S.** 1997. Human zoonotic infections transmitted by dogs and cats. *Arch. Intern. Med.* **157:**1933–1943.

Malassezia pachydermatis
1. **Aizawa, T., R. Kano, Y. Nakamura, S. Watanabe, and A. Hasegawa.** 1999. Molecular heterogeneity in clinical isolates of *Malassezia pachydermatis* from dogs. *Vet. Microbiol.* **70:**67–75.
2. **Akerstedt, J., and I. Vollset.** 1995. *Malassezia pachydermatis* with special reference to canine skin disease. *Br. Vet. J.* **152:**269–281.
3. **Bond, R., C. M. Elwood, R. M. Littler, L. Pinter, and D. H. Lloyd.** 1998. Humoral and cell-mediated responses to *Malassezia pachydermatis* in healthy dogs and dogs with *Malassezia* dermatitis. *Vet. Rec.* **143:**381–384.
4. **Bond, R., E. A. Ferguson, C. F. Curtis, J. M. Craig, and D. H. Lloyd.** 1996. Factors associated with elevated cutaneous *Malassezia pachydermatis* populations in dogs with pruritic skin disease. *J. Small Anim. Pract.* **37:**103–107.
5. **Bond, R., A. I. Lamport, and D. H. Lloyd.** 2000. Colonisation status of *Malassezia pachydermatis* on the hair and in the hair follicle of healthy beagle dogs. *Res. Vet. Sci.* **68:**291–293.
6. **Bond, R., L. E. Saijonmaa-Koulumies, and D. H. Lloyd.** 1995. Population sizes and frequency of *Malassezia pachydermatis* at skin and mucosal sites on healthy dogs. *J. Small Anim. Pract.* **36:**147–150.
7. **Chang, H. J., H. L. Miller, N. Watkins, M. J. Arduino, D. A. Ashford, G. Midgley, S. M. Aguero, R. Pinto-Powell, C. F. von Reyn, W. Edwards, M. M. McNeil, and W. R. Jarvis.** 1998. An epidemic of *Malassezia pachydermatis* in an intensive care nursery associated with colonization of health care workers' dogs. *N. Engl. J. Med.* **338:**706–711.
8. **Coutinho, S. D., and C. R. Paula.** 2000. Proteinase, phospholipase, hyaluronidase, and chondroitin-sulphatase production by *Malassezia pachydermatis*. *Med. Mycol.* **38:**73–76.
9. **Gabal, M. A.** 1988. Preliminary studies on the mechanism of infection and characterization of *Malassezia pachydermatis* in association with canine otitis externa. *Mycopathologia* **104:**93–98.
10. **Gedek, B., K. Brutzel, R. Gerlach, F. Netzer, H. Rocken, H. Unger, and J. Symoens.** 1979. The role of *Pityrosporum pachydermatis* in otitis externa of dogs: evaluation of a treatment with miconazole. *Vet. Rec.* **104:**138–140.
11. **Kennis, R. A., E. J. Rosser, Jr., N. B. Olivier, and R. W. Walker.** 1996. Quantity and distribution of *Malassezia* organisms on the skin of clinically normal dogs. *J. Am. Vet. Med. Assoc.* **208:**1048–1051.
12. **Kiss, G., S. Radvanyi, and G. Szigeti.** 1996. Characteristics of *Malassezia pachydermatis* strains isolated from canine otitis externa. *Mycoses* **39:**313–321.
13. **Mancianti, F., A. Rum, S. Nardoni, and M. Corazza.** 2000. Extracellular enzymatic activity of *Malassezia* spp. isolates. *Mycopathologia* **149:**131–135.
14. **Masuda, A., T. Sukegawa, N. Mizumoto, H. Tani, T. Miyamoto, K. Sasai, and E. Baba.** 2000. Study of lipid in the ear canal in canine otitis externa with *Malassezia pachydermatis*. *J. Vet. Med. Sci.* **62:**1177–1182.
15. **Masuda, A., T. Sukegawa, H. Tani, T. Miyamoto, K. Sasai, Y. Morikawa, and E. Baba.** 2001. Attachment of *Malassezia pachydermatis* to the ear dermal cells in canine otitis externa. *J. Vet. Med. Sci.* **63:**667–669.
16. **Morris, D. O.** 1999. *Malassezia* dermatitis and otitis. *Vet. Clin. North Am. Small Anim. Pract.* **29:**1303–1310.
17. **Morris, D. O., D. J. Clayton, K. J. Drobatz, and P. J. Felsburg.** 2002. Response to *Malassezia pachydermatis* by peripheral blood mononuclear cells from clinically normal and atopic dogs. *Am. J. Vet. Res.* **63:**358–362.
18. **Morris, D. O., N. B. Olivier, and E. J. Rosser.** 1998. Type-1 hypersensitivity reactions to *Malassezia pachydermatis* extracts in atopic dogs. *Am. J. Vet. Res.* **59:**836–841.
19. **Plant, J. D., W. S. Rosenkrantz, and C. E. Griffin.** 1992. Factors associated with and prevalence of high *Malassezia pachydermatis* numbers on dog skin. *J. Am. Vet. Med. Assoc.* **201:**879–882.
20. **Romano, A., E. Segal, and M. Blumenthal.** 1978. Canaliculitis with isolation of *Pityrosporum pachydermatis*. *Br. J. Ophthalmol.* **62:**732–734.
21. **Salkin, I. F., W. B. Stone, and M. A. Gordon.** 1980. Association of *Malassezia* (*Pityrospo-*

rum) pachydermatis with sarcoptic mange in New York State. *J. Wildl. Dis.* **16**:509–514.
22. **Takahashi, M., T. Ushijima, and Y. Ozaki.** 1984. Biological activity of *Pityrosporum*. I. Enhancement of resistance in mice stimulated by *Pityrosporum* against *Salmonella typhimurium*. *Immunology* **51**:697–702.
23. **Takahashi, M., T. Ushijima, and Y. Ozaki.** 1986. Biological activity of *Pityrosporum*. II. Antitumor and immune stimulating effect of *Pityrosporum* in mice. *J. Natl. Cancer Inst.* **77**:1093–1097.

PARASITES

Demodex canis
1. **Baker, K. P.** 1970. Observations on the epidemiology, diagnosis and treatment of demodicosis in dogs. *Vet. Rec.* **86**:90–91.
2. **Barriga, O. O., N. W. al-Khalidi, S. Martin, and M. Wyman.** 1992. Evidence of immunosuppression by *Demodex canis*. *Vet. Immunol. Immunopathol.* **32**:37–46.
3. **Barta, O., C. Waltman, P. P. Oyekan, R. K. McGrath, and T. N. Hribernik.** 1983. Lymphocyte transformation suppression caused by pyoderma—failure to demonstrate it in uncomplicated mange. *Comp. Immunol. Microbiol. Infect. Dis.* **6**:9–18.
4. **Brockis, D. C.** 1994. Otitis externa due to *Demodex canis*. *Vet. Rec.* **135**:409–410.
5. **Burrows, A. K.** 2000. Generalised demodicosis in the dog: the unresponsive or recurrent case. *Aust. Vet. J.* **78**:244–246.
6. **Caswell, J. L., J. A. Yager, W. M. Parker, and P. F. Moore.** 1997. A prospective study of the immunophenotype and temporal changes in the histologic lesions of canine demodicosis. *Vet. Pathol.* **34**:279–287.
7. **Day, M. J.** 1997. An immunohistochemical study of the lesions of demodicosis in the dog. *J. Comp. Pathol.* **116**:203–216.
8. **DeBoer, D. J., P. J. Ihrke, and A. A. Stannard.** 1988. Circulating immune complex concentrations in selected cases of skin disease in dogs. *Am. J. Vet. Res.* **49**:143–146.
9. **Gothe, R.** 1989. Demodicosis of dogs—a factorial disease? *Berl. Muench. Tieraerztl. Wochenschr.* **102**:293–297.
10. **Greve, J. H., and S. M. Gaafar.** 1966. Natural transmission of *Demodex canis* in dogs. *J. Am. Vet. Med. Assoc.* **148**:1043–1045.
11. **Hirsh, D. C., B. B. Baker, N. Wiger, S. G. Yaskulski, and B. I. Osburn.** 1975. Suppression of in vitro lymphocyte transformation by serum from dogs with generalized demodicosis. *Am. J. Vet. Res.* **36**:1591–1595.
12. **Hsu, W. H., and D. D. Schaffer.** 1988. Effects of topical application of amitraz on plasma glucose and insulin concentrations in dogs. *Am. J. Vet. Res.* **49**:130–131.
13. **Kraiss, A.** 1987. Proliferating ability of the lymphocytes of demodectic dogs during immune cell-stimulating therapy. *Tieraerztl. Prax.* **15**:63–66.
14. **Latimer, K.S ., K. W. Prasse, E. A. Mahaffey, D. L. Dawe, M. D. Lorenz, and J. R. Duncan.** 1983. Neutrophil movement in selected canine skin disease. *Am. J. Vet. Res.* **44**:601–605.
15. **Lemarie, S. L., C. S. Foil, and D. W. Horohov.** 1994. Evaluation of interleukin-2 production and interleukin-2 receptor expression in dogs with generalized demodicosis. *Proc. Am Acad. Vet. Dermatol.* **10**:26–27.
16. **Nayak, D. C., S. B. Tripathy, P. C. Dey, S. K. Ray, D. N. Mohanty, G. S. Parida, S. Biswal, and M. Das.** 1997. Prevalence of canine demodicosis in Orissa (India). *Vet. Parasitol.* **73**:347–352.
17. **Paulik, S., J. Mojzisova, V. Bajova, D. Baranova, and I. Paulikova.** 1996. Evaluation of canine lymphocyte blastogenesis prior and after in vitro suppression by dog demodicosis serum using ethidium bromide fluorescence assay. *Vet. Med. (Praha)* **41**:7–12.
18. **Paulik, S., J. Mojzisova, V. Bajova, D. Baranova, and I. Paulikova.** 1996. Lymphocyte blastogenesis to concanavalin A in dogs with localized demodicosis according to duration of clinical disease. *Vet. Med. (Praha)* **41**:245–249.
19. **Shaw, S. E., and A. P. Foster.** 2000. Treatment of canine adult-onset demodicosis. *Aust. Vet. J.* **78**:243–244.
20. **Shipstone, M.** 2000. Generalised demodicosis in dogs, clinical perspective. *Aust. Vet. J.* **78**:240–242.
21. **Sischo, W. M., P. J. Ihrke, and C. E. Franti.** 1989. Regional distribution of ten common skin diseases in dogs. *J. Am. Vet. Med. Assoc.* **195**:752–756.
22. **Tamura, Y., Y. Kawamura, I. Inoue, and S. Ishino.** 2001. Scanning electron microscopy description of a new species of *Demodex canis* spp. *Vet. Dermatol.* **12**:275–278.
23. **Toman, N., M. Svoboda, J. Rybnicek, J. Krejci, M. Faldyna, and O. Barta.** 1997. Immunosuppression in dogs with pyoderma and/or demodicosis. *Vet. Med. (Praha)* **42**:299–306.
24. **White, S. D.** 1986. Facial dermatosis in four dogs with hyperadrenocorticism. *J. Am. Vet. Med. Assoc.* **188**:1441–1444.
25. **Wilkie, B. N., R. J. Markham, and C. Hazlett.** 1979. Deficient cutaneous response to

PHA-P in healthy puppies from a kennel with a high prevalence of demodicosis. *Can J. Comp. Med.* **43**:415–419.

Dirofilaria immitis (heartworm)
1. **Abbot, P. K.** 1961. *Dirofilaria immitis* in the peritoneal cavity. *Aust. Vet. J.* **37**:467.
2. **Bowman, D.** 1999. *Georgis' Parasitology for Veterinarians,* 7th ed. W.B. Saunders Co., Philadelphia, Pa.
3. **Busch, D. S., and J. O. Noxon.** 1992. Pneumothorax in a dog infected with *Dirofilaria immitis. J. Am. Vet. Med. Assoc.* **201**:1893.
4. **Cooley, A. J., R. M. Clemmons, and T. L. Gross.** 1987. Heartworm disease manifested by encephalomyelitis and myositis in a dog. *J. Am. Vet. Med. Assoc.* **190**:431–432.
5. **Crissman, R. S., and J. N. Ross, Jr.** 1983. Electron microscopy of intimal lesions in the pulmonary trunk of a dog with *Dirofilaria immitis. J. Submicrosc. Cytol.* **15**:509–517.
6. **Dalton, G. O., Jr., L. A. Bruce, and T. L. Huber.** 1971. Effect of *Dirofilaria immitis* on renal function in the dog. *Am. J. Vet. Res.* **32**:2087–2089.
7. **Donahoe, J. M., and E. A. Holzinger.** 1974. *Dirofilaria immitis* in the brains of a dog and a cat. *J. Am. Vet. Med. Assoc.* **164**:518–519.
8. **Eaton, K. A., and T. J. Rosol.** 1989. Caval syndrome in a *Dirofilaria immitis*-infected dog treated with dichlorvos. *J. Am. Vet. Med. Assoc.* **195**:223–224.
9. **Elwood, C.** 2001. The cardiovascular system, p. 117–128. *In* I. Ramsey and B. Tennant (ed.), *Manual of Canine and Feline Infectious Diseases.* British Small Animal Veterinary Association, Gloucester, England.
10. **Frank, J. R., F. B. Nutter, A. E. Kyles, C. E. Atkins, and R. K. Sellon.** 1997. Systemic arterial dirofilariasis in five dogs. *J. Vet. Intern. Med.* **11**:189–194.
11. **Gbakima, A. A., W. el-Sadr, and B. M. Greene.** 1986. Delayed isotype switching in *Dirofilaria immitis* infection. *Trans. R. Soc. Trop. Med. Hyg.* **80**:305–308.
12. **Goggin, J. M., D. S. Biller, C. M. Rost, B. M. DeBey, and C. L. Ludlow.** 1997. Ultrasonographic identification of *Dirofilaria immitis* in the aorta and liver of a dog. *J. Am. Vet. Med. Assoc.* **210**:1635–1637.
13. **Grauer, G. F., C. A. Culham, R. R. Dubielzig, S. L. Longhofer, and R. B. Grieve.** 1989. Experimental *Dirofilaria immitis*-associated glomerulonephritis induced in part by *in situ* formation of immune complexes in the glomerular capillary wall. *J. Parasitol.* **75**:585–593.
14. **Henry, C. J.** 1992. Salivary mucocele associated with dirofilariasis in a dog. *J. Am. Vet. Med. Assoc.* **200**:1965–1966.
15. **Lavers, D. W., D. M. Spratt, and C. Thomas.** 1969. *Dirofilaria immitis* from the eye of a dog. *Aust. Vet. J.* **45**:284–286.
16. **Liu, S. K., K. M. Das, and R. J. Tashjian.** 1966. Adult *Dirofilaria immitis* in the arterial system of a dog. *J. Am. Vet. Med. Assoc.* **148**:1501–1507.
17. **Lok, J. B., D. H. Knight, G. T. Wang, M. E. Doscher, T. J. Nolan, M. J. Hendrick, W. Steber, and K. Heaney.** 2001. Activity of an injectable, sustained-release formulation of moxidectin administered prophylactically to mixed-breed dogs to prevent infection with *Dirofilaria immitis. Am. J. Vet. Res.* **62**:1721–1726.
18. **Mason, R. W., and A. R. Tait.** 1969. *Dirofilaria immitis*-posterior caval syndrome in a dog. *Aust. Vet. J.* **45**:435–436.
19. **Matsumoto, H., T. Yamada, N. Takemura, T. Sako, H. Koyama, S. Motoyoshi, and T. Inada.** 1996. Detection of circulating immune complexes in dog sera by immune adherence hemagglutination method. *J. Vet. Med. Sci.* **58**:272–230.
20. **Newton, W. L.** 1968. Longevity of an experimental infection with *Dirofilaria immitis* in a dog. *J. Parasitol.* **54**:187–188.
21. **Patton, C. S., and F. M. Garner.** 1970. Cerebral infarction caused by heartworms (*Dirofilaria immitis*) in a dog. *J. Am. Vet. Med. Assoc.* **156**:600–605.
22. **Rawlings, C. A.** 1980. Cardiopulmonary function in the dog with *Dirofilaria immitis* infection: during infection and after treatment. *Am. J. Vet. Res.* **41**:319–325.
23. **Scott, D. W.** 1979. Nodular skin disease associated with *Dirofilaria immitis* infection in the dog. *Cornell Vet.* **69**:233–240.
24. **Seavers, A.** 1998. Cutaneous syndrome possibly caused by heartworm infestation in a dog. *Aust. Vet. J.* **76**:18–20.
25. **Shah, M. K.** 1999. Human pulmonary dirofilariasis: review of the literature. *South. Med. J.* **92**:276–279.
26. **Skidmore, J. P., P. D. Dooley, and C. DeWitt.** 2000. Human extrapulmonary dirofilariasis in Texas. *South. Med. J.* **93**:1009–1010.
27. **Slonka, G. F., W. Castleman, and S. Krum.** 1977. Adult heartworms in arteries and veins of a dog. *J. Am. Vet. Med. Assoc.* **170**:717–719.
28. **Tanaka, K. I., and R. B. Atwell.** 1993. Immunohistological observations on pulmonary tissues from dogs infected with *Dirofilaria immitis. Vet. Res. Commun.* **17**:109–117.
29. **Todd, K. S., and T. P. Howland.** 1983. Transplacental transmission of *Dirofilaria immitis* microfilariae in the dog. *J. Parasitol.* **69**:371

30. van Heerden, J., A. Verster, and D. J. Gouws. 1980. Neostigmine-responsive weakness and glomerulonephritis associated with heartworm *Dirofilaria immitis* infestation in a dog. *J. S. Afr. Vet. Assoc.* **51**:251–253.

Fleas
1. Bowman, D. 1999. *Georgis' Parasitology for Veterinarians,* 7th ed. W.B. Saunders Co., Philadelphia, Pa.
2. Cadiergues, M. C., C. Caubet, and M. Franc. 2001. Comparison of the activity of selamectin, imidacloprid and fipronil for the treatment of dogs infested experimentally with *Ctenocephalidies canis* and *Ctenocephalides felis felis*. *Vet. Rec.* **149**:704–706.
3. Cheeseman, M. T. 1998. Characterization of apyrase activity from the salivary glands of the cat flea *Ctenocephalides felis*. *Insect Biochem. Mol. Biol.* **28**:1025–1030.
4. Cheeseman, M. T., P. A. Bates, and J. M. Crampton. 2001. Preliminary characterization of esterase and platelet-activating factor (PAF)-acetylhydrolase activities from cat flea (*Ctenocephalides felis*) salivary glands. *Insect Biochem. Mol. Biol.* **31**:157–164.
5. Dryden, M.W., and M.K. Rust. 1994. The cat flea: biology, ecology and control. *Vet. Parasitol.* **52**:1–19.
6. Greene, W. K., R. L. Carnegie, S. E. Shaw, R. C. Thompson, and W. J. Penhale. 1993. Characterization of allergens of the cat flea, *Ctenocephalides felis:* detection and frequency of IgE antibodies in canine sera. *Parasite Immunol.* **15**:69–74.
7. Halliwell, R. E., J. F. Preston, and J. G. Nesbitt. 1987. Aspects of the immunopathogenesis of flea allergy dermatitis in dogs. *Vet. Immunol. Immunopathol.* **17**:483–494.
8. Lee, S. E., I. P. Johnstone, R. P. Lee, and J. P. Opdebeeck. 1999. Putative salivary allergens of the cat flea, *Ctenocephalides felis felis*. *Vet. Immunol. Immunopathol.* **69**:229–237.
9. Mason, I., R. Bond, D. A. Gunn-Moore, and A. Sparkes. 2001. The skin, p. 197–218. *In* I. Ramsey and B. Tennant (ed.), *Manual of Canine and Feline Infectious Diseases*. British Small Animal Veterinary Association, Gloucester, England.
10. McDermott, M. J., E. Weber, S. Hunter, K. E. Stedman, E. Best, G. R. Frank, R. Wang, J. Escudero, J. Kuner, and C. McCall. 2000. Identification, cloning, and characterization of a major cat flea salivary allergen (Cte f1). *Mol. Immunol.* **37**:361–375.
11. Payne-Johnson, M., T. P. Maitland, J. Sherington, D. J. Shanks, P. J. Clements, M. G. Murphy, A. McLoughlin, A. D. Jernigan, and T. G. Rowan. 2000. Efficacy of selamectin administered topically to pregnant and lactating female dogs in the treatment and prevention of adult roundworm (*Toxocara canis*) infections and flea (*Ctenocephalides felis felis*) infestations in the dams and their pups. *Vet. Parasitol.* **91**:347–358.
12. Zakson-Aiken, M., L. M. Gregory, P. T. Meinke, and W. L. Shoop. 2001. Systemic activity of the avermectins against the cat flea (Siphonaptera: Pulicidae). *J. Med. Entomol.* **38**:576–580.

Intestinal nematodes
1. Baker, D. G., and D. R. Strombeck. 1985. Intestinal parasitism in dogs from a Placer County, California, animal control facility. *Calif. Vet.* **39**:32–36.
2. Bowman, D. 1999. *Georgis' Parasitology for Veterinarians,* 7th ed. W.B. Saunders Co., Philadelphia, Pa.
3. Dubinsky, P., K. Havasiova-Reiterova, B. Petko, I. Hovorka, and O. Tomasovicova. 1995. Role of small mammals in the epidemiology of toxocariasis. *Parasitology* **110**:187-193.
4. Hayes, H. M., Jr., M. M. Morin, and D. A. Rubenstein. 1983. Canine biliary carcinoma: epidemiological comparisons with man. *J. Comp. Pathol.* **93**:99–107.
5. Loukas, A., A. Doedens, M. Hintz, and R. M. Maizels. 2000. Identification of a new C-type lectin, TES-70, secreted by infective larvae of *Toxocara canis*, which binds to host ligands. *Parasitology* **121**:545–554.
6. Overgaauw, P. A. 1997. Aspects of *Toxocara* epidemiology: toxocarosis in dogs and cats. *Crit. Rev. Microbiol.* **23**:233–251.
7. Verine, H. J., J. P. Gevrey, and J. E. Murat. 1969. *Toxocara canis* as a support for cholelithiasis in the dog. *Vet. Rec.* **85**:98–99.
8. Visco, R. J., R. M. Corwin, and L. A. Selby. 1977. Effect of age and sex on the prevalence of intestinal parasitism in dogs. *J. Am. Vet. Med. Assoc.* **170**:835–837.

Intestinal protozoa
1. Allen, P. C., and R. H. Fetterer. 2000. Effect of *Eimeria acervulina* infections on plasma L-arginine. *Poult. Sci.* **79**:1414–1417.
2. Aumont, G., P. Yvore, and A. Esnault. 1986. Experimental coccidiosis in goats. 2. Effect of parasitism on nutritional balances and some blood parameters. *Ann. Rech. Vet.* **17**:191–196.
3. Bowman, D. 1999. *Georgis' Parasitology for Veterinarians,* 7th ed, W.B. Saunders Co., Philadelphia, Pa.
4. Byrnes, S., R. Eaton, and M. Kogut. 1993. In vitro interleukin-1 and tumor necrosis factor-

α production by macrophages from chickens infected with either *Eimeria maxima* or *Eimeria tenella*. *Int. J. Parasitol.* **23:**639-645.

5. **Dubey, J. P., A. Koestner, and R. C. Piper.** 1990. Repeated transplacental transmission of *Neospora caninum* in dogs. *J. Am. Vet. Med. Assoc.* **197:**857–860.

6. **Dubey, J. P., S. E. Weisbrode, and W. A. Rogers.** 1978. Canine coccidiosis attributed to an Isospora ohioensis-like organism: a case report. *J. Am. Vet. Med. Assoc.* **173:**185–191.

7. **Hyun, C. S., C. W. Chen, N. L. Shinowara, T. Palaia, F. S. Fallick, L. A. Martello, M. Mueenuddin, V. M. Donovan, and S. Teichberg.** 1995. Morphological factors influencing transepithelial conductance in a rabbit model of ileitis. *Gastroenterology* **109:**13–23.

8. **Innes, E. A., D. Buxton, S. Maley, S. Wright, J. Marks, I. Esteban, A. Rae, A. Schock, and J. Wastling.** 2000. Neosporosis. Aspects of epidemiology and host immune response. *Ann. N. Y. Acad. Sci.* **916:**93–101.

9. **Kogut, M. H., and K. C. Powell.** 1993. Preliminary findings of alterations in serum alkaline phosphatase activity in chickens during coccidial infections. *J. Comp. Pathol.* **108:**113–119.

10. **Licois, D., and P. Mongin.** 1980. An hypothesis of the pathogenesis of diarrhea in the rabbit based on a study of intestinal contents. *Reprod. Nutr. Dev.* **20:**1209–1216.

11. **Mohammed, R. A., O. A. Idris, S. M. el Sanousi, and E. B. Abdelsalam.** 2000. The effect of coccidian infection on the gut microflora of Nubian goat kids. *Dtsch. Tieraerztl. Wochenschr.* **107:**414–416.

12. **Odin, M., and J. P. Dubey.** 1993. Sudden death associated with *Neospora caninum* myocarditis in a dog. *J. Am. Vet. Med. Assoc.* **203:**831–833.

13. **Perl, S., S. Harrus, C. Satuchne, B. Yakobson, and D. Haines.** 1998. Cutaneous neosporosis in a dog in Israel. *Vet. Parasitol.* **79:**257–261.

14. **Peters, M., F. Wagner, and G. Schares.** 2000. Canine neosporosis: clinical and pathological findings and first isolation of *Neosporum caninum* in Germany. *Parasitol. Res.* **86:**1–7.

15. **Qin, Z. R., A. Arakawa, E. Baba, T. Fukata, T. Miyamoto, K. Sasai, and G. S. Withanage.** 1995. *Eimeria tenella* infection induces recrudescence of previous *Salmonella enteritidis* infection in chickens. *Poult. Sci.* **74:**1786–1792.

16. **Qin, Z. R., T. Fukata, E. Baba, and A. Arakawa.** 1995. Effects of *Eimeria tenella* infections on *Salmonella enteritidis* infection in chickens. *Poult. Sci.* **74:**1–7.

17. **Ruehlmann, D., M. Podell, M. Oglesbee, and J. P. Dubey.** 1995. Canine neosporosis: a case report and literature review. *J. Am. Anim. Hosp. Assoc.* **31:**174–183.

18. **Ruff, M. D., M. A. Abdel Nabi, R. N. Clarke, M. Mobarak, and M. A. Ottinger.** 1988. Effect of coccidiosis on reproductive maturation of male Japanese quail. *Avian Dis.* **32:**41–45.

19. **Uggla, A., J. P. Dubey, G. Lundmark, and P. Olson.** 1989. Encephalomyelitis and myositis in a boxer puppy due to a *Neospora*-like infection. *Vet. Parasitol.* **32:**255–260.

PATHOGENS OF SWINE

10

INTRODUCTION

The domestic pig (*Sus scrofa domestica*) has assumed a significant role in biomedical research. To some extent, the domestic pig has replaced the dog and cat as the nonrodent model of choice. The impetus for this switch has come from several sources, including the increasing costs of purpose-bred dogs and cats relative to generic pigs and concerns about the use of "pet" animals in biomedical research, and from a growing appreciation of the many physiologic and anatomic similarities between humans and swine. The pig serves as an animal model for research involving the dermal, cardiopulmonary, gastrointestinal, renal, and other body systems. In addition, swine have been used extensively in nutritional research as models in which to study the physiology of addictions, such as to alcohol and tobacco. Lastly, swine have become the organ donor of choice in xenotransplantation experiments.

Many pigs used in biomedical research are purpose bred by commercial vendors. This is certainly true in cases where genetic and physiologic uniformity are necessary. These pigs tend to be relatively free of primary pathogens, and experience few serious infections throughout life so long as animal housing and care remain at high levels. However, there remains a large number of "farm" pigs purchased from private, small-scale operations. Many of these pigs are used in studies that can tolerate animals from less controlled environments, or in teaching laboratories where genetic and physiologic uniformity are less important.

To an even greater extent than noted in the chapters covering other large animal species, very few reports directly describe the research-altering effects of pathogens on their porcine hosts. It would seem that for many projects, greater effort should be made to determine the microbiologic status of the research swine involved. Yet often this does not seem to be the case. There appears to be a level of acceptance of "background" infections in research pigs that would not be accepted in laboratory rodents. Once again, the literature covering natural case reports and experimental infections has been reviewed to allow a reasonable synthesis of the known and potential physiologic effects these pathogens may have on the porcine research subject. For the reader interested in more complete discussions of virtually all diseases of swine, the reader is referred to the excellent text by the same title, diseases of swine. It is heavily referenced in this section. This author acknowledges great indebtedness to the writers of that comprehensive work.

VIRUSES

Encephalomyocarditis virus

Agent

Encephalomyocarditis virus (EMCV) is a single-stranded RNA (ssRNA) virus in the family *Picornaviridae*. These are small viruses with great importance in human and veterinary medicine. Examples of medically important picornaviruses include poliomyelitis virus and the virus of foot-and-mouth disease. EMCV is in the genus *Cardiovirus*. Several strains of the virus have been isolated. There is considerable strain-to-strain variation in virulence (8, 11).

Epidemiology

Incidence of EMCV infection is low, although outbreaks have been reported in pigs from many parts of the world (7). Rodents are thought to be the natural hosts of EMCV, but young pigs, as well as several other mammals, are also susceptible to infection. Pig-to-pig transmission occurs (5), but does not appear to constitute a major reservoir of infection (16). Likewise, transplacental transmission has been demonstrated in naturally and experimentally infected cases, but may not play a significant role epidemiologically (2, 9, 11). Rats, and to a possibly greater extent, mice, appear to represent the primary sources of infection. Rodents succumb to infection and their carcasses contain high levels of virus. In addition, rodents excrete virus in their feces and urine, and may expose pigs through contaminated feed or drinking water.

Clinical signs

Clinical signs of EMCV infection vary with viral strain and host age (8, 11). Nursing piglets are most susceptible to disease caused by EMCV. When present, premonitory signs of EMCV include fever, anorexia, listlessness, dyspnea, staggering, trembling, and paralysis (7). However, premonitory signs are uncommon. Rather, affected piglets die suddenly due to myocardial failure. Mortality may be quite high. Clinical signs in older pigs are much less common and may be limited to respiratory distress (4). Infected sows may experience reproductive failure, which is evidenced by abortions and mummified or stillborn fetuses (1, 4, 9).

Pathology

Viremia occurs within days of oral inoculation, is transient, and is followed by fecal excretion of virus through the ninth day postinfection (3, 7). Excretion beyond the period of viremia is suggestive of viral replication in the gut (7). Large viral loads may be found in lymphoid tissues, including the spleen and mesenteric lymph nodes, as well as from myocardium. Virus can also be recovered from other visceral organs. Pigs dying of EMCV have relatively few pathologic lesions. The spleen may be found devoid of blood. The heart is enlarged, soft, and pale (7). Myocardial lesions appear as necrotic streaks or splotches consisting of mononuclear cell infiltration with or without calcification. Edematous changes in the pericardium and lungs may also be present (6, 12, 14). Pulmonary lesions may be the only lesions detected in young pigs (4). Fetal or neonatal pigs may also develop encephalitis, meningitis, and neuronal degeneration (7).

Interference with research

Natural infection of research swine with EMCV will at a minimum compromise studies involving the cardiovascular, enterohepatic, lymphoreticular, musculoskeletal, nervous, reproductive, and respiratory systems. However, because viral replication occurs in multiple visceral organs, most body systems may be affected. Also, the high mortality of young pigs will obviously negatively affect any study in which pigs are bred.

Diagnosis and control

A diagnosis of EMCV infection may be suspected with a history of reproductive failure and high neonatal mortality. Disease in older pigs may be more difficult to recognize clinically. Finding characteristic myocardial lesions at necropsy supports a diagnosis of EMCV infection, but must be differentiated from vitamin E and selenium deficiency (7). Confirmation of infection has historically relied on virus isolation from myocardium. This may be supported by immunohistochemistry. More recently, reverse transcriptase (RT)-PCR assays have been developed that provide more rapid results (15). Serologic testing of fluids from dead fetuses may reveal primary antibody (1, 10). However, in general, testing of neonatal pigs dying acutely is not appropriate because death often occurs prior to development of a detectable serologic response (13). There is no treatment available for EMCV infection. Control efforts should focus on elimination of rodents.

Hemagglutinating encephalomyelitis virus

Agent
Hemagglutinating encephalomyelitis virus (HEV) is an enveloped, ssRNA virus in the family *Coronaviridae,* genus *Coronavirus* (9). It is antigenically related to bovine coronavirus. The name is derived from the fact that HEV hemagglutinates erythrocytes of several species. Only one serotype has been identified. There are however, strain differences, as noted below.

Epidemiology
Infection with HEV occurs in most swine producing areas of the world. Many pigs may be unapparent carriers, indicating that the disease is of relatively little economic importance. Indeed, serologic studies indicate that seroprevalence rates commonly range from 30 to 90%, although seronegative herds can also occasionally be found. Transmission occurs when naive pigs contact or inhale nasal secretions. Viral excretion typically occurs for 8 to 10 days after infection (8).

Clinical signs
Most infections with HEV are asymptomatic. This is due to passively acquired immunity, which persists until the development of an age-related resistance to clinical disease. However, in newborn piglets, HEV may be associated with either of two clinical conditions. Viral strain determines which disease pattern develops. In the first case, HEV causes "vomiting and wasting disease" (VWD). This occurs in piglets less than 2 to 3 weeks of age, and is characterized by sneezing, coughing, tooth grinding, retching and vomiting, dehydration, constipation, weight loss or runting, depression, and death, or eventual death due to starvation or secondary bacterial infection (3, 8). In contrast, other viral strains cause encephalomyelitis, also in newborn piglets. A mild form of VWD may develop, but this is then overshadowed by signs indicative of central nervous system (CNS) dysfunction. These may include muscle tremors, hyperesthesia, gait abnormalities, backward walking, dog sitting, weakness, paddling, blindness, opisthotonus, nystagmus, and finally, prostration, dyspnea, coma, and death (6, 8, 10). Mortality may approach 100%, but piglets that recover do so completely, except for lagging weight gains. For both clinical presentations, pigs infected as adults show milder signs, and almost always recover.

Pathology
Following infection, often by the oronasal route, viral replication occurs in epithelial cells of the respiratory tract, and to a lesser extent, tonsils and small intestine (2). Virus rapidly spreads by peripheral nerves to many regions of the CNS, as well as to peripheral nerve plexuses (5). Gross pathologic changes are generally limited to a mild catarrhal rhinitis in cases of encephalomyelitis, and gastroenteritis with gas distension in cases of VWD. Microscopically, one observes lesions in the CNS, tonsils, lungs, and stomach. CNS lesions consist of nonsuppurative encephalomyelitis. Tonsilar lesions include epithelial degeneration and lymphocytic infiltration. Pulmonary lesions consist of interstitial peribronchiolar pneumonia, while gastric lesions include degeneration of the stomach ganglia and peri-

vascular cuffing, most prominently in the pyloric region (4, 8, 10). A humoral immune response to HEV infection develops quickly in sows, is passively transferred to their offspring, and limits disease in affected piglets until the development of age-related immunity is adequate to further prevent clinical disease (7).

Interference with research
Other than descriptions of clinical and pathologic changes induced by HEV, there is almost no literature indicating the potential effects that HEV may have on research involving infected swine. Andries (1) demonstrated that gastric emptying is delayed following viral infection of intestinal plexuses. However, on the basis of the clinicopathologic findings, one can assume that studies involving the enterohepatic, hematopoietic, lymphoreticular, musculoskeletal, nervous, and respiratory systems could be markedly affected when very young pigs are used. The extent to which these same systems would be affected immediately following infection of older pigs is unknown. It is possible that natural infection of older pigs more commonly used in research would also transiently compromise studies involving those body systems listed, necessitating their removal from the study. It is unlikely that seropositive young adult or adult pigs would be compromised.

Diagnosis and control
HEV infection may be suspected from the clinical signs, when present. These are not likely to be obvious in older pigs. Confirmation requires laboratory diagnostic testing. Diagnosis has historically been based on viral isolation from the tonsils, brain, and lung; rising antibody titer; or immunohistochemistry. It is likely that molecular methods, including RT-PCR, will become commercially available and commonly used. However, given the relatively short period of viral excretion, serology is currently the most reliable confirmatory test. There is no treatment for HEV infection. It is likely that many types of research involving adult pigs will not be affected by HEV, since adult pigs are frequently seropositive and asymptomatic. However, the decision to cull should be made with the investigator. There are no HEV vaccines commercially available. Like other coronaviruses, HEV is easily inactivated by harsh environmental conditions and most commonly used disinfectants.

Porcine circovirus

Agent
Porcine circovirus (PCV) is a small, circular, nonenveloped, relatively recently discovered ssDNA virus. Because of rather unique genetic structural properties, it was placed in a new family, the *Circoviridae* (1). At least two virus types, 1 and 2, have been reported. Of these, type 2 is of greater clinical importance (6).

Epidemiology
While the global range of PCV is yet to be determined, it appears that the virus has worldwide distribution in the production swine population (1). Seropositive swine have been identified in research colonies (29). Longitudinal studies suggest that piglets become infected by around 11 to 13 weeks of age. This corresponds to time of movement to the fattening unit in production programs (4). Transmission appears to be primarily horizontal, although the full range of means of transmission have yet to be determined. Infected boars shed virus particles in their semen for up to 47 days; however, replication competent virus has not been demonstrated (11, 14). Transplacental transmission has also been documented, but may be of relatively little importance (1, 2, 5). An early report suggested that some exposed humans seroconverted (27), but this has not been confirmed by others (9). At this point, PCV is not considered zoonotic.

Clinical signs
Most infections with PCV are asymptomatic; however, on occasion, clinical signs are observed. In fact, the range of clinical signs associated with PCV infection continues to

widen. PCV was first reported to cause congenital tremors in nursing piglets. Affected pigs show varying degrees of involvement, both in number of pigs affected, and in severity of symptoms. Skeletal muscle tremors may be induced by noises or chilling, are bilateral, and when severe, may result in starvation due to the inability to nurse. Pigs that survive generally recover within 3 weeks (15). Recently, PCV has been associated with postweaning multisystemic wasting syndrome (PMWS) in weanling pigs 6 to 8 weeks of age. In these cases, clinical signs include weight loss, loss of condition, cardiorespiratory distress, icterus, lymphadenopathy, diarrhea, coughing, and CNS disturbances (1). Morbidity is low but mortality may be high. It should be noted that the full expression of PMWS may require dual infection with PCV and porcine parvovirus, or porcine reproductive and respiratory syndrome virus (1, 7, 10). Additional studies are needed to determine the respective roles of these viruses in PMWS. Lastly, PCV has been implicated in cases of sow abortion, and in porcine dermatitis and nephropathy syndrome (19, 21). Infections with PCV are asymptomatic in adult pigs. However, disease severity can be accentuated following nonspecific immune stimulation, as occurs with vaccination (12).

Pathology

Following infection, virus replicates in most lymphoid tissues, as well as nasal mucosa, lung, liver, the CNS, and small intestine (2, 21, 26). On entry into a new host, PCV utilizes the host's cellular enzymatic machinery for its own replication, in an obligatory manner. PCV is known to replicate inside monocytes, macrophages, hepatocytes (1, 22), and in cases of congenital tremors, neurons of the central nervous system (26). Microscopic lesions observed in cases of congenital tremor are limited to abnormal myelin, and retardation in myelin deposition in the spinal cord (13, 26). In contrast, gross pathologic findings in PMWS include muscle wasting; skin and lymph node pallor; lymphoid, including splenic, enlargement; and firm, rubbery, and consolidated lungs. Variable findings include alveolar hemorrhage, icterus, hepatic mottling and atrophy, enlarged and mottled kidneys, mottling of the cecum, and petechiation of the mucosa of the spiral colon (1, 3). The most prominent gross and histologic lesions result from pronounced lymphocytic-histiocytic infiltrations. Additional microscopic lesions include lymphohistiocytic to granulomatous interstitial pneumonia, hepatitis, nephritis, myocarditis, enteritis, pancreatitis, and loss of B-cell follicles with expansion of T-cell areas in lymphoid organs (1, 21, 25). PCV has a similarly wide organ and tissue distribution pattern in cases of porcine dermatitis and nephropathy syndrome, with the addition of dermal infection (19, 22). Following experimental infection, virus persists in vivo for at least a month (16). Virus-neutralizing antibodies develop slowly, and are unapparent until 28 days postinfection (20).

Interference with research

PCV infection clearly would invalidate most research involving young pigs. In addition to cytoarchitectural changes in most organs, PCV specifically up-regulates major histocompatibility complex (MHC) class I antigen and reduces the number of cells expressing class II antigen, decreases antigen presentation by macrophages, induces $CD4^+$ and B-lymphocyte depletion in lymphoid tissues, and increases numbers of monocytes and immature granulocytes (8, 17, 23, 24, 25). Therefore, young pigs infected with PCV are unsuitable for research involving the cardiovascular, dermal, enterohepatic, hematopoietic, lymphoreticular, musculoskeletal, nervous, respiratory, and urinary systems. The reproductive system would be affected in breeding pigs. It is certain that much additional information will be reported on this pathogen.

Diagnosis and control

A preliminary diagnosis of PCV may be made on the basis of clinical signs, with confirmation achieved by virus isolation or immunostaining. More recently, molecular methods have been developed. While PCR is rapid and sensitive, in situ hybridization better correlates the presence of virus, with characteristic lesions (6). For distinguishing clinical from subclinical infections, immunohistochemistry, quantitative virus isolation, and antigen-capture enzyme-linked immunosorbent assay (ELISA) are more accurate (18). Lastly, serologic methods are particularly useful for screening herds (28). Pigs showing clinical signs of infection are not useful as research subjects, and should be euthanized. However, the laboratory animal veterinarian and principal investigator may agree that using older, seropositive pigs may be suitable for specific research purposes. PCV is highly resistant to environmental stresses, including acidic and thermal environments. This, along with the high prevalence of infection, render eradication difficult. Efforts should be directed toward preventing entry of the virus into the facility. To facilitate this goal, research pigs should only be purchased from herds known to be free of PCV. Where space, facilities, and project objectives will allow, an "all-in-all-out" approach to research pig management will also minimize the risk of virus establishment in the facility. Information is lacking regarding the epidemiology and pathophysiology of PCV. This knowledge would facilitate development of rational control programs.

Porcine enteroviruses

Agents
Swine are susceptible to a number of enteroviruses in the family *Picornaviridae*. These are small, ssRNA viruses. At least 11 serotypes of porcine enterovirus have been described (6). Serotypes 1 and 9 are associated with Teschen/Talfan disease and swine vesicular disease, respectively. In many parts of the world, including the United States, these are reportable diseases. Their unlikely discovery in a research animal facility would naturally result in depopulation. Therefore, they will not be discussed further. The focus of this text is on those enteroviruses that may occur in laboratory animal facilities. While there are currently roughly a dozen serotypes, it should be noted that newly developed molecular classification schemes may eventually result in reclassification of individual serotypes into new genera (9).

Epidemiology
Porcine enteroviruses are common in commercial swine operations (10). Research animal facilities purchasing pigs from these sources are likely to introduce enteroviruses into their facility. Some have reported a seasonality to enterovirus infection, with infections detected more frequently in the spring and summer (7). Definitive information is lacking concerning transmission of enteroviruses; however, virus may be excreted in the feces, persisting up to a month after infection (12). Direct contact is therefore likely an important means of transmission. Pregnant sows orally inoculated with enterovirus have failed to transmit the infection to their gestating fetuses (12). So, while enterovirus has been shown to enter blastomeres (3), it is doubtful that this mechanism is clinically significant.

Clinical signs
Many, if not most, infections with porcine enteroviruses are asymptomatic. Disease syndromes associated with swine enteroviruses include poliomyelitis (serotypes 1, 2, 3, and 5), diarrhea (serotypes 1, 2, 3, 5, and 8), pneumonia (serotypes 1, 2, 3, and 8), myocardial or pericardial disease (serotypes 2 and 3), and quite commonly, reproductive disorders (serotypes 1, 3, 6, and 8). Poliomyelitis is characterized by CNS dysfunction, including paralysis, paresis, convulsions, and gait abnormalities (1). Diarrhea occurs in young pigs, and results in loss of condition (8). Myocardial or pericardial disease often accompanies nervous system disease (13). Reproductive dysfunction resulting from infection with porcine enteroviruses is one of the more common clinical sequelae, and has been given the acronym "SMEDI." This stands for stillbirth, mummification, embryonic death, and infer-

tility. These terms accurately describe the clinical effects of viral infection. Gestational age is an important factor in determining the outcome of infection in individual sows (14).

Pathology

Within a day of infection, virus is detectable in the respiratory and gastrointestinal systems, and in the mesenteric lymph nodes. Within 5 days of infection, primary viremia disseminates virus to other systems, including the CNS. Virus localizes in the CNS. Peak viral loads are found on postinfection day 6. Also, because of a developing immune response, virus is rapidly cleared from the circulation, generally by postinfection days 6 to 11. Thereafter, neuropathology develops quickly (1). Most serotypes have a tropism for intestinal tissues, particularly the spiral colon and ileum (14). However, depending on strain, virus may also be detected in virtually all visceral organs, lymphoid tissue, turbinates, diaphragm, and the CNS. For example, serotype 3 causes myocarditis and pericarditis, in addition to CNS lesions, within 3 to 7 days of infection. Myocarditis and pericarditis may be due to upregulation of nitric oxide production (13). Other serotypes have been associated primarily with pneumonitis (11). Immunity is primarily humoral (5). In contrast, cellular immune mechanisms appear to be weak, localized, and not associated with significant antiviral activity (4).

Interference with research

It should be clear that clinical cases of porcine enterovirus infection could markedly interfere with studies involving the cardiovascular, enterohepatic, musculoskeletal, nervous, reproductive, and respiratory systems (13). Specific viral strains with predilections for other visceral organs may also interfere with studies involving those target organs. Unfortunately, little direct information exists to guide investigators and veterinarians concerning the significance of asymptomatic infections. Enteroviruses have been shown to alter periparturient steroid hormone levels in farrowing sows (2). Studies involving young or reproducing pigs should exclude pigs infected with enterovirus.

Diagnosis and control

Porcine enterovirus infection should be suspected when any of the above-mentioned syndromes are observed. Definitive diagnosis may be accomplished using a number of testing modalities, including serology, immunohistochemistry, viral isolation, and more recently, RT-PCR assay. Control of porcine enteroviruses is complicated by high prevalence. Swine intended for research should be tested serologically prior to entry into the facility. Facility veterinarians should carefully consider whether exclusion of this virus is necessary in light of the intended use of the animals.

Porcine parvovirus

Agent

Porcine parvovirus (PPV) is a nonenveloped, ssDNA virus of the family *Parvoviridae*. Many features of the biology of this virus are similar to those of parvoviruses in other species. Although there are genetic and biological similarities between PPV and parvoviruses of other species, PPV is antigenically distinct. Only one serotype of PPV is known to exist (21). In 1987, Japanese investigators isolated a DNA virus with physicochemical similarities to PPV. This new virus was associated with diarrhea in suckling pigs (20). Additional information is needed before the relationships of these viruses can be stated with certainty.

Epidemiology

Parvoviral disease is common among commercially raised swine (11). Animal facilities that purchase pigs from these sources may thereby import PPV. PPV is highly infectious, and is transported from one location to another with remarkable speed and ease. Acutely or chronically infected pigs shed virus in the oral secretions and in the feces. Transmission is primarily by oronasal exposure. Transmission is facilitated by direct contact, contaminated fomites, and biological vectors such as animal caretakers. In this regard, contaminated premises represent the primary reservoir of infection for other pigs. Transplacental infection is also common and is further discussed below. Lastly, it remains uncertain if episodic or prolonged viral shedding occurs in the semen of boars (4, 18).

Clinical signs
Many infections with PPV are asymptomatic. However, clinical signs are largely dependent on age of infection and previous exposure (5, 19). Reproductive failure is the most common sequela to PPV infection, and occurs when gilts or primiparous sows are infected prior to 56 days of gestation (13). In these cases, dams return to estrus 3 to 8 weeks after breeding, or deliver stillborn or mummified fetuses. In fact, PPV infection is the most important cause of fetal loss in swine worldwide (12). In facilities where PPV is endemic, most sows have seroconverted by their third pregnancy (5). Piglets farrowed by dams infected later in gestation are often weak and/or runted. Litters are also smaller because some fetal death will have occurred. Other, less common clinical presentations include low fertility in boars, neonatal systemic disease, vesicular disease of the feet and mouth in piglets, and respiratory disease (8, 9, 15).

Pathology
Following oral or intranasal inoculation, viremia is noted from day 2 to about day 6 postinfection, resulting in distribution of the virus to virtually all organs. Virus also infects lymphocytes, monocytes, and macrophages, which are in turn destroyed (16). By about postinfection day 15 in pregnant sows, virus reaches the fetus. Histologic evidence of infection is nearly always absent from adult pigs, but includes mononuclear cell infiltration, and necrosis of many visceral organs in the fetus. Most prominently, lesions are noted in the liver, heart, kidney, myocardium, and cerebrum (21). Immunity is primarily humoral and develops within 5 or 6 days of infection. Virus-neutralizing antibody is passed to piglets by the colostrum, and is protective for up to 24 weeks post partum (21). Fetuses infected after about 70 days gestation may remain persistently infected for life but it is unlikely that they excrete virus (3). These pigs also develop an immune response, which may be useful diagnostically. Despite the development of an immune response, circumstantial evidence suggests that PPV may persist chronically in individual pigs. While this occurs to some extent in parvovirus infections of other host species, PPV may be particularly suited to persistent infection (11).

Interference with research
Again, the reader is referred to chapter 9 for information concerning potential and documented effects of parvovirus on the canine host. It is likely that some of these effects occur in swine infected with PPV, although differences in primary sites of organ involvement (enteric versus reproductive) suggest that caution is warranted in extrapolating from other species. In the pig, natural or experimental PPV infection has been shown to induce leukocytosis (16), alter reproductive hormone levels (14), and contaminate cell cultures. Concerning the latter, cell cultures may be freed of infection by the addition of homologous viral antiserum to their nutrient media (10). There is no question that research studies involving reproduction would be compromised by infection with PPV. In addition, studies involving the cardiovascular, dermal, endocrine, hematopoietic, lymphoreticular, nervous, respiratory, and urinary systems would be compromised, particularly in very young pigs. It is likely that natural infection of older pigs with PPV would have fewer confounding effects.

Diagnosis and control
Immunologically based methods for diagnosing PPV have predominated for many years. The ELISA and the indirect immunofluorescence assay (IFA) utilizing fetal tissues are

rapid and moderately reliable, and detect current infections (6). In contrast, traditional serology is of limited value in diagnosing immediate cause of porcine reproductive disease because of the high prevalence of seropositive pigs in many herds. Recently, PCR assays have been developed (17). These will likely take on an increasingly important role in PPV diagnosis. There is no treatment for reproductive failure due to PPV infection. An effective control program includes purchase of pigs from reputable vendors, and, where pigs will be bred in a research facility potentially contaminated with PPV, vaccination of gilts prior to breeding. One may also expose gilts to seropositive sows to facilitate natural infection of the gilts. Not all gilts will become infected, however, leaving some to experience clinical disease if infected during pregnancy (11). It is imperative that the laboratory animal veterinarian be familiar with the vaccination and local disease history and health status of pigs to be brought into the facility. The veterinarian must communicate with the investigator to match the microbial profile of the pigs, with their intended research use. Like other parvoviruses, PPV is highly resistant to environmental stresses, including heat, pH extremes, dessication, and chemicals whose virucidal action involves destruction of the viral envelope (2). Parvoviruses are inactivated by bleach (1:30) but not by quaternary ammonium compounds (1, 7). Protective clothing worn while working with infected pigs or in contaminated areas should be thoroughly disinfected, or disposed of, along with all other contaminated materials.

Porcine reproductive and respiratory syndrome virus

Agent
Porcine reproductive and respiratory syndrome virus (PRRSV) is an enveloped, ssRNA virus in the family *Arteriviridae* (37). North American and European isolates of PRRSV differ markedly in genotype, antigenicity, phenotype, and virulence (26). This appears to be due to a relatively high mutation rate, typical of RNA viruses.

Epidemiology
The clinical syndrome associated with PRRSV was first observed in the United States in 1987. Serologic surveys of archival samples reveal that PRRSV was present in Canada almost a decade before it was recognized in the United States. Thereafter, PRRSV spread rapidly to most of the rest of the swine-producing regions of the world (4). PRRSV is highly infectious but not highly contagious (44). Virus is present primarily in the saliva and blood, and rarely in urine and feces (30, 43). PRRSV is known to be transmitted orally (22), transplacentally (8), by aerosol (24), by injection (28), in the milk (41), and via semen (12). The main routes of viral excretion and the primary modes of transmission for PRRSV appear to be vertical from dam to offspring, and horizontal from infected pigs to their uninfected herd mates (24). Horizontal transmission likely occurs via nose-to-nose contact, and through contact with blood and/or saliva during fighting. Typically, more than half of the herds surveyed in a region will be positive for virus (24). Once established within a herd, the infection rate within the herd rises as the pigs age (4).

Clinical signs
The scope of clinical signs observed with PRRSV is broader than for many other swine diseases. The clinical presentation is greatly influenced by virus strain, host age, management factors, and herd immunity. PRRSV is considered a component of the porcine respiratory disease complex. In brief, PRRSV causes reproductive loss of fetuses, followed by respiratory disease in surviving piglets. Both morbidity and mortality tend to be high. Gilts or sows infected during pregnancy experience systemic disease which manifests as fever; anorexia; a blue discoloration of the snout, ears, and vulva; agalactia; late-term abortion; premature births; and birth of dead or mummified fetuses (4). Piglets born alive are weak and

over half will die with respiratory disease during the first postpartum week, while additional pigs will succumb from nursing through weaning (23, 29). Clinical signs of infection include conjunctivitis, emaciation, listlessness, watery diarrhea, tremors, paddling, and a splay-legged posture. Boars, grower, and finishing pigs infected from herd mates may also show systemic clinical signs following initial infection, although these are generally less severe (4). In all cases, secondary bacterial and other viral infections may contribute to clinical disease and pathogenesis. In this regard, PRRSV is often found as a copathogen, along with *Mycoplasma hyopneumoniae, Pasteurella multocida,* porcine circovirus type 2, swine influenza virus, and other pathogens (4, 42).

Pathology
Following infection, PRRSV binds to cells of monocyte-macrophage lineage by a heparin-like receptor molecule located on the host cell surface (15). Replication occurs within macrophages found in mucosal surfaces such as the tonsils, nasal mucosa, spleen, and lungs (5, 40). Transport to regional lymph nodes is rapidly followed by viremia, resulting in widespread organ distribution of the virus. Virus is most often found in the thymus, tonsils, and lymph nodes of pre- or postnatal pigs. This distribution again reflects viral predilection for lymphoid tissue (8). It should be noted that since infected macrophages may be found in every organ of the body, inflammatory lesions may also be observed in virtually all organ systems. However, these occur most prominently in the respiratory, reproductive, lymphoreticular, and central nervous systems; and less commonly, the urinary and cardiovascular systems (13, 14, 31, 33). In this regard, infected suckling piglets develop interstitial pneumonia, lymphoid hyperplasia, lymphoplasmacytic rhinitis, encephalitis, myocarditis, and gastric myositis. Infected adult pigs develop inflammatory lesions primarily in the reproductive organs. (4, 31). Infected pigs may excrete virus for prolonged periods. The maximum period of viral excretion is unknown, but a carrier state has been found to extend up to about 150 days, with virus persisting in the tonsils and other tissues of the oropharyngeal region (1, 19). Immunity to PRRSV involves both cellular and humoral components. Cellular responses develop at about 4 weeks postinfection, peak at about 7 weeks, and decline after 11 weeks (3). Viral infection simultaneously induces a polyclonal activation of B cells in the tonsils and an exaggerated and prolonged specific antibody response due to persistent infection in lymphoid organs (21). An adequate humoral response is not reached until 10 or more weeks after infection, but then is long lived and contributes to eventual viral clearing and protection against reinfection (4, 20, 34).

Interference with research
As noted above, PRRSV primarily infects macrophages. These cells distribute to all organs of the body. Therefore, PRRSV infection has the potential of compromising swine research covering a wide range of organ systems. Specifically, PRRSV induces tumor necrosis factor α (TNF-α) production in alveolar macrophages, resulting in apoptosis of infected macrophages and uninfected bystander cells, thereby compromising studies involving the immune system (11, 39). Relatedly, PRRSV has also been shown to decrease bactericidal and phagocytic activity of macrophages, resulting in increased susceptibility to other pathogens, most notably *Streptococcus suis* (17, 39), and possibly *Salmonella choleraesuis* (43), *Haemophilus parasuis* (36), and *Escherichia coli* (25). PRRSV, in combination with *Bordetella bronchiseptica,* increases the severity of *P. multocida* infection (7). PRRSV has also been shown to increase secretion of matrix metalloproteases in the lungs (18). These enzymes are important in cleavage of the extracellular matrix and subsequent infiltration of T cells, monocytes, and neutrophils into tissues as part of the inflammatory process. In a *M. hyopneumoniae*-PRRSV coinfection study, single infection with PRRSV increased expression of mRNA for the proinflammatory cytokines interleukin 1α (IL1α), IL1β, and

IL8 in tracheal ring explants (39). The authors suggested that these cytokines may play a role in the pulmonary pathology caused by these agents. PRRSV has also been shown to alter reactive oxygen and prostaglandin E2 production in alveolar macrophages (10); increase the number of cytotoxic T cells and natural killer cells in the lungs (32); increase serum IL6 and haptoglobin concentrations (2); compromise spermatogenesis by replicating inside spermatids and spermatocytes, causing apoptosis (38); and cause thrombocytopenia, anemia, and transient lymphocytopenia (4). In summary, studies involving the cardiovascular, enterohepatic, hematopoietic, lymphoreticular, musculoskeletal, nervous, reproductive, and respiratory systems could be impacted by natural infection with PRRSV.

Diagnosis and control
PRRSV should be suspected on the basis of history and clinical signs. However, because these vary markedly, definitive diagnosis of PRRSV infection relies on laboratory methods. Diagnosis has traditionally been accomplished using virus isolation, ideally from moribund live piglets. Unfortunately, cell-culture requirements for isolation of PRRSV are fairly stringent, and virus is readily inactivated in tissues if they are not refrigerated or frozen soon after collection (4). These factors compromise the reliability of virus isolation. Reliance on serology is complicated by cross-reactivity with PRRSV vaccine-induced antibodies. In cases where vaccination has not occurred, IFA, ELISA, and other serologic tests are reliable only for identifying previous exposure. Recently, the molecular-based assay, RT-PCR has been used for diagnosis, as well as differentiation of isolates (9, 16). In this regard, RT-PCR on oropharyngeal scrapings has proven most reliable for identifying infected animals and for distinguishing carrier from noncarrier animals (19). There is no treatment available for PRRSV. Infected pigs should be destroyed. While commercial vaccines are available, their use should be carefully considered. Attenuated vaccines have generally proven more efficacious than inactivated vaccines. On the other hand, the propensity for genetic drift among strains of PRRSV may result in vaccine strains not protecting against challenge with field isolates. In addition, modified live viruses may be transmitted to naive pigs and cause disease, persist for long periods, only slowly induce immunity, and may cross the placenta and cause congenital infection in fetal pigs (4, 6, 24). Lastly, there has been at least one report of reversion of a vaccine strain to virulence, with associated disease (27). Only inactivated vaccines are safe for use in virus-free herds. Prevention should be focused on obtaining only seronegative pigs, and on husbandry and management practices that will keep them that way. PRRSV does not survive for long periods in the environment, and is inactivated by low pH and high temperatures, but remains infectious for up to 6 days at room temperature, and much longer at cooler temperatures, including freezing. Like many other enveloped viruses, PRRSV is readily inactivated by commonly used detergents, and disinfectants such as dilute bleach, iodine, and quaternary ammonium compound (35).

Porcine rotavirus

Agent
Porcine rotavirus is a nonenveloped, double-stranded RNA (dsRNA) virus of the family *Reoviridae* and genus *Rotavirus*. To date, seven distinct serogroups have been identified. Pigs may be infected with rotaviruses in groups A, B, D, and E (18). Group A porcine rotavirus is of greatest clinical concern. Several strains of porcine rotavirus A have been reported and many contain multiple serotypes (4, 11).

Epidemiology
Historically, porcine rotaviruses have been extremely common in commercial pig herds (3). More current prevalence data is lacking. Studies indicate that porcine rotavirus moves quickly through a herd, until virtually all pigs have been infected (10). It is therefore

likely that research facilities purchasing pigs from producers will readily import rotavirus-infected pigs into the facility, unless specific steps are taken to exclude the virus. Transmission is fecal-oral. Immune sows represent the primary source of infective virus for their offspring at a time when piglets are most susceptible to infection (2). On average, pigs farrowed by nonimmune dams become infected before 5 weeks of age (6). Usually, virus is excreted in the feces for just over a week (1), but shedding may recur up to 3 to 4 weeks later (6). It has been reported that many immune, adult pigs do not excrete virus in their feces (6). However, as noted previously, seropositive sows have been demonstrated to excrete virus around farrowing (2). Therefore, the assertion that many immune, adult pigs do not excrete virus in their feces appears incorrect. This issue has not been adequately addressed. Immune adult pigs likely do represent a continuing source of infection for naive pigs. Virus remains infective in the environment for many months at cool temperatures (20).

Clinical signs
The clinical symptoms induced by porcine rotavirus infection are largely dependent on immune status, age of infection, viral inoculum, swine management and husbandry practices, and virus strain. Although the clinical signs associated with experimental infections in gnotobiotic pigs will be described, it should be noted that this is unlike the situation in most animal facilities, where infection with rotavirus may be endemic. In the latter cases, clinical signs will be unapparent or much less severe, because some level of herd and individual immunity will exist. Clinical signs are most severe in pigs infected prior to 1 week of age. In these cases, pigs rapidly become listless, anorexic, and occasionally vomit (24). Weight gain is delayed (23). Affected pigs quickly develop watery, yellowish diarrhea, which lasts for 3 to 5 days. During this time, pigs become dehydrated, and many die (23). With each additional week of age, experimentally infected pigs show fewer and less severe clinical signs (22). Pigs infected after about 6 weeks of age typically do not show clinical signs of disease. (18). Naturally infected pigs show milder clinical signs than their age-matched gnotobiotic and experimentally infected counterparts. Pigs infected after weaning often do not show clinical signs, unless they are concurrently infected with other enteric pathogens, most notably enterotoxigenic *E. coli* or transmissible gastroenteritis virus. Less is known of the clinical effects of porcine rotaviruses of other serogroups. While group C viruses appear to produce clinical signs similar to those produced by group A virus, group B and E viruses are less pathogenic (15). It should be noted, however, that mixed infections with different groups or strains are common (11, 14, 16).

Pathology
Within hours following infection, porcine rotavirus colonizes and replicates in the distal small intestinal villous enterocytes. Viral attachment or entry, rather than replication, results in cell dysfunction and death, leading to ballooning degeneration of enterocytes, mild villous atrophy, blunting, and epithelial desquamation (17, 21, 24). While clinical signs are more severe in younger pigs, enterocytes of older pigs are just as heavily infected as those of young pigs. The low mitotic index in neonatal pigs, compared with adults, results in prolonged enterocyte replacement after virus-associated enterocyte destruction. Therefore, age-related differences in enterocyte infection cannot explain differences in severity of disease (8). Whatever the determining influences, the degree of enterocyte damage is a primary factor in determining the severity of the infection. Villous damage precludes adequate digestion and absorption of nutrients, resulting in an osmotic diarrhea and changes in intestinal permeability (23, 25). In surviving pigs, epithelial cytoarchitecture returns to normal within 1 to 2 weeks, depending on pig age at infection (18, 22). Older pigs recover more quickly. Effective immunity is primarily humoral and local, rather than systemic (9, 26). When gilts or sows are immune,

antibodies are passed in the colostrum but decline rapidly (1, 13). Colostral antibodies protect the piglets from disease, but not from infection, for up to about 3 to 5 weeks (9).

Interference with research

Clearly, natural infection of suckling, and possibly recently weaned, research pigs with porcine rotavirus would compromise studies involving the enterohepatic system. In addition, studies in which growth or other nutritional parameters were measured would likely also be affected. Porcine rotavirus has been shown to reduce digestive enzyme production through loss of enterocytes, to decrease small intestinal Na^+K^+-ATPase activity and glucose-coupled Na^+ absorption, and to otherwise alter permeability of Na^+, K^+, Ca^{2+}, and other electrolytes (18, 19). Similar effects on electrolyte transport have been noted in rotavirus infection of rabbit intestinal cells (12). In humans, rotavirus infection induces prostaglandin release, which may exacerbate the inflammatory process (27), and alters actin cytoskeleton regulation through inducing changes in intracellular calcium concentrations (5). It is unlikely that pigs infected as adults would be affected to such an extent that they should be excluded from research studies. However, there are no data addressing this question.

Diagnosis and control

Diagnosis may be accomplished using fecal samples and a variety of virus detection methods, such as immunologically based methods, virus isolation, electron microscopy, and more recently, RT-PCR and other molecular assays (7). Electron microscopy remains the "gold standard." However, that position will likely be supplanted by molecular methods. It is essential to obtain fecal samples for diagnosis as soon after onset of diarrhea as possible, since viral shedding is short-lived (18). There is no direct treatment for porcine rotavirus infection. Clinically affected pigs should be isolated. If the decision is made to retain affected pigs, therapy is supportive, and includes fluid and electrolyte replacement, antibiotic administration to prevent secondary bacterial infections, and provision of warmth (18). In addition to being nearly ubiquitous, porcine rotaviruses are extremely stable under adverse conditions, and are resistant to commonly used disinfectants. These factors make it nearly impossible to permanently exclude or eliminate virus from a contaminated facility. Control efforts should focus on reducing the environmental virus load and facilitating development of immunity in gilts (18). Effective immunization against porcine rotavirus is difficult because immunity tends to be strain specific. However, use of appropriate modified live vaccines will reduce clinical signs in young pigs. The decision to vaccinate should be made on the basis of the age and source of pigs to be used, history of the facility, and intended body systems to be studied.

Swine herpesvirus (pseudorabies)

Agent

Swine herpesvirus, or pseudorabies virus (PRV), is a dsDNA virus in the alphavirus subfamily of the family *Herpesviridae*. The alphaviruses are distinguished from other subfamilies by having very short (<24 h) lytic replication cycles and the propensity to establish latent infections in sensory ganglia and lymphoid tissue (28). While only one serotype of PRV is recognized, several strains of PRV have been isolated, and are differentiated by a variety of features, including antigenicity, nucleic acid sequences, and virulence (27). Both virulence and immunogenicity appear to be influenced by specific, and different, envelope glycoproteins.

Epidemiology

The pig is the only natural host of PRV, although livestock of many other species may become infected. The infection causes rapid death prior to viral excretion in these aberrant hosts. Thus, introduction of the virus by aberrant hosts is not likely to occur in laboratory animal facilities. Aggressive and laudable efforts on the part of producers, veterinarians, and governmental agencies in several swine-producing states has resulted in the near eradication of PRV from farm-raised pigs in the United States. While infection persists in wild-pig populations, efforts to keep these from infecting commercially raised pigs have been quite successful. Transmission is primarily through the introduction of virus-positive pigs, and occurs by aerosolization of oral and nasal secretions, but also occurs transplacentally, transmammary, during exchange of body fluids during copulation, and by fomites (15). Aerosol transmission may occur across many miles (3, 4).

Clinical signs

The introduction of PRV into a naive herd results in rapid spread of the virus. Most infections are asymptomatic (9, 24). The appearance of clinical disease is most evident in those herds with young pigs, since clinical signs are more severe in younger pigs. However, virus strain and inoculum also affect disease severity. Clinical signs are best understood in the context of predilection of the virus for tissues of the respiratory and nervous systems (15). Younger pigs tend to show dysfunction of the nervous system, while older pigs show more respiratory signs. For example, neonatal pigs become listless, anorexic, and febrile within 2 to 4 days of infection. CNS signs quickly follow, and include trembling, hypersalivation, nystagmus, seizures, postural and gait abnormalities, and high death rates. Weaned pigs tend to show similar, although less severe signs with lower mortality, and may also develop respiratory signs including nasal discharge with sneezing, dyspnea, and cough. Those pigs that survive are stunted. Grower pigs show primarily respiratory signs, characterized by rhinitis, coughing, and pneumonia. Respiratory pathology is accompanied by a general decline in body condition and activity. Adult pigs also develop fever and respiratory signs, but generally recover, while pregnant gilts or sows may reabsorb or abort fetuses. In one study, 5 of 12 pregnant gilts, experimentally infected by the intranasal route, died (14). Other clinical signs include vomiting, pruritus, and ophthalmic symptoms (13, 14, 16, 24). Clinical signs may be exacerbated by secondary bacterial or viral infections, including *Actinobacillus pleuropneumoniae, P. multocida* or porcine influenza virus (8, 15). Following an explosive outbreak, latent infection is established in the survivors, with few subsequent clinical signs. However, stress may facilitate recurrence of milder forms of the disease.

Pathology

Following infection, in general, by the oral or inhalational route, virus replicates in the nasopharyngeal and tonsillar epithelium (17). Lymphatic spread to local nodes quickly follows. More virulent strains tend not only to spread more easily to the CNS via cranial nerve extension, but also are more likely to disseminate systemically by the circulation (23). All strains appear to share tropism for the upper respiratory tract, in addition to the CNS. Gross necropsy findings include rhinitis, tonsillitis, pneumonia, hepatitis, splenitis, keratoconjunctivitis, vasculitis, orchitis, endometritis, vaginitis, placentitis, and occasionally, enteritis in young pigs (1, 10, 20, 24). Histologic changes in the CNS include meningoencephalitis, ganglioneuritis, mononuclear cell perivascular cuffing, and glial nodules (15, 27). Intranuclear inclusions are usually, although not always, found within cells of the CNS and tonsils. Histologic changes in the upper tonsils and respiratory tract include epithelial necrosis, mononuclear inflammation, bronchitis, and alveolitis. Respiratory pathology is more severe in pigs with superimposed bacterial infection (8). Focal lesions consisting of necrosis, intranuclear inclusions, and mononuclear cell infiltration are found in other affected organs as well (1, 6, 10, 22). Within a week of infection, virus is shed in essentially all body secretions. Immunity to PRV is primarily humoral (18, 19). As immunity develops, virus becomes latent in neural ganglia and, to a lesser extent, in the tonsils (2). Physiologic stress may cause viral recrudescence (15).

Interference with research
There is a surprising paucity of information directly describing the physiologic effects of PRV. In this regard, PRV has been shown to inhibit macrophage function (7, 11, 12) and exacerbate infection with *M. hyopneumoniae* (26), *H. parasuis* serovar 4 (21), or *S. suis* type 2 (12). In addition, much can be inferred about the potential research effects of PRV from reports describing natural or experimental infections with PRV. Certainly, natural infection of newborn pigs with PRV would alter research involving multiple organ systems, including the cardiovascular, enterohepatic, lymphoreticular, musculoskeletal, nervous, reproductive, and respiratory systems. Natural infections of older pigs would likely not compromise such a wide range of studies. However, the discovery of PRV should be reported to state animal health authorities and would likely result in the elimination of the herd.

Diagnosis and control
Natural infection with PRV may be suspected on the basis of history and clinical signs. However, laboratory confirmation is required, and is most reliably accomplished simply by pathologic examination. Gross and histopathologic findings may be augmented by immunohistologic viral detection (fluorescent antibody testing) and virus isolation. More recently, PCR assays have proven highly reliable and will likely assume an increasing role in the diagnostic approach to PRV infection (5). Serology is useful for evaluating overall herd status and for assessing the infection history of individual pigs, but is not reliable for detection of an acute outbreak, since antibodies may not yet be detectable. In the laboratory setting, treatment of affected pigs is unlikely to result in the salvage of useful research animals, and is at odds with state eradication efforts. Effective modified live and gene-deleted vaccines are available, but the goal should be a PRV-free research herd. PRV may be eradicated from a herd by serologic testing and elimination of positive animals, segregation of pigs by age, all-in/all-out management systems, reestablishment of the herd with virus-free pigs, and strict attention to sanitation (15). PRV survives on many fomites for approximately a week (25), but is susceptible to inactivation by drying, sunlight, and common disinfectants (15).

Swine influenza virus

Agent
Swine influenza virus (SIV) is an ssRNA virus in the family *Orthomyxoviridae*. SIV is designated a type A influenza virus. Type designations are based on antigenic differences in viral proteins. Type A influenza viruses infect humans, swine, birds, and horses. Further, multiple subtypes have been identified. These are distinguished by host of origin, geographic origin, strain number, and year of isolation, as well as by specific combinations of hemagglutinin (H) and neuraminidase (N) surface glycoprotein variants (1).

Epidemiology
SIV is one of the most studied of swine viral pathogens. It has a worldwide distribution and high prevalence, and is therefore of concern to swine producers and researchers globally. A large literature links humans, swine, and birds (particularly ducks and turkeys) in epidemiological relationships. These studies indicate that SIV may pass between species, allowing one species to serve as a reservoir of new viral strains capable of infecting the others (6, 7). Transmission of SIV is primarily by aerosol exposure to infectious droplets. Most outbreaks are reported in the fall and winter months, and occur soon after the introduction of new pigs into a susceptible herd (2). In these cases, clinical disease is promoted by environmental stresses, such as freezing tem-

peratures and rain, and the presence of a susceptible population. The presence of a true carrier state has not been documented satisfactorily.

Clinical signs
SIV causes acute respiratory disease. Symptoms are severe in very young pigs from nonimmune dams, but are generally mild to moderate in older animals and in piglets from immune dams (4). More severe clinical signs accompany concurrent infection with pathogens such as *A. pleuropneumoniae, P. multocida, H. parasuis, S. suis* type 2, *M. hyopneumoniae,* and porcine reproductive and respiratory syndrome virus (5, 11). Many if not most cases of SIV are asymptomatic. When present, clinical signs of SIV infection include nasal discharge, sneezing, fever, painful coughing, labored breathing, anorexia, weakness, reluctance to move, and prostration. In nearly all cases, weight loss occurs or weight gain is interrupted (1, 12). Uncomplicated cases tend to recover within a matter of days, whereas those complicated by secondary bacterial infection recover more slowly if at all. It is likely that few cases are truly uncomplicated by opportunistic pathogens.

Pathology
Following infection, viral replication occurs primarily in the lungs (8), although virus can be isolated from most visceral organs in fatal cases. In this regard, virus has been isolated from the lungs, nasal secretions, spleen, heart, liver, kidneys, brain, and gonads (4). Gross findings in SIV infection include reddened mucosa of the upper respiratory tract, enlarged cervical lymph nodes, emphysematous and consolidated lung lobes, enlarged spleen, and reddened gastric mucosa. Histologically, one observes rhinitis, conjunctivitis, pulmonary edema, and bronchopneumonia. In some reports of experimental infection, a humoral immune response was detectable within 8 days of infection, and peaked a week later (3), while others report that antibodies did not develop until a month after infection (4). Cellular responses have also been detected within 2 weeks of infection (3).

Interference with research
SIV primarily infects the lungs and therefore causes most of its deleterious effects in that organ system. However, secondary effects may influence research involving other organ systems as well. For example, SIV has been shown to induce the proinflammatory cytokines alpha interferon (IFN-α), TNF-α, and IL-1 (12) and cause degranulation and aggregation of platelets (9). Therefore, studies involving the respiratory and lymphoreticular systems would be compromised by natural infection with SIV, as would studies involving weight gain, activity levels, and other parameters associated with nutrition and behavior. In addition, viral replication within organs of the cardiovascular, enterohepatic, lymphoreticular, nervous, reproductive, and urinary systems may confound studies involving those systems. It is certain that older pigs, including those more commonly used in biomedical research, would experience less organ compromise than newborn piglets. However, definitive information on this issue is lacking.

Diagnosis and control
A presumptive diagnosis of SIV may be based on acute onset of characteristic clinical signs, but laboratory confirmation is essential. Definitive diagnosis historically has required viral isolation or rising serologic titers. It should be noted that false-negative serology may result when pigs are coinfected with other viral agents. More recently, RT-PCR assays have been developed and will surely replace traditional diagnostic methods (10). The decision to treat or cull affected research pigs should be made on the basis of the particular needs of the research study. If instituted, treatment is primarily supportive, and includes optimal housing conditions, as well as adequate high-quality feed and water. Antibiotic therapy may help prevent secondary bacterial infections. Killed vaccines are available, but their usefulness in the research setting is questionable.

Research swine should be obtained from virus-free herds. Swine should be protected from exposure to other potential reservoir hosts such as birds. Likewise, personnel known or suspected of carrying influenza virus should not be allowed to care for or work around research swine (13).

Transmissible gastroenteritis virus

Agent
Transmissible gastroenteritis virus (TGEV) is an enveloped, ssRNA virus of the family *Coronaviridae*. The biology of TGEV is typical of the family. Only one serotype is recognized. However, multiple strains have been isolated that differ in virulence (18).

Epidemiology
TGEV is globally distributed, with a high prevalence in most swine-producing areas of the world. Incidence of disease is highest in the winter and early spring (29). Recovered or otherwise asymptomatic and fecal virus-shedding pigs appear to serve as reservoirs of infection for incoming, susceptible pigs (21). Transmission is by oral exposure to contaminated feces. Birds and insects may likewise vector the pathogen to susceptible herds (12, 25). Fomites may also facilitate spread of the virus within a facility (31). Lastly, TGEV may be shed in the milk of infected sows (17), and remains infective in frozen, contaminated carcases (11).

Clinical signs
TGEV causes explosive outbreaks of diarrheal disease in suckling pigs. Additional clinical signs include vomiting, weight loss, dehydration, and death within a week of onset of clinical signs (23). As pigs age, clinical signs become more variable. Most cases are mild or unapparent. However, exceptions arise, where even adult pigs present with vomiting, diarrhea, fever, anorexia, agalactia, and even death (23). Therefore, in the research animal facility, where investigators tend to utilize weaned, or even adult pigs, the animal care staff must remain watchful for signs of TGEV. In those settings where there is a continual influx of susceptible pigs, an enzootic pattern of disease may result, where clinical signs are observed most frequently in weaned pigs as maternal antibody wanes (23).

Pathology
Following ingestion, virus traverses the stomach, surviving the acid environment, and replicates primarily in the small intestine, particularly the jejunum. Infection of intestinal epithelial cells results in cell death, villus atrophy, and subsequent replacement by immature cells lacking mature enzymatic and ion-transport capabilities. Incomplete digestion of sugars and electrolyte imbalances contribute to the resulting osmotic diarrhea. Gross lesions include gastrointestinal distension with yellowish fluid, and a thinned intestinal wall. Microscopically, there is epithelial necrosis and villus atrophy. Crypt cells are spared (22). Virus has also been found to replicate in mammary tissue (27). Immunity to TGEV is both cellular and humoral (2). Increased susceptibility of neonatal pigs and periparturient sows is explained in part by immaturity of the cytotoxic capabilities of effector lymphocytes (5). Of the antibody isotypes produced in response to infection, secretory IgA is of greatest importance (28).

Interference with research
Few studies have directly investigated the physiologic effects of TGEV on the swine host. Review of the available literature reveals that TGEV causes intestinal enzymatic deficiencies (29); altered sodium and chloride ion transport (4, 15); early, transient increased jejunal permeability to some macromolecules (16); increased intestinal phospholipase B activity (13); intestinal protein loss (26); an influx and stimulation of intestinal intraepithelial and mesenteric lymphocytes (1, 8, 30); and hypoglycemia, metabolic acidosis, and other biochemical indicators of intestinal dysfunction (9, 10). TGEV has been shown to induce IFN-α production in pig blood mononuclear

cells (6, 7, 24). Natural infection of research pigs with TGEV would compromise studies involving the enterohepatic system, including growth, nutrition, and serum analytes. In addition, TGEV may compromise studies involving the lymphoreticular system by altering lymph node architecture and inducing cytokine production.

Diagnosis and control

An outbreak of TGEV can be suspected with the appearance of vomiting and diarrhea. However, laboratory confirmation is necessary, and has traditionally been accomplished using virus isolation, immunofluorescence staining of cell cultures or intestinal sections, electron microscopy on feces or intestinal contents, histology, and serology (31). Serology is only useful for previously naive herds, or when paired sera are available in previously seropositive herds (29). More recently, RT-PCR assays have been developed and will surely assume a major role in the diagnosis of TGEV because they are rapid, accurate, and cost effective (19, 20). Affected pigs do not respond well to treatment. However, supportive care including fluid and electrolyte supplementation, antibiotic therapy, and provision of warm, dry housing should be provided if the pigs are to be retained. One should critically evaluate whether it is wise to retain infected pigs for use in research, since they are compromised physiologically, and because they serve as sources of infection for susceptible pigs on other studies. There may be cases where the pigs remain useful for specific types of projects, but should be euthanized immediately on completion of the study. In previously naive herds, serologic testing, followed by culling of seropositive pigs has proven successful in eradicating the pathogen (14). TGEV is readily inactivated by commonly used disinfectants, especially those with lipid-dissolving properties (3). A number of killed and modified live vaccines are available, but it is preferable to obtain research swine from herds known to be free of TGEV, and then practice husbandry standards that maximize pathogen exclusion.

Porcine respiratory coronavirus

Agent

Porcine respiratory coronavirus (PRCV) is an enveloped, ssRNA virus of the family *Coronaviridae*. PRCV is a deletion mutant of TGEV, but with respiratory rather than enteric tropism (8). Except for this distinction, PRCV is biologically similar to TGEV (9). Therefore, the interested reader is referred to the preceding section for additional information on the biology of these viruses.

Epidemiology

PRCV was first identified in Europe. It has since been found in most swine-producing regions of the world. PRCV is shed primarily in nasal secretions, and is therefore transmitted by aerosol and by direct contact. Other epidemiologic features are similar to TGEV.

Clinical signs

Most cases of PRCV are subclinical, or are limited to mild to moderate respiratory disease and decreased weight gains (2, 13). However, strains differ in virulence, and occasionally, severe signs develop (9). Recently, PRCV has become recognized as a contributor to the porcine respiratory disease complex (12).

Pathology

The pathogenesis of PRCV infection is similar to that of TGEV, except that the primary target organ is the respiratory tract. In this regard, PRCV infects epithelial cells of the nares, trachea, bronchi, bronchioles, and alveoli, as well as in the tonsils, intestinal tract, and pulmonary alveolar macrophages (4, 6, 7). As a result, mild, diffuse, interstitial pneumonia is a common, although not universal, pathologic finding (6, 12). Immunity to PRCV involves mechanisms similar to those of TGEV infection. In fact, piglets nursing sows immune to PRCV (10), and nursing or weaned pigs previously exposed to PRCV (2, 13), are protected against severe disease following challenge exposure to TGEV. These studies confirm the high antigenic relatedness and substantial cross protectiveness of these viruses.

Interference with research

The extent to which the more specific physiologic effects of TGEV are shared by PRCV is incompletely known. PRCV stimulates bronchial lymph nodes (1) and elevates bronchial alveolar lavage IFN-α levels (11). In one study, bronchoalveolar lavage IFN-α levels were elevated in only one of six pigs experimentally infected with PRCV (12). At this point it can be asserted that natural infection of research swine with PRCV will compromise research involving the lymphoreticular and respiratory systems, and those studies where growth parameters are evaluated.

Diagnosis and control

Diagnosis of PRCV infection is similar to that described for TGEV. It is possible to distinguish TGEV from PRCV using either blocking ELISA (3) or RT-PCR (5). There is scant information on the specific control and eradication of PRCV. It is likely that approaches used for TGEV are also effective for PRCV.

BACTERIA

Actinobacillus pleuropneumoniae

Agent

Actinobacillus pleuropneumoniae is an encapsulated, gram-negative coccobacillus. At least 15 serotypes of *A. pleuropneumoniae* have been identified. These differ in virulence and other traits. Most contain R plasmids encoding resistance to multiple antibiotics (5).

Epidemiology

A. pleuropneumoniae, like other members of the genus, is a common commensal inhabitant of mucous membranes, primarily of the respiratory tract. Crowded conditions and poor ventilation facilitate spread of clinical disease. Transmission is by aerosol and contact exposure to infectious secretions of chronically infected pigs (21).

Clinical signs

A. pleuropneumoniae is the cause of porcine pleuropneumonia. Disease occurs most commonly in 2- to 6-month-old pigs. Clinical signs include fever, vomiting, inappetence, coughing, difficult and rapid breathing, and occasional death (24). Affected sows may abort. Weight gains of surviving pigs lag behind those of uninfected pigs by about a week (28). Piglets nursing immune sows can still become colonized with *A. pleuropneumoniae* (8).

Pathology

Following infection, *A. pleuropneumoniae* colonizes the tonsils, then descends and attaches to the epithelial lining of the lower respiratory tract (12). Several *A. pleuropneumoniae* virulence factors have been identified. These contribute to pathogenesis, and include pili and lipopolysaccharide (LPS), which facilitate adherence to terminal airways; repeats in toxin (RTX)-type pore-forming hemolysins, including *Actinobacillus pleuropneumoniae* toxins (Apx) I to IV, which are capable of killing macrophages and neutrophils at high concentration, and stimulate an oxidative burst at low concentration; transferrin-binding proteins; urease, which may impair local immune responses; and others (3, 6, 25). Increased activity of phagocytic cells, along with bacterial LPS, may damage surrounding tissue, resulting in additional inflammation with release of proinflammatory enzymes and cytokines, including nitric oxide synthase 2 and TNFα (9). In addition, an antiphagocytic capsule may contribute to virulence of the organism (5). Gross necropsy findings in *A. pleuropneumoniae* infection include petechial hemorrhages, distended interlobular septa, consolidation, and fibrinous pleuritis. Microscopic lesions include coagulative necrosis, necrotizing pleuropneumonia, and focal abscessation (24). Less common pathologic findings associated with *A. pleuropneumoniae* include fibrinopurulent arthritis, necrotizing osteomyelitis, nephritis, and meningitis (20, 26). Effective immune responses to *A. pleuropneumoniae* involve neutralizing antibody (14), and phagocytosis and killing by neutrophils and macrophages (10, 13). Cross protection between serotypes is only partial (11, 23).

Interference with research
A. pleuropneumoniae has been reported to increase neutrophil chemotaxis (31) and cytokine release from blood and tissue leukocytes (2, 18, 22, 31), impair local immune responses (4, 7), induce acute-phase protein release (1, 16, 17), decrease serum zinc and iron concentrations (1), induce thymic necrosis (29), and suppress oxidative hepatic biotransformation (27). Some of these immune-modulating effects have been demonstrated even in subclinically infected pigs (22). Natural infections with *A. pleuropneumoniae* may render pigs permanently unsuitable for research involving the enterohepatic, hematopoietic, lymphoreticular, musculoskeletal, nervous, reproductive, respiratory, and urinary systems. In addition, studies in which growth rates are to be measured will likely also be compromised by natural infection. Prior to purchasing pigs for research use, the laboratory animal veterinarian should contact the vendor and inquire concerning pathogen history and status. Some swine herds are certified pleuropneumonia free. If pigs are not purchased from these certified pathogen-free vendors, it is likely that, in many cases, investigators will be utilizing pigs that may be asymptomatic carriers of *A. pleuropneumoniae*. The investigator and laboratory animal veterinarian should consider whether this may confound particular research studies. It is likely that, in most cases, carrier pigs will remain useful as research subjects.

Diagnosis and control
Herd monitoring for infection with *A. pleuropneumoniae* is commonly performed serologically. Acute cases are diagnosed by nasal swab culture, recalling that *A. pleuropneumoniae* requires nicotinamide adenine dinucleotide for growth on blood agar. More recently, PCR assays utilizing tonsillar swab samples have been developed. These are more sensitive than serology for detecting subclinically infected animals (8). Antibiotic treatment will speed recovery of clinical illness and minimize loss of piglets (30). Swine-breeding colonies can be cleared of *A. pleuropneumoniae*, using a combination of vaccination, antibiotic treatment, herd management approaches, and sanitation, but it is laborious and costly (19). A number of commercially available disinfectants have been found useful against *A. pleuropneumoniae* (15). Among them, the quaternary ammonium compounds were highly effective. Sodium hypochlorite was less effective in the presence of organic matter. For many commercial vendors of research-quality swine, vaccination of pigs against *A. pleuropneumoniae* is part of the routine health program.

Bordetella bronchiseptica

Agent
Bordetella bronchiseptica is a motile, aerobic, gram-negative coccobacillus commonly found inhabiting the ciliated respiratory epithelium of swine and many other mammals. Strains isolated from pigs appear to be host specific, in contrast to those of some other host species. The extent to which strain differences of *B. bronchiseptica* affect lesion development remains in question (14). It is likely that both strain differences and environmental factors affect clinical outcome of infection.

Epidemiology
Virtually all conventionally managed swine herds are infected with *B. bronchiseptica* (4). Prevalence of the pathogen is widespread, but is of relatively minor economic importance. Transmission of *B. bronchiseptica* is by aerosol and direct contact from infected young pigs and carrier sows. Over the course of several months, the prevalence of infection declines in carrier pigs. Management practices that ex-

pose pigs to increased stress, such as crowding, high production, frequent movement and mixing of pigs, poor ventilation, inadequate temperature control, and poor hygiene favor transmission and disease development (4).

Clinical signs

Most swine harboring *B. bronchiseptica* are asymptomatic. However, toxigenic strains of *B. bronchiseptica* cause a condition known as nonprogressive atrophic rhinitis (NPAR). In addition, *B. bronchiseptica* contributes to progressive atrophic rhinitis (PAR), a much more serious condition for which the primary pathogen is toxigenic *P. multocida* (2). Where clinical signs occur, they include mild nasal turbinate bone hypoplasia resulting in varying degrees of snout and facial distortion. In severe cases, this may interfere with respiration. Affected pigs may sneeze, snuffle, or cough and have excessive nasal discharge. Sneezing rarely results in nasal hemorrhaging. The age at which infection occurs in large part determines the clinical outcome. Newborn pigs are most susceptible to infection and lesion development. Susceptibility declines markedly by 6 weeks of age (4). Growing pigs infected later in life may also experience turbinate hypoplasia when *B. bronchiseptica* enters a susceptible herd, but this tends to be transient, with resumed and complete growth of the facial structures (4). In addition to NPAR, *B. bronchiseptica* may depress appetite and weight gains, and occasionally cause pneumonia in newborn piglets (3, 5, 9, 13, 16).

Pathology

Following infection, *B. bronchiseptica* attaches to and colonizes the tonsils and ciliated epithelium of the upper respiratory tract. There, the pathogen proliferates. Pathogenic strains of *B. bronchiseptica* produce a number of virulence factors. Among them, a thermolabile, dermonecrotic cytotoxin that diffuses into and interferes with the physiology of local osteoblasts. This leads to hypoplasia of the turbinates and facial malformation (7). Hypoplasia is generally mild, but can be complete. In most cases, turbinates are not completely damaged by infection. In these cases, turbinate regeneration begins within a month of infection, and results in normal facial conformation (16). Affected pigs are found to have varying degrees of catarrhal rhinitis. Pathogenic *B. bronchiseptica* also produce an iron-binding siderophore that robs the host of iron (12). Dermonecrotic toxin is also necessary for the development of bronchopneumonia (3). Pulmonary lesions of bronchopneumonia associated with primary respiratory infections of *B. bronchiseptica* are characterized by regional reddening and consolidation of the lungs, principally in the apical and cardiac lobes. Microscopically, one finds vasculitis followed by vascular endothelial hyperplasia, alveolar hemorrhage, necrosis, interlobular edema, perivascular and peribronchiolar fibrosis, and infiltration of neutrophils (6, 9). In addition, administration of *B. bronchiseptica* dermonecrotic toxin to specific pathogen-free pigs has been shown to cause lesions in the stomach, liver, kidney, and lymphoid organs (6, 7, 11). Colostral immunity protects piglets against developing NPAR, but not against infection (10), and vaccination of sows delays infection of offspring.

Interference with research

In the research setting, most investigators purchase pigs that are beyond the age at which they would be clinically affected by *B. bronchiseptica*. However, swine purchased with conformational malformations due to earlier infection with *B. bronchiseptica* may not be useful for particular research studies involving the musculoskeletal system. Prior to purchasing swine for research studies involving the respiratory system, the buyer should inquire about the *B. bronchiseptica* status of the herd. When uninfected and pregnant sows are purchased, or a breeding herd is established, natural infection with *B. bronchiseptica* could compromise the usefulness of offspring intended for use in respiratory research. In these cases, pregnant gilts or sows should be vaccinated with *B. bronchiseptica* bacterin (4). Pulmonary infection of research pigs with *B. bronchiseptica* will certainly compromise studies involving the lymphoreticular and respiratory systems, and those in which growth parameters are measured. In addition, *B. bronchiseptica* has been shown to decrease, and then increase alkaline phosphatase levels in locally affected bone (15); increase serum lactic dehydrogenase and total protein levels in acutely affected pigs (1); reduce serum haptoglobin levels (8); and reduce lymphocyte numbers (11). Lastly, *B. bronchiseptica* may interfere with studies involving the enterohepatic and urinary systems through induction of cytoarchitectural changes.

Diagnosis and control
B. bronchiseptica is readily isolated in nasal swab or lung lavage cultures on blood and MacConkey agar. Assigning microbial responsibility to atrophic rhinitis lesions is not a simple matter. This is addressed more fully in the discussion of *P. multocida*. It is likely that PCR assays developed for detection of *B. bronchiseptica* infections in other species will also be used for diagnosis of *B. bronchiseptica* in swine. NPAR caused by *B. bronchiseptica* cannot be resolved by treatment. Individual pigs with *B. bronchiseptica* pneumonia should be euthanized, or treated with potentiated sulfonamides or oxytetracycline (4). The decision to euthanize or treat should be made in light of the intended use of the pigs. In reality, thorough control measures are multifactorial. The interested reader is referred elsewhere for excellent discussions on control in a herd situation (4). *B. bronchiseptica* is susceptible to common disinfectants, but otherwise survives for prolonged periods in the environment. Once present in the research environment, eradication of *B. bronchiseptica* is probably impossible without resorting to rederivation and expensive barrier housing. The goal should be reduction in bacterial load in the environment. This may be accomplished with thorough cleaning and disinfection of the premises, isolation or elimination of shedding pigs identified by nasal swab culture, prophylactic use of antibiotics in the feed, and vaccination of sows with bacterin (4).

Clostridium perfringens type C

Agent
Swine may become infected with a number of clostridial agents. Among the most common is *Clostridium perfringens* type C, an invasive, nonmotile, encapsulated, spore-forming, gram-positive rod (2). There are five types of *C. perfringens*. These are differentiated by their repertoire of toxin production. Swine may be infected with type C, which produces α, β, and to a lesser extent, δ toxins (2, 9).

Epidemiology
C. perfringens type C occurs commonly in most swine-producing regions of the world. Asymptomatic adult pigs often serve as carriers of *C. perfringens* (6). Once contaminated with infectious spores, the environment may remain contaminated for many months, providing a reservoir of infection for susceptible pigs. Transmission is by ingestion of contaminated soil or feces. In newborn pigs, this may occur within minutes of birth.

Clinical signs
C. perfringens type C produces hemorrhagic enterotoxemia in newborn pigs. Affected pigs are often less than 24 h old, and almost always less than one week old (4, 6). Consumption of a protein- and calorie-rich diet, such as sow's milk, predisposes to clinical disease in nursing pigs. Carbohydrate composition appears to influence toxin production, with simple sugars increasing production (7). Clinical signs are absent in older carrier pigs. On occasion, disease occurs in weaned pigs on high protein/calorie diets. Overeating of rich diets by weaned pigs allows undigested feed to pass through the intestinal tract. This supports bacterial overgrowth, while excessive food consumption slows gut motility, allowing for toxin absorption. Each of these factors facilitates disease (2, 9). When present, clinical signs develop rapidly, vary in severity depending on

age and immune status, and may include depression, weakness, anorexia, abdominal pain, dehydration, fever, hemorrhagic diarrhea, and death. Mortality rates may approach 100% in the progeny of nonimmune sows (4, 6). In peracute cases, newborn piglets are simply found dead. Less severe cases also occur in which mortality is lower or is slower in coming. Chronic infection may occur with only mild diarrhea and failure to gain weight (9).

Pathology
Following infection, *C. perfringens* colonizes jejunal villi. Pathologic changes are due primarily to β-toxin production and release. β-toxin forms pores in cell membranes, resulting in electrolyte diffusion and cell death (8). Toxemia may occur within 12 h, and may affect a variety of organs. In this regard, extraintestinal lesions caused by necrotoxins include polioencephalomalacia, meningitis, adrenal cortical necrosis, hemorrhagic nephrosis, gastritis, edematous and hyperemic or hemorrhagic lymphadenopathy, peritoneal exudates and fibrinous peritonitis, pericardial exudation, cardiomyopathy, hepatic congestion, splenic enlargement, subcutaneous edema, myositis, hematuria, pleural effusion, and pulmonary edema (5, 9). Young pigs are particularly susceptible to disease because their immature intestinal mucosa lacks enzymes that would inactivate toxin. In addition, sow colostrum contains antitrypsin activity that removes the protective effect of trypsin (2). At necropsy, gross findings include intensely reddened small intestinal loops filled with red-brown, liquid contents, and blood-stained fluid in the abdominal cavity (9). The microscopic hallmark of *C. perfringens* is necrosis of small intestinal villi (1, 6). Specifically, histologic findings include complete desquamation of enterocytes and hemorrhagic necrosis of the small intestinal villus lamina propria and beyond, occasionally affecting tissue layers through to the serosa. Lesions are centered in the jejunum, but may extend from the stomach to the ileum. Organisms may penetrate the intestinal wall and cause gaseous, necrotic lesions in organs such as the peritoneum, adjacent musculature, and draining mesenteric lymph nodes (9). Immunity to *C. perfringens* is primarily antibody mediated, and is directed against the toxins (1).

Interference with research
Young pigs clinically affected by *C. perfringens* type C will be unusable for most research studies. In addition to intestinal damage, lesions may occur in a multitude of organs, thereby compromising research involving the cardiovascular, dermal, endocrine, hematopoietic, lymphoreticular, musculoskeletal, nervous, respiratory, and urinary systems. Also, growth will be stunted. Reports of specific effects of *C. perfringens* type C on host physiology are rare. *C. perfringens* has been shown to cause hypoglycemia, elevated blood urea nitrogen, and alterations in red and white blood cell parameters, including anemia and leukopenia (4). Natural infection of research pigs with *C. perfringens* will likely necessitate the euthanasia and replacement of the pigs. However, older pigs experiencing less severe disease may remain useful for specific purposes unrelated to the organ systems potentially affected. The decision to cull or retain previously affected pigs should be made after careful consideration by the investigator and laboratory animal veterinarian.

Diagnosis and control
C. perfringens infection may be presumed on the basis of clinical signs and histologic findings. However, definitive diagnosis requires laboratory confirmation. This may be accomplished in freshly killed pigs by simply gram-staining small intestinal contents and examining for large numbers of clostridia-like bacilli. However, rapid bacterial overgrowth limits the usefulness of this technique to the immediate postmortem period. Thereafter, specialized laboratory tests are required to detect and differentiate clostridial toxins. Many of these tests rely on bioassay in rodents and incorporate toxin-specific antisera. Differentiation of toxins is important, since simply

recovering bacteria by anaerobic culture will not confirm primary clostridial disease. More recently, multiplex PCR assays have been developed which profile for multiple *C. perfringens* toxin-encoding genes (10). The toxin gene profile indicates clostridial type present and rules in or rules out *C. perfringens* as a likely cause of disease. In general, treatment of affected pigs is unrewarding (6), because clinical signs are due to toxin production, which is not eliminated by antibiotic therapy. The organism is nearly impossible to eliminate from contaminated environments unless housing areas can be chemically disinfected. Whether or not there is a history of *C. perfringens* infection, breeding gilts and sows should be actively immunized. Additional control measures include prevention of overeating by weaned pigs, improved sanitation, prophylactic antibiotic use, and other, more intensive steps. Lastly, it is important to purchase pigs without a history of *C. perfringens* enteritis and reared by toxoid-immunized sows (3, 9).

Erysipelothrix rhusiopathiae

Agent
Erysipelothrix rhusiopathiae is a gram-positive, nonmotile rod. At least 23 serotypes of *E. rhusiopathiae* have been identified. These differ in the composition of specific proteins and proteinases (11).

Epidemiology
E. rhusiopathiae is commonly found in the environment wherever pigs are raised. At least 80 other species of vertebrates have been found infected, most asymptomatically. The list includes humans, in which the corresponding disease is referred to as "erysipeloid." This wide range of susceptible species highlights the potential for reservoirs of infection for research pigs. However, the most important reservoir of infection is asymptomatic carrier pigs, where infection of the tonsils is common. In fact, it is estimated that 30 to 50% of apparently healthy or convalescing pigs harbor *E. rhusiopathiae* in their tonsils or other lymphoid tissues (7, 14). Transmission occurs primarily through ingestion of soil, or fecal contamination of feed or water, but may also occur by inhalation or wound contamination, including use of contaminated tattooing devices (5).

Clinical signs
Because of the nearly ubiquitous presence of this pathogen around swine, and the active immunity that results from infection, most cases of infection with *E. rhusiopathiae* are asymptomatic. Factors favoring development of clinical disease include environmental stressors, dietary changes, and subclinical aflatoxicosis (2, 14). Young pigs less than 3 months of age are often protected due to passive immunity from the sow. Likewise, pigs older than 3 years generally are actively immune. When present, clinical signs include fever, anorexia, depression, vomiting, stiff gait, reduced growth rates, and reluctance to walk (1, 10, 14). Some pigs develop pink to purple "diamond-shaped" urticarial lesions on the skin. Over the course of about a week, the discoloration resolves, or the involved skin sloughs, usually with pigs recovering. On occasion, skin involvement can be extensive and severe. In these cases, the prognosis for recovery is poor (11). In addition, hematogenous spread to other organ systems may allow for the development of additional and varying clinical signs. These may include signs of cardiac insufficiency or sudden death, abortion and other causes of reduced fecundity, and encephalitis (6, 14).

Pathology
Following entry into the body, local colonization allows proliferation of the pathogen. Shortly thereafter, some pigs become septicemic. Hematogenous dispersal of *E. rhusiopathiae* results in vasculitis and other local pathologic changes in a variety of organs. Cellular damage is due to neuraminidase, which cleaves sialic acid from cell surfaces and causes hyaline thrombus formation (14). Necropsy of

pigs dying from acute infection with *E. rhusiopathiae* reveals hemorrhagic changes in the gastric serosa, skeletal and cardiac musculature, skin, and renal cortex. Congestion may be observed in the lungs, liver, spleen, lymph nodes, and urinary bladder. Affected joints contain fibrinous exudation and erosions of articular cartilage. Later, chronic immune stimulation from persistent antigen in the joint tissue results in articular changes and lameness (4). In the heart, bacterial emboli cause valvular endocarditis, and elsewhere, renal infarctions. Petechial and ecchymotic hemorrhages may be noted on the epicardium and in the atrial musculature (11, 15). The characteristic diamond-shaped skin lesions are due to thromboembolism of small arteries supplying the integument, leading to ischemic necrosis. Immunity is primarily humoral, with opsonization and phagocytosis by macrophages having important terminal roles. In this regard, partial immunity appears to be an important factor in the development of skin lesions (14).

Interference with research
Natural infection of research pigs with *E. rhusiopathiae* is likely to compromise research involving a variety of body systems. Compromise of the animals may be chronic and subtle, due to the chronic nature of the infection. The investigator may not appreciate the degree of compromise until after the study is completed and the animals are necropsied. This results in considerable waste of resources. Potentially worse is the case in which pigs are used for sophisticated research studies but then not necropsied, leaving the investigator clueless as to the degree of compromise. Studies most likely to be compromised by natural infection with *E. rhusiopathiae* include those involving the cardiovascular and musculoskeletal systems, but may also include those involving the dermal, enterohepatic, hematopoietic, lymphoreticular, nervous, reproductive, respiratory, and urinary systems. Specific physiologic changes attributed to *E. rhusiopathiae* include induction of a transient (3 to 5 day) lymphocytosis, relative eosinophilia, decreased red blood cell indicators, hypoglycemia, elevated liver enzymes (14); elevated acid phosphatase, β-glucuronidase, and β-acetylglucosaminidase activity in synovial cells (12); increased circulating antibody and complement levels (13); and induction of intercellular adhesion molecule-1 on chondrocytes from affected joints (3).

Diagnosis and control
Infection with *E. rhusiopathiae* may be suspected on the basis of clinical signs, particularly when the skin form ("diamond skin disease") occurs. Laboratory confirmation is by gram staining of lesioned tissue or blood smears, or by culture of the same (11). Chronic lesions are less often rewarding. More recently, PCR assays using arthritic joint samples, with or without broth enrichment, have been developed (8, 9). Acutely affected pigs can be treated successfully with penicillin (1). However, treatment must be evaluated in light of the future utility of the research subjects. *E. rhusiopathiae* is remarkably environmentally resistant, surviving for many months in feces, and for shorter periods in soil. Therefore, once contaminated, animal facilities will require thorough disinfecting prior to restocking. Vaccination is recommended when there is a history of erysipelas, but protection is often incomplete (14). Disease prevention is accomplished through optimal sanitation and nutrition, stress reduction, and careful evaluation of incoming stock.

Haemophilus parasuis

Agent
Haemophilus parasuis is a pleomorphic, gram-negative rod in the family *Pasteurellaceae*. Like most other members of the genus, *H. parasuis* has special growth requirements. *H. parasuis* requires nicotinamide adenine dinucleotide, formerly termed, "V factor," for growth on blood agar. At least 15 serotypes are recognized. These may differ markedly in virulence (6). Serovars 5, 4, and 13 are most prevalent globally (2, 9).

Epidemiology
H. parasuis usually inhabits and can be recovered from the nasopharyngeal mucous membranes of swine, and is therefore ubiquitous in swine-raising areas of the world. Only the most rigidly controlled herds are free from infection. Where endemic, infection likely occurs shortly after birth. Exposure of older naive animals often occurs with the introduction of pigs from infected herds. Transmission occurs by aerosol and contact exposure.

Clinical signs
Clinical outcome of *H. parasuis* infection is dependent on bacterial strain, immune status of the host, and other undetermined factors. Most infections with *H. parasuis* are asymptomatic, and pigs live as healthy, actively immune carriers. Clinical disease occurs following introduction of the pathogen into naive herds. Disease may also follow exposure of pigs to environmental stresses such as weaning, transport, and other suboptimal management practices (10). Lastly, disease may accompany primary viral infection, such as swine influenza virus, pseudorabies virus (5), or porcine reproductive and respiratory syndrome virus (12); or primary bacterial infection, as with *Mycoplasma hyorhinis*. Therefore, while *H. parasuis* is often an opportunistic pathogen, primary infections do occur in immunologically naive herds. Clinical disease caused by *H. parasuis* typically occurs in recently weaned, stressed pigs, and may be limited to the respiratory tract, or may be systemic, and known as polyserositis, or Glässer's disease. Signs of systemic illness develop within a week, and are referable to inflammation of serous membranes. Therefore, clinical signs may include fever, anorexia, depression, nasal discharge, cyanosis, respiratory distress, abdominal pain, swollen joints, lameness and reluctance to walk, tremor, incoordination, and death (2, 9, 10, 15).

Pathology
Following aerosol inoculation, *H. parasuis* colonizes the nasal and tracheal mucosa, prior to septicemic spread to other organs (14). Like other members of the genus, *H. parasuis* produces a LPS toxin that binds to LPS receptors and induces release of proinflammatory cytokines IL-1 and TNF from macrophages. In addition, the bacterial capsule is antiphagocytic. As a result, *H. parasuis* infection is associated with pus production at serosal surfaces. Gross lesions are therefore typical of acute fibrinopurulent inflammation of the serosal surfaces, and include rhinitis, bronchopneumonia, pleuritis, peritonitis, pericarditis, polyarthritis, and meningitis (1, 9, 10), in addition to other lesions such as renal glomerular thrombosis (8). Immunity is primarily humoral. Although serotypes differ, considerable protective cross-reactivity also exists between them (6, 13). The role, if any, of cell-mediated immunity has yet to be elucidated.

Interference with research
Little direct information has been published describing host physiologic changes following clinical infection with *H. parasuis*. Direct information is limited to reports of host iron acquisition by *H. parasuis* (3); elevation of acute-phase proteins (11); cleavage and metabolism of sialic acid (4); and altered hematologic, serum chemistry, and coagulation system parameters as pigs approached death (1, 15). Obviously, these latter changes are reflective of disseminated intravascular coagulation and endotoxic shock, and cannot be assumed to occur in asymptomatic or mildly infected pigs. However, given the propensity of the organism to infect serosal surfaces, one can anticipate some degree of compromise in projects involving the cardiovascular, lymphoreticular, musculoskeletal, and nervous systems. In addition, peritonitis will surely affect studies of nearly any kind. Lastly, *H. parasuis* infection may influence studies involving the urinary system; and the lymphoreticular system, through stimulation of proinflammatory cytokines. Of course, if *H. parasuis* is a secondary pathogen, the research project may also be compromised by whatever primary pathogen is present. It is more difficult to state with certainty whether the more common asymptomatic, or "subclinical" infections will

interfere with experimental studies. It is likely that they will not. However, the point at which an infection becomes "clinical" in even the mildest sense of the word is not known with certainty for any pathogen, including *H. parasuis*.

Diagnosis and control
H. parasuis may be suspected on the basis of herd history, clinical signs, and necropsy findings, and is confirmed by culture and identification of the organism if that effort is successful. *H. parasuis* can usually, but not always, be recovered from affected tissues. Failure to isolate the organism is generally due to mishandling after collection. More recently, PCR assays have been developed for the rapid diagnosis of *H. parasuis* infection (7). Affected pigs can be treated with a number of antibiotics, including penicillins, cephalosporins, potentiated sulfonamides, and fluoroquinolones. *H. parasuis* is susceptible to environmental stressors, and so dies quickly when outside the animal host. Disinfection of the premises following an outbreak will therefore greatly reduce the environmental load of the organism, but will not eradicate it, since the primary reservoir is the asymptomatic adult pig. It is common practice among vendors of research pigs to vaccinate for *H. parasuis*. This practice should be encouraged, since passively transferred maternal immunity protects piglets from clinical disease, while not interfering with development of active immunity (13).

Lawsonia intracellularis

Agent
Lawsonia intracellularis is a slender, curved, gram-negative rod in the family *Desulfovibrionaceae*. It is closely related to the campylobacters. It was formerly called ileal symbiont intracellularis, and is an obligate intracellular pathogen (4).

Epidemiology
L. intracellularis has an unusually wide host range, which includes the fox, deer, dog, guinea pig, hamster, horse, monkey, rabbit, rat, pig, emu, and ostrich (4). *L. intracellularis* is globally distributed, infecting an estimated 30 to 40% of pig herds, with up to 50% of pigs affected during outbreaks (5). *L. intracellularis* is known to be a central component of a complex of acute and chronic conditions that fall under the category of "porcine proliferative enteropathies." Uncomplicated, "classical" chronic infections with *L. intracellularis* are referred to as "chronic proliferative enteropathy" (CPE), or "porcine intestinal adenomatosis." Susceptible pigs are infected through direct or indirect ingestion of contaminated feces. Introduction of *L. intracellularis* into a naive herd most often occurs with the introduction of asymptomatic contaminator pigs (4, 9).

Clinical signs
In herds endemically infected with *L. intracellularis,* many pigs can be found to be asymptomatic fecal shedders. Pigs of all ages may become infected, with the majority of infections being found in growing to finishing pigs 8 to 16 weeks of age. Clinical signs are first observed 8 to 10 days after exposure, peak in severity by 2 to 3 weeks, and often become chronic, with spontaneous remission of signs occurring 4 to 10 weeks after initial appearance. Clinical signs may be mild, and include only minor weight loss or failure to gain. Moderate signs of infection include anorexia, diarrhea, dullness, and apathy. In the most severe cases, there is scouring, wasting, and death. In more acute cases, pigs may experience small intestinal hemorrhaging, revealed as anemia, pallor, and excretion of black, tarry feces. About half of these pigs will die. Pregnant females usually abort (1, 4, 5).

Pathology
Following exposure, colonization of the intestinal mucosa occurs through association with the host cell membrane, and induced phagocytosis. *L. intracellularis* survives and multiplies free within the host cell cytoplasm. By yet undetermined mechanisms, normal processes of cell growth and differentiation of host cells are disrupted (6). Instead, the cell

continues to undergo multiple mitotic events, resulting in formation of a hyperplastic, or "adenomatous" mucosa. Development of hyperplasia may involve IFN-γ (10). Mucosal hyperplasia can be so extensive as to result in loss of protein into the feces, and interference with nutrient absorption (7). *L. intracellularis* is uniformly identified within these mucosal lesions. Alteration of mucosal cytoarchitecture may be so severe as to lead to inflammatory changes ranging from superficial fibrinous reactions, to extensive, deep, coagulative necrosis, followed by production of granulation tissue (5). Some pigs develop more acute changes, including necrotizing enteritis, granulomatous regional ileitis, or acute hemorrhagic proliferative enteropathy (5, 8, 9). Lesions are most commonly observed in the distal small intestine and proximal colon, but may spread to local mesenteric lymph nodes (5, 9). Lesions are not observed in recovered pigs, or in pigs more than 2 years of age, presumably due to the development of active immunity, although immune mechanisms are not well characterized (9).

Interference with research
There is scant published information on the direct effects of *L. intracellularis* on host physiology. Clearly, natural infection of research swine with *L. intracellularis* will compromise studies involving the enterohepatic system, and those studies where growth or feed-intake measurements are to be evaluated. In addition, studies involving the lymphoreticular system may be compromised because of *L. intracellularis*-associated changes in tissue leukocyte phenotypes. Lastly, the hematopoietic system may be stimulated to increase blood-cell production in those cases where intestinal blood loss is significant.

Diagnosis and control
Diagnosis of *L. intracellularis* has traditionally relied on demonstration of the organism in feces or affected intestinal tissue, either by direct staining with modified Ziehl-Neelsen or Giminez stains (tissue impression smears), immunohistochemistry, or more recently, through PCR assay (3). Serologic assays correlate well with lesion development, but are unlikely to reveal subclinical infection in endemically infected herds. *L. intracellularis* has not been grown in artificial media, eliminating routine bacterial culture methods from the diagnostic arsenal. *L. intracellularis* can be grown in cell cultures, but this is impractical for routine use, and with the availability of more reliable methods, is not necessary. Of these methods, immunohistochemistry appears to be the most sensitive for fecal analysis (2). Affected pigs can be treated with tylosin, oxytetrcycline, and others (5). However, careful consideration of the utility of affected pigs should be given prior to initiating treatment. Long-term antibiotic therapy can also be useful to prevent development of lesions while pigs are on study. *L. intracellularis* is capable of surviving in the environment for remarkably long periods, considering that it is an obligate intracellular pathogen. It is also quite resistant to commonly used disinfectants, but is inactivated by quaternary ammonium and iodine-based compounds (5). Eradication depends on thorough cleanup and disinfection.

Leptospira spp.

Agent
Leptospires are thin, spiral, motile, gram-negative rods. While DNA-based taxonomic studies indicate that there are eight species, leptospires have traditionally been classified into 23 serogroups containing more than 200 serovars. Among the most important in swine are: *L. pomona, L. icterohaemorrhagiae, L. canicola, L. tarassovi, L. bratislava,* and *L. muenchen* (7).

Epidemiology
Leptospires are globally distributed in many host animal species, with swine, humans, and other mammals commonly infected. Such wide host ranges provide ample sources of infection for unprotected, susceptible animals. Asymptomatic rodent and porcine hosts con-

stitute the major reservoir of infection for susceptible research pigs. *Leptospira* spp. are shed in the urine and genital secretions. Leptospires survive in mild, moist environmental conditions. Transmission is by ingestion or inhalation of infectious urine or urine-contaminated feed, water, or soil; or through contact with infectious reproductive secretions during breeding (4).

Clinical signs
Infections of swine with swine-adapted serovars are generally asymptomatic. Disease results when these serovars are introduced into susceptible herds, or when atypical (non-host-adapted) species infect research swine. In acute clinical cases, signs are compatible with bacteremia, and include fever, anorexia, listlessness, and less commonly, jaundice. Young pigs tend to be affected more severely. More commonly, infection is endemic in a herd, and clinical signs are compatible with chronic disease. In these cases, signs are primarily associated with reproductive failure. It is common to observe abortions and the birth of dead or weak pigs, although clinical signs are substantially influenced by infecting serovar. Because it is relatively uncommon for pigs to be bred in the research setting, bacteremic disease in young pigs may be encountered more frequently (4).

Pathology
Following colonization of the oral or genital mucous membranes, *Leptospira* spp. disseminate hematogenously, ultimately affecting numerous organs, and colonizing primarily the liver and kidneys. Most infections are asymptomatic. Pathologic changes result from the cytopathic effects of *Leptospira* spp. endotoxin, which interferes with cellular electrolyte balance (10). The primary pathologic event at the tissue level is vascular endothelial damage, resulting in vascular damage and blood leakage (3). Secondary changes include icterus due to liver damage and destruction of red blood cells, and nephritis due to renal tubular injury. Grossly, there is multiorgan petechial or ecchymotic hemorrhaging. Microscopic lesions consist of renal tubular necrosis, focal hepatic necrosis, lymphocytic infiltration of the adrenal glands, and meningoencephalitis with perivascular lymphocytic infiltration (2, 4). Other organs affected include the lungs and mammary glands. Within about 2 weeks of infection, humoral immunity effectively terminates bacteremia. Renal infection is more slowly eliminated, often persisting from several months to a few years. Thereafter, pigs tend to be immune from reinfection with the original serovar (1, 4).

Interference with research
Virtually nothing has been published that would indicate direct effects of *Leptospira* spp. on swine physiology, other than lesion descriptions. In other species, *Leptospira* spp. have been shown to stimulate superoxide dismutase activity (6), induce mononuclear procoagulant activity (8), and activate B lymphocytes (5). Natural infection of research swine with *Leptospira* spp. will compromise research involving most organ systems, most assuredly the endocrine, enterohepatic, hematopoietic, nervous, reproductive, respiratory, and urinary systems. Studies in which weight gains or feed intake are determined will also be affected. It is currently unknown whether research involving asymptomatically infected adult swine will be affected by these infections. If pigs are to be used in research not involving the organ systems named above, it would seem reasonable to continue to utilize them as research subjects, after full clinical and hematologic recovery from infection.

Diagnosis and control
Infection with *Leptospira* spp. may be suspected on the basis of clinical signs. Definitive diagnosis requires laboratory confirmation. This has been accomplished historically using serology (paired samples), dark-field microscopy, bacterial culture, animal inoculation, and specialized stains of various bodily fluids and tissues (7). Urine sediment and kidney sections are the most rewarding diagnostically.

Serovars have traditionally been determined serologically. More recently, however, PCR assays have proven highly reliable for diagnosis, and can be used to determine serovar (9). If treatment is begun early in the course of infection, affected animals may be successfully treated with penicillin, fluoroquinolones, tetracylines, and others. Prior to treating infected pigs, the investigator and laboratory animal veterinarian should discuss the potential effects of *Leptospira* spp. infection on host physiology to determine whether the swine have been compromised as research subjects. It is prudent to initiate prophylactic treatment when bringing susceptible pigs into a facility with a history of *Leptospira* spp. infection. When administered annually, bacterins prevent clinical disease in a serovar-specific manner, but not bacterial colonization. Leptospires are easily inactivated by environmental temperature extremes, and by essentially all commonly used disinfectants. Therefore, contaminated premises should be thoroughly disinfected prior to repopulation with research swine. The potential exposure history of newly purchased swine should be carefully evaluated to determine whether prophylactic antibiotic, or bacterin administration, is warranted. Lastly, rodent control is important for pigs housed outdoors or in conventional swine-housing units.

Mycoplasma hyopneumoniae

Agent

Mycoplasma hyopneumoniae is a pleomorphic, gram-negative bacterium. In addition to *M. hyopneumoniae,* several other members of the genus also infect swine, including *M. hyorhinis*, *M. hyosynoviae*, *M. flocculare*, *M. sualvi,* and *M. hyopharyngis* (13). Because of its more prominent role as a pathogen of swine, this discussion will be limited to *M. hyopneumoniae*. All *Mycoplasma* spp. lack a cell wall. Instead, organelles are bound by a cellular membrane.

Epidemiology

M. hyopneumoniae is found in all swine-producing regions of the world. Within herds, infection rates can reach nearly 100% (9). The natural reservoir of infection is the pig. Asymptomatically infected swine carry organisms on the mucous membranes, and represent the most common source of infection for naive pigs. Transmission is primarily by direct contact between animals through contact with infectious respiratory secretions. Environmental stressors and poor husbandry facilitate the development of disease (16).

Clinical signs

M. hyopneumoniae has recently been recognized as a significant copathogen with PRRSV. *M. hyopneumoniae* is therefore a component of porcine respiratory disease complex (PRDC). In addition, most cases of enzootic pneumonia involving *M. hyopneumoniae* are actually mixed infections with other copathogens, including viral, bacterial, or nematode agents. The term "enzootic pneumonia" itself conveys considerable information regarding the epidemiologic and clinical picture. Clinical signs are associated with chronic respiratory disease, and include a nonproductive cough, and weight loss or failure to gain weight. Clinical disease has been reported in pigs as young as 2 weeks of age. In fact, signs may develop within 2 weeks of infection. More typically, however, clinical signs are observed in pigs 3 to 6 months of age, because the disease spreads slowly and so is often not immediately recognized (12, 13).

Pathology

Following colonization of the upper respiratory mucosa, *M. hyopneumoniae* quickly spreads to the trachea, bronchi, and bronchioles. In those locations, pathologic changes are thought to be caused by a series of processes, including attachment and colonization of ciliated epithelium, cytotoxicity, competition for nutrients, and evasion or modulation of the host immune response (13). Grossly, lungs are edematous, atelectatic, and contain scattered, well-demarcated areas of consolidation (6). Microscopic lesions include ciliary and epithelial damage, and peribronchial and perivascular lymphoreticular hyperplasia. The latter are thought to be exacerbated by the host immune response. In this regard, immunity to *M. hyopneumoniae* is relatively ineffectual. Immunity involves both innate and acquired components, including the mucociliary escalator, complement activation, and humoral and cellular components (8). Some components of the immune response are themselves associated with pathologic changes. For example, complement activation results in inflammation and contributes to morbidity. Also, pronounced antibody responses are associated with pneumonic lesion development (16).

Interference with research
Like other members of the genus, *M. hyopneumoniae* may have profound effects on specific aspects of host health and physiology. *M. hyopneumoniae* is known to predispose the host to disease caused by other respiratory pathogens, including *P. multocida* and *A. pleuropneumoniae* (1); alter respiratory function, blood gas, and pH values (6); cause ependymal cell cytopathology (15); increase intracellular Ca^{2+} release (11); increase sulfated mucin in bronchial goblet cells (5); serve as a B-cell mitogen (10); alter pulmonary macrophage and neutrophil function (2, 4); and immune suppress the host (7). Natural infection of research swine with *M. hyopneumoniae* clearly will compromise studies involving the lymphoreticular, nervous, and respiratory systems, as well as studies in which weight gain or body condition are evaluated.

Diagnosis and control
Diagnosis of *M. hyopneumoniae* infection relies on laboratory methods, including bacterial culture; special staining techniques; serology-based assays such as agglutination assays, immunohistochemistry, and immunofluorescence, and more recently, PCR assay and other molecular methods (3, 13). Antibiotic therapy may clear *M. hyopneumoniae* from infected pigs (14). However, treatment often fails to completely eliminate the pathogen, leaving the host a chronic carrier. For this reason, before deciding to treat or cull, careful consideration must be given to the intended research use of infected pigs, and to their potential to serve as a source of infection for other pigs. Prevention of disease is highly dependent on minimizing environmental stresses and preventing the introduction of other pathogens, including PRRSV. Pigs are routinely vaccinated against *M. hyopneumoniae*, with variable success (8). However, it is far preferable to obtain, maintain, and utilize *M. hyopneumoniae*-free pigs in biomedical research, than to find oneself in a situation where vaccination is required to reduce losses. Even without a cell wall, *M. hyopneumoniae* is susceptible to environmental extremes and to commonly used disinfectants. It does survive well, however, in cool, moist environments. Therefore, *M. hyopneumoniae* may be difficult to clear from open environments.

Pasteurella multocida

Agent
Pasteurella multocida is a gram-negative, nonmotile, facultatively anaerobic rod. Both avirulent and toxigenic strains have been isolated and studied. *P. multocida* has five capsular serotypes: A. B, C, D, and E. Of these, A, B, and D have been isolated from swine. Serotypes A and D are much more common than serotype B, which is restricted to Asia (11).

Epidemiology
P. multocida is a common commensal organism wherever swine are found. Within herds, carrier rates may be extremely high if not absolute. Therefore, while many animal hosts have been identified, the primary reservoir remains the nasal mucosa and tonsils of asymptomatic carrier pigs. Introduction of carrier swine into a susceptible population or herd is a common means of disease establishment. Transmission is by nose-to-nose contact, inhalation, ingestion, or wound inoculation. Transmission and/or clinical disease are enhanced by crowding, poor ventilation, inadequate temperature control, dusty or hand-delivered feed, unsanitary conditions, and bacterial strain virulence (5, 8, 11).

Clinical signs
The majority of *P. multocida* infections are asymptomatic. However, *P. multocida* has been associated with at least two clinical conditions. The first is PAR, caused by toxigenic strains of *P. multocida*. PAR may be exacerbated by coinfection with *B. bronchiseptica*. The clinical picture is dependent on several variables, including bacterial strain, host genetics, immune status, management and husbandry factors, ammonia and dust exposure, and the amount of toxin absorbed locally. In turn, the latter is highly dependent on host age (5, 8). The condition occurs most commonly in young pigs 3 weeks to 7 months of age. Destruction of the turbinates results in poor growth, malformed facial structure, sneezing, snuffling, epistaxis, and staining of the face with tears, as tear ducts become obstructed. Secondarily, loss of functional turbinates facilitates establishment of *P. multocida* and *B. bronchiseptica* pneumonia, thereby exacerbating clinical disease. In addition to PAR, *P. multocida* is associated with another clinical condition; pneumonic pasteurellosis. This is the final stage of a syndrome known as PRDC. Clinical signs include fever; cough; exercise intolerance; abdominal breathing; extreme weight loss; and less commonly, otitis and abortion. Death is uncommon (11). Serotype A is more frequently isolated from pigs with pneumonic pasteurellosis than serotype D (13, 20).

Pathology
Members of the genus *Pasteurella* produce a number of pathogenic compounds, including LPS, outer-membrane proteins, adhesins, leukotoxins, and enzymes such as hyaluronidase and neuraminidase. Specific substances are antiphagocytic, protect against complement-mediated lysis, facilitate adherence to target cells, are directly cytotoxic, or have mitogenic properties (11). Among these, dermonecrotic toxin, also called *P. multocida* toxin (Pmt), is a potent virulence factor in swine infections. Following infection, *P. multocida* colonizes the nasal mucosa and tonsils (1). Bacterial Pmt is directly cytotoxic, and causes osteoclastic bone resorption, likely through stimulation of IL-6 release from fibroblasts (6, 14, 16, 19). In combination with the irritation of the nasal mucosa caused by elevated ammonia and *B. bronchiseptica* dermonecrotic toxin, the net effect of Pmt activity is nasal turbinate hypoplasia. Gross findings of PAR include small to absent turbinates, and facial distortion. Microscopic findings in PAR include fibrous replacement of the bony plates primarily of the ventral conchae, nasal turbinate epithelial hyperplasia or metaplasia, mucosal gland atrophy, mucosal inflammation, and osteolysis (5). Following resolution of acute infection, some degree of turbinate recovery often occurs as animals age. *P. multocida* is also responsible for lesions associated with pneumonic pasteurellosis (13). Lesion development is highly dependent on bacterial strain. However, there are clearly additional, as yet unknown factors associated with disease development, since experimental inoculation of pigs with toxigenic strains frequently does not result in disease. This observation is made so often that some have concluded that *P. multocida* is not a primary pathogen, but is simply opportunistic (11). Once established, *P. multocida* causes anteroventral consolidation; bronchopneumonia; and with highly virulent strains, pleuritis, pericarditis, and abscessation (12, 13). Secondary or less common lesions may include disseminated focal nephritis (3), otitis media and interna (10), acute septicemia (17), and abortion (4). Immunity is primarily humoral, although antigenic stimulation by *P. multocida* is weak (2, 18).

Interference with research
Other than those reporting direct pathologic findings, few studies have reported on host physiologic changes caused by *P. multocida*, that would indicate reduced usefulness of pigs as research subjects. Experimental administration and in vitro studies of Pmt reveal that this toxin is capable of a wide range of host effects, including lymphopenia, liver dysfunction, possibly renal impairment (19), and IL-6 release (14). The extent to which these effects

also occur in vivo is unknown. Experimental infection has also been shown to increase proteins associated with an acute-phase reaction, such as serum haptoglobin (7). This author does not advise the automatic culling of pigs found to be carrying *P. multocida*. Most infections are asymptomatic. In addition, development of pneumonia usually requires turbinate lesions associated with PAR. Therefore, pigs lacking clinical evidence of turbinate damage are unlikely to have compromised pulmonary systems. Such pigs are likely to remain valid research subjects. If, on the other hand, clinical signs of PAR occur, or there is a history of pneumonic pasteurellosis, pigs from these herds are certainly unsuitable for research involving the respiratory system. In addition, research involving the cardiovascular, reproductive, and urinary systems may also be compromised. Lastly, studies wherein growth rates are evaluated would also be affected.

Diagnosis and control
Diagnosis of toxigenic *P. multocida* infection may be suspected on the basis of clinical presentation. However, given the multifactorial nature of PAR, and the multiple causes of porcine pneumonia, laboratory confirmation is essential. This may be accomplished by bacterial culture of nasal or tonsilar swabs, tracheal washings, or lung samples (15). More recently, PCR assays have been developed for rapid and reliable diagnosis of toxigenic strains of *P. multocida* (9). It should be noted, however, that *P. multocida* is usually isolated from asymptomatic swine. Therefore, the decision to keep, treat, or cull pigs carrying *P. multocida* is not "cut and dry." Acute infections with *P. multocida* have historically responded to a variety of antimicrobials. More recently, however, an increasing number of isolates have been shown to be resistant to multiple antibiotics. Therefore, sensitivity testing should be performed to aid antimicrobial selection. More permanent solutions to controlling any clinical condition associated with *P. multocida* must include significant management and husbandry changes that reduce stress and pathogen exposure. These include maintaining closed colonies, housing fewer pigs together, and minimizing reassortment of pigs once social hierarchies have been established (11). Husbandry practices should include vaccination of sows with bacterin. *P. multocida* is rapidly inactivated by commonly used disinfectants, as well as by heat or ultraviolet light (5). Commercial vendors of research swine are certainly aware of the infection status of their herds. Prior to purchase of research swine intended for use in pulmonary studies, the vendor should be asked to supply information concerning the herd history of PAR and pneumonia. Newly purchased pigs should be carefully examined for conformational evidence of PAR. Because *P. multocida* is considered zoonotic, personnel working with infected or potentially infected research swine should exercise a high degree of personal protection.

Streptococcus suis

Agent
Pigs may be infected with a number of *Streptococcus* spp. Among these are *S. suis*, *S. intestinalis*, *S. hyointestinalis*, *S. alactolyticus*, *S. porcinus*, *S. dysgalactiae,* and *S. bovis*. This discussion will focus on *S. suis*. However, the interested reader is directed elsewhere for excellent coverage of streptococcal diseases of swine (4). *S. suis* is a gram-positive, facultatively anaerobic coccus which occurs in chains. Swine isolates fall within the Lancefield groups R, S, RS, and T (4).

Epidemiology
S. suis may be found wherever swine are produced. Many swine commonly carry *S. suis* in the upper respiratory tract, specifically the tonsils and nasal cavity, lower genital tract, and intestinal tract (3, 10). In fact, many pigs are infected with *S. suis* by the time of weaning (9). The vast majority of these infections are asymptomatic. In addition, many other species of animals may serve as reservoir hosts of *S.*

suis. These include dogs, cats, cattle, sheep, goats, deer, horses, and ducks and other birds (4). This extensive reservoir is not likely to be of concern in research pigs housed indoors, but may have an impact on programs where pigs are housed outside, or are purchased from vendors whose pigs are at risk of infection from other animals. Concerning the latter, *S. suis* generally enters a susceptible swine herd via carrier pigs. Transmission occurs primarily through inhalation or ingestion, but may also occur at birth, during mating, or by contact with contaminated fomites. Lastly, flies have been shown to vector *S. suis* (4).

Clinical signs
Few clinical signs are observed in endemically infected colonies. While infection rates may reach 100%, clinical disease is rarely found in more than 5% of the herd. However, on entry into a susceptible population, *S. suis* may cause disease in weaner pigs, frequently those between 5 and 10 weeks of age. Environmental, management, and husbandry stressors will greatly increase the appearance of clinical disease (3). In these cases a wide range of clinical signs may be observed. These include fever, respiratory distress, cyanosis, nasal and vaginal discharge, abortions, incoordination and other CNS signs, inappetence, depression, and shifting lameness (2). The latter signs are due to septicemia. Peracute cases may die of meningitis, without showing premonitory signs.

Pathology
Following colonization of mucous membranes, *S. suis* disseminates throughout the animal by mechanisms that are incompletely understood. Hematogenous spread is clearly an important means of dissemination within the host. This results in pathologic changes in a variety of organ systems. Pathologic findings include histologic evidence of meningitis, a hallmark feature (10). Endocarditis is also frequently noted (1). Other, less common or less pronounced findings include conjunctivitis, arthritis and polyserositis, bronchopneumonia, rhinitis, and vaginitis (4, 6). It should be noted, however, that pathologic changes are highly dependent on bacterial strain, and therefore vary among geographical locations. Immunity to *S. suis* depends on IgM and IgG antibodies directed against bacterial surface antigens (5).

Interference with research
Like other members of the genus, and indeed most bacteria capable of septicemic spread, *S. suis* is capable of profound effects on host physiology. Unfortunately, little scientific effort has been directed toward elucidating those effects. *S. suis* has been shown to induce release of proinflammatory cytokines from cells of mononuclear lineage (7). Research swine asymptomatically infected with *S. suis* are likely to remain valid research subjects for most types of studies. However, a history of *S. suis* infection in purchased swine should be carefully considered when evaluating the proposed research applications. Clearly, pigs that have experienced clinical streptococcosis are unsuitable for research involving the cardiovascular and nervous systems, and may also be unusable for studies involving the enterohepatic, lymphoreticular, musculoskeletal, reproductive, and respiratory systems.

Diagnosis and control
Presumptive diagnosis of *S. suis* infection is based on clinical signs and pathologic findings. However, laboratory confirmation is necessary. This is best accomplished by culture of cerebrospinal fluid, lung, and other target tissues. Serology is not very useful for anything other than determination of vaccination efficacy, or for surveying pathogen-free herds. Serotyping should be performed as a matter of epidemiologic significance. More recently, PCR assays have been developed for both diagnosis and strain typing (11). If treatment is planned, antibiotic sensitivity testing should be performed prior to antibiotic selection. *S. suis* survives in the environment for relatively long periods. However, most commonly used disinfectants effectively inactivate the organism, unless organic material reduces compound ac-

tivity. It is labor intensive, costly, and unrealistic to attempt eradication of *S. suis* from a research swine herd, unless all pigs can be removed and the premises thoroughly disinfected. If this is not possible, one may settle for disease prevention. Key components of such efforts include prevention of overcrowding, providing adequate ventilation and sanitation, minimizing temperature fluctuations, not mixing swine with age spreads exceeding 2 weeks, and generally keeping stress to a minimum (3). Vaccination programs continue to be met with mixed success. Alternatively, at the time of arrival of new pigs, and for a few weeks thereafter, it may be advantageous to treat with oral antibiotics until the pigs have acclimated. In these cases, amoxicillin would seem a reasonable choice. Because *S. suis* has caused serious infections in persons working with or around swine (8), personnel working with research swine should exercise a high degree of personal protection.

PARASITES

Ascaris suum

Agent
Commonly referred to as the "large roundworm," *Ascaris suum* is a nematode parasite of the small intestinal tract of swine. Male *A. suum* may reach 25 cm in length, while females may reach 40 cm. Female worms are oviparous, capable of producing enormous numbers of eggs.

Epidemiology
Globally, *A. suum* remains the most common worm parasite of swine. Herd infection rates vary greatly, but even fairly recently, have been approximately 70% (3). Among age groups, infection is more common among growing versus adult pigs. Large numbers of unembryonated eggs are released and pass in the feces. Embryonation occurs in the environment within about 3 weeks. Eggs are "sticky" and readily adhere to boots, clothing, arthropod vectors, cleaning utensils, etc., and are thereby easily transported within a facility. Infective eggs survive for extended periods under even moderately harsh conditions, thereby serving as a source of infection for many years to come. Infective eggs are ingested by a pig. Following hatching, second-stage larvae penetrate the wall of the cecum and colon, enter the hepatic portal system, and arrive at the liver. There, larvae molt to the third larval stage, and are transported to the lungs by the venous blood. Larvae penetrate the bronchioles, are coughed up and swallowed, and arrive back in the small intestine approximately 2 weeks postinfection. Subsequent molts result in fertile adults roughly 50 days after infection. Most adult worms die and are expelled within 6 months of infection, and nearly all are lost within a year of infection (3, 9).

Clinical signs
Swine infected with low numbers of *A. suum* may not show evidence of infection. However, even low-level infection depresses feed intake and weight gain. At higher levels, feed conversion is also decreased (5), and pigs present with fever, chronic cough ("thumps"), and labored breathing (3).

Pathology
Larval migration through the liver and lungs represents the primary pathologic events of ascariasis. In the liver, migrating larvae cause focal hemorrhaging, eosinophil infiltration, lymphatic enlargement ("milk spots"), and fibrotic changes. In the lungs, larval migration results in verminous pneumonia, characterized by focal hemorrhaging, edema, emphysema, and secondary bacterial infections. Ascarid infection also enhances the pathogenicity of pulmonary viral infections. Adult worms are also pathogenic, since they rob the host of nutrients and interfere with normal digestive and absorptive processes (8). Adult worms may obstruct the bile duct, causing icterus, or in very heavy infections, obstruct the movement of intestinal contents and cause fatal rupture of the small intestine. Immunity to *A. suum* is

pronounced, typical of ascarid infections, primarily humoral, and is induced by intense and continued systemic exposure to worm products released by all life-cycle stages found in the host. Regional immune responses occur, and are specific to the life-cycle stages present in specific organs (6).

Interference with research
Surprisingly few reports have focused on the physiologic effects of infection with *A. suum*. In the pig, *A. suum* interferes with nitrogen metabolism (5) and alters concentrations of specific hormones, enzymes, electrolytes, minerals, and vitamins in serum. These include serum albumin, iron, thyroxin, vitamins A and E, nonesterified fatty acids, inorganic phosphorus, selected corticosteroids and others (2, 4). Many of these physiologic changes occur during specific stages of infection, and are not evident throughout the entire course of infection. In other host species, *A. suum* or its products decrease levels of available pancreatic digestive enzymes (11), while increasing their concentrations in serum (12), alter basophil numbers in bone marrow (1), and suppress IgE and IgG antibody responses (10). In addition, there is a body of literature describing the effects of *A. suum* extracts on the respiratory system. These are used as models of IgE-mediated allergic airway disease. Lastly, extracts from the closely related human ascarid, *Ascaris lumbricoides*, have been shown to interfere with coagulation and fibrinolysis in vitro (7). Concerning these latter effects, it has yet to be demonstrated that these also occur in pigs infected with *A. suum*. It is difficult to indicate the number of migrating larvae needed to compromise research involving the endocrine, enterohepatic, hematopoietic, lymphoreticular, and respiratory systems, since this will depend on the amount of tissue recovery or regeneration that occurs, and the specific research applications in question. Heavy infections clearly could seriously compromise the validity of studies involving these systems. Less severe infections will also compromise studies in which feed conversion, weight gain, or other nutritional parameters are measured. For these reasons, ascarid infections should be minimized.

Diagnosis and control
A. suum infection should be assumed present in pigs. Diagnosis is made by observing the characteristic eggs in fecal flotation preparations. Finding liver "milk spots" at necropsy also suggests the occurrence of infection, but must be differentiated from lesions caused by migrating larvae of the kidney worm, *Stephanurus dentatus*. Treatment for removal of adult and developing worms is by administration of pyrantel tartrate at 22 mg/kg body weight, given as a powdered premix (3). Other anthelmintics, such as piperazine, are also active against adult worms, but are less so against developing larvae. Infective eggs are remarkably resistant to commonly used disinfectants. Steam and direct sunlight will inactivate them. In general, prevention of contamination is far more easily accomplished than eradication once environmental contamination with eggs has occurred. Therefore, research pigs should be housed on sealed surfaces that can be steam cleaned at least weekly, feces should be removed daily, and pigs should be administered pyrantel tartrate on entry into the facility. *A. suum* infects humans, although the entire life cycle is not completed. Therefore, personnel working with swine should practice personal hygiene to avoid zoonotic infection.

Isospora suis

Agent
Swine may be infected with a large number of protozoal agents. Among these, *Eimeria* spp. are the most common. However, these are nonpathogenic even when administered by the millions (14). In contrast, *Isospora suis* may be highly pathogenic. In fact, *I. suis* is without question the most clinically and economically important protozoal pathogen of swine. *I. suis* is an Apicomplexan parasite, and is the causative agent of swine coccidiosis.

Epidemiology

Infection rates for *I. suis* are high wherever swine are raised in confinement. The life cycle of *I. suis* is direct, with unsporulated oocysts released in the feces. Sporulation occurs within 12 h under ideal conditions, although 2 to 3 days is more typical (3). The sporulated oocyst represents the infectious stage for a susceptible pig. Following ingestion of contaminated feed or water, oocysts excyst, releasing sporozoites which infect cells of the intestinal epithelium, primarily in the jejunum and ileum. Several rounds of asexual reproduction (schizogony) occur. These are followed by gametogony, the production of sexual stages, which unite and develop into unsporulated oocysts. The entire life cycle requires about 5 days postinfection (17). The source of infection for nursing piglets remains somewhat of a mystery. Clearly, the sow is not the primary source. Once established, it is likely that contaminated fomites, such as farrowing crates, represent the primary source of infection for newborn piglets (14).

Clinical signs

Infections of weaned and adult pigs are nearly always asymptomatic. In contrast, nursing piglets exposed to even modest inoculations develop severe disease between 7 and 11 days of age. The most prominent clinical sign is yellowish to grayish diarrhea, which becomes increasingly fluid over time. Piglets continue to nurse, but develop a rough hair coat, dehydration, slowed weight gain, and lose condition. Death is uncommon, unless the clinical condition is worsened by concurrent infections with other enteric pathogens (15). Some have suggested that postweaning stress may reactivate neonatally acquired infections, but this appears to be uncommon (16).

Pathology

Following ingestion and excystation, sporozoites preferentially infect epithelial cells of the villous tips. The extent of pathologic change in the intestine is directly dependent on the infecting dose. Gross lesions found in heavily infected pigs include fibrinonecrotic membranes in the jejunum and ileum. Microscopic lesions include villous atrophy and fusion, crypt hyperplasia, epithelial metaplasia, and necrotic enteritis (14, 17). Villous lesions reduce epithelial function, leading to malabsorption and osmotic diarrhea, which explains the fluid loss and increased gut motility. Maturation of nonspecific components of the immune system play more important roles in resistance to infection, than does acquired immunity (5). However, in addition to innate mechanisms, pigs develop strong immune responses to *I. suis,* such that once pigs recover from a primary infection, recurrence of disease does not occur (18).

Interference with research

Coccidia are known to affect host physiology in a number of ways. Most of these relate to the enteric system. In swine, *I. suis* has been shown to reduce mucus synthesis in small intestinal goblet cells (9), alter ratios of enterocytes and goblet cells (13), and alter activity levels of several enteric enzymes, including dehydrogenases, monoamine oxidase, alkaline phosphatase, β-D-glucosidase, 5-nucleotide phosphohydrolase, phosphoglucomutase, and acid phosphotase (6, 7, 8, 10, 11, 12). Infection has also been shown to lower serum β-globulin concentrations (4). In some cases, loss of enzyme activity is also associated with changes in the muscularis mucosae (7). These alterations will certainly interfere with research involving the enterohepatic system, and with other studies in which nutritional or growth parameters are measured. In addition, *I. suis* may interfere with experimental infection of pigs with other enteric pathogens under study (1).

Diagnosis and control

Coccidiosis caused by *I. suis* may be suspected when nursing pigs present with diarrhea that is unresponsive to antibiotic therapy, although *Strongyloides ransomi* infection may present with similar signs. Confirmation of infection is usually possible by demonstrating large numbers of characteristic *I. suis* oocysts in diarrheic feces 1 to 3 days after the start of signs. On occasion, pigs will die prior to shedding of oocysts, so a diagnosis of coccidiosis cannot be ruled out simply because oocysts are not found. In these cases, examination of feces from several piglets will often reveal the cause. Because sows are not the primary source of infection for newborn piglets, prophylactic treatment of sows does not prevent clinical disease in newborns. Prophylactic treatment of newborn piglets with the antiprotozoal toltrazuril (Baycox®, Bayer Corporation) greatly reduces oocyst shedding and incidence of diarrhea (2). Unfortunately, toltrazuril is not currently available in the United States, but *can be legally imported under the personal use importation rule*. Because it is difficult if not impossible to find swine herds free of *I. suis* infection, efforts should be directed toward prevention of clinical disease. These efforts are most likely to succeed when strict attention is given to sanitation. Housing areas should be thoroughly cleaned, then disinfected with concentrated (50%) bleach or ammonia compounds. These should be allowed several hours of contact time, followed by steam cleaning. Secondarily, management and husbandry practices that reduce physiologic stress should also be utilized (14).

Sarcoptes scabiei var. *suis*

Agent
Sarcoptes scabiei is a burrowing mite of the family *Sarcoptidae*. It is easily recognized as such by the possession of short, stumpy legs that extend only a short distance beyond the margins of the body. *S. scabiei* var. *suis* is the causative agent of sarcoptic acariasis or "mange" in swine.

Epidemiology
S. scabiei var. *suis* is found wherever swine are produced. Herd prevalence often exceeds 50%, while animal prevalence ranges from 20 to 95%, with 20% more typical (1). The life cycle of *S. scabiei* consists of egg, larva, nymph, and adult. All these permanently inhabit the epidermis in tunnels created by digesting away and feeding on epidermal cells. Female mites release eggs within the tunnels. Eggs hatch within 3 to 5 days. Developing larvae molt to the nymph stage, which continue development and molt to the adult stage within the tunnels. The entire life cycle requires 10 to 25 days (1). Most mite activity is confined to the inside surfaces of the ear pinnae. In fact, this site in older pigs represents the primary reservoir of infestation for other pigs. Transmission is by direct contact. Environmental contamination is of lesser importance, but has been documented (1).

Clinical signs
Most pigs infested with *S. scabiei* var. *suis* are asymptomatic. However, a significant number of pigs develop clinical symptoms. Sarcoptic acariasis occurs in two forms. First, common mange is characterized by an initial increase in mite population, with mite-filled encrustations forming in the ears. This is followed by reddening of the skin, intense pruritus, and a dramatic decline in the number of recoverable mites. This progression of signs suggests the development of an effective type 1 hypersensitivity reaction (2). As pruritus increases, pigs seek relief through scratching and rubbing. This results in depressed growth rates, hair loss, abrasions, and thickening of the skin (4). Second, chronic, or hyperkeratotic mange is less common, and is most frequently observed in older swine, in particular, in sows after two or three litters. Clinical signs of chronic mange include "asbestos-like" scabs loosely attached to the skin. The scabs contain numerous mites. The specific form of acariasis developing in any individual pig is strongly influenced by host genetics and nutrition. Concerning the latter, diets low in protein and iron promote the development of hyperkeratotic acariasis, since these pigs are less capable of mounting an effective immune response (1, 2).

Pathology
Swine follow a pattern of cutaneous hypersensitivity to *S. scabiei* that is typical of the

TABLE 10-1. Body systems known or likely to be affected by pathogen indicated

Pathogen	Cardio-vascular	Dermal	Endocrine	Entero-hepatic	Hema-topoietic	Lympho-reticular	Musculo-skeletal	Nervous	Reproductive	Respiratory	Urinary
Encephalomyocarditis virus	X							X	X	X	
Hemagglutinating encephalomyelitis virus				X	X		X	X		X	
Porcine circovirus	X	X		X	X	X	X	X	X	X	
Porcine enteroviruses	X	X	X	X			X	X	X	X	X
Porcine parvovirus	X	X	X	X	X	X	X	X	X	X	X
Porcine reproductive and respiratory syndrome virus	X			X	X	X	X	X	X	X	
Porcine rotavirus				X							
Swine herpesvirus (pseudorabies)	X			X		X	X	X	X	X	
Swine influenza virus				X		X			X	X	X
Transmissible gastroenteritis virus	X		X	X		X	X	X			
Porcine respiratory coronavirus						X		X		X	
Actinobacillus pleuropneumoniae				X	X	X	X	X	X	X	X
Bordetella bronchiseptica		X		X		X	X	X		X X	X X
Clostridium perfringens type C	X		X	X	X		X X	X		X	X
Erysipelothrix rhusiopathiae	X	X		X	X	X	X	X	X	X	X
Haemophilus parasuis	X				X X	X X	X	X		X	X
Lawsonia intracellularis			X	X		X					
Leptospira spp.								X	X		X
Mycoplasma hyopneumoniae							X X	X X	X	X X	X
Pasteurella multocida	X X									X X	
Streptococcus suis	X			X	X	X X		X	X X	X X	X
Ascaris suum			X	X		X X				X	
Isospora suis				X	X						
Sarcoptes scabiei var. suis		X									

PATHOGENS OF SWINE ■ 319

mammalian host response to ectoparasite infestation. This pattern is one of (i) induction, (ii) delayed hypersensitivity, (iii) delayed and immediate hypersensitivity, (iv) immediate hypersensitivity only, and (v) desensitization (3). Each phase is associated with specific components of immune responsiveness, including both cellular and humoral components. Common mange is characterized by focal erythema and urticaria, with extensive infiltration by eosinophils, mast cells, and lymphocytes, but few, if any, mites. Dermatitis results when pigs scratch and rub. In contrast, hyperkeratotic acariasis causes the formation of thick, scabs that are loosely attached to the skin. These contain very high numbers of mites. Lesions are most common on the ear pinnae, but may spread to the head and neck (2, 6, 8).

Interference with research
There is a relative paucity of information describing the physiologic effects of S. scabiei var. suis on the swine host. S. scabiei var. suis infestation causes increased total protein and γ-globulin levels in infested pigs (9). In other host species, S. scabiei has been shown to mildly alter blood leukocyte profiles (7), although this has not been reproduced in pigs infested with S. scabiei var. suis (10). Natural infestation of research swine with S. scabiei var. suis has the potential to interfere with virtually any research study, but particularly those involving the dermal and lymphoreticular systems. The pruritus associated with common mange can be incapacitating, since affected pigs will spend much of their waking hours seeking relief through scratching and rubbing. In addition, infestation can reduce feed utilization efficiency and weight gains, thereby interfering with studies in which these parameters are directly or indirectly measured.

Diagnosis and control
Sarcoptic mange may be suspected based on clinical signs alone. Laboratory confirmation consists of visually observing mites among the debris adhering to the inner surfaces of the ear pinnae. Further confirmation is obtained by microscopic demonstration of mites in skin scrapings that have been partially dissolved with 10% KOH (1). Scrapings from the inner surfaces of the ear pinnae consistently yield the highest numbers of mites. Several treatments are available for not only the treatment of clinical disease, but for the eradication of mites from a facility (1, 5). Mites are rapidly killed by desiccation or direct sunlight, and do not survive more than a few days off the host.

REFERENCES
VIRUSES
Encephalomyocarditis virus
1. **Christianson, W. T., H. S. Kim, H. S. Joo, and D. M. Barnes.** 1990. Reproductive and neonatal losses associated with possible encephalomyocarditis virus infection in pigs. *Vet. Rec.* **126:**54–57.
2. **Christianson, W. T., H. S. Kim, I. J. Yoon, and H. S. Joo.** 1992. Transplacental infection of porcine fetuses following experimental challenge inoculation with encephalomyocarditis virus. *Am. J. Vet. Res.* **53:**44–47.
3. **Craighead, J. E., P. H. Peralta, T. G. Murnane, and A. Shelokov.** 1963. Oral infection of swine with the encephalomyocarditis virus. *J. Infect. Dis.* **112:**205–212.
4. **Dea, S., R. Bilodeau, R. Sauvageau, and G. P. Martineau.** 1991. Outbreaks in Quebec pig farms of respiratory and reproductive problems associated with encephalomyocarditis virus. *J. Vet. Diagn. Investig.* **3:**275–282.
5. **Foni, E., G. Barigazzi, L. Sidoli, P. S. Marcato, G. Sarli, L. Della Salda, and M. Spinaci.** 1993. Experimental encephalomyocarditis virus infection in pigs. *Zentbl. Vetmed. Reihe B* **40:**347–352.
6. **Glastonbury, J. R.** 1977. Preweaning mortality in the pig. Pathological findings in piglets dying between birth and weaning. *Aust. Vet. J.* **53:**310–314.
7. **Joo, H. S.** 1999. Encephalomyocarditis virus, p. 139–144. *In* B. E. Straw, S. D'Allaire, W. L. Mengeling, and D. J. Taylor (ed.), *Diseases of Swine*, 8th ed. Iowa State University Press, Ames.
8. **Kim, H. S., W. T. Christianson, and H. S. Joo.** 1989. Pathogenic properties of encephalomyocarditis virus isolates in swine fetuses. *Arch. Virol.* **109:**51–57.
9. **Kim, H. S., H. S. Joo, and M. E. Bergeland.** 1989. Serologic, virologic, and histopathologic observations of encephalomyocarditis virus infec-

tion in mummified and stillborn pigs. *J. Vet. Diagn. Investig.* **1**:101–104.
10. **Kim, H. S., H. S. Joo, W. T. Christianson, and R. B. Morrison.** 1991. Evaluation of serologic methods for the detection of antibodies to encephalomyocarditis virus in swine fetal thoracic fluids. *J. Vet. Diagn. Investig.* **3**:283–286.
11. **Koenen, F., and H. Vanderhallen.** 1997. Comparative study of the pathogenic properties of a Belgian and a Greek encephalomyocarditis virus (EMCV) isolate for sows in gestation. *Zentbl. Vetmed. Reihe B* **44**:281–286.
12. **Marcato, P. S., G. Sarli, L. Della Salda, G. Barigazzi, E. Foni, L. Sidoli, and M. Spinaci.** 1992. Ultrastructural study of experimental myocarditis induced by cardiovirus (SMCV-M) in swine. *J. Submicrosc. Cytol. Pathol.* **24**:371–379.
13. **Stott, J. L.** 1999. Picornaviridae, p. 371–378. *In* D. C. Hirsh and Y. C. Zee (ed.), *Veterinary Microbiology*. Blackwell Science, Inc., Malden, Mass.
14. **Tsangaris, T., S. Lekkas, and G. Kanakoudis.** 1989. Changes in the myocardium in encephalomyocarditis of pigs. *Dtsch. Tieraerztl. Wochenschr.* **96**:301–303.
15. **Vanderhallen, H., and F. Koenen.** 1997. Rapid diagnosis of encephalomyocarditis virus infections in pigs using a reverse transcriptase-polymerase chain reaction. *J. Virol. Methods* **66**:83–89.
16. **Zimmerman, J., K. Schwartz, H. T. Hill, M. C. Meetz, R. Simonson, and J. H. Carlson.** 1993. Influence of dose and route on transmission of encephalomyocarditis virus to swine. *J. Vet. Diagn. Investig.* **5**:317–321.

Hemagglutinating encephalomyelitis virus
1. **Andries, K.** 1982. Pathogenese en epizoötiologie van "vomiting and wasting disease," een virale infektie bij het varken. Ph.D. dissertation. Med. Fac. Diergeneeskd. Rijksuniv., Ghent, Belgium.
2. **Andries, K., and M. B. Pensaert.** 1980. Immunofluroescence studies on the pathogenesis of hemagglutinating encephalomyelitis virus after oronasal inoculation. *Am. J. Vet. Res.* **41**:1372–1378.
3. **Andries, K., M. Pensaert, and P. Callebaut.** 1978. Pathogenicity of hemagglutinating encephalomyelitis (vomiting and wasting disease) virus of pigs, using different routes of inoculation. *Zentbl. Vetmed. Reihe B* **25**:461–468.
4. **Cutlip, R. C., and W. L. Mengeling.** 1972. Lesions induced by hemagglutinating encephalomyelitis virus strain 67N in pigs. *Am. J. Vet. Res.* **33**:2003–2009.
5. **Hirano, N., K. Tohyama, and H. Taira.** 1998. Spread of swine hemagglutinating enceph-

alomyelitis virus from peripheral nerves to the CNS. *Adv. Exp. Med. Biol.* **440**:601–607.
6. **Mengeling, W. L., and R. C. Cutlip.** 1976. Pathogenicity of field isolates of hemagglutinating encephalomyelitis virus for neonatal pigs. *J. Am. Vet. Med. Assoc.* **168**:236–239.
7. **Paul, P. S., and W. L. Mengeling.** 1984. Persistence of passively acquired antibodies to hemagglutinating encephalomyelitis virus in swine. *Am. J. Vet. Res.* **45**:932–934.
8. **Pensaert, M. B.** 1999. Hemagglutinating encephalomyelitis virus, p. 151–157. *In* B. E. Straw, S. D'Allaire, W. L. Mengeling, and D. J. Taylor (ed.), *Diseases of Swine,* 8th ed. Iowa State University Press, Ames.
9. **Stott, J. L.** 1999. Coronaviridae, p. 418–429. *In* D. C. Hirsh and Y. C. Zee (ed.), *Veterinary Microbiology*. Blackwell Science, Inc., Malden, Mass.
10. **Werdin, R. E., D. K. Sorensen, and W. C. Stewart.** 1976. Porcine encephalomyelitis caused by hemagglutinating encephalomyelitis virus. *J. Am. Vet. Med. Assoc.* **168**:240–246.

Porcine circovirus
1. **Allan, G. M., and J. A. Ellis.** 2000. Porcine circovirus: a review. *J. Vet. Diagn. Investig.* **12**:3–14.
2. **Allan, G. M., F. McNeilly, J. P. Cassidy, G. A. C. Reilly, B. M. Adair, W. A. Ellis, and M. S. McNulty.** 1995. Pathogenesis of porcine circovirus: Experimental infections of colostrum-deprived piglets and examination of pig foetal material. *Vet. Microbiol.* **44**:49–64.
3. **Allan, G. M., F. McNeilly, S. Kennedy, B. Daft, E. G. Clarke, J. A. Ellis, D. M. Haines, B. M. Meehan, and B. M. Adair.** 1998. Isolation of porcine circovirus-like viruses from pigs with a wasting disease in the USA and Europe. *J. Vet. Diagn. Investig.* **10**:3–10.
4. **Allan, G. M., K. V. Phenix, D. Todd, and B. M. Adair.** 1994. Some biological and physico-chemical properties of porcine circovirus. *J. Vet. Med.* **41**:17–26.
5. **Bogdan, J., K. West, E. Clark, C. Konoby, D. Haines, G. Allan, F. McNeilly, B. Meehan, S. Krakowka, and J. A. Ellis.** 2001. Association of porcine circovirus 2 with reproductive failure in pigs: a retrospective study, 1995–1998. *Can. Vet. J.* **42**:548–550.
6. **Calsamiglia, M., J. Segales, J. Quintana, C. Rosell, and M. Domingo.** 2002. Detection of porcine circovirus types 1 and 2 in serum and tissue samples of pigs with and without postweaning multisystemic wasting syndrome. *J. Clin. Microbiol.* **40**:1848–1850.
7. **Choi, C., and C. Chae.** 2000. Distribution of porcine parvovirus in porcine circovirus 2-

infected pigs with postweaning multisystemic wasting syndrome as shown by in-situ hybridization. *J. Comp. Pathol.* **123:**302–305.

8. **Darwich, L., J. Segales, M. Domingo, and E. Mateu.** 2002. Changes in CD4(+), CD8(+), CD 4(+) CD8(+), and immunoglobulin M-positive peripheral blood mononuclear cells of postweaning multisystemic wasting syndrome-affected pigs and age-matched uninfected wasted and healthy pigs correlate with lesions and porcine circovirus type 2 load in lymphoid tissues. *Clin. Diagn. Lab. Immunol.* **9:**236–242.

9. **Ellis, J. A., B. M. Wiseman, G. Allan, C. Konoby, S. Krakowka, B. M. Meehan, and F. McNeilly.** 2000. Analysis of seroconversion to porcine circovirus 2 among veterinarians from the United States and Canada. *J. Am. Vet. Med. Assoc.* **217:**1645–1646.

10. **Kennedy, S., D. Moffett, F. McNeilly, B. Meehan, J. Ellis, S. Krakowka, and G. M. Allan.** 2000. Reproduction of lesions of postweaning multisystemic wasting syndrome by infection of conventional pigs with porcine circovirus type 2 alone or in combination with porcine parvovirus. *J. Comp. Pathol.* **122:**9–24.

11. **Kim, J., D. U. Han, C. Choi, and C. Chae.** 2001. Differentiation of porcine circovirus (PCV)-1 and PCV-2 in boar semen using a multiplex nested polymerase chain reaction. *J. Virol. Methods* **98:**25–31.

12. **Kyriakis, S. C., K. Saoulidis, S. Lekkas, C. C. Miliotis, P. A. Papoutsis, and S. Kennedy.** 2002. The effects of immuno-modulation on the clinical and pathological expression of postweaning multisystemic wasting syndrome. *J. Comp. Pathol.* **126:**38–46.

13. **Lamar, C. H.** 1971. Characterization of peculiar cellular structures in the spinal cords of pigs affected with myoclonia congenita. M.S. thesis. Purdue University.

14. **Larochelle, R., A. Bielanski, P. Muller, and R. Magar.** 2000. PCR detection and evidence of shedding of porcine circovirus type 2 in boar semen. *J. Clin. Microbiol.* **38:**4629–4632.

15. **Lukert, P. D., and G. M. Allan.** 1999. Porcine circovirus, p. 119–124. *In* B. E. Straw, S. D'Allaire, W. L. Mengeling, and D. J. Taylor (ed.), *Diseases of Swine,* 8th ed. Iowa State University Press, Ames.

16. **Magar, R., R. Larochelle, S. Thibault, and L. Lamontagne.** 2000. Experimental transmission of porcine circovirus type 2 (PCV2) in weaned pigs: a sequential study. *J. Comp. Pathol.* **123:**258–269.

17. **McNeilly, F., G. M. Allan, J. C. Foster, B. M. Adair, and M. S. McNulty.** 1996. Effect of porcine circovirus on porcine alveolar macrophage function. *Vet. Immunol. Immunopathol.* **49:**295–306.

18. **McNeilly, F., I. McNair, M. O'Connor, S. Brockbank, D. Gilpin, C. Lasagna, G. Boriosi, G. Meehan, J. Ellis, S. Krakowka, and G. M. Allan.** 2002. Evaluation of a porcine circovirus type 2-specific antigen-capture enzyme-linked immunosorbent assay for the diagnosis of postweaning multisystemic wasting syndrome in pigs: comparison with virus isolation, immunohistochemistry, and the polymerase chain reaction. *J. Vet. Diagn. Investig.* **14:**106–112.

19. **Meehan, B. M., F. McNeilly, I. McNair, I. Walker, J. A. Ellis, S. Krakowka, and G. M. Allan.** 2001. Isolation and characterization of porcine circovirus 2 from cases of sow abortion and porcine dermatitis and nephropathy syndrome. *Arch. Virol.* **146:**835–842.

20. **Pogranichnyy, R. M., K. J. Yoon, P. A. Harms, S. L. Swenson, J. J. Zimmerman, and S. D. Sorden.** 2000. Characterization of immune response of young pigs to porcine circovirus type 2 infection. *Viral Immunol.* **13:**143–153.

21. **Rosell, C., J. Segales, J. A. Ramos-Vera, J. M. Folch, G. M. Rodriguez-Arrioja, C. O. Duran, M. Balasch, J. Plana-Duran, and M. Domingo.** 2000. Identification of porcine circovirus in tissues of pigs with porcine dermatitis and nephropathy syndrome. *Vet. Rec.* **146:**40–43.

22. **Rosell, C., J. Segales, and M. Domingo.** 2000. Hepatitis and staging of hepatic damage in pigs naturally infected with porcine circovirus type 2. *Vet. Pathol.* **37:**687–692.

23. **Sarli, G., L. Mandrioli, M. Laurenti, L. Sidoli, C. Cerati, G. Rolla, and P. S. Marcato.** 2001. Immunohistochemical characterization of the lymph node reaction in pig post-weaning multisystemic wasting syndrome (PMWS). *Vet. Immunol. Immunopathol.* **83:**53–67.

24. **Segales, J., F. Alonso, C. Rosell, J. Pastor, F. Chianini, E. Campos, L. Lopez-Fuertes, J. Quintana, G. Rodriguez-Arrioja, M. Calsamiglia, J. Pujols, J. Dominguez, and M. Domingo.** 2001. Changes in peripheral blood leukocyte populations in pigs with natural postweaning multisystemic wasting syndrome (PMWS). *Vet. Immunol. Immunopathol.* **81:**37–44.

25. **Shibahara, T., K. Sato, Y. Ishikawa, and K. Kadota.** 2000. Porcine circovirus induces B lymphocyte depletion in pigs with wasting disease syndrome. *J. Vet. Med. Sci.* **62:**1125–1131.

26. **Stevenson, G. W., M. Kiupel, S. K. Mittal, J. Choi, K. S. Latimer, and C. L. Kanitz.** 2000. Tissue distribution and genetic typing of porcine circoviruses in pigs with naturally occur-

ring congenital tremors. *J. Vet. Diagn. Investig.* **13**:57–62.
27. **Tischer, I., L. Bode, J. Apodaca, H. Timm, D. Peters, R. Rasch, S. Pociuli, and E. Gerike.** 1995. Presence of antibodies reacting with porcine circovirus in sera of humans, mice, and cattle. *Arch. Virol.* **140**:1427–1439.
28. **Tischer, I., L. Bode, D. Peters, S. Pociuli, and B. Germann.** 1995. Distribution of antibodies to porcine circovirus in swine populations of different breeding farms. *Arch. Virol.* **140**:737–743.
29. **Tischer, I., W. Mields, D. Wolff, M. Vagt, and W. Griem.** 1986. Studies on epidemiology and pathogenicity of porcine circovirus. *Arch. Virol.* **91**:271–276.

Porcine enteroviruses
1. **Baba, S. P., E. H. Bohl, and R. C. Meyer.** 1966. Infection of germfree pigs with a porcine enterovirus. *Cornell Vet.* **56**:386–394.
2. **Bielaaski, A., and J. I. Raeside.** 1977. Plasma concentrations of steroid hormones in sows infected experimentally with *Leptospira pomona* or porcine enterovirus strain T1 in late gestation. *Res. Vet. Sci.* **22**:28–34.
3. **Bolin, S. R., J. J. Turek, L. J. Runnels, and D. P. Gustafson.** 1983. Pseudorabies virus, porcine parvovirus, and porcine enterovirus interactions with the zona pelucida of the porcine embryo. *Am. J. Vet. Res.* **44**:1036–1039.
4. **Brundage, L. J., J. B. Derbyshire, and B. N. Wilkie.** 1980. Cell mediated responses in a porcine enterovirus infection in piglets. *Can. J. Comp. Med.* **44**:61–69.
5. **Hazlett, D. T., and J. B. Derbyshire.** 1977. The protective effect of two porcine enterovirus vaccines in swine. *Can. J. Comp. Med.* **41**:264–273.
6. **Honda, E., A. Kimata, I. Hattori, T. Kumagai, T. Tsuda, and T. Tokui.** 1990. A serological comparison of 4 Japanese isolates of porcine enteroviruses with the international reference strains. *Nippon Juigaku Zasshi* **52**:49–54.
7. **Kemeny, L. J.** 1981. Isolation of transmissible gastroenteritis virus, pseudorabies virus, and porcine enterovirus from pharyngeal swabs taken from market-weight-swine. *Am. J. Vet. Res.* **42**:1987–1989.
8. **Kresse, J. I., M. L. Snyder, P. H. Fynskov, and W. C. Stewart.** 1977. Isolation of a new porcine enterovirus in the United States. *Can. J. Comp. Med.* **41**:355–356.
9. **Krumbholz, A., M. Dauber, A. Henke, E. Birch-Hirschfeld, N. J. Knowles, A. Stelzner, and R. Zell.** 2002. Sequencing of porcine enterovirus groups II and III reveals unique features of both virus groups. *J. Virol.* **76**:5813–5821.
10. **McCormick, B. M., S. J. Driesen, I. D. Connaughton, and R. P. Monckton.** 1986. Prevalence of enteroviral and parvoviral antibodies in pig sera. *Res. Vet. Sci.* **41**:397–401.
11. **Meyer, R. C., G. T. Woods, and J. Simon.** 1966. Pneumonitis in an enterovirus infection in swine. *J. Comp. Pathol.* **76**:397–405.
12. **Pensaert, M., and W. de Meurichy.** 1973. A porcine Enterovirus causing fetal death and mummification. II. Experimental infection of pregnant sows. *Zentbl. Vetmed. Reihe B* **20**:760–762.
13. **Shin, T., S. Cho, and C. Lee.** 2001. Detection of inducible nitric oxide synthase- and nitrotyrosine-positive cells in the lesions of pericarditis induced by porcine enterovirus serotype 3 infection. *J. Vet. Med. Sci.* **63**:1017–1019.
14. **Stott, J. L.** 1999. Picornaviridae, p. 371–378. *In* D. C. Hirsh and Y. C. Zee (ed.), *Veterinary Microbiology*. Blackwell Science, Inc., Malden, Mass.

Porcine parvovirus
1. **Brown, T. T., Jr.** 1981. Laboratory evaluation of selected disinfectants as virucidal agents against porcine parvovirus, pseudorabies virus, and transmissible gastroenteritis virus. *Am. J. Vet. Res.* **42**:1033–1036.
2. **Gordon, J. C., and E. J. Angrick.** 1986. Canine parvoviruses: environmental effects on infectivity. *Am. J. Vet. Res.* **47**:1464–1467.
3. **Gradil, C. M., H. S. Joo, and T. W. Molitor.** 1990. Persistence of porcine parvovirus in swine infected in utero and followed through maturity. *Zentbl. Vetmed. Reihe B* **37**:309–316.
4. **Gradil, C., T. Molitor, M. Harding, and B. Crabo.** 1990. Excretion of porcine parvovirus through the genital tract of boars. *Am. J. Vet. Res.* **51**:359–362.
5. **Huysman, C. N., L. A. van Leengoed, M. C. de Jong, and A. L. van Osta.** 1992. Reproductive failure associated with porcine parvovirus in an enzootically infected pig herd. *Vet. Rec.* **131**:503–506.
6. **Jenkins, C. E.** 1990. An enzyme-linked immunosorbent assay for detection of porcine parvovirus in fetal tissue. *J. Virol. Methods* **39**:179–184.
7. **Kennedy, M. A., V. S. Mellon, G. Caldwell, and L. N. Potgieter.** 1995. Virucidal efficacy of the newer quaternary ammonium compounds. *J. Am. Anim. Hosp. Assoc.* **31**:254–258.
8. **Kresse, J. I., W. D. Taylor, W. W. Stewart, and K. A. Eernisse.** 1985. Parvovirus infection in pigs with necrotic and vesicle-like lesions. *Vet. Microbiol.* **10**:525–531.
9. **Lager, K. M., and W. L. Mengeling.** 1994. Porcine parvovirus associated with cutaneous lesions in piglets. *J. Vet. Diagn. Investig.* **6**:357–359.

10. Mengeling, W. L. 1978. Elimination of porcine parvovirus from infected cell cultures by inclusion of homologous antiserum in the nutrient medium. *Am. J. Vet. Res.* **39:**323–324.
11. Mengeling, W. L. 1999. Porcine parvovirus, p. 187–200. *In* B. E. Straw, S. D'Allaire, W. L. Mengeling, and D. J. Taylor (ed.), *Diseases of Swine,* 8th ed. Iowa State University Press, Ames.
12. Mengeling, W. L., K. M. Lager, and A. C. Vorwald. 2000. The effect of porcine parvovirus and porcine reproductive and respiratory syndrome virus on porcine reproductive performance. *Anim. Reprod. Sci.* **60–61:**199–210.
13. Mengeling, W. L., and P.-S. Paul. 1981. Reproductive performance of gilts exposed to porcine parvovirus at 56 or 70 days of gestation. *Am. J. Vet. Res.* **42:**2074–2076.
14. Meyers, P. J., R. M. Liptrap, R. B. Miller, and J. Thorsen. 1987. Hormonal changes in sows after induced porcine parvovirus infection in early pregnancy. *Am. J. Vet. Res.* **48:**621–626.
15. Murphy, F. A., E. P. J. Gibbs, M. C. Horzinek, and M. J. Studdert. 1999. *Veterinary Virology,* 3rd ed. Academic Press, Inc., San Diego, Calif.
16. Paul, P. S., W. L. Mengeling, and T. T. Brown, Jr. 1979. Replication of porcine parvovirus in peripheral blood lymphocytes, monocytes, and peritoneal macrophages. *Infect. Immun.* **25:**1003–1007.
17. Soares, R. M., E. L. Durigon, J. G. Bersano, and L. J. Richtzenhain. 1999. Detection of porcine parvovirus DNA by the polymerase chain reaction assay using primers to the highly conserved nonstructural protein gene, NS-1. *J. Virol. Methods* **78:**191–198.
18. Thacker, B. J., H. S. Joo, N. L. Winkelman, A. D. Leman, and D. M. Barnes. 1987. Clinical, virologic, and histopathologic observations of induced porcine parvovirus infection in boars. *Am. J. Vet. Res.* **48:**763–767.
19. Too, H. L., and R. J. Love. 1986. Some epidemiological features and effects on reproductive performance of endemic porcine parvovirus infection. *Aust. Vet. J.* **63:**50–53.
20. Yasuhara, H., M. Yamanaka, A. Izumida, T. Hirahara, M. Nakai, and Y. Inaba. 1995. Experimental infection of pigs with a parvovirus isolated from the diarrheic feces of a pig. *J. Vet. Med. Sci.* **57:**629–634.
21. Zee, Y. C. 1999. Parvoviridae, p. 333–339. *In* D. C. Hirsh and Y. C. Zee (ed.), *Veterinary Microbiology.* Blackwell Science, Inc., Malden, Mass.

Porcine reproductive and respiratory syndrome virus

1. Allende, R., W. W. Laegreid, G. F. Kutish, J. A. Galeota, R. W. Wills, and F. A. Osorio. 2000. Porcine reproductive and respiratory syndrome virus: description of persistence in individual pigs upon experimental infection. *J. Virol.* **74:**10834–10837.
2. Asai, T., M. Mori, M. Okada, K. Uruno, S. Yazawa, and I. Shibata. 1999. Elevated serum haptoglobin in pigs infected with porcine reproductive and respiratory syndrome virus. *Vet. Immunol. Immunopathol.* **70:**143–148.
3. Bautista, E. M., and T. W. Molitor. 1997. Cell-mediated immunity to porcine reproductive and respiratory syndrome virus in swine. *Viral Immunol.* **10:**83–94.
4. Benfield, D. A., J. E. Collins, S. A. Dee, P. G. Halbur, H. S. Joo, K. M. Lager, W. L. Mengeling, M. P. Mutraugh, K. D. Rossow, G. W. Stevenson, and J. J. Zimmerman. 1999. Porcine reproductive and respiratory syndrome, p. 201–232. *In* B. E. Straw, S. D'Allaire, W. L. Mengeling, and D. J. Taylor (ed.), *Diseases of Swine,* 8th ed. Iowa State University Press, Ames.
5. Beyer, J., D. Fichtner, H. Schirrmeier, U. Polster, E. Weiland, and H. Wege. 2000. Porcine reproductive and respiratory syndrome virus (PRRSV): kinetics of infection in lymphatic organs and lung. *J. Vet. Med. Ser. B* **47:**9–25.
6. Bøtner, A., B. Standbygaard, K. J. Sorensen, P. Have, K. G. Madsen, S. Madsen, and S. Alexandersen. 1997. Appearance of acute PRRS-like symptoms in sow herds after vaccination with a modified live PRRS vaccine. *Vet. Rec.* **141:**497–499.
7. Brockmeier, S. L., M. V. Palmer, S. R. Bolin, and R. B. Rimler. 2001. Effects of intranasal inoculation with *Bordetella bronchiseptica,* porcine reproductive and respiratory syndrome virus, or a combination of both organisms on subsequent infection with *Pasteurella multocida* in pigs. *Am. J. Vet. Res.* **62:**521–525.
8. Cheon, D. S., and C. Chae. 2001. Distribution of porcine reproductive and respiratory syndrome virus in stillborn and liveborn piglets from experimentally infected sows. *J. Comp. Pathol.* **124:**231–237.
9. Cheon, D. S., and C. Chae. 2001. Polymerase chain reaction-based restriction fragment length polymorphism pattern of porcine reproductive and respiratory syndrome virus directly from lung tissues without virus isolation in Korea. *J. Vet. Med. Sci.* **63:**567–571.
10. Chiou, M. T., C. R. Jeng, L. L. Chueh, C. H. Cheng, and V. F. Pang. 2000. Effects of porcine reproductive and respiratory syndrome virus (isolate tw91) on porcine alveolar macrophages in vitro. *Vet. Microbiol.* **71:**9–25.

11. Choi, C., and C. Chae. 2002. Expression of tumour necrosis factor-a is associated with apoptosis in lungs of pigs experimentally infected with porcine reproductive and respiratory syndrome virus. *Res. Vet. Sci.* **72**:45–49.

12. Christopher-Hennings, J., L. D. Holler, D. A. Benfield, and E. A. Nelson. 2001. Detection and duration of porcine reproductive and respiratory syndrome virus in semen, serum, peripheral blood mononuclear cells, and tissues from Yorkshire, Hampshire, and Landrace boars. *J. Vet. Diagn. Investig.* **13**:133–142.

13. Cooper, V. L., R. A. Hesse, and A. R. Doster. 1997. Renal lesions associated with experimental porcine reproductive and respiratory syndrome virus (PRRSV) infection. *J. Vet. Diagn. Investig.* **9**:198–201.

14. Darbes, J., A. Hafner, W. Breuer, T. Hanichen, E. Banholzer, and W. Hermanns. 1996. Histopathological findings in pigs of various ages suffering from spontaneous infection with the porcine reproductive and respiratory syndrome virus (PRRSV). *Zentbl. Vetmed. Reihe A* **43**:353–363.

15. Delputte, P. L., N. Vanderheijden, H. J. Nauwynck, and M. B. Pensaert. 2002. Involvement of the matrix protein in attachment of porcine reproductive and respiratory syndrome virus to a heparinlike receptor on porcine alveolar macrophages. *J. Virol.* **76**:4312–4320.

16. Egli, C., B. Thur, L. Liu, and M. A. Hofmann. 2001. Quantitative TaqMan RT-PCR for the detection and differentiation of European and North American strains of porcine reproductive and respiratory syndrome virus. *J. Virol. Methods.* **98**:63–75.

17. Feng, W., S. M. Laster, M. Tompkins, T. Brown, J. S. Xu, C. Altier, W. Gomez, D. Benfield, and M. B. McCaw. 2001. In utero infection by porcine reproductive and respiratory syndrome virus is sufficient to increase susceptibility of piglets to challenge by *Streptococcus suis* type II. *J. Virol.* **75**:4889–4895.

18. Girard, M., P. Cleroux, P. Tremblay, S. Dea, and Y. St.-Pierre. 2001. Increased proteolytic activity and matrix metalloprotease expression in lungs during infection by porcine reproductive and respiratory syndrome virus. *J. Gen. Virol.* **82**:1253–1261.

19. Horter, D. C., R. M. Pogranichniy, C. C. Chang, R. B. Evans, K. J. Yoon, and J. J. Zimmerman. 2002. Characterization of the carrier state in porcine reproductive and respiratory syndrome virus infection. *Vet. Microbiol.* **86**:213–228.

20. Lager, K. M., W. L. Mengeling, and S. L. Brockmeier. 1997. Duration of homologous porcine reproductive and respiratory syndrome virus immunity in pregnant swine. *Vet. Microbiol.* **58**:127–133.

21. Lamontagne, L., C. Page, R. Larochelle, D. Longtin, and R. Magar. 2001. Polyclonal activation of B cells occurs in lymphoid organs from porcine reproductive and respiratory syndrome virus (PRRSV)-infected pigs. *Vet. Immunol. Immunopathol.* **82**:165–182.

22. Magar, R., Y. Robinson, C. Dubuc, and R. Larochelle. 1995. Isolation and experimental oral transmission in pigs of a porcine reproductive and respiratory syndrome virus isolate. *Adv. Exp. Med. Biol.* **380**:139–144.

23. Mengeling, W. L., K. M. Lager, and A. C. Vorwald. 1998. Clinical effects of porcine reproductive and respiratory syndrome virus on pigs during the early postnatal interval. *Am. J. Vet. Res.* **59**:52–55.

24. Mortensen, S., H. Stryhn, R. Sogaard, A. Boklund, K. D. Stark, J. Christensen, and P. Willeberg. 2002. Risk factors for infection of sow herds with porcine reproductive and respiratory syndrome (PRRS) virus. *Prev. Vet. Med.* **53**:83–101.

25. Nakamine, M., Y. Kono, S. Age, C. Hoshino, J. Shirai, and T. Ezaki. 1998. Dual infection with enterotoxigenic *Escherichia coli* and porcine reproductive and respiratory syndrome virus observed in weaning pigs that died suddenly. *J. Vet. Med. Sci.* **60**:555–561.

26. Nelsen, C. J., M. P. Murtaugh, and K. S. Faaberg. 1999. Porcine reproductive and respiratory syndrome virus comparison: divergent evolution on two continents. *J. Virol.* **73**:270–280.

27. Nielsen, H. S., M. B. Oleksiewicz, R. Forsberg, T. Stadejek, A. Bøtner, and T. Storgaard. 2001. Reversion of a live porcine reproductive and respiratory syndrome virus vaccine investigated by parallel mutations. *J. Gen. Virol.* **82**:1263–1272.

28. Otake, S., S. A. Dee, K. D. Rossow, H. S. Joo, J. Deen, T. W. Molitor, and C. Pijoan. 2002. Transmission of porcine reproductive and respiratory syndrome virus by needles. *Vet. Rec.* **150**:114–115.

29. Pejsak, Z., T. Stadejek, and I. Markowska-Daniel. 1997. Clinical signs and economic losses caused by porcine reproductive and respiratory syndrome virus in a large breeding herd. *Vet. Microbiol.* **55**:317–322.

30. Rossow, K. D., E. M. Bautista, S. M. Goyal, T. W. Molitor, M. P. Murtaugh, R. B. Morrison, D. A. Benfield, and J. E. Collins. 1994. Experimental porcine reproductive and respiratory syndrome virus infection in one-, four-, and 10-week-old pigs. *J. Vet. Diagn. Investig.* **6**:3–12.

31. **Rossow, K. D., J. L. Shivers, P. E. Yeske, D. D. Polson, R. R. Rowland, S. R. Lawson, M. P. Murtaugh, E. A. Nelson, and J. E. Collins.** 1999. Porcine reproductive and respiratory syndrome virus infection in neonatal pigs characterized by marked neurovirulence. *Vet. Rec.* **144:**444–448.

32. **Samson, J. N., T. G. de Bruin, J. J. Voermans, J. J. Meulenberg, J. M. Pol, and A. T. Bianchi.** 2000. Changes of leukocyte phenotype and function in the broncho-alveolar lavage fluid of pigs infected with porcine reproductive and respiratory syndrome virus: a role for $CD8^+$ cells. *J. Gen. Virol.* **82:**497–505.

33. **Scruggs, D. W., and S. D. Sorden.** 2001. Proliferative vasculopathy and cutaneous hemorrhages in porcine neonates infected with the porcine reproductive and respiratory syndrome virus. *Vet. Pathol.* **38:**339–342.

34. **Shibata, I., M. Mori, and S. Yazawa.** 2000. Experimental reinfection with homologous porcine reproductive and respiratory syndrome virus in SPF pigs. *J. Vet. Med. Sci.* **62:**105–108.

35. **Shirai, J., T. Kanno, Y. Tsuchiya, S. Mitsubayashi, and R. Seki.** 2000. Effects of chlorine, iodine, and quaternary ammonium compound disinfectants on several exotic disease viruses. *J. Vet. Med. Sci.* **62:**85–92.

36. **Solano, G. I., E. Bautista, T. W. Molitor, J. Segales, and C. Pijoan.** 1998. Effect of porcine reproductive and respiratory syndrome virus infection on the clearance of *Haemophilus parasuis* by porcine alveolar macrophages. *Can. J. Vet. Res.* **62:**251–256.

37. **Stott, J. L.** 1999. Coronaviridae, p. 418–429. *In* D. C. Hirsh and Y. C. Zee (ed.), *Veterinary Microbiology*. Blackwell Science, Inc., Malden, Mass.

38. **Sur, J. H., A. R. Doster, J. S. Christian, J. A. Galeota, R. W. Wills, J. J. Zimmerman, and F. A. Osorio.** 1997. Porcine reproductive and respiratory syndrome virus replicates in testicular germ cells, alters spermatogenesis, and induces germ cell death by apoptosis. *J. Virol.* **71:**9170–9179.

39. **Thanawongnuwech, R., P. G. Halbur, and E. L. Thacker.** 2000. The role of pulmonary intravascular macrophages in porcine reproductive and respiratory syndrome virus infection. *Anim. Health Res. Rev.* **1:**95–102.

40. **Van Reeth, K.** 1997. Pathogenesis and clinical aspects of a respiratory porcine reproductive and respiratory syndrome virus infection. *Vet. Microbiol.* **55:**223–230.

41. **Wagstrom, E. A., C. C. Chang, K. J. Yoon, and J. J. Zimmerman.** 2001. Shedding of porcine reproductive and respiratory syndrome virus in mammary gland secretions of sows. *Am. J. Vet. Res.* **62:**1876–1880.

42. **Wills, R. W., J. T. Gray, P. J. Fedorka-Cray, K. J. Yoon, S. Ladely, and J. J. Zimmerman.** 2000. Synergism between porcine reproductive and respiratory syndrome virus (PRRSV) and *Salmonella choleraesuis* in swine. *Vet. Microbiol.* **71:**177–192.

43. **Wills, R. W., J. J. Zimmerman, K. J. Yoon, S. L. Swenson, L. J. Hoffman, M. J. McGinley, H. T. Hill, and K. B. Platt.** 1997. Porcine reproductive and respiratory syndrome virus: routes of excretion. *Vet. Microbiol.* **57:**69–81.

44. **Yoon, K. J., J. J. Zimmerman, C. C. Chang, S. Cancel-Tirado, K. M. Harmon, and M. J. McGinley.** 1999. Effect of challenge dose and route on porcine reproductive and respiratory syndrome virus (PRRSV) infection in young swine. *Vet. Res.* **30:**629–638.

Porcine rotavirus

1. **Askaa, J., B. Bloch, G. Bertelsen, and K. O. Rasmussen.** 1983. Rotavirus associated diarrhoea in nursing piglets and detection of antibody against rotavirus in colostrum, milk and serum. *Nord. Vet. Med.* **35:**441–447.

2. **Benfield, D. A., I. Stotz, R. Moore, and J. P. McAdaragh.** 1982. Shedding of rotavirus in feces of sows before and after farrowing. *J. Clin. Microbiol.* **16:**186–190.

3. **Bridger, J. C., and J. F. Brown.** 1985. Prevalence of antibody to typical and atypical rotaviruses in pigs. *Vet. Rec.* **116:**50.

4. **Bridger, J. C., B. Burke, G. M. Beards, and U. Desselberger.** 1992. The pathogenicity of two porcine rotaviruses differing in their *in vitro* growth characteristics and genes 4. *J. Gen. Virol.* **73:**3011–3015.

5. **Brunet, J. P., J. Cotte-Laffitte, C. Linxe, A. M. Quero, M. Geniteau-Legendre, and A. Servin.** 2000. Rotavirus infection induces an increase in intracellular calcium concentration in human intestinal epithelial cells: role in microvillar actin alteration. *J. Virol.* **74:**2323–2332.

6. **Debouck, P., and M. Pensaert.** 1983. Rotavirus excretion in suckling pigs followed under field circumstances. *Ann. Rech. Vet.* **14:**447–448.

7. **Elschner, M., J. Prudlo, H. Hotzel, P. Otto, and K. Sachse.** 2002. Nested reverse transcriptase-polymerase chain reaction for the detection of group A rotaviruses. *J. Vet. Med. Ser. B* **49:**77–81.

8. **Gelberg, H. B.** 1992. Studies on the age resistance of swine to group A rotavirus infection. *Vet. Pathol.* **29:**161–168.

9. **Gelberg, H. B., J. S. Patterson, and G. N. Woode.** 1991. A longitudinal study of rotavirus

antibody titers in swine in a closed specific pathogen-free herd. *Vet. Microbiol.* **28**:231–242.
10. **Gelberg, H. B., G. N. Woode, T. S. Kniffen, M. Hardy, and W. F. Hall.** 1991. The shedding of group A rotavirus antigen in a newly established closed specific pathogen-free swine herd. *Vet. Microbiol.* **28**:213–229.
11. **Geyer, A., T. Sebata, I. Peenze, and A. Steele.** 1995. A molecular epidemiological study of porcine rotaviruses. *J. S. Afr. Vet. Assoc.* **66**:202–205.
12. **Halaihel, N., V. Lievin, J. M. Ball, M. K. Estes, F. Alvarado, and M. Vasseur.** 2000. Direct inhibitory effect of rotavirus NSP4(114-135) peptide on the Na$^+$-D-glucose symporter of rabbit intestinal brush border membrane. *J. Virol.* **74**:9464–9470.
13. **Hess, R. G., and P. A. Bachmann.** 1981. Distribution of antibodies to rotavirus in serum and lacteal secretions of naturally infected swine and their suckling pigs. *Am. J. Vet. Res.* **42**:1149–1152.
14. **Janke, B. H., J. K. Nelson, D. A. Benfield, and E. A. Nelson.** 1990. Relative prevalence of typical and atypical strains among rotaviruses from diarrheic pigs in conventional swine herds. *J. Vet. Diagn. Investig.* **2**:308–311.
15. **Kim, Y., K. O. Chang, B. Straw, and L. J. Saif.** 1999. Characterization of group C rotaviruses associated with diarrhea outbreaks in feeder pigs. *J. Clin. Microbiol.* **37**:1484–1488.
16. **Magar, R., Y. Robinson, and M. Morin.** 1991. Identification of atypical rotaviruses in outbreaks of preweaning and postweaning diarrhea in Quebec swine herds. *Can. J. Vet. Res.* **55**:260–263.
17. **Narita, M., A. Fukusho, S. Konno, and Y. Shimizu.** 1982. Intestinal changes in gnotobiotic piglets experimentally inoculated with porcine rotavirus. *Natl. Inst. Anim. Health Q.* **22**:54–60.
18. **Paul, P. S., and G. W. Stevenson.** 1999. Rotavirus and reovirus, p. 255–275. *In* B. E. Straw, S. D'Allaire, W. L. Mengeling, and D. J. Taylor (ed.), *Diseases of Swine*, 8th ed. Iowa State University Press, Ames.
19. **Perez, J. F., M. C. Ruiz, M. E. Chemello, and F. Michelangeli.** 1999. Characterization of a membrane calcium pathway induced by rotavirus infection in cultured cells. *J. Virol.* **73**:2481–2490.
20. **Ramos, A. P., C. C. Stefanelli, R. E. Linhares, B. G. de Brito, N. Santos, V. Gouvea, R. de Cassia Lima, and C. Nozawa.** 2000. The stability of porcine rotavirus in feces. *Vet. Microbiol.* **71**:1–8.
21. **Shaw, R. D., S. J. Hempson, and E. R. Mackow.** 1995. Rotavirus diarrhea is caused by nonreplicating viral particles. *J. Virol.* **69**:5946–5950.
22. **Shaw, D. P., L. G. Morehouse, and R. F. Solorzano.** 1989. Experimental rotavirus infection in three-week-old pigs. *Am. J. Vet. Res.* **50**:1961–1965.
23. **Svensmark, B., J. Askaa, C. Wolstrup, and K. Nielsen.** 1989. Epidemiological studies of piglet diarrhea in intensively managed Danish sow herds. IV. Pathogenicity of porcine rotavirus. *Acta Vet. Scand.* **30**:71–76.
24. **Theil, K. W., E. H. Bohl, R. F. Cross, E. M. Kohler, and A. G. Agnes.** 1978. Pathogenesis of porcine rotaviral infection in experimentally inoculated gnotobiotic pigs. *Am. J. Vet. Res.* **39**:213–220.
25. **Vellenga, L., H. J. Egberts, T. Wensing, J. E. van Dijk, J. M. Mouwen, and H. J. Breukink.** 1992. Intestinal permeability in pigs during infection. *Am. J. Vet. Res.* **53**:1180–1183.
26. **Ward, L. A., E. D. Rich, and T. E. Besser.** 1996. Role of maternally derived circulating antibodies in protection of neonatal swine against porcine group A rotavirus. *J. Infect. Dis.* **174**:276–282.
27. **Yamashiro, Y., T. Shimizu, S. Oguchi, and M. Sato.** 1989. Prostaglandins in the plasma and stool of children with rotavirus gastroenteritis. *J. Pediatr. Gastroenterol. Nutr.* **9**:322–327.

Swine herpesvirus (pseudorabies)
1. **Bolin, C. A., S. R. Bolin, J. P. Kluge, and W. L. Mengeling.** 1985. Pathologic effects of intrauterine deposition of pseudorabies virus on the reproductive tract of swine in early pregnancy. *Am. J. Vet. Res.* **46**:1039–1042.
2. **Cheung, A. K.** 1995. Investigation of pseudorabies virus DNA and RNA in trigeminal ganglia and tonsil tissues of latently infected swine. *Am. J. Vet. Res.* **56**:45–50.
3. **Christensen, L. S., S. Mortensen, A. Botner, S. B. Strandbygaard, L. Ronsholt, C. A. Henriksen, and J. B. Andersen.** 1993. Further evidence of long distance airborne transmission of Aujesky's disease (pseudorabies) virus. *Vet. Rec.* **132**:317–321.
4. **Christensen, L. S., J. Mousing, S. Mortensen, K. J. Sorensen, S. B. Strandbygaard, C. A. Henriksen, and J. B. Andersen.** 1990. Evidence of long distance airborne transmission of Aujesky's disease (pseudorabies) virus. *Vet. Rec.* **127**:471–474.
5. **Echeverria, M. G., M. R. Pecoraro, N. B. Pereyra, C. L. Pidone, C. M. Galosi, M. E. Etcheverrigaray, and E. O. Nosetto.** 2000. Rapid diagnosis of pseudorabies virus infection in swine tissues using the polymerase chain reaction (PCR). *Rev. Argent. Microbiol.* **32**:109–115.

6. Ezura, K., Y. Usami, K. Tajima, H. Komaniwa, S. Nagai, M. Narita, and K. Kawashima. 1995. Gastrointestinal and skin lesions in piglets naturally infected with pseudorabies virus. *J. Vet. Diagn. Investig.* **7**:451–455.
7. Fuentes, M. C., and C. Pijoan. 1986. Phagocytosis and intracellular killing of *Pasteurella multocida* by porcine alveolar macrophages after infection with pseudorabies virus. *Vet. Immunol. Immunopathol.* **13**:165–172.
8. Fuentes, M. C., and C. Pijoan. 1987. Pneumonia in pigs induced by intranasal challenge exposure with pseudorabies virus and *Pasteurella multocida*. *Am. J. Vet. Res.* **48**:1446–1448.
9. Grant, R. A. 1975. Pseudorabies: clinical manifestations. *J. Am. Med. Assoc.* **167**:257.
10. Hsu, F. S., R. M. Chu, R. C. Lee, and S. H. Chu. 1980. Placental lesions caused by pseudorabies virus in pregnant sows. *J. Am. Vet. Med. Assoc.* **177**:636–641.
11. Iglesias, G., C. Pijoan, and T. Molitor. 1989. Interactions of pseudorabies virus with swine alveolar macrophages. Effects of virus infection on cell functions. *J. Leukoc. Biol.* **45**:410–415.
12. Iglesias, G., C. Pijoan, and T. Molitor. 1992. Effects of pseudorabies virus infection upon cytotoxicity and antiviral activities of porcine alveolar macrophages. *Comp. Immunol. Microbiol. Infect. Dis.* **15**:249–259.
13. Iglesias, J. G., and J. W. Harkness. 1988. Studies of transplacental and perinatal infection with two clones of a single Aujeszky's disease (pseudorabies) virus isolate. *Vet. Microbiol.* **16**:243–254.
14. Kluge, J. P., and C. J. Maré. 1974. Swine pseudorabies: abortion, clinical disease, and lesions in pregnant gilts infected with pseudorabies virus (Aujeszky's disease). *Am. J. Vet. Res.* **35**:911–915.
15. Kluge, J. P., G. W. Beran, H. T. Hill, and K. B. Platt. 1999. Pseudorabies (Aujeszky's disease), p. 233–246. *In* B. E. Straw, S. D'Allaire, W. L. Mengeling, and D. J. Taylor (ed.), *Diseases of Swine,* 8th ed. Iowa State University Press, Ames.
16. Larsen, R. E., R. E. Shope, Jr., A. D. Leman, and H. J. Kurtz. 1980. Semen changes in boars after experimental infection with pseudorabies virus. *Am. J. Vet. Res.* **41**:733–739.
17. Masic, M., M. Ercegan, and M. Petrovic. 1965. Die Bedeutung der tonsillen für die pathogenese und diagnose der Aujeszkyschen krankheit bie schweinen. *Zentbl. Vetmed.* **12**:398–405.
18. McFerran, J. B. 1975. Studies on immunity to Aujeszky's disease (pseudorabies) virus infection in pigs. *Dev. Biol. Stand.* **28**:563–570.
19. Narita, M., T. Imada, M. Haritani, and H. Kawamura. 1989. Immunohistologic study of pulmonary and lymphatic tissues from gnotobiotic pigs inoculated with ara-T-resistant strain of pseudorabies virus. *Am. J. Vet. Res.* **50**:1940–1945.
20. Narita, M., S. Inui, and Y. Schimizu. 1984. Tonsillar changes in pigs given pseudorabies (Aujeszky's disease) virus. *Am. J. Vet. Res.* **45**:247–251.
21. Narita, M., K. Kawashima, S. Matsuura, A. Uchimura, and Y. Miura. 1994. Pneumonia in pigs infected with pseudorabies virus and *Haemophilus parasuis* serovar 4. *J. Comp. Pathol.* **110**:329–339.
22. Narita, M., Y. M. Zhao, K. Kawashima, S. Arai, H. Hirose, S. Yamada, and K. Ezura. 1998. Enteric lesions induced by different pseudorabies (Aujeszky's disease) virus strains inoculated into closed intestinal loops of pigs. *J. Vet. Diagn. Invest.* **10**:36–42.
23. Pol, J. M., A. L. Gielkens, and J. T. van Oirschot. 1989. Comparative pathogenesis of three strains of pseudorabies virus in pigs. *Microb. Pathog.* **7**:361–371.
24. Schneider, W. J., and J. A. Howarth. 1973. Clinical course and histopathologic features of pseudorabies virus-induced keratoconjunctivitis in pigs. *Am. J. Vet. Res.* **34**:393–401.
25. Schoenbaum, M. A., J. D. Freund, and G. W. Beran. 1991. Survival of pseudorabies virus in the presence of selected diluents and fomites. *J. Am. Vet. Med. Assoc.* **198**:1393–1397.
26. Shibata, I., M. Okada, K. Urono, Y. Samegai, M. Ono, T. Sakano, and S. Sato. 1998. Experimental dual infection of cesarean-derived, colostrum-deprived pigs with *Mycoplasma hyopneumoniae* and pseudorabies virus. *J. Vet. Med. Sci.* **60**:295–300.
27. Veselinova, A. 1981. Comparative pathomorphological studies of piglets infected with different strains of the pseudorabies virus. *Vet. Med. Nauki* **18**:17–24.
28. Wheeler, J. G., and F. A. Osorio. 1991. Investigation of sites of pseudorabies virus latency, using polymerase chain reaction. *Am. J. Vet. Res.* **52**:1799–1803.

Swine influenza virus
1. Ardans, A. A. 1999. Orthomyxoviridae, p. 396–402. *In* D. C. Hirsh and Y. C. Zee (ed.), *Veterinary Microbiology*. Blackwell Science, Inc., Malden, Mass.
2. Chapman, M. S., P. H. Lamont, and J. W. Harkness. 1978. Serological evidence of continuing infection of swine in Great Britain with an influenza A virus (H3N2). *J. Hyg.* **80**:415–422.

3. **Charley, B.** 1977. Local immunity in the pig respiratory tract. I. Cellular and humoral immune responses following swine influenza infection. *Ann. Microbiol. (Paris)* **128B:**95–107.
4. **Easterday, B. C.** 1972. Immunologic considerations in swine influenza. *J. Am. Vet. Med. Assoc.* **160:**645–648.
5. **Easterday, B. C., and K. Van Reeth.** 1999. Swine influenza, p. 277–290. In B. E. Straw, S. D'Allaire, W. L. Mengeling, and D. J. Taylor (ed.), *Diseases of Swine,* 8th ed. Iowa State University Press, Ames.
6. **Hinshaw, V. S., R. G. Webster, and B. Turner.** 1978. Novel influenza A viruses isolated from Canadian feral ducks: including strains antigenically related to swine influenza (Hsw1N1) viruses. *J. Gen. Virol.* **41:**115–127.
7. **Lipkind, M., Y. Weisman, and E. Shihmanter.** 1984. Isolation of viruses antigenically related to the swine influenza virus from an outbreak of respiratory disease in turkey farms in Israel. *Vet. Rec.* **114:**426–428.
8. **Mensik, J., L. Valicek, and Z. Pospisil.** 1971. Pathogenesis of swine influenza infection produced experimentally in suckling piglets. 3. Multiplication of virus in the respiratory tract of suckling piglets in the presence of colostrum-derived specific antibody in their blood stream. *Zentbl. Vetmed. Reihe B* **18:**665–678.
9. **Rivard, G. E., and M. Potier.** 1977. Platelet aggregation induced by swine influenza vaccine. *Lancet* **2:**302.
10. **Schorr, E., D. Wentworth, and V. S. Hinshaw.** 1994. Use of polymerase chain reaction to detect swine influenza virus in nasal swab specimens. *Am. J. Vet. Res.* **55:**952–956.
11. **Thacker, E. L., B. J. Thacker, and B. H. Janke.** 2001. Interaction between *Mycoplasma hyopneumoniae* and swine influenza virus. *J. Clin. Microbiol.* **39:**2525–2530.
12. **Van Reeth, K., and H. Nauwynck.** 2000. Proinflammatory cytokines and viral respiratory disease in pigs. *Vet. Res.* **31:**187–213.
13. **Wentworth, D. E., M. W. McGregor, M. D. Macklin, V. Newmann, and V. S. Hinshaw.** 1997. Transmission of swine influenza virus to humans after exposure to experimentally infected pigs. *J. Infect. Dis.* **175:**7–15.

Transmissible gastroenteritis virus

1. **Brim, T. A., J. L. VanCott, J. K. Lunney, and L. J. Saif.** 1994. Lymphocyte proliferation responses of pigs inoculated with transmissible gastroenteritis virus or porcine respiratory coronavirus. *Am. J. Vet. Res.* **55:**494–501.
2. **Brim, T. A., J. L. VanCott, J. K. Lunney, and L. J. Saif.** 1995. Cellular immune responses of pigs after primary inoculation with porcine respiratory coronavirus or transmissible gastroenteritis virus and challenge with transmissible gastroenteritis virus. *Vet. Immunol. Immunopathol.* **48:**35–54.
3. **Brown, T. T., Jr.** 1981. Laboratory evaluation of selected disinfectants as virucidal agents against porcine parvovirus, pseudorabies virus, and transmissible gastroenteritis virus. *Am. J. Vet. Res.* **42:**1033–1036.
4. **Butler, D. G., D. G. Gall, M. H. Kelly, and J. R. Hamilton.** 1974. Transmissible gastroenteritis: mechanisms responsible for diarrhea in an acute enteritis in piglets. *J. Clin. Invest.* **53:**1335–1342.
5. **Cepica, A., and J. B. Derbyshire.** 1984. Antibody-dependent and spontaneous cell-mediated cytotoxicity against transmissible gastroenteritis virus infected cells by lymphocytes from sows, fetuses and neonatal piglets. *Can. J. Comp. Med.* **48:**258–261.
6. **Charley, B., and L. Lavenant.** 1990. Characterization of blood mononuclear cells producing IFN alpha following induction by coronavirus-infected cells (porcine transmissible gastroenteritis virus). *Res. Immunol.* **141:**141–151.
7. **Charley, B., L. Lavenant, and F. Lefèvre.** 1994. Coronavirus transmissible gastroenteritis virus-mediated induction of IFNa-mRNA in porcine leukocytes requires prior synthesis of soluble proteins. *Vet. Res.* **25:**29–36.
8. **Chu, R. M., R. D. Glock, and R. F. Ross.** 1982. Changes in gut-associated lymphoid tissues of the small intestine of eight-week-old pigs infected with transmissible gastroenteritis virus. *Am. J. Vet. Res.* **43:**67–76.
9. **Cornelius, L. M., B. E. Hooper, and E. O. Haelterman.** 1968. Changes in fluid and electrolyte balance in baby pigs with transmissible gastroenteritis. *Am. J. Clin. Pathol.* **2:**105–113.
10. **Drolet, R., M. Morin, and M. Fontaine.** 1984. Hypoglycemia: a factor associated with low survival rate of neonatal piglets infected with transmissible gastroenteritis virus. *Can. J. Comp. Med.* **48:**282–285.
11. **Forman, A. J.** 1991. Infection of pigs with transmissible gastroenteritis virus from contaminated carcasses. *Aust. Vet. J.* **68:**25–27.
12. **Gough, P. M., and R. D. Jorgenson.** 1983. Identification of porcine transmissible gastroenteritis virus in house flies (*Musca domestica* Linneaus). *Am. J. Vet. Res.* **44:**2078–2082.
13. **Goven, A. J., and E. V. DeBuysscher.** 1985. Intestinal phopholipase B activity in pigs inoculated with transmissible gastroenteritis virus. *Am. J. Vet. Res.* **46:**1503–1505.

14. Gunn, H. M. 1996. Elimination of transmissible gastroenteritis virus from a pig farm by culling and serological surveillance. *Vet. Rec.* **138:**196–198.
15. Homaidan, F. R., A. Torres, M. Donowitz, and G. W. Sharp. 1991. Electrolyte transport in piglets infected with transmissible gastroenteritis virus. Stimulation by verapamil and clonidine. *Gastroenterology* **101:**895–901.
16. Keljo, D. J., D. G. Butler, and J. R. Hamilton. 1985. Altered jejunal permeability to macromolecules during viral enteritis in the piglet. *Gastroenterology* **88:**998–1004.
17. Kemeny, L. J., and R. D. Woods. 1977. Quantitative transmissible gastroenteritis virus shedding patterns in lactating sows. *Am. J. Vet. Res.* **38:**307–310.
18. Kim, B., and C. Chae. 2002. Experimental infection of piglets with transmissible gastroenteritis virus: a comparison of three strains (Korean, Purdue and Miller). *J. Comp. Pathol.* **126:**30–37.
19. Kim, L., K. O. Chang, K. Sestak, A. Parwani, and L. J. Saif. 2000. Development of a reverse transcriptase-nested polymerase chain reaction assay for differential diagnosis of transmissible gastroenteritis virus and porcine respiratory coronavirus from feces and nasal swabs of infected pigs. *J. Vet. Diagn. Investig.* **12:**385–388.
20. Kim, S. Y., D. S. Song, and B. K. Park. 2001. Differential detection of transmissible gastroenteritis virus and porcine epidemic diarrhea virus by duplex RT-PCR. *J. Vet. Diagn. Investig.* **13:**516–520.
21. Morin, M., R. F. Solorzano, L. G. Morehouse, and L. D. Olson. 1978. The postulated role of feeder swine in the perpetuation of the transmissible gastroenteritis virus. *Can. J. Comp. Med.* **42:**379–384.
22. Moxley, R. A., and L. R. Olson. 1989. Lesions of virus infection in experimentally inoculated pigs suckling immunized sows. *Am. J. Vet. Res.* **50:**708–716.
23. Murphy, F. A., E. P. J. Gibbs, M. C. Horzinek, and M. J. Studdert. 1999. *Veterinary Virology,* 3rd ed. Academic Press, Inc., San Diego, Calif.
24. Naidoo, D., and J. B. Derbyshire. 1992. Interferon induction in porcine leukocytes with transmissible gastroenteritis virus. *Vet. Microbiol.* **30:**317–327.
25. Pilchard, E. I. 1965. Experimental transmission of transmissible gastroenteritis virus by starlings. *Am. J. Vet. Res.* **26:**1177–1179.
26. Prochazka, Z., J. Hampl, M. Sedlacek, J. Maasek, and J. Stepanek. 1975. Protein loss in piglets infected with transmissible gastroenteritis virus. *Zentbl. Vetmed Reihe B* **22:**138–146.
27. Saif, L. J., and E. H. Bohl. 1983. Passive immunity to transmissible gastroenteritis virus: Intramammary viral inoculation of sows. *Ann. N.Y. Acad. Sci.* **409:**708–723.
28. Saif, L. J., J. L. van Cott, and T. A. Brim. 1994. Immunity to transmissible gastroenteritis virus and porcine respiratory coronavirus infections in swine. *Vet. Immunol. Immunopathol.* **43:**89–97.
29. Saif, L. J., and R. D. Wesley. 1999. Transmissible gastroenteritis and porcine respiratory coronavirus, p. 295–325. *In* B. E. Straw, S. D'Allaire, W. L. Mengeling, and D. J. Taylor (ed.), *Diseases of Swine,* 8th ed. Iowa State University Press, Ames.
30. Shimizu, M., and Y. Shimizu. 1979. Lymphocyte proliferative response to viral antigen in pigs infected with transmissible gastroenteritis virus. *Infect. Immun.* **23:**239–243.
31. Stott, J. L. 1999. Coronaviridae, p. 418–429. *In* D. C. Hirsh and Y. C. Zee (ed.), *Veterinary Microbiology.* Blackwell Science, Inc., Malden, Mass.

Porcine respiratory coronavirus
1. Brim, T. A., J. L. VanCott, J. K. Lunney, and L. J. Saif. 1994. Lymphocyte proliferation responses of pigs inoculated with transmissible gastroenteritis virus or porcine respiratory coronavirus. *Am. J. Vet. Res.* **55:**494–501.
2. Brim, T. A., J. L. VanCott, J. K. Lunney, and L. J. Saif. 1995. Cellular immune responses of pigs after primary inoculation with porcine respiratory coronavirus or transmissible gastroenteritis virus and challenge with transmissible gastroenteritis virus. *Vet. Immunol. Immunopathol.* **48:**35–54.
3. Carman, S., G. Josephson, B. McEwen, B. Maxie, G. Maxie, M. Antochi, K. Eernisse, G. Nayar, P. Halbur, G. Erickson, and E. Nilsson. 2002. Field validation of a commercial blocking ELISA to differentiate antibody to transmissible gastroenteritis virus (TGEV) and porcine respiratory coronavirus and to identify TGEV-infected swine herds. *J. Vet. Diagn. Investig.* **14:**97–105.
4. Cox, E., J. Hooyberghs, and M. B. Pensaert. 1990. Sites of replication of a porcine respiratory coronavirus related to transmissible gastroenteritis virus. *Res. Vet. Sci.* **48:**165–169.
5. Kim, L., K. O. Chang, K. Sestak, A. Parwani, and L. J. Saif. 2000. Development of a reverse transcriptase-nested polymerase chain reaction assay for differential diagnosis of transmissible gastroenteritis virus and porcine respiratory coronavirus from feces and nasal swabs of infected pigs. *J. Vet. Diagn. Investig.* **12:**385–388.
6. O'Toole, D., I. Brown, A. Bridges, and S. F. Cartwright. 1989. Pathogenicity of experi-

mental infection with "pneumotropic" porcine coronavirus. *Res. Vet. Sci.* **47**:23–29.
7. Pensaert, M., P. Callebaut, and J. Vergote. 1986. Isolation of a porcine respiratory, nonenteric coronavirus related to transmissible gastroenteritis. *Vet. Q.* **8**:257–261.
8. Rasschaert, D., M. Duarte, and H. Laude. 1990. Porcine respiratory coronavirus differs from transmissible gastroenteritis virus by a few genomic deletions. *J. Gen. Virol.* **71**:2599–2607.
9. Saif, L. J., and R. D. Wesley. 1999. Transmissible gastroenteritis and porcine respiratory coronavirus, p. 295–325. *In* B. E. Straw, S. D'Allaire, W. L. Mengeling, and D. J. Taylor (ed.), *Diseases of Swine*, 8th ed. Iowa State University Press, Ames, Iowa.
10. Sestak, K., I. Lanza, S. K. Park, P. A. Weilnau, and L. J. Saif. 1996. Contribution of passive immunity to porcine respiratory coronavirus to protection against transmissible gastroenteritis virus challenge exposure in suckling pigs. *Am. J. Vet. Res.* **57**:664–671.
11. Van Reeth, K., G. Labarque, H. Nauwynck, and M. Pensaert. 1999. Differential production of proinflammatory cytokines in the pig lung during different respiratory virus infections: correlations with pathogenicity. *Res. Vet. Sci.* **67**:47–52.
12. Van Reeth, K., H. Nauwynck, and M. Pensaert. 2000. A potential role for tumour necrosis factor-alpha in synergy between porcine respiratory coronavirus and bacterial lipopolysaccharide in the induction of respiratory disease in pigs. *J. Med. Microbiol.* **49**:613–620.
13. Wesley, R. D., and R. D. Woods. 1996. Induction of protective immunity against transmissible gastroenteritis virus after exposure of neonatal pigs to porcine respiratory coronavirus. *Am. J. Vet. Res.* **57**:157–162.

BACTERIA

Actinobacillus pleuropneumoniae

1. Baarsch, M. J., D. L. Foss, and M. P. Murtaugh. 2000. Pathophysiologic correlates of acute porcine pleuropneumonia. *Am. J. Vet. Res.* **61**:684–690.
2. Balaji, R., K. J. Wright, J. L. Turner, C. M. Hill, S. S. Dritz, B. Fenwick, J. A. Carrollt, M. E. Zannelli, L. A. Beausang, and J. E. Minton. 2002. Circulating cortisol, tumor necrosis factor-α, interleukin-1β, and interferon-γ in pigs infected with *Actinobacillus pleuropneumoniae*. *J. Anim. Sci.* **80**:202–207.
3. Baltes, N., I. Hennig-Pauka, and G. F. Gerlach. 2002. Both transferrin binding proteins are virulence factors in *Actinobacillus pleuropneumoniae* serotype 7 infection. *FEMS Microbiol. Lett.* **209**:283–287.
4. Baltes, N., W. Tonpitak, G. F. Gerlach, I. Hennig-Pauka, A. Hoffmann-Moujahid, M. Ganter, and H. J. Rothkotter. 2001. *Actinobacillus pleuropneumoniae* iron transport and urease activity: effects on bacterial virulence and host immune response. *Infect. Immun.* **69**:472–478.
5. Biberstein, E. L., and D. C. Hirsh. 1999. Actinobacillus, p. 141–143. *In* D. C. Hirsh and Y. C. Zee (ed.), *Veterinary Microbiology*. Blackwell Science, Inc., Malden, Mass.
6. Bosse, J. T., H. Janson, B. J. Sheehan, A. J. Beddek, A. N. Rycroft, J. Simon Kroll, and P. R. Langford. 2002. *Actinobacillus pleuropneumoniae*: pathobiology and pathogenesis of infection. *Microb. Infect.* **4**:225–235.
7. Caruso, J. P., and R. F. Ross. 1990. Effects of *Mycoplasma hyopneumoniae* and *Actinobacillus* (*Haemophilus*) *pleuropneumoniae* infections on alveolar macrophage functions in swine. *Am. J. Vet. Res.* **51**:227–231.
8. Chiers, K., E. Donne, I. Van Overbeke, R. Ducatelle, and F. Haesebrouck. 2002. *Actinobacillus pleuropneumoniae* infections in closed swine herds: infection patterns and serological profiles. *Vet. Microbiol.* **85**:343–352.
9. Cho, W. S., and C. Chae. 2002. Expression of nitric oxide synthase 2 and tumor necrosis factor alpha in swine naturally infected with *Actinobacillus pleuropneumoniae*. *Vet. Pathol.* **39**:27–32.
10. Cruijsen, T. L., L. A. Van Leengoed, T. C. Dekker-Nooren, E. J. Schoevers, and J. H. Verheijden. 1992. Phagocytosis and killing of *Actinobacillus pleuropneumoniae* by aleolar macrophages and polymorphonuclear leukocytes isolated from pigs. *Infect. Immun.* **60**:4867–4871.
11. Cruijsen, T., L. A. van Leengoed, M. Ham-Hoffies, and J. H. Verheijden. 1995. Convalescent pigs are protected completely against infection with a homologous *Actinobacillus pleuropneumoniae* strain but incompletely against a heterologous-serotype strain. *Infect. Immun.* **63**:2341–2343.
12. Dom, P., F. Haesebrouck, R. Ducatelle, and G. Charlier. 1994. In vivo association of *Actinobacillus pleuropneumoniae* serotype 2 with the respiratory epithelium of pigs. *Infect. Immun.* **62**:1262–1267.
13. Dom, P., F. Haesebrouck, E. M. Kamp, and M. A. Smits. 1992. Influence of *Actinobacillus pleuropneumoniae* serotype 2 and its cytolysins on porcine neutrophil chemiluminescence. *Infect. Immun.* **60**:4328–4334.
14. Furesz, S. E., B. A. Mallard, J. T. Bosse, S. Rosendal, B. N. Wilkie, and J. I. MacInnes. 1997. Antibody- and cell-mediated immune re-

sponses of *Actinobacillus pleuropneumoniae*-infected and bacterin-vaccinated pigs. *Infect. Immun.* **65**:358–365.
15. **Gutierrez, C. B., J. I. Rodriguez Barbosa, J. Suarez, O. R. Gonzalez, R. I. Tascon, and E. F. Rodriguez Ferri.** 1995. Efficacy of a variety of disinfectants against *Actinobacillus pleuropneumoniae* serotype 1. *Am. J. Vet. Res.* **56**:1025–1029.
16. **Hall, W. F., T. E. Eurell, R. D. Hansen, and L. G. Herr.** 1992. Serum haptoglobin concentration in swine naturally or experimentally infected with *Actinobacillus pleuropneumoniae*. *J. Am. Vet. Med. Assoc.* **201**:1730–1733.
17. **Heegaard, P. M., J. Klausen, J. P. Nielsen, N. Gonzalez-Ramon, M. Pineiro, F. Lampreave, and M. A. Alava.** 1998. The porcine acute phase response to infection with *Actinobacillus pleuropneumoniae*. Haptoglobin, C-reactive protin, major acute phase protein and serum amyloid A protein are sensitive indicators of infection. *Comp. Biochem. Physiol. Part B Comp. Biochem. Mol. Biol.* **119**:365–373.
18. **Huang, H., A. A. Potter, M. Campos, F. A. Leighton, P. J. Willson, D. M. Haines, and W. D. Yates.** 1999. Pathogenesis of porcine *Actinobacillus pleuropneumoniae*, part II: roles of proinflammatory cytokines. *Can. J. Vet. Res.* **63**:69–78.
19. **Hunneman, W. A., P. C. Vasseur, and C. J. Kuiper.** 1989. Study of the possibility of breeding serologically negative animals from a breeding farm infected with serotype 2 *Actinobacillus pleuropneumoniae*. *Tijdschr. Diergeneeskd.* **114**:1039–1045.
20. **Jensen, T. K., M. Boye, T. Hagedorn-Olsen, H. J. Riising, and O. Angen.** 1999. *Actinobacillus pleuropneumoniae* osteomyelitis in pigs demonstrated by fluorescent in situ hybridization. *Vet. Pathol.* **36**:258–261.
21. **Jobert, J. L., C. Savoye, R. Cariolet, M. Kobisch, and F. Madec.** 2000. Experimental aerosol transmission of *Actinobacillus pleuropneumoniae* to pigs. *Can. J. Vet. Res.* **64**:21–26.
22. **Johansson, E., C. Fossum, L. Fuxler, and P. Wallgren.** 2001. Effects of an experimental infection with *Actinobacillus pleuropneumoniae* on the interferon-α and interleukin-6 producing capacity of porcine peripheral blood mononuclear cells stimulated with bacteria, virus or plasmid DNA. *Vet. Microbiol.* **79**:171–182.
23. **Jolie, R. A., M. H. Mulks, and B. J. Thacker.** 1995. Cross-protection experiments in pigs vaccinated with *Actinobacillus pleuropneumoniae* subtypes 1A and 1B. *Vet. Microbiol.* **45**:383–391.
24. **Liggett, A. D., L. R. Harrison, and R. L. Farrell.** 1987. Sequential study of lesion development in experimental *Haemophilus pleuropneumonia*. *Res. Vet. Sci.* **42**:204–212.
25. **Maier, E., N. Reinhard, R. Benz, and J. Frey.** 1996. Channel-forming activity and channel size of the RTX toxins ApxI, ApxII, and ApxIII of *Actinobacillus pleuropneumoniae*. *Infect. Immun.* **64**:4415–4423.
26. **Madsen, L. W., M. Boye, T. K. Jensen, and B. Svensmark.** 2001. *Actinobacillus pleuropneumoniae* demonstrated in situ in exudative meningitis and nephritis. *Vet. Rec.* **149**:746–747.
27. **Monshouwer, M., R. F. Witkamp, S. M. Nijmeijer, A. Pijpers, J. H. Verheijden, and A. S. Van Miert.** 1995. Selective effects of a bacterial infection (*Actinobacillus pleuropneumoniae*) on the hepatic clearance of caffeine, antipyrine, paracetamol, and indocyanine green in the pig. *Xenobiotica* **25**:491–499.
28. **Rohrbach, B. W., R. F. Hall, and J. P. Hitchcock.** 1993. Effect of subclinical infection with *Actinobacillus pleuropneumoniae* in commingled feeder swine. *J. Am. Vet. Med. Assoc.* **202**:1095–1098.
29. **Stine, D. L., M. J. Huether, R. A. Moxley, and S. Srikmaran.** 1991. *Actinobacillus pleuropneumoniae*-induced thymic lesions in mice and pigs. *Infect. Immun.* **59**:2885–2891.
30. **Stipkovits, L., D. Miller, R. Glavits, L. Fodor, and D. Burch.** 2001. Treatment of pigs experimentally infected with *Mycoplasma hyopneumoniae*, *Pasteurella multocida*, and *Actinobacillus pleuropneumoniae* with various antibiotics. *Can. J. Vet. Res.* **65**:213–222.
31. **Wang, F. I., J. W. Yang, S. Y. Hung, and I. J. Pan.** 2001. In vitro migratory responses of swine neutrophils to *Actinobacillus pleuropneumoniae*. *Exp. Anim.* **50**:139–145.

Bordetella bronchiseptica
1. **Baetz, A. L., L. J. Kemeny, and C. K. Graham.** 1974. Blood chemical changes in growing pigs exposed to aerosol of *Bordetella bronchiseptica*. *Am. J. Vet. Res.* **35**:451–453.
2. **Brockmeier, S. L., M. V. Palmer, S. R. Bolin, and R. B. Rimler.** 2001. Effects of intranasal inoculation with *Bordetella bronchiseptica*, porcine reproductive and respiratory syndrome virus, or a combination of both organisms on subsequent infection with *Pasteurella multocida* in pigs. *Am. J. Vet. Res.* **62**:521–525.
3. **Brockmeier, S. L., K. B. Register, T. Magyar, A. J. Lax, G. D. Pullinger, and R. A. Kunkle.** 2002. Role of the dermonecrotic toxin of *Bordetella bronchiseptica* in the pathogenesis of respiratory disease in swine. *Infect. Immun.* **70**:481–490.

4. de Jong, M. F. 1999. Progressive and nonprogressive atrophic rhinitis, p. 355–384. *In* B. E. Straw, S. D'Allaire, W. L. Mengeling, and D. J. Taylor, *Diseases of Swine*, 8th ed. Iowa State University Press, Ames.
5. **Drummond, J. G., S. E. Curtis, R. C. Meyer, J. Simon, and H. W. Norton.** 1981. Effects of atmospheric ammonia on young pigs experimentally infected with *Bordetella bronchiseptica*. *Am. J. Vet. Res.* **42**:963–968.
6. **Duncan, J. R., F. K. Ramsey, and W. P. Switzer.** 1966. Pathology of experimental *Bordetella bronchiseptica* infection in swine: pneumonia. *Am. J. Vet. Res.* **27**:467–472.
7. **Elias, B., G. Boros, M. Albert, S. Tuboly, P. Gergely, L. Papp, I. Barna Vetro, P. Rafai, and E. Molnar.** 1990. Clinical and pathological effects of the dermonecrotic toxin of *Bordetella bronchiseptica* and *Pasteurella multocida* in specific-pathogen-free piglets. *Nippon Juigaku Zasshi.* **52**:677–688.
8. **Francisco, C. J., T. R. Shryock, D. P. Bane, and L. Unverzagt.** 1996. Serum haptoglobin concentration in growing swine after intranasal challenge with *Bordetella bronchiseptica* and toxigenic *Pasteurella multocida* type D. *Can. J. Vet. Res.* **60**:222–227.
9. **Janetschke, P., H. Gunther, P. Kielstein, J. Martin, and W. Schonherr.** 1977. *Bordetella bronchiseptica* pneumonia in the swine. *Arch. Exp. Vet. Med.* **31**:289–298.
10. **Kono, Y., S. Suzuki, T. Mukai, K. Okazaki, E. Honda, and T. Yamashiro.** 1994. Detection of specific systemic and local IgG and IgA antibodies of pigs after infection with *Bordetella bronchiseptica* by ELISA. *J. Vet. Med. Sci.* **56**:249-253.
11. **Magyar, T., and R. Glavits.** 1990. Immunopathological changes in mice caused by *Bordetella bronchiseptica* and *Pasteurella multocida*. *Acta Vet. Hung.* **38**:203–210.
12. **Register, K. B., T. F. Ducey, S. L. Brockmeier, and D. W. Dyer.** 2001. Reduced virulence of a *Bordetella bronchiseptica* siderophore mutant in neonatal swine. *Infect. Immun.* **69**:2137–2143.
13. **Runge, M., M. Ganter, F. Delbeck, W. Hartwick, A. Ruffer, B. Franz, and G. Amtsberg.** 1996. Demonstration of pneumonia in swine as a constant problem: culture and immunofluorescence microscopic studies of bronchoalveolar lavage (BAL) and serological findings. *Berl. Muench. Tieraerztl. Wochenschr.* **109**:101–107.
14. **Rutter, J. M., L. M. Francis, and B. F. Sansom.** 1982. Virulence of *Bordetella bronchiseptica* from pigs with or without atrophic rhinitis. *J. Med. Microbiol.* **15**:105–116.
15. **Silveira, D., N. Edington, and I. M. Smith.** 1982. Alkaline phosphatase activity in the turbinates of pigs infected with *Bordetella bronchiseptica*. *J. Comp. Pathol.* **92**:621–627.
16. **Underdahl, N. R., T. E. Socha, and A. R. Doster.** 1982. Long-term effect of *Bordetella bronchiseptica* infection in neonatal pigs. *Am. J. Vet. Res.* **43**:622–625.

Clostridium perfringens **type C**
1. **Bergeland, M. E.** 1972. Pathogenesis and immunity of *Clostridium perfringens* type C enteritis in swine. *J. Am. Vet. Med. Assoc.* **160**:568–571.
2. **Biberstein, E. L., and D. C. Hirsh.** 1999. The clostridia, p. 233–245. *In* D. C. Hirsh and Y. C. Zee (ed.), *Veterinary Microbiology*. Blackwell Science, Inc., Malden, Mass.
3. **Ganovski, D., T. Dikova, and K. Shoilev.** 1984. Anaerobic dysentery in pigs. *Vet. Med. Nauki* **21**:34–39.
4. **Högh, P.** 1967. Necrotizing infectious enteritis in piglets, caused by *C. perfringens* type C. II. Incidence and clinical features. *Acta Vet. Scand.* **8**:301–323.
5. **Högh, P.** 1969. Necrotizing infectious enteritis in piglets, caused by *C. perfringens* type C. III. Pathological changes. *Acta Vet. Scand.* **10**:57–83.
6. **Morin, M., J. B. Phaneuf, and R. Malo.** 1981. *Clostridium perfringens* type C enteritis in a Quebec swine herd. *Can. Vet. J.* **22**:58.
7. **Sakurai, J., and C. L. Duncan.** 1979. Effect of carbohydrates and control of culture pH on beta toxin production by *Clostridium perfringens* type C. *Microbiol. Immunol.* **23**:313–318.
8. **Shatursky, O., R. Bayles, M. Rogers, B. J. Jost, J. G. Songer, and R. K. Tweten.** 2000. *Clostridium perfringens* beta-toxin forms potential-dependent, cation-selective channels in lipid bilayers. *Infect. Immun.* **68**:5546–5551.
9. **Taylor, D. J.** 1999. Clostridial infections, p. 395–412. *In* B. E. Straw, S. D'Allaire, W .L. Mengeling, and D. J. Taylor (ed.), *Diseases of Swine*, 8th ed. Iowa State University Press, Ames.
10. **Yoo, H. S., S. U. Lee, K. Y. Park, and Y. H. Park.** 1997. Molecular typing and epidemiological survey of prevalence of *Clostridium perfringens* types by multiplex PCR. *J. Clin. Microbiol.* **35**:228–232.

Erysipelothrix rhusiopathiae
1. **Amass, S. F., and D. A. Scholz.** 1998. Acute nonfatal erysipelas in sows in a commercial farrow-to-finish operation. *J. Am. Vet. Med. Assoc.* **212**:708–709.
2. **Cysewski, S. J., R. L. Wood, A. C. Pier, and A. L. Baetz.** 1978. Effects of aflatoxin on the development of acquired immunity to swine erysipelas. *Am. J. Vet. Res.* **39**:445–448.

3. Davies, M. E., A. Horner, and B. Franz. 1994. Intercellular adhesion molecule-1 (ICAM-1) and MHC class II on chondrocytes in arthritic joints from pigs experimentally infected with *Erysipelothrix rhusiopathiae*. *FEMS Immunol. Med. Microbiol.* **9:**265–272.
4. Franz, B., M. E. Davies, and A. Horner. 1995. Localization of viable bacteria and bacterial antigens in arthritic joints of *Erysipelothrix rhusiopathiae*-infected pigs. *FEMS Immunol. Med. Microbiol.* **12:**137–142.
5. Harrington, R., Jr. 1973. Transmission of *Erysipelothrix rhusiopathiae* in swine by a slap tattoo instrument. *Am. J. Vet. Res.* **34:**1109–1110.
6. Hoffmann, C. W., and G. Bilkei. 2002. Case study: chronic erysipelas of the sow- a subclinical manifestation of reproductive problems. *Reprod. Domest. Anim.* **37:**119–120.
7. Okolo, M. I. 1986. Isolation of *Erysipelothrix rhusiopathiae* from apparently healthy pigs reared under intensive and free range systems of management. *Microbios* **47:**29–35.
8. Shimoji, Y., Y. Mori, K. Hyakutake, T. Sekizaki, and Y. Tokomizo. 1998. Use of an enrichment broth cultivation-PCR combination assay for rapid diagnosis of swine erysipelas. *J. Clin. Microbiol.* **36:**86–89.
9. Takeshi, K., S. Makino, T. Ikeda, N. Takada, A. Nakashiro, K. Nakanishi, K. Oguma, K. Katoh, H. Sunagawa, and T. Ohyama. 1999. Direct and rapid detection by PCR of *Erysipelothrix* sp. DNAs prepared from bacterial strains and animal tissues. *J. Clin. Microbiol.* **37:**4093–4098.
10. Wabacha, J. K., G. K. Gitau, J. M. Nduhiu, A. G. Thaiya, P. M. Mbithi, and S. J. Munyua. 1998. An outbreak of urticarial form of swine erysipelas in a medium-scale piggery in Kiambu District, Kenya. *J. S. Afr. Vet. Assoc.* **69:**61–63.
11. Walker, R. 1999. Erysipelothrix, p. 229–232. *In* D. C. Hirsh and Y. C. Zee (ed.), *Veterinary Microbiology*. Blackwell Science, Inc., Malden, Mass.
12. Winkelmann, J., G. Trautwein, W. Leibold, W. Drommer, and R. Weiss. 1978. Enzyme, enzyme-histochemical and immunohistochemical studies in chronic erysipelas polyarthritis of swine. *Z. Rheumatol.* **37:**67–80.
13. Winkelmann, J., G. Trautwein, R. Muller-Peddinghaus, W. Drommer, W. Leibold, and K. H. Bohm. 1983. Immunopathologic aspects of chronic erysipelas polyarthritis in swine. *Z. Rheumatol.* **42:**91–100.
14. Wood, R. L. 1999. Erysipelas, p. 419–430. *In* B. E. Straw, S. D'Allaire, W. L. Mengeling, and D. J. Taylor (ed.), *Diseases of Swine*, 8th ed. Iowa State University Press, Ames.
15. Wouda, W., J. M. Snijders, M. J. van den Broek, E. Gruys, J. G. van Logtestijn. 1987. Endocarditis and meat inspection in slaughtering pigs. 1. Clinical, pathological and microbiological aspects. *Tijdschr. Diergeneeskd.* **112:**1226–1235.

Haemophilus parasuis
1. Amano, H., M. Shibata, K. Takahashi, and Y. Sasaki. 1997. Effects of endotoxin pathogenicity in pigs with acute septicemia of *Haemophilus parasuis* infection. *J. Vet. Med. Sci.* **59:**451–455.
2. Biberstein, E. L. 1999. *Haemophilus* spp., p. 144–147. *In* D. C. Hirsh and Y. C. Zee (ed.) *Veterinary Microbiology*. Blackwell Science, Inc., Malden, Mass.
3. Charland, N., C. G. D'Silva, R. A. Dumont, and D. F. Niven. 1995. Contact-dependent acquisition of transferrin-bound iron by two strains of *Haemophilus parasuis*. *Can. J. Microbiol.* **41:**70–74.
4. Lichtensteiger, C. A., and E. R. Vimr. 1997. Neuraminidase (sialidase) activity of *Haemophilus parasuis*. *FEMS Microbiol. Lett.* **152:**269–274.
5. Narita, M., K. Kawashima, S. Matsuura, A. Uchimura, and Y. Miura. 1994. Pneumonia in pigs infected with pseudorabies virus and *Haemophilus parasuis* serovar 4. *J. Comp. Pathol.* **110:**329–339.
6. Nielsen, R. 1993. Pathogenicity and immunity studies of *Haemophilus parasuis* serotypes. *Acta Vet. Scand.* **34:**193–198.
7. Oliveira, S., L. Galina, and C. Pijoan. 2001. Development of a PCR test to diagnose *Haemophilus parasuis* infections. *J. Vet. Diagn. Investig.* **13:**495–501.
8. Peet, R. L., J. Fry, J. Lloyd, J. Henderson, J. Curran, and D. Moir. 1983. *Haemophilus parasuis* septicaemia in pigs. *Aust. Vet. J.* **60:**187.
9. Rapp-Gabrielson, V. J. 1999. *Haemophilus parasuis*, p. 475–481. *In* B. E. Straw, S. D'Allaire, W. L. Mengeling, and D. J. Taylor (ed.), *Diseases of Swine*, 8th ed. Iowa State University Press, Ames.
10. Riley, M. G., E. G. Russell, and R. B. Callinan. 1977. *Haemophilus parasuis* infection in swine. *J. Am. Vet. Med. Assoc.* **171:**649–651.
11. Schrodl, W., R. Kunze, and M. Kruger. 1998. Determination of C-reactive protein and neopterin in serum of diseased and bacterially infected swine. *Berl. Muench. Tieraerztl. Wochenschr.* **111:**321–325.
12. Solano, G. I., E. Bautista, T. W. Molitor, J. Segales, and C. Pijoan. 1998. Effect of porcine reproductive and respiratory syndrome virus infection on the clearance of *Haemophilus parasuis* by porcine alveolar macrophages. *Can. J. Vet. Res.* **62:**251–256.

13. Solano-Aguilar, G. I., C. Pijoan, V. Rapp-Gabrielson, J. Collins, L. F. Carvalho, and N. Winkelman. 1999. Protective role of maternal antibodies against *Haemophilus parasuis* infection. *Am. J. Vet. Res.* **60**:81–87.
14. Vahle, J. L., J. S. Haynes, and J. J. Andrews. 1997. Interaction of *Haemophilus parasuis* with nasal and tracheal mucosa following intranasal inoculation of cesarean derived colostrum deprived (CDCD) swine. *Can. J. Vet. Res.* **61**:200–206.
15. Wiegland, M., P. Kielstein, D. Pohle, and A. Rassbach. 1997. Examination of primary SPF swine after experimental infection with *Haemophilus parasuis*. Clinical symptoms, changes in hematological parameters and in the parameters of the cerebrospinal fluid. *Tieraerztl. Prax.* **25**:226–232.

Lawsonia intracellularis
1. Gogolewski, R. P., R. W. Cook, and E. S. Batterham. 1991. Suboptimal growth associated with porcine intestinal adenomatosis in pigs in nutritional studies. *Aust. Vet. J.* **68**:406–408.
2. Guedes, R. M., C. J. Gebhart, N. L. Winkelman, R. A. Mackie-Nuss, T. A. Marsteller, and J. Deen. 2002. Comparison of different methods for diagnosis of porcine proliferative enteropathy. *Can. J. Vet. Med.* **66**:99–107.
3. Kim, J., C. Choi, W. S. Cho, and C. Chae. 2000. Immunohistochemistry and polymerase chain reaction for the detection of *Lawsonia intracellularis* in porcine intestinal tissues with proliferative enteropathy. *J. Vet. Med. Sci.* **62**:771–773.
4. Lawson, G. H. K., and C. J. Gebhart. 2000. Proliferative enteropathy. *J. Comp. Pathol.* **122**:77–100.
5. McOrist, S., and C. J. Gebhart. 1999. Porcine proliferative enteropathies, p. 521–534. *In* B. E. Straw, S. D'Allaire, W. L. Mengeling, and D. J. Taylor (ed.), *Diseases of Swine,* 8th ed. Iowa State University Press, Ames.
6. McOrist, S., L. Roberts, S. Jasni, A. C. Rowland, G. H. Lawson, C. J. Gebhart, and B. Bosworth. 1996. Developed and resolving lesions in porcine proliferative enteropathy: possible pathogenetic mechanisms. *J. Comp. Pathol.* **115**:35–45.
7. Rowan, T. G., and T. L. Lawrence. 1982. Amino acid digestibility in pigs with signs of porcine intestinal adenomatosis. *Vet. Rec.* **110**:306–307.
8. Rowland, A. C., and G. H. K. Lawson. 1975. Porcine intestinal adenomatosis: A possible relationship with necrotic enteritis, regional ileitis and proliferative haemorrhagic enteropathy. *Vet. Rec.* **97**:178–181.
9. Smith, D. G., and G. H. Lawson. 2001. *Lawsonia intracellularis:* getting inside the pathogenesis of proliferative enteropathy. *Vet. Microbiol.* **82**:331–345.
10. Smith, D. G., S. C. Mitchell, T. Nash, and S. Rhind. 2000. Gamma interferon influences intestinal epithelial hyperplasia caused by *Lawsonia intracellularis* infection in mice. *Infect. Immun.* **68**:6737–6743.

Leptospira spp.
1. Ballard, S. A., B. Adler, B. D. Millar, R. J. Chappel, R. T. Jones, and S. Faine. 1984. The immunoglobin response of swine following experimental infection with *Leptospira interrogans* serovar pomona. *Zentbl. Bakteriol. Mikrobiol. Hyg. Ser. A* **256**:510–517.
2. Cheville, N. F., R. Huhn, and R. C. Cutlip. 1980. Ultrastructure of renal lesions in pigs with acute leptosprosis caused by *Leptospira pomona*. *Vet. Pathol.* **17**:338–351.
3. De Brito, T., G. M. Bohm, and P. H. Yasuda. 1979. Vascular damage in acute experimental leptospirosis of the guinea-pig. *J. Pathol.* **128**:177–182.
4. Ellis, W. A. 1999. Leptospirosis, p. 483–493. *In* B. E. Straw, S. D'Allaire, W. L. Mengeling, and D. J. Taylor (ed.), *Diseases of Swine,* 8th ed. Iowa State University Press, Ames.
5. Isogai, E., H. Isogai, N. Fujii, and K. Oguma. 1990. Biological effects of leptospiral lipopolysaccharide to mouse B, T and NK cells. *Nippon Juigaku Zasshi* **52**:923–930.
6. Kim, Y. G., D. Y. Jeon, and M. K. Yang. 1997. Superoxide dismutase activity and lipid peroxidation in the liver of guinea pig infected with *Leptospira interrogans*. *Free Radic. Res.* **26**:1–6.
7. LeFebvre, R. L. 1999. Leptospirae, p. 185–189. *In* D. C. Hirsh and Y. C. Zee (ed.), *Veterinary Microbiology*. Blackwell Science, Inc., Malden, Mass.
8. Miragliotta, G., and D. Fumarola. 1983. In vitro effect of *Leptospira icterohaemorrhagiae* on human mononuclear leukocytes procoagulant activity: comparison of virulent with nonvirulent strain. *Can. J. Comp. Med.* **47**:70–72.
9. Savio, M. L., C. Rossi, P. Fusi, S. Tagliabue, and M. L. Pacciarini. 1994. Detection and identification of *Leptospira interrogans* serovars by PCR coupled with restriction endonuclease analysis of amplified DNA. *J. Clin. Microbiol.* **32**:935–941.
10. Younes-Ibrahim, M., B. Buffin-Meyer, L. Cheval, P. Burth, M. V. Castro-Faria, C. Barlet-Bas, S. Marsy, and A. Doucet. 1997. Na, K-ATPase: a molecular target for *Leptospira*

interrogans endotoxin. *Braz. J. Med. Biol. Res.* **30:** 213–223.

Mycoplasma hyopneumoniae
1. **Amass, S. F., L. K. Clark, W. G. van Alstine, T. L. Bowersock, D. A. Murphy, K. E. Knox, and S. R. Albregts.** 1994. Interaction of *Mycoplasma hyopneumoniae* and *Pasteurella multocida* infections in swine. *J. Am. Vet. Med. Assoc.* **204:**102–107.
2. **Asai, T., M. Okada, Y. Yokomizo, S. Sato, and Y. Mori.** 1996. Suppressive effect of bronchoalveolar lavage fluid from pigs infected with *Mycoplasma hyopneumoniae* on chemiluminescence of porcine peripheral neutrophils. *Vet. Immunol. Immunopathol.* **51:**325–31.
3. **Calsamiglia, M., J. E. Collins, and C. Pijoan.** 2000. Correlation between the presence of enzootic pneumonia lesions and detection of *Mycoplasma hyopneumoniae* in bronchial swabs by PCR. *Vet. Microbiol.* **76:**299 303.
4. **Caruso, J. P., and R. F. Ross.** 1990. Effects of *Mycoplasma hyopneumoniae* and *Actinobacillus* (*Haemophilus*) *pleuropneumoniae* infections on alveolar macrophage functions in swine. *Am. J. Vet. Res.* **51:**227–231.
5. **DeBey, M. C., C. D. Jacobson, and R. F. Ross.** 1992. Histochemical and morphologic changes of porcine airway epithelial cells in response to infection with *Mycoplasma hyopneumoniae*. *Am. J. Vet. Res.* **53:**1705–1710.
6. **Intraraksa, Y., R. L. Engen, and W. P. Switzer.** 1984. Pulmonary and hematologic changes in swine with *Mycoplasma hyopneumoniae* pneumonia. *Am. J. Vet. Res.* **45:**474–477.
7. **Kishima, M., and R. F. Ross.** 1985. Suppressive effect of nonviable *Mycoplasma hyopneumoniae* on phytohemagglutinin-induced transformation of swine lymphocytes. *Am. J. Vet. Res.* **46:**2366–2368.
8. **Kristensen, B., P. Paroz, J. Nicolet, M. Wanner, and A. L. de Weck.** 1981. Cell-mediated and humoral immune response in swine after vaccination and natural infection with *Mycoplasma hyopneumoniae*. *Am. J. Vet. Res.* **42:**784–788.
9. **Lium, B. M., and M. Falk.** 1991. An abattoir survey of pneumonia and pleuritis in slaughter weight swine from 9 selected herds. I. Prevalence and morphological description of gross lung lesions. *Acta Vet. Scand.* **32:**55–65.
10. **Messier, S., and R. F. Ross.** 1991. Interactions of *Mycoplasma hyopneumoniae* membranes with porcine lymphocytes. *Am. J. Vet. Res.* **52:**1497–1502.
11. **Park, S. C., S. Yibchok-Anun, H. Cheng, T. F. Young, E. L. Thacker, F. C. Minion, R. F. Ross, and W. H. Hsu.** 2002. *Mycoplasma hyopneumoniae* increases intracellular calcium release in porcine ciliated tracheal cells. *Infect. Immun.* **70:**2502–2506.
12. **Rautiainen, E., A. M. Virtala, P. Wallgren, and H. Saloniemi.** 2000. Varying effects of infections with *Mycoplasma hyopneumoniae* on the weight gain recorded in three different multisource fattening pig herds. *J. Vet. Med. Ser. B* **47:** 461–469.
13. **Ross, R. F.** 1999. Mycoplasmal diseases, p. 495–509. *In* B. E. Straw, S. D'Allaire, W. L. Mengeling, and D. J. Taylor (ed.), *Diseases of Swine*, 8th ed. Iowa State University Press, Ames.
14. **Stipkovits, L., D. Miller, R. Glavits, L. Fodor, and D. Burch.** 2001. Treatment of pigs experimentally infected with *Mycoplasma hyopneumoniae*, *Pasteurella multocida*, and *Actinobacillus pleuropneumoniae* with various antibiotics. *Can. J. Vet. Res.* **65:**213–222.
15. **Williams, P. P., and J. E. Gallagher.** 1981. Effects of *Mycoplasma hyopneumoniae* and *M. hyorhinis* on ependymal cells of the porcine lateral ventricles as observed by scanning and transmission electron microscopy. *Scanning Electron Microsc.* **4:**133–140.
16 **Yagihashi, T., S. Kazama, and M. Tajima.** 1993. Seroepidemiology of mycoplasmal pneumonia of swine in Japan as surveyed by an enzyme-linked immunosorbent assay. *Vet. Microbiol.* **34:**155–166.

Pasteurella multocida
1. **Ackermann, M. R., M. C. DeBay, K. B. Register, D. J. Larson, and J. M. Kinyon.** 1994. Tonsil and turbinate colonization by toxigenic and nontoxigenic strains of *Pasteurella multocida* in conventionally raised swine. *J. Vet. Diagn. Investig.* **6:**375–377.
2. **Berndt, A., and G. Muller.** 1997. Heterogeneity of porcine alveolar macrophages in experimental pneumonia. *Vet. Immunol. Immunopathol.* **57:**279–287.
3. **Butonschon, J.** 1991. Statistical evidence for a link between pleuropneumonia and disseminated focal nephritis in pigs. *Zentbl. Vetmed. Reihe A* **38:**287–299.
4. **Carter, G. R., and J. B. Biddy.** 1966. *Pasteurella multocida* recovered from aborted swine foetuses. *Vet. Rec.* **78:**884.
5. **de Jong, M. F.** 1999. Progressive and nonprogressive atrophic rhinitis, p. 355–384. *In* B. E. Straw, S. D'Allaire, W. L. Mengeling, and D. J. Taylor (ed.), *Diseases of Swine*, 8th ed. Iowa State University Press, Ames.
6. **Elias, B., G. Boros, M. Albert, S. Tuboly, P. Gergely, L. Papp, I. Barna Vetro, P. Ra-**

fai, and E. Molnar. 1990. Clinical and pathological effects of the dermonecrotic toxin of *Bordetella bronchiseptica* and *Pasteurella multocida* in specific-pathogen-free piglets. *Nippon Juigaku Zasshi.* **52:**677–688.
7. **Francisco, C. J., T. R. Shryock, D. P. Bane, and L. Unverzagt.** 1996. Serum haptoglobin concentration in growing swine after intranasal challenge with *Bordetella bronchiseptica* and toxigenic *Pasteurella multocida* type D. *Can. J. Vet. Res.* **60:**222–227.
8. **Hamilton, T. D., J. M. Roe, C. M. Hayes, P. Jones, G. R. Pearson, and A. J. Webster.** 1999. Contributory and exacerbating roles of gaseous ammonia and organic dust in the etiology of atrophic rhinitis. *Clin. Diagn. Lab. Immunol.* **6:**199–203.
9. **Lichtensteiger, C. A., S. M. Steenbergen, R. M. Lee, D. D. Polson, and E. R. Vimr.** 1996. Direct PCR analysis for toxigenic *Pasteurella multocida*. *J. Clin. Microbiol.* **34:**3035–3039.
10. **Olson, L. D.** 1981. Gross and microscopic lesions of middle and inner ear infections in swine. *Am. J. Vet. Res.* **42:**1433–1440.
11. **Pijoan, C.** 1999. Pneumonic pasteurellosis, p. 511–520. *In* B. E. Straw, S. D'Allaire, W. L. Mengeling, and D. J. Taylor, *Diseases of Swine,* 8th ed. Iowa State University Press, Ames.
12. **Pijoan, C., and M. Fuentes.** 1987. Severe pleuritis associated with certain strains of *Pasteurella multocida* in swine. *J. Am. Vet. Med. Assoc.* **191:**823–826.
13. **Pijoan, C., A. Lastra, C. Ramirez, and A. D. Leman.** 1984. Isolation of toxigenic strains of *Pasteurella multocida* from lungs of pneumonic swine. *J. Am. Vet. Med. Assoc.* **185:**522–523.
14. **Rosendal, S., P. L. Frandsen, J. P. Nielsen, and R. Gallily.** 1995. *Pasteurella multocida* toxin induces IL-6, but not IL-1a or TNFa in fibroblasts. *Can. J. Vet. Res.* **59:**154–156.
15. **Schoss, P., and M. Alt.** 1995. Are nasal swabs for swine appropriate for the diagnosis of bacterial pneumonia agents? *Dtsch. Tieraerztl. Wochenschr.* **102:**427–430.
16. **Sterner-Kock, A., B. Lanske, S. Uberschar, and M. J. Atkinson.** 1995. Effects of the *Pasteurella multocida* toxin on osteoblastic cells in vitro. *Vet. Pathol.* **32:**274–279.
17. **Townsend, K. M., D. O'Boyle, T. T. Phan, T. X. Hanh, T. G. Wijewardana, I. Wilkie, N. T. Trung, and A. J. Frost.** 1998. Acute septicemic pasteurellosis in Vietnamese pigs. *Vet. Microbiol.* **63:**205–215.
18. **van Diemen, P. M., G. de Vries Reileingh, and H. K. Parmentier.** 1994. Immune reponses of piglets to *Pasteurella multocida* toxin and toxoid. *Vet. Immunol. Immunopathol.* **41:**307–321.
19. **Williams, P. P., M. R. Hall, and R. B. Rimler.** 1990. Host response to *Pasteurella multocida* turbinate atrophy toxin in swine. *Can. J. Vet. Res.* **54:**157–163.
20. **Zhao, G., C. Pijoan, and M. P. Murtaugh.** 1993. Epidemiology of *Pasteurella multocida* in a farrow-to-finish swine herd. *Can. J. Vet. Res.* **57:**136–138.

Streptococcus suis
1. **Akkermans, J. P., and U. Vecht.** 1994. Streptococcal infections as cause of death in pigs brought in for necropsy. *Tijdschr. Diergeneeskd.* **119:**123–128.
2. **Clifton-Hadley, F. A., T. J. L. Alexander, M. R. Enright, and J. Guise.** 1984. Monitoring herds for *Streptococcus suis* type 2 by sampling tonsils of slaughter pigs. *Vet. Rec.* **115:**562–564.
3. **Dee, S. A., A. R. Carlson, N. L. Winkelman, and M. M. Corey.** 1993. Effect of management practices on the *Streptococcus suis* carrier rate in nursery swine. *J. Am. Vet. Med. Assoc.* **203:**295–299.
4. **Higgins, R., and M. Gottschalk.** 1999. Streptococcal diseases, p. 563–578. *In* B. E. Straw, S. D'Allaire, W. L. Mengeling, and D. J. Taylor (ed.), *Diseases of Swine,* 8th ed. Iowa State University Press, Ames.
5. **Holt, M. E., M. R. Enright, and T. J. Alexander.** 1989. Studies of the protective effect of different fractions of sera from pigs immune to *Streptococcus suis* type 2 infection. *J. Comp. Pathol.* **100:**435–442.
6. **Iglesias, J. G., M. Trujano, and J. Xu.** 1992. Inoculation of pigs with *Streptococcus suis* type 2 alone or in combination with pseudorabies virus. *Am. J. Vet. Res.* **53:**364–367
7. **Segura, M., N. Vadeboncoeur, and M. Gottschalk.** 2002. CD14-dependent and -independent cytokine and chemokine production by human THP-1 monocytes stimulated by *Streptococcus suis* capsular type 2. *Clin. Exp. Immunol.* **127:**243–254.
8. **Strangmann, E., H. Froleke, and K. P. Kohse.** 2002. Septic shock caused by *Streptococcus suis:* case report and investigation of a risk group. *Int. J. Hyg. Environ. Health* **205:**385–392.
9. **Torremorell, M., M. Calsamiglia, and C. Pijoan.** 1998. Colonization of suckling pigs by *Streptococcus suis* with particular reference to pathogenic serotype 2 strains. *Can. J. Vet. Res.* **62:**21–26.
10. **van Leengoed, L. A., U. Vecht, and E. R. Verheyen.** 1987. *Streptococcus suis* type 2 infections in pigs in the Netherlands (Part two). *Vet. Q.* **9:**111–117.

11. **Wisselink, H. J., J. J. Joosten, and H. E. Smith.** 2002. Multiplex PCR assays for simultaneous detection of six major serotypes and two virulence-associated phenotypes of *Streptococcus suis* in tonsillar specimens from pigs. *J. Clin. Microbiol.* **40:**2922–2929.

PARASITES

Ascaris suum

1. **Chan, B. S.** 1965. Quantitative changes in the basophil cells of guinea-pig bone marrow following the administration of *Ascaris* body fluid. *Immunology* **8:**566–577.
2. **Chroustova, E., J. Raszyk, I. Herzig, M. Toulova, M. Dvorak, and J. Urbanova.** 1986. Influence of the migration of *Ascaris suum* larvae on blood parameters in the pig. *Angew. Parasitol.* **27:**15–22.
3. **Corwin, R. M., and T. B. Stewart.** 1999. Internal parasites, p. 713–730. *In* B. E. Straw, S. D'Allaire, W. L. Mengeling, and D. J. Taylor (ed.), *Diseases of Swine,* 8th ed. Iowa State University Press, Ames.
4. **Feder, H., A. Dey-Hazra, and K. Enigk.** 1972. Changes in plasma enzymes, blood electrolytes, and mineral concentrations associated with the migration of larvae of *Ascaris suum* in the liver of the pig. *Z. Prakt. Anasth. Wiederbeleb. Intensivther.* **23:**17–24.
5. **Hale, O. M., T. B. Stewart, and O. G. Marti.** 1985. Influence of an experimental infection of *Ascaris suum* on performance of pigs. *J. Anim. Sci.* **60:**220–225.
6. **Jungersen, G., L. Eriksen, P. Nansen, P. Lind, T. Rasmussen, and E. N. Meeusen.** 2001. Regional immune responses with stage-specific antigen recognition profiles develop in lymph nodes of pigs following *Ascaris suum* larval migration. *Parasite Immunol.* **23:**185–194.
7. **Kadlubowski, R., and A. Ochecka.** 1982. Effect of proteolysis inhibitors from *Ascaris lumbricoides* on the coagulation and fibrinolysis of human plasma. *Angew. Parasitol.* **23:**78–82.
8. **Martin, J., D. W. Crompton, E. Carrera, and M. C. Nesheim.** 1984. Mucosal surface lesions in young protein-deficient pigs infected with *Ascaris suum* (Nematoda). *Parasitology* **88:**333–340.
9. **Murrell, K. D., L. Eriksen, P. Nansen, H. C. Slotved, and T. Rasmussen.** 1997. *Ascaris suum*: a revision of its early migratory path and implications for human ascariasis. *J. Parasitol.* **83:**255–260.
10. **Soares, M. F., M. S. Macedo, and I. Mota.** 1987. Suppressive effect of an *Ascaris suum* extract on IgE and IgG antibody responses in mice. *Braz. J. Med. Biol. Res.* **20:**203–211.
11. **Zoltowska, K., J. Dziekonska-Rynko, and Z. Jablonowski.** 1989. Trypsin and α-amylase activity in the pancreas of guinea pigs. I. The influence of infective dose and duration of infection by *Ascaris suum* Goeze, 1782. *Wiad. Parazytol.* **35:**565–570.
12. **Zoltowska, K., and Z. Jablonowski.** 1989. α-amylase activity in serum and some organs of guinea pigs with larval ascariasis. *Wiad. Parazytol.* **35:**559–563.

Isospora suis

1. **Baba, E., and S. M. Gaafar.** 1985. Interfering effect of *Isospora suis* infection on *Salmonella typhimurium* infection in swine. *Vet. Parasitol.* **17:**271–278.
2. **Driesen, S. J., V. A. Fahy, and P. G. Carland.** 1995. The use of toltrazuril for the prevention of coccidiosis in piglets before weaning. *Aust. Vet. J.* **72:**139–141.
3. **Ernst, J. V., D. S. Lindsay, J. A. Jarvinen, K. S. Todd, Jr., and D. P. Bane.** 1986. The sporulation time of *Isospora suis* oocysts from different sources. *Vet. Parasitol.* **22:**1–8.
4. **Jarvinen, J. A., G. L. Zimmerman, D. J. Schons, and C. Guenther.** 1988. Serum proteins of neonatal pigs orally inoculated with *Isospora suis* oocysts. *Am. J. Vet. Res.* **49:**380–385.
5. **Koudela, B., and S. Kucerova.** 1999. Role of acquired immunity and natural age resistance on course of *Isospora suis* coccidiosis in nursing piglets. *Vet. Parasitol.* **82:**93–99.
6. **Kudweis, M., Z. Lojda, and I. Julis.** 1991. Histochemistry of acid phosphatase in small intestine mucosa in experimental coccidiosis in suckling piglets. *Vet. Med. (Praha)* **36:**93–105.
7. **Kudweis, M., Z. Lojda, and I. Julis.** 1991. Histochemistry of nucleoside phosphatases and phosphoglucomutase in the small intestine during coccidiosis in piglets. *Vet. Med. (Praha)* **36:**153–163.
8. **Kudweis, M., Z. Lojda, and I. Julis.** 1991. β-D-glucosidase in the microvillus zone of small intestine enterocytes in experimental coccidiosis in suckling piglets. *Vet. Med. (Praha)* **36:**225–234.
9. **Kudweis, M., Z. Lojda, I. Julis, and J. Vitovec.** 1989. Mucus synthesis in the goblet cells of the small intestine in experimental infection with the coccidium *Isospora suis* in piglets. *Vet. Med. (Praha)* **34:**727–734.
10. **Kudweis, M., Z. Lojda, I. Julis, J. Vitovec, and B. Koudela.** 1990. Alkaline phosphatase activity in goblet cells in the small intestine of piglets experimentally infected with the coccidium *Isospora suis*. *Vet. Med. (Praha)* **35:**275–284.
11. **Kudweis, M., Z. Lojda, I. Julis, J. Vitovec, and B. Koudela.** 1990. Densitometric analysis

of aminopeptidase M activity in small intestine mucosa in piglets experimentally infected with *Isospora suis*. *Vet. Med. (Praha)* **35**:679–694.
12. Kudweis, M., Z. Lojda, J. Vitovec, and B. Koudela. 1989. Activity of selected dehydrogenases and monoamine oxidases in the small intestine of gnotobiotic piglets infected with the coccidium *Isospora suis*. *Vet. Med. (Praha)* **34**:287–296.
13. Kudweis, M., Z. Lojda, J. Vitovec, B. Koudela, and J. Sterba. 1989. The ratio of enterocytes and goblet cells in the mucosa of the small intestine in experimental infection of piglets with the coccidium *Isospora suis*. *Vet. Med. (Praha)* **34**:33–38.
14. Lindsay, D. S., B. L. Blagburn, and J. P. Dubey. 1999. Coccidia and other protozoa, p. 655–667. *In* B. E. Straw, S. D'Allaire, W. L. Mengeling, and D. J. Taylor (ed.), *Diseases of Swine*, 8th ed. Iowa State University Press, Ames.
15. Lindsay, D. S., W. L. Current, and J. R. Taylor. 1985. Effects of experimentally induced *Isospora suis* infection on morbidity, mortality, and weight gains in nursing pigs. *Am. J. Vet. Res.* **46**:1511–1512.
16. Nilsson, O. 1988. *Isospora suis* in pigs with post weaning diarrhoea. *Vet. Rec.* **122**:310–311.
17. Robinson, Y., M. Morin, C. Girard, and R. Higgins. 1983. Experimental transmission of intestinal coccidiosis to piglets: clinical, parasitological and pathological findings. *Can. J. Comp. Med.* **47**:401–407.
18. Stuart, B. P., D. B. Sisk, D. M. Bedell, and H. S. Gosser. 1982. Demonstration of immunity against *Isospora suis* in swine. *Vet. Parasitol.* **9**:185–191.

Sarcoptes scabiei **var.** *suis*

1. Cargill, C., and P. R. Davies. 1999. External parasites, p. 669–683. *In* B. . Straw, S. D'Allaire, W. L. Mengeling ,and D. J. Taylor (ed.), *Diseases of Swine*, 8th ed. Iowa State University Press, Ames.
2. Cargill, C. F., and K. J. Dobson. 1979. Experimental *Sarcoptes scabiei* infestation in pigs: (1) Pathogenesis. *Vet. Rec.* **104**:11–14.
3. Davis, D. P., and R. D. Moon. 1990. Dynamics of swine mange: a critical review of the literature. *J. Med. Entomol.* **27**:727–737.
4. Elbers, A. R., P. G. Rambags, H. M. van der Heijden, and W. A. Hunneman. 2000. Production performance and pruritic behaviour of pigs naturally infected by *Sarcoptes scabiei* var. *suis* in a contact transmission experiment. *Vet. Q.* **22**:145–149.
5. Firkins, L. D., C. J. Jones, D. P. Keen, J. J. Arends, L. Thompson, V. L. King, and T. L. Skogerboe. 2001. Preventing transmission of *Sarcoptes scabiei* var. *suis* from infested sows to nursing piglets by a prefarrowing treatment with doramectin injectable solution. *Vet. Parasitol.* **99**:323–330.
6. Hollanders, W., and J. Vercruysse. 1990. Sarcoptic mite hypersensitivity: a cause of dermatitis in fattening pigs at slaughter. *Vet. Rec.* **126**:308–310.
7. Lowenstein, M., G. Loupal, W. Baumgartner, and E. Kutzer. 1996. Histology of the skin and determination of blood and serum parameters during the recovery phase of sarcoptic mange in cattle after avermectin (Ivomec) treatment. *Appl. Parasitol.* **37**:77–86.
8. Morsy, G. H., and S. M. Gaafar. 1989. Responses of immunoglobulin-secreting cells in the skin of pigs during *Sarcoptes scabiei* infestation. *Vet. Parasitol.* **33**:165–175.
9. Sheahan, B. J. 1975. Pathology of *Sarcoptes scabiei* infection in pigs. 1. Naturally occurring and experimentally induced lesions. *J. Comp. Pathol.* **85**:87–95.
10. Wooten, E. L., F. Blecha, A. B. Broce, and D. S. Pollmann. 1986. The effect of sarcoptic mange on growth performance, leukocytes and lymphocyte proliferative responses in pigs. *Vet. Parasitol.* **22**:315–324.

PATHOGENS OF NONHUMAN PRIMATES

11

INTRODUCTION

Because of their physiologic similarities to humans, nonhuman primates, here simply referred to as primates, continue to hold a very important position within biomedical research. Primates still serve as relevant models for research involving reproductive physiology, infectious diseases, toxicology, cognitive function, neurophysiology, and others. In some countries, including the United States, pharmaceutical products intended for human use are tested in primates prior to release on the human market.

During the past few decades, growing concern for the plight of wild populations of primates has led to legislation that has greatly reduced the number of wild-caught primates exported from range countries. This decrease has been of such a magnitude that comparatively few wild-caught primates are currently used in biomedical research. In the future, all primates used in research are likely to be captive bred. One result of this change in animal source has been a dramatic decline in the breadth and prevalence of pathogens encountered in the primate research facility. Of course reduced infection rates have also been facilitated by improvements in animal husbandry, pathogen surveillance, and veterinary care. Previously, it could be safely assumed that all wild-caught primates were infected with some pathogen(s). While this appears to no longer be the case, a significant percentage of laboratory primates are infected with primary or opportunistic pathogens. Except for some of the viral infections, remarkably little has been published on the effects of these pathogens on host physiology. This information is of course necessary for one to understand the potential effects that infection can have on research. In this chapter, the most commonly identified primate pathogens are introduced. When any of these pathogens are diagnosed, the laboratory animal veterinarian and the scientific investigator should discuss the infection in light of the intended use of the animal(s). The reader interested in historically significant but currently less common pathogens, pathogens reportable to governmental authorities, and/or those requiring immediate euthanasia of affected animals, is referred to other scholarly sources for that information (1, 2, 3, 4).

It is an especially difficult task to assess retrospectively the effects of pathogens on primate physiology. This is because of the common and apparently long-standing infection of primates with a variety of viral agents, many of which themselves alter host physiology. It is difficult to go back in time and sort out the effects caused by identified pathogens, when the primates under study might have also been infected with then unknown viral agents. However, every effort has been made by this author to do so.

VIRUSES

Hepatitis B virus

Agent
Hepatitis B virus (HBV) is an enveloped DNA virus in the family *Hepadnaviridae*. The genome is circular and consists of a complete strand and an incomplete, complementary strand. While humans appear to be the natural host, multiple strains have been identified in wild chimpanzees, and appear to infect geographically distinct chimpanzee subspecies (4). Globally, HBV is an important cause of hepatitis in humans. HBV is one of several important hepatitis viruses known to infect, and to be named after, specific animal hosts such as woodchucks, ducks, and ground squirrels.

Epidemiology
Several species of primates have been found seropositive for HBV infection. These include the chimpanzee, gibbon, orangutan, baboon, patas monkey, vervet monkey, mangabey, langur, Celebes ape, several species of macaques, and several New World monkeys (11). Recovery or demonstration of virus has been limited to chimpanzees, white-handed gibbons, and less commonly, cynomolgus macaques (1, 2). It has been proposed that the primary route of transmission may be from mother to infant during parturition (9). In addition, transmission likely occurs by exchange of body fluids (12). Infected primates often show no clinical signs, yet are persistently infected and excreting virus. These animals likely serve as important reservoirs of infection for other primates, as well as for their human caretakers. Concerning the latter, relatively little is known about zoonotic HBV infection.

Clinical signs
Naturally infected animals generally show no clinical signs of infection. Experimental infection has variably resulted in anorexia, lethargy, abdominal tenderness, and rarely, jaundice (13). In one report, 1 of 19 cynomolgus monkeys developed similar signs, and also developed hepatomegaly (6).

Pathology
Following infection, virus colonizes and replicates in the liver and spleen (8). Incubation time is long, generally about 3 to 4 months (2). Grossly, the liver may be congested, enlarged, and fatty. Microscopic lesions are variable but, in general, consist of nonsuppurative lymphocytic inflammation and hepatocellular necrosis (2). Infected hepatocytes take on a "ground glass" appearance and contain viral antigen. Infected cells are attacked and killed by cytotoxic lymphocytes (5). Lymphoid stimulation is also evident in the spleen and local lymph nodes (6). In some animals, an effective immune response consisting of cytopathic, humoral, and noncytopathic antiviral mechanisms may almost completely clear virus from acutely infected chimpanzees, allowing histologic recovery over 3 to 4 months (2, 3).

Interference with research
In all but the mildest cases, it should be assumed that HBV will complicate studies involving the enterohepatic and lymphoreticular systems, as well as studies where nutritional parameters are measured. These parameters might include feed intake, food preferences, weight gain or loss, and others. HBV has been shown to elevate serum alanine aminotransferase and alkaline phosphatase activities, as well as serum bilirubin concentration (2, 6); and to inhibit immune responsiveness (7).

Diagnosis and control
Diagnosis of HBV is complicated by the lack of clinical signs. Infection may be suspected on the basis of necropsy findings. Infection can be confirmed serologically. In this regard,

the HBV-core and HBV-e antigen, and antibody status of chimpanzees should be known, both for veterinary, as well as human health considerations. Because HBV is zoonotic, appropriate personal protection should be exercised. An equally great concern, however, is the transmission of HBV from infected caretakers to susceptible chimpanzees and cynomolgus monkeys. Caretakers and other persons who will have contact with laboratory primates should be found to be HBV-free prior to entry into the animal facility. It is recommended that animal care personnel working with laboratory primates be vaccinated against HBV as part of the occupational health program. Primates known to be infected with HBV should be cared for under animal biosafety level (ABSL)-2 conditions. There is no effective treatment for eradicating HBV from infected primates. Prednisolone has been shown to reduce hepatic inflammation (6). Before initiating treatment, the scientific value of the animal subject should be reviewed. It may be possible to transfer the animal to studies that would not be affected by HBV infection. Newborn chimpanzees have been successfully immunized against HBV infection (10).

Herpesvirus

Agent

Several herpesviruses have been recovered from primates. These DNA viruses are all in the family *Herpesviridae,* and are grouped in the subfamilies *Alphaherpesvirinae, Betaherpesvirinae,* and *Gammaherpesvirinae.* While these subfamilies differ in important biological properties, they share features common to the family. Because Asian macaques represent the majority of primates used in biomedical research, this review will focus on *Cercopithecine herpesvirus*-1 (CHV-1), also known as *Herpesvirus simiae.* CHV-1 shares features with other members of the subfamily Alphaherpesvirinae, including the closely related *Herpesvirus hominus* (herpes simplex) of humans. These features include transmission by secretions associated with mucosal surfaces; restriction of lesions to mucosal surfaces of the enteric, respiratory, dermal, and reproductive systems; and formation of vesicles and pustules which eventually rupture, leaving ulcers.

Epidemiology

CHV-1 commonly infects several species of Asian macaques, including *Macaca arctoides, M. cyclopis, M. fascicularis, M. fuscata, M. mulatta,* and *M. radiata* (3). Infection rates are low in infants, and increase dramatically as monkeys reach sexual maturity (6). Viral transmission occurs through exchange of bodily fluids. This occurs most frequently by blood and saliva contact during fighting, but also during sexual contact. Monkeys are infected for life, and periodically shed the virus in oral or genital secretions. Virus can be found in mucosal lesions, but virus shedding may also occur without clinical signs.

Clinical signs

CHV-1 rarely causes more than mild clinical disease in natural hosts. When present, clinical signs most often consist of oral and genital vesicles, pustules, and ulcers. These lesions generally resolve within 10 to 14 days. Development of clinical disease, or reappearance of signs in previously asymptomatic infection, are thought to be brought on by stress. Stress may include that of concurrent medical conditions, and other direct or indirect causes of immune suppression. In this regard, Carlson and coworkers reported on two cases of B virus infection that appeared to have been considerably worsened by concurrent infection with retrovirus (1). Stress is also thought to be involved in reactivation of virus shedding. In some studies, however, monkeys subjected to quarantine, parturition, or breeding did not resume virus shedding (8). Additional studies are clearly needed in this area to elucidate the triggers for recrudescence of disease and/or virus shedding. Disseminated infection occurs rarely, and is generally fatal (4).

Clinical signs of disseminated disease vary, complicating diagnosis. This is particularly true when the clinical episode arises slowly (3). Infections in nonmacaque species, both Old and New World, are rare, but uniformly fatal.

Pathology
Following infection, viral replication occurs at the site of inoculation, inducing localized inflammation. Thereafter, virus moves in a retrograde manner, to the sensory ganglion serving the infected body region, where latent infection is established. Pathologic findings of infected epithelia include ballooning degeneration, coagulative necrosis, and eosinophilic intranuclear inclusion bodies at the site of inoculation. Disseminated infection is accompanied by widespread, hemorrhagic necrosis in the liver, spleen, lung, brain, uterus, adrenal gland, pancreas, and lymphoid organs (4). Resolution of clinical signs, but not clearing of infection, follows the development of an antibody response.

Interference with research
Natural infection of primates with CHV-1 limits the usefulness of affected animals. Infected animals constitute a serious risk to human health, and so their retention in the animal program should be based on institutional policy. More directly, monkeys infected with CHV-1 may be unsuitable for research involving the dermal, endocrine, enterohepatic, lymphoreticular, nervous, reproductive, and respiratory systems. The occurrence of clinical signs may also preclude their use in studies involving behavioral observations. While rare, monkeys with disseminated infection are likely to die and so will be unusable for any purpose. Lastly, infected monkeys may not be appropriate for studies in which there is an increased likelihood for research or animal care personnel to contact bodily fluids.

Diagnosis and control
A diagnosis of CHV-1 infection may be strongly suspected by observing typical mucosal lesions. Confirmation of infection is based on serologic testing. To ascertain the potential hazard to humans, virus isolation should be attempted by swabbing the lesions and submitting samples to a qualified diagnostic laboratory. Determination of infection status in asymptomatic monkeys is much more challenging because of the common occurrence of false-negative tests and variable seroconversion among primates (5). Effective flow charts have been devised to guide accurate diagnosis of CHV-1 infection. Diagnostic tests incorporated into the paradigm include enzyme-linked immunosorbent assay (ELISA) and Western blots (5). In addition, PCR assay has been used to demonstrate latent infection in neural tissues and has proven highly reliable (7). No therapeutic means of eliminating B virus from individual monkeys exists. In addition, treatment of affected monkeys represents an unacceptable risk to personnel. Each institution must establish policies regarding the holding of animals known to be infected. Eradication of the virus from the facility is a long and arduous process, and relies on repeated testing, followed by culling of infected animals (5). It is recommended that where possible, institutions purchase only B-virus-free monkeys. This will likely not be possible in large institutions using many monkeys. CHV-1 infection is often fatal in humans. Fortunately, infection does not appear to be highly contagious, since remarkably few cases of human infection have occurred. In this regard, most human infections are acquired by bites or scratches from virus-shedding monkeys, rather than through other forms of direct or indirect contact. However, humans have been known or suspected of acquiring infection by splash exposure to body fluids of infected laboratory primates. Infection causes vesiculopustular lesions at the site of infection, followed by ascending paralysis, encephalitis, and death in humans. Personnel working around macaques must abide by ABSL-2 standard operating procedures. These procedures will limit the potential for human exposures, and will ensure appropriate responses when

potential instances of exposure occur. Guidelines for exposure prevention and postexposure actions have been developed (2).

Respiratory syncytial virus

Agent
Respiratory syncytial virus (RSV), also known as "chimpanzee coryza," is a single-stranded RNA (ssRNA) virus in the family Paramyxoviridae, subfamily Pneumovirinae. Many different strains have been isolated. These appear to have a broad host range (7).

Epidemiology
RSV is a common cause of respiratory disease in children. In this regard, humans represent the natural reservoir host. Of the primates, chimpanzees are most commonly found infected. However, several species of Old and New World monkeys have been experimentally infected. These include rhesus and bonnet macaques, African green monkeys, squirrel monkeys, owl monkeys, and cebus monkeys. RSV is highly contagious and spreads easily by inhalation of aerosolized droplets.

Clinical signs
Many RSV infections in monkeys are asymptomatic. Other cases are mild and result in increased respiratory rate, fever, and increased lung sounds (9). On occasion, more severe cases occur and affected primates develop sneezing, coughing, and mucopurulent nasal discharge, in addition to the signs listed above (1). Young chimpanzees have rarely died from RSV infection (3).

Pathology
Following inhalation, RSV infection of respiratory epithelial cells is enhanced by surfactant protein A (4). RSV replicates throughout the respiratory tract, eliciting a strong immune response, which primarily consists of a secretory immunoglobulin A (IgA) antibody. In contrast, IgG is nonprotective, and may predispose to the formation of immune complexes within pulmonary vessels, peribronchiolar inflammation, and pneumonitis (11). Grossly, the nasopharyngeal mucosa, as well as the tonsils, and local and bronchial lymph nodes appear reddened and prominent. The lungs are consolidated and reddened. Microscopically, lesions consist of bronchiolitis, periarteritis, focal alveolitis, bronchopneumonia, intracytoplasmic inclusion bodies, and syncytial giant cell formation (1, 3, 14). It has been suggested that in humans, childhood infection with RSV results in reduced lung function later in life. However, other evidence suggests that an underlying deficit in pulmonary function is to blame (6, 10). Additional studies are needed to resolve this issue. It is similarly unknown whether residual effects occur following RSV infection of monkeys.

Interference with research
In vitro studies indicate that RSV alters the distribution of proteins within host respiratory epithelial cell membranes (2), inhibits mitogen-induced proliferation of lymphocytes through the action of the fusion protein (13), increases cytokine expression (8), accelerates ribavirin metabolism (15), and reduces bacterial killing by virus-infected monocytes (12). In other species, RSV stimulates neutrophil degranulation and chemokine release (5), and induces substance P release, which contributes to development of bronchiolitis (16). Clearly, primates naturally infected with RSV will be unsuitable for research involving the lymphoreticular, nervous, or respiratory systems. In addition, studies in which parameters associated with growth and activity levels may be temporarily affected.

Diagnosis and control
RSV infection may be suspected on the basis of clinical presentation. However, laboratory confirmation is necessary, since a number of other viral and bacterial pathogens can cause similar clinical signs. Confirmation of infection in humans, monkeys, and other susceptible species, is accomplished using serology, electron microscopy, and increasingly, reverse transcriptase (RT)-PCR assay. There is no ef-

fective chemotherapy for RSV infection, although on an experimental basis, intranasally administered monoclonal IgA rapidly reduces viral shedding (17). Treatment should be directed toward symptomatic relief and prevention of opportunistic bacterial infections. Prevention involves isolating monkeys showing signs of infection, and keeping infected personnel away from susceptible primates. In this regard, animal care and research personnel must understand the risks of transmitting RSV to susceptible chimpanzees. Persons showing signs of potential RSV infection should avoid contact with susceptible animals.

Rotavirus

Agents
Simian rotavirus is a naked double-stranded RNA (dsRNA) virus in the family *Reoviridae*. Rotaviruses are divided into groups A-G on the basis of antigenic differences in capsid protein VP6 (5). Laboratory primates are susceptible to at least two primate-specific strains, as well as to infection with human rotaviruses (7, 15). Rotaviruses naturally infecting infant rhesus macaques are type A rotaviruses, similar to the type A rotavirus of humans.

Epidemiology
Several Old and New World primate species have been found seropositive for rotavirus infection (10). So, while few studies have investigated the incidence of rotavirus infection in laboratory monkeys, it is thought that infection may be common. Transmission is through ingestion of feces containing infectious virus particles. As a nonenveloped virus, rotavirus survives for extended periods in the environment.

Clinical signs
Rotaviruses commonly cause severe diarrhea in their natural hosts. In contrast, primates rarely show clinical signs of rotavirus infection. On occasion, infant primates infected with rotavirus develop profuse, watery diarrhea which begins within 48 h, peaks 72 h after infection, and lasts for several days. Appetite and weight gain are usually not affected (5, 10).

Pathology
Following infection, rotavirus replicates in the epithelium lining the distal third of the intestinal villus tip. Infection results in death of these cells. Pathologic findings appear to be limited to epithelial cell necrosis, ballooning degeneration, and villous atrophy. Loss of digestive and absorptive potential results in diarrhea (3). Immunity is primarily humoral, with secretory IgA providing local protection. Specific antibody lessens the severity of subsequent infection, and limits the duration of diarrhea (2).

Interference with research
Remarkably little has been published concerning the effects of rotavirus infection on primate physiology. In this case, much can be learned from literature related to other host species, including mice, humans, and cattle. That information can then be cautiously extrapolated to monkeys. Even at that, essentially all evidence of the confounding effects of rotavirus infection come from in vitro experiments. The extent to which these effects occur in vivo is unknown. Rotavirus has been shown to increase cellular permeability to Ca^{2+}, thereby augmenting its cytopathic effects (6). Rotavirus has also been shown to interfere with sodium-coupled transport of D-glucose and L-leucine (1), alter intestinal epithelial cell lipid composition (4), and interfere with cytoskeletal organization (13). Also, rotavirus nonstructural glycoprotein NSP4 functions as an enterotoxigenic peptide when secreted from rotavirus-infected cells (16). Lastly, there is disagreement on whether rotavirus infection acts synergistically with other enteric pathogens to worsen diarrheal disease (11, 12). Differences in findings may be due to differences in host species studied. It is probable that natural rotavirus infection will have limited effects on research involving primates. Studies involving the enterohepatic sys-

tem of newborn primates would likely be affected, as would studies where other nutritional parameters are measured.

Diagnosis and control
Rotavirus infection may be suspected in young monkeys with diarrhea. However, a plethora of other pathogens cause similar clinical signs. Diagnosis is accomplished by virus isolation from diarrheic stools, immunoelectron microscopy, polyacrylamide gel electrophoresis, RT-PCR assay, and use of commercially available kits (5, 14). The latter will detect type A rotaviruses. There is no specific treatment for rotavirus infection. Affected monkeys should receive supportive treatment, including fluid and electrolyte therapy, supplemental nutrition, and prophylactic antibiotics. Rotaviruses are stable over a wide range of humidity but are inactivated at high temperature (8) and by radiation, dilute bleach, peroxide, concentrated alcohol, and phenolic compounds (9). Considerable additional information concerning the prevalence of rotavirus infection is needed. This information would facilitate development of strategies to prevent infection in laboratory primates.

Simian hemorrhagic fever virus

Agent
Simian hemorrhagic fever virus (SHFV) is a ssRNA virus of the family *Arteriviridae*. It is closely related to equine arteritis virus, porcine reproductive and respiratory syndrome virus, lactate dehydrogenase-elevating virus of mice, and others. Several strains of SHFV have been identified. These differ in pathogenicity, in vitro growth, and other features (3).

Epidemiology
SHFV has been shown to naturally infect a wide range of primates without causing disease. These include patas monkeys, African green monkeys, and baboons. These species may be persistently infected and shed virus, thereby serving as potential sources of infection for more susceptible species. Essentially all macaque species have either been shown to be, or are assumed to be, highly susceptible to infection. Patas monkeys are the most likely natural reservoir host, and appear to be commonly and chronically infected (4, 5). SHFV is highly contagious, and is transmitted by aerosol, direct contact, or fomites. However, initial crossover from less susceptible to more susceptible species may require transfer of contagious body fluids, e.g., blood. This may occur by contaminated multidose vials, tattooing needles, and other potentially contaminated instruments (5, 8).

Clinical signs
Where known to infect primate species other than macaques, SHFV infection is most often asymptomatic. In patas monkeys, for example, clinical signs are uncommon, but are also dependent on viral strain. Less virulent strains are uniformly asymptomatic. However, infection by more virulent strains causes acute onset of fever, anorexia, lethargy, facial edema, dehydration, and occasionally, small subcutaneous hemorrhages (3, 5). In contrast, macaques infected with SHFV rapidly develop fever, followed shortly by bleeding diatheses; that is bleeding from multiple sites, including the gastrointestinal tract, renal system, nose, and subcutaneous locations. Subcutaneous bleeding may appear as pinpoint spots or large bruises. Affected macaques also show signs of depression, dehydration, light avoidance (photophobia), cyanosis, and abortion (4, 7).

Pathology
Pathologic findings largely depend on host species and virus strain. Patas monkeys infected with avirulent strains usually do not develop pathologic lesions, and may become persistently infected. Those encountering more virulent strains develop milder versions of the hemorrhagic lesions described below. In these cases, infection induces a strong humoral immune response, which effectively terminates the infection. In macaques, SHFV replicates inside macrophages. Virus may therefore reach virtually all organs. Gross le-

sions include severe reddening of the proximal duodenum and splenic enlargement. Microscopic lesions include congestion, hemorrhaging, and necrosis of the intestinal mucosa. Similar lesions may be found elsewhere in the intestinal tract, in virtually all lymphoid tissue, and in other visceral organs. In addition, lesions indicative of disseminated intravascular coagulation may occur in the liver, renal glomeruli, and lung. In some cases, lymphohistiocytic meningoencephalitis develops. Changes in serum biochemistry profiles include elevation of liver enzymes and blood urea nitrogen, proteinuria, and hematuria. In addition, coagulation disorders result in increased fibrin degradation products, thrombocytopenia, and elevated clotting times (1, 3, 6, 8).

Interference with research
Relatively little has been published describing physiologic changes in primates naturally infected with SHFV. The severity of disease associated with natural infection of patas monkeys, baboons, and African green monkeys will vary with virus strain virulence. Infection may at least temporarily compromise research involving a range of body systems, depending on the extent and severity of vascular and visceral organ involvement. At a minimum, studies involving the cardiovascular, dermal, enterohepatic, hematopoietic, lymphoreticular, nervous, reproductive, respiratory, and urinary systems may be compromised. Certainly, studies involving measurement of serum proteins, clotting factors, and potentially other analytes, would also be affected. Lastly, behavioral studies would be affected to the degree that appetite and activity levels declined. Morphogenesis of the arteriviruses occurs in the golgi region. Accordingly, others have shown induction of autoimmune (anti-golgi antigen) antibodies in animals infected with arteriviruses (9). It remains to be determined whether similar autoantibodies are induced in primates infected with SHFV. Macaques infected with SHFV should be euthanized. Therefore, infection with SHFV will indirectly compromise any research involving macaques.

Diagnosis and control
SHFV may be suspected on the basis of clinical signs coupled with necropsy findings. However, given the extremely serious nature of hemorrhagic diseases of primates, macaques showing signs of epizootic hemorrhagic disease should be immediately euthanized. The entire facility should be quarantined and disinfected to protect the remaining monkeys as well as to protect personnel (8). Confirmation of SHFV is accomplished using virus isolation and indirect immunofluorescence assay. Both of these methods have their disadvantages. Recently, improved diagnostic capability for SHFV infection has been achieved through the development of a quantitative ELISA. This assay can be used to distinguish active infections from historical titers from previous exposure (2). No treatment is available for SHFV infection. Mildly affected patas and African green monkeys could be treated symptomatically. However, that decision should involve facility administrators, clinical veterinarians, and the principal investigator. Prevention of SHFV infection includes separation of primate species, particularly patas monkeys, from macaques.

Simian immunodeficiency viruses

Agent
The simian immunodeficiency viruses (SIVs) constitute a group of closely related ssRNA virus isolates in the family *Retroviridae* and genus *Lentivirus*. These isolates are designated according to the natural host species. Four isolates are associated with immune deficiency disease in Old World primates. These virus isolates are also closely related to human immunodeficiency virus-1 (HIV-1) and HIV-2, the causative agents of human AIDS. For this reason, SIV infection has been a valuable model of human HIV infection. Together, these ten viruses have been placed into five distinct genetic groupings (6).

Epidemiology

SIV infection is common in primates, both wild and laboratory (9). Sexual transmission appears to account for most cases of naturally acquired infection. In addition, transmission occurs by contact with other bodily fluids, through intrauterine passage, and in the laboratory setting, through inoculation or implantation of contaminated cells or tissues. Naturally infected species include rhesus macaque (*Macaca mulatta* = SIVmac), African green monkey (*Cercopithecus aethiops* = SIVagm), cynomolgus monkey (*Macaca fascicularis* = SIVcyn), sooty mangabey (*Cercocebus torquatus atys* = SIVsm), pig-tailed macaque (*Macaca nemestrina* = SIVmne), stump-tailed macaque (*Macaca arctoides* = SIVstm), mandrill (*Mandrillus sphinx* = SIVmnd), chimpanzee (*Pan troglodytes* = SIVcpz), and Syke's monkey (*Cercopithecus mitis* = SIVsyk). Unconfirmed serologic evidence of infection has also been reported for other Old World primate species. Although virus isolates can pass between host species, in general, this does not appear to occur (16). Natural infection of New World primates has not been reported, although common marmosets and cotton-topped tamarins are susceptible to experimental infection with HIV-2, and may therefore also be susceptible to SIV (18).

Clinical signs

Natural SIV infection in reservoir hosts, including African green monkeys, sooty mangabeys, Syke's monkeys, mandrills, or chimpanzees causes no clinical disease. In contrast, macaques infected with host-specific isolates of SIV experience profound immune suppression. The most consistent clinical signs of SIV infection in macaques are malabsorptive diarrhea and wasting. These may represent primary SIV enteropathy, or may be due to secondary, opportunistic infection with agents similar to those causing enteritis and wasting in patients with AIDS (17). Opportunistic infections may result in other clinical signs as well. Those will depend largely on the offending agent(s). SIV-infected macaques frequently also develop signs of central nervous system (CNS) dysfunction, pulmonary distress, and skin rashes, compatible with the principal pathologic changes accompanying infection (16). Death usually occurs within 4 months to 3 years.

Pathology

Following exposure, SIV infects $CD4^+$ cells through interaction between the viral glycoprotein gp120, the CD4 molecule, and the coreceptor CCR5 (5). Susceptible cells therefore include helper T lymphocytes, cells of the monocyte/macrophage lineage, and antigen-presenting dendritic cells. Infection is followed by reverse transcription of viral RNA, resulting in the production of DNA copies. Progeny virus is produced by transcription of viral DNA. These bud from the surface of infected lymphocytes. By mechanisms that are as yet poorly understood, viral infection results in the depletion of affected $CD4^+$ T cells. In contrast, viral progeny are formed intracytoplasmically within macrophages. These cells are not depleted, and may serve to disseminate virus throughout the body. Favorite sites of viral replication and accumulation include the spleen and lymph nodes. No lesions have been noted in nonmacaque species. Instead, these species are persistently and asymptomatically infected. The pathologic presentation is quite different in macaques. In these hosts, pathologic findings are variable, and are due to a wide phylogenetic range of opportunistic pathogens, including viral, fungal, bacterial, and parasitic agents. In addition, SIV is a direct cause of lesion development (13). Pathologic changes in the lymphoreticular system include at least six different patterns, which may occur simultaneously. These include normal morphology, follicular hyperplasia, follicular involution with or without paracortical changes, depletion of follicular and paracortical regions, granulomatous lymphadenitis, and generalized lymphoproliferation. Thymic atrophy is common (3). Nervous system involvement consistently includes meningoencephalitis. Encephalitic changes occur in both the gray and white matter of the spinal cord and brain, optic neuropathy develops, and widespread neuronal atrophy occurs (20, 27). In the gastrointestinal system, lesions may be absent, may include fulminant necrohemorrhagic gastroenteritis, or may lie somewhere in between (10, 12). It has been proposed that the intestinal tract is a primary target system for SIV because of the large population of mucosal lymphocytes and macrophages in that organ (16). SIV infection also causes cardiopulmonary lesions (25). Most prominent is a severe pulmonary arteritis. There is pronounced medial and intimal proliferation of the pulmonary arteries, resulting in vascular thrombosis and pulmonary infarction. The pathogenesis of these lesions is unknown but may arise from primary endothelial injury (4). Retroviral interstitial pneumonia is also common (2). Dermal lesions include transient exanthema characterized by perivascular lymphocytic dermatitis associated with infiltration by $CD8^+$ cytotoxic T cells. In addition, SIV causes hepatitis similar to that developing in AIDS patients, with periportal inflammation, focal biliary damage, and duct proliferation (7). SIV has also been associated with renal glomerulosclerosis (1), testicular atrophy, degeneration, and azoospermia secondary to orchitis (19), and cachexia (22).

Interference with research

Host species that do not develop immunodeficiency disease following SIV infection will likely remain useful as subjects in most types of research. However, it should not be assumed that host species are free of physiologic changes that might compromise the research value of such animals. For example, although chimpanzees infected with a HIV-1-like lentivirus (SIVcpz-ant) are asymptomatic, they develop thrombocytopenia, reduction of $CD8^+$ T lymphocytes, and alterations in natural killer cell activity. At a minimum, these changes may influence immunologic studies (11). More obviously, natural infection of host species susceptible to immunodeficiency disease will render affected animals unfit for most types of research. In particular, studies involving the cardiovascular, dermal, enterohepatic, hematopoietic, nervous, reproductive, respiratory, and urinary systems will be compromised. In addition, studies wherein body weight, activity levels, cognitive function, and potentially other phenotypic indices are evaluated, will also be affected. Of course opportunistic infections may invalidate research involving other organ systems as well. Specific physiologic changes associated with SIV infection in macaques include profound changes in relative populations of lymphocyte subsets, altered cytokine production profiles (26), impaired natural killer cell activity (23), altered dendritic cell homeostasis (28), down-regulation of major histocompatibility complex (MHC) class I expression (21), reduced cardiac output (25), changes in texture of cerebral white matter (24), decreased cognitive ability (8), and depressed digestive enzyme activities (10).

Diagnosis and control

Infection of macaques with SIV may be suspected on the basis of clinical signs, in particular, where unusual, opportunistic infections occur. Confirmation of infection in macaques may be achieved using direct and indirect serology-based methods, virus isolation, electron microscopy, Northern blotting, and RT-PCR, according to defined paradigms (15). Infected animals should be culled. Diagnosis of infection in nonmacaque species requires diagnostic methods that do not rely on demonstration of antibody, since these animals do not seroconvert. There is no treatment available for eradicating SIV infection. Prevention includes separation of macaques from other Old World primate species. Personnel working with Old World primates should practice meticulous personal protection to avoid accidental exposure to SIV as well as other primate zoonoses (14). While disease has not resulted from accidental human SIV infection, persons have seroconverted, and in some cases, virus has been isolated from the patients (14). The long-term effects of zoonotic SIV infection are unknown. It is therefore wise to avoid infection.

Simian retrovirus type D

Agent
Primates are susceptible to a growing list of retroviruses. Among them, and clearly the most significant from the perspective of primate health, is Simian retrovirus type D (SRV/D). SRV/D is a member of the family *Retroviridae,* subfamily *Oncovirinae.* SRV/D is actually a group of closely related viruses. While a few are endogenous, the more common and significant are exogenous viruses. These include SRV/D types 1 to 5, all of which are infective to *Macaca* spp. (7).

Epidemiology
SRV/D is highly contagious, so infection is common in Asian macaques. Serologic surveys of captive populations reveal prevalence rates from 0% to more than 90%. Transmission is through exposure to infectious body fluids, including saliva and blood. It is noteworthy that SRV/D may be recovered from the saliva of healthy carrier animals. Therefore, biting, with inoculation of body fluids, is a common route of transmission. Mother-to-offspring transmission, both pre- and postpartum, also facilitates establishment and maintenance of infection within the animal colony (14). In this regard, in utero infection is thought to result in a chronic, seronegative carrier state (9).

Clinical signs
Many animals infected with SRV/D are asymptomatic, yet excreting virus. Others develop an immune response adequate for clearing of the infection. These also show no signs of disease. Still others develop generalized disease evidenced by a collection of clinical signs. These include weight loss or failure to gain weight, fever, depression, lethargy, necrotizing gingivitis and stomatitis, and chronic diarrhea (3). Death may occur within a few months of onset of fulminating immune deficiency (5). In addition to these signs, many macaques develop subcutaneous or retroperitoneal fibromatosis. While the subcutaneous form generally causes no clinical signs, advanced cases of the retroperitoneal form may interfere with normal gastrointestinal function, resulting in for example, intestinal obstruction (2). Finally, in some cases of SRV/D infection, resulting immune suppression facilitates infection with a wide range of opportunistic pathogens. In this regard, SRV/D is similar to SIV, although the types of opportunistic pathogens are somewhat different. Specifically, SRV/D is more often associated with pyogenic bacterial infections, while SIV is more commonly associated with *Mycobacterium avium, Pneumocystis carinii,* Simian virus 40, and adenovirus. Both diseases share other opportunistic infections in common (7). Opportunistic infection seems less common in cynomolgus monkeys versus other macaque species (3). Infants born to viremic mothers exhibit low birth weight, prematurity, high perinatal mortality, and increased incidence of simian acquired immunodeficiency syndrome (SAIDS) (14).

Pathology
Following infection, SRV/D infects both B and T lymphocytes, as well as macrophages, epithelial cells, and cells of the choroid plexus (6, 8). Asymptomatic animals may be found incidentally to have generalized lymphadenopathy, with expansion of both $CD4^+$ and $CD8^+$ T cell populations (3). By mechanisms that remain largely unknown, infection eventually results in loss of infected immune system cells. Thereafter, the hallmark pathologic finding is profound depletion of lymphocytes from virtually all lymphoid tissues (3, 10, 16). The subsequent profound immune compromise allows for infection with opportunistic pathogens, particularly pyogenic bacteria. These are accompanied by pathologic changes associated with those organisms. In addition to these, SRV/D is associated with the development of subcutaneous or retroperitoneal fibromatosis, possibly with interleukin 6 (IL-6) as an auto-

crine growth factor (12). In the retroperitoneal form, the mesentery, mesenteric lymph nodes, and gastrointestinal organs become progressively covered and entrapped by a disseminated infiltration of fibrous connective tissue. As the condition progresses, other organs within the abdominal cavity may become involved, although the lesion rarely infiltrates organ parenchyma (2). Other lesions associated with SRV/D infection include immunoblastic lymphoma (11), and follicular lymphoid infiltration of various organs, particularly the brain, bone marrow, and salivary glands of viremic animals (3).

Interference with research
While asymptomatic macaques naturally infected with SRV/D will likely continue to be useful for most purposes, their presence in the colony jeopardizes the health of the remaining, uninfected animals, although direct contact is required for transmission. Macaques that have mounted an effective immune response and have cleared the virus should likewise be suitable for most research applications. Clearly, natural infection of laboratory macaques with SRV/D will result in clinically affected animals being unsuitable for most research applications. Specific effects on host physiology are surprisingly few, except for reports of alterations within the lymphoreticular system (16). Clinicopathologic changes associated with SRV/D infection include pancytopenia, that is, decreased numbers of essentially all red and white blood cells (3). SRV/D has also been shown to cause neutrophil dysfunction (1), increased cytokine (IL-6) production (12), and increased cerebrospinal fluid (CSF) concentrations of the excitotoxin quinolinic acid (4). Therefore, SRV/D-infected macaques may be unsuitable for research involving the enterohepatic, hematopoietic, lymphoreticular, nervous, and reproductive systems. In addition, studies in which weight gain, activity levels, or cognitive function are measured may be compromised. Naturally, studies involving other immune-suppressive viruses, or any other infectious disease, would also be negated by SRV/D infection.

Diagnosis and control
SRV/D infection may be suspected on the basis of clinical signs, most prominently retroperitoneal fibromatosis. Evidence of opportunistic infections suggestive of profound immune suppression should also raise suspicion, although immune suppression can be caused by a number of other viruses in addition to SRV/D. Diagnosis may be confirmed serologically in those animals that mount a humoral response. However, a significant portion of infected animals are seronegative. In these cases, virus isolation and in situ hybridization techniques are diagnostic. More recently, RT-PCR assay has proven to be a reliable indicator of infection (15). Guidelines for testing and removal of infected animals have been reported elsewhere (13). If followed explicitly, these should facilitate the derivation of a virus-free colony. While challenging, this approach must be taken to develop a colony of animals suitable for biomedical research. Once the colony is free of SRV/D, it should be closed to new arrivals.

Simian T-cell leukemia virus

Agent
Simian T-cell leukemia virus-1 (STLV-1) is a type C oncovirus in the family *Retroviridae*. It is among the most significant of a group of closely related oncogenic viruses. STLV-1 serves as a model of human T-cell leukemia virus type 1 (HTLV-1) infection, which causes adult T-cell leukemia/lymphoma (ATLL) and tropical spastic paraparesis, a neurologic disorder. Several STLV-1 isolates have been recovered. These have been clustered into seven virus clades, on the basis of genetic relatedness. Cross-species transmission may be common and appears to be limited only by geographic proximity of host species (11). There is no conclusive evidence that STLV-1 is infectious to humans, although genetic re-

latedness of T-lymphotropic viruses isolated from humans and other primates suggest that primate-to-human transmission has occurred (2).

Epidemiology

Among laboratory primates, STLV-1 infection is common in some geographically isolated groups of wild and captive baboons, macaques, and African green monkeys (6, 10). Serologic evidence of infection has been found in 33 species of primates (7). Among baboons, seroprevalence and clinical signs are more common in females (3). The full spectrum of routes of transmission is unknown. Transmission is thought to be primarily through exchange of body fluids, including blood, saliva, and reproductive secretions. Vertical transmission is considered less important than for SIV or SRV/D.

Clinical signs

Most infections with STLV-1 are asymptomatic. However, in some animals, STLV-1 is associated with lymphoproliferative disorders, most commonly occurring in baboons. Clinical disease manifests as depression, anorexia, low body weight, anemia, respiratory difficulty, nodular skin lesions, and regional or generalized lymphadenopathy and hepatosplenomegaly similar to ATLL of humans. Pulmonary involvement, with resulting respiratory distress, is common. Cutaneous involvement, presenting as nodular skin lesions, is less frequent (3).

Pathology

The pathogenesis of lymphoid disorder associated with STLV-1 infection is incompletely known. It appears that a portion of the pathology is due to integration of viral genes into that of T lymphocytes, while exogenous alterations on control of T-cell proliferation are also active. Regardless, expansion of T-lymphocyte, and rarely B-lymphocyte, populations result in the development of non-Hodgkin's lymphoma and leukemia (3).

The primary immune system organs, including lymph nodes, spleen, and liver, are generally involved, as are the lungs, skin, and heart. These organs contain pale tan to white space-occupying foci typical of proliferative lymphoid tissue (3). Leukemia occurs in more than 50% of cases (8). Pulmonary findings include peribronchiolar and/or perivascular accumulations of monomorphic to pleomorphic neoplastic lymphocytes, multinucleated giant cells, congestion, consolidation, edema, necrosis, inflammation, and pleural thickening, in addition to the lymphoid foci previously mentioned. Dermal nodules are 3 to 5 mm in diameter and are located primarily over the abdomen and hands (3). Infected animals usually develop anti-STLV-1 antibodies. However, infected animals have remained seronegative for up to 43 months (5).

Interference with research

It is known that STLV-1 causes hypercalcemia (uncommonly), and leukocytosis with circulating multilobulated neoplastic cells (3, 9). Clearly, whether or not clinical signs are present, natural infection of laboratory primates with STLV-1 would render host animals unsuitable for research involving the cardiovascular, enterohepatic, hematopoietic, and lymphoreticular systems. Clinically affected animals should also be excluded from studies involving the dermal and respiratory systems, and studies in which weight gain and behavior are evaluated.

Diagnosis and control

Diagnosis of STLV-1 infection is often made at necropsy or physical examination, as a result of routine checks of peripheral blood smears, or may be revealed radiographically with pulmonary involvement (3). Laboratory tests, including serology and RT-PCR, are confirmatory. There is no treatment for STLV-1 infection. Infected animals should be eliminated from the colony. Effective test and removal strategies based on serology and RT-PCR have been developed (4). While an

HTLV-1 subunit vaccine has proven effective in preventing STLV-1 infection of pig-tailed macaques, vaccination of a colony would complicate serologic diagnosis (1). Prevention is based on establishment and maintenance of a virus-free colony.

Simian virus 40

Agent

Simian virus 40 (SV40), also known as polyomavirus, is a small, naked dsDNA virus of the family *Papovaviridae*. Members of this family share structural and chemical properties, but the different genera are genetically unrelated and cause markedly different clinical diseases. The SV40 genome encodes two DNA-binding proteins that facilitate transcription of late viral genes. These genes have proven useful in the development of transgenic animals.

Epidemiology

SV40 is common as a latent infection of wild and captive Asian macaques, including those species most commonly used in research (4). Little information is available on modes of transmission. SV40 has been found contaminating cell cultures, and occasionally gains initial access into primates receiving cell implants. It is likely that transmission is by contact with infectious body fluids, particularly urine. However, additional research is needed to determine the range and importance of different natural routes of transmission.

Clinical signs

While infection is common in macaques, clinical disease is rare. Clinical disease is always secondary to immune suppression, most often due to retroviral infection. For example, concurrent infection with SIV has been consistently associated with clinical SV40 infection (2). Because clinical disease generally accompanies severe immune suppression, concurrent infection with other pathogens is common. Signs of infection with these secondary pathogens predominate.

Pathology

Following infection, virus disseminates hematogenously. In immune-competent hosts, latent infection is established. The site of latent infection is currently unknown. On the basis of studies with SV40, and with related polyomaviruses of humans, likely candidates include the kidney, the CNS, and possibly peripheral blood mononuclear cells (5, 6). Disease occurs when immune-suppressed animals become infected with SV40. In these cases, primary infection may result in meningoencephalitis without demyelination. In latently infected hosts, immune suppression reactivates infection, leading to enhanced viral replication and lesion formation in the brain, lung, and kidney (6). Microscopic lesions during recrudescent infection include focal to widespread cerebral demyelination and progressive multifocal leukoencephalopathy; interstitial pneumonia; and nonsuppurative renal tubulointerstitial nephritis, fibrosis, glomerulosclerosis, and atrophy, with tubular cast formation (2, 6). Intranuclear viral inclusions are observed in all affected tissues.

Interference with research

SV40 has been extensively studied precisely for its ability to transform cells in vitro and to produce neoplasia in vivo. In this regard, SV40 is known to be oncogenic in nonhost animals, and has occasionally been associated with tumors in macaques (3). It is difficult to separate the concurrent effects of other pathogens, such as SIV, from the effects of SV40. Possibly for this reason, very little is known definitively about the effects of SV40 on host physiology. Macaques infected with SIV and concurrently infected with SV40 develop anemia and elevated blood urea nitrogen (BUN) (4). Elevated BUN is related to renal injury. It is likely that SV40 infection in immune-competent monkeys will not compromise their usefulness. However, monkeys coinfected with SIV and SV40 will not be suitable for research involving the nervous, respiratory, and urinary systems. It remains to be determined what, if any, effect infection may have on the lymphoreticular system.

Diagnosis and control
Because SV40 does not produce a characteristic clinical syndrome, diagnosis must rely on laboratory testing. Traditionally, demonstration of virions by electron microscopy was considered diagnostic. More recently, molecular methods, such as in situ hybridization and PCR assay have become more widely used (5, 6). There is no treatment for SV40 infection, although the antiviral drug cidofovir has shown some promise (1). However, when clinical signs trigger testing that results in a diagnosis of SV40 infection, animals are likely to have other, more serious concurrent infections. These infections should be the focus of any attempts at treatment. Because infection with SV40 is so common in the research primate population, it will be difficult to obtain animals free of infection. For now, it appears that investigators will have to contend with SV40 as a potential research variable. Prevention of infection with other pathogens, particularly immune-suppressive viruses, will help ensure that SV40 does not adversely affect host physiology.

BACTERIA

Campylobacter spp.

Agent
Campylobacter spp. are gram-negative, slender, curved, microaerophilic rods. Several species infect primates. These include *C. jejuni*, *C. coli*, *C. fetus*, *C. laridis*, *C. sputorum*, and *C. hyointestinalis*. Among these, *C. jejuni* is most common, with *C. coli* less common, and the others uncommon. This discussion will focus on *C. jejuni*.

Epidemiology
Campylobacters are known to infect a wide range of host species, including both Old and New World primates. Both *C. jejuni* and *C. coli* are zoonotic. These wide host ranges provide the potential for laboratory primates to become infected from multiple reservoir hosts, including humans. Prevalence studies have revealed infection rates as high as 100% for *C. jejuni* and *C. coli*. Increasing rates of infection are associated with time in captivity, although this appears to vary with host species and study (6), and is likely indicative of different institutional management approaches. Transmission of infection is strictly through direct or indirect ingestion of feces.

Clinical signs
Most infections with *Campylobacter* spp. are associated with poorly virulent bacterial strains and so are asymptomatic (6). Infections with more virulent strains of *C. jejuni* cause serious disease. Disease is most severe in infant monkeys. In these hosts, infection results in clinical disease within 24 to 32 h (12). Diarrhea is the hallmark of campylobacteriosis. In this regard, the particular presentation, whether bloody, invasive-type diarrhea or watery, secretory diarrhea, depends on the spectrum of toxins produced (7). Watery diarrhea is much more common. Additional clinical signs include anorexia, weight loss, and failure to gain weight. In these young animals, diarrhea lasts about 10 days (11, 13). *C. jejuni* localizes in the liver and gall bladder, and continues to be excreted intermittently in the feces for 2 to 3 weeks (4, 11). Infection of older monkeys generally does not result in clinical signs, although bacterial shedding follows about the same course as in younger animals (6). The interested reader is referred elsewhere for additional coverage of several case reports of campylobacteriosis in different primate species (6).

Pathology
Various isolates of *C. jejuni* produce proteins with cytotonic or cytotoxic activity. In this regard, *C. jejuni* produces toxins similar to cholera toxin and the heat-labile toxin of *Escherichia coli*. Cytotoxins include a hemolysin, a protein that increases intracellular cAMP followed by cell death, a hepatotoxin, and others. *C. jejuni* also produces an adhesin,

through which it binds to target cells. Most, although not all of these toxins have been shown to play some role in pathogenesis. Following ingestion, *C. jejuni* adheres to mucosal epithelial cells of the distal small intestine and colon. It is thought that the heat-labile toxin disrupts normal cAMP balance and eicosanoid production, leading to osmotic diarrhea (3). In addition, some strains are directly invasive, penetrating host epithelial cells and causing the eventual death and sloughing of the cell. Apoptosis is accelerated and degenerative changes follow (6, 12). Gross lesions include thinning of the bowel wall, distension of the intestines with pasty-to-fluid yellow-gray feces, profound weight loss; and in some cases, congestion of the intestinal mucosa, overlaid with blood and mucus. Regional lymph nodes are enlarged and watery to slightly bloody fluid (serosanguinous transudate) may be present in the abdominal cavity (6). Microscopically, *C. jejuni* causes enteritis and colitis, characterized by inflammatory cell infiltration, necrosis, loss of columnar epithelium, villus blunting, and dilated lacteals (6, 11). Characteristically comma-shaped bacteria may be seen on the mucosal surface and within the lamina propria following silver staining (6). Antibodies are produced within days of infection. These effectively eliminate and prevent the reoccurrence of clinical signs. Despite this, immunity is inadequate to prevent reinfection. Milk IgA protects neonates against diarrheal disease (14).

Interference with research
There is little direct information concerning the physiologic effects of *Campylobacter* spp. on primate physiology. Clinicopathologic changes associated with campylobacteriosis include leukocytosis and severe electrolyte imbalance (5, 12). In other host species, *Campylobacter jejuni* or its products impair fetal development (9), induce anxiety in otherwise asymptomatic mice (8), activate macrophages, and induce cytokine production (10). It is unknown whether similar effects occur in primates. It is likely that asymptomatic monkeys remain useful research subjects. However, that remains to be determined. Certainly, clinically affected monkeys would not be suitable for studies involving the enterohepatic and lymphoreticular, or where body weight gain and/or food consumption were measured. It is unknown what effects on intestinal pathologic cytoarchitecture might appear later in life, in primates infected as infants.

Diagnosis and control
Campylobacteriosis may be suspected when infant monkeys develop acute diarrhea. However, since other pathogens may cause similar signs, laboratory confirmation is necessary. This has traditionally been accomplished by special staining of fecal or intestinal smears, by dark-field or phase-contrast microscopy examination for motile forms, and by bacterial culture followed by biochemical testing. Bacterial culture is somewhat complicated by the fact that *Campylobacter* spp. require special growth conditions, including special media and atmospheric conditions (increased CO_2 and decreased O_2). Some species, such as *C. jejuni*, are thermophilic, and grow best at 42°C. This growth characteristic is useful for isolating the organism from other bacteria. More recently, PCR assays have been developed for rapid and accurate diagnosis of campylobacteriosis (2). It is likely that PCR will replace bacterial culture, or will more frequently be used in conjunction with culture. Several antibiotic regimens have been developed for effective treatment of acute campylobacteriosis in particular species of primates. These generally involve oral administration of erythromycin (30 to 50 mg/kg/day for 7 to 10 days) or oxytetracyline (900 mg/liter in drinking water for 10 days) (6). In addition, supportive therapy should be provided, including fluid and electrolyte replacement, prophylactic antibiotics, and provision of supplemental heat if needed. An experimental vaccine has been developed that is efficacious in rhesus macaques (1). However, its routine use in a laboratory animal facility is probably not warranted. Prevention of infection de-

pends on strict adherence to hygienic practices, both for the facility and the personnel.

Shigella flexneri

Agent
Shigella flexneri is a nonmotile, aerobic, and facultatively anaerobic gram-negative rod. Like other members of the genus, *S. flexneri* constitutes a serogroup, and is itself divided into subserotypes that vary in virulence.

Epidemiology
S. flexneri is among the most common bacterial pathogens of captive primates. *S. flexneri* has been recovered from a wide range of both Old and New World primates (2, 5). It is apparent that few wild primates are infected with *S. flexneri*, but that infection rates climb rapidly on entry into captive populations. Because *S. flexneri* survives for only a few days outside of the host, asymptomatic carriers constitute the most important reservoir of endemic infection. Transmission is fecal-oral. *S. flexneri* may be transported by arthropod vectors, as well as on fomites. Because antibody responses are relatively weak, reinfection is common (5).

Clinical signs
Many primates infected with *S. flexneri* are asymptomatic. Factors that facilitate development of clinical disease are incompletely known. Hypovitaminosis C is thought to be a predisposing factor. Virulence factors which promote bacterial invasion and intracellular replication certainly play a role. The hallmark of *S. flexneri* infection is diarrhea. The character of the stool ranges from watery, to pasty, mucoid, bloody, or combinations thereof. Diarrhea may persist for several days. Other common clinical signs include depression, dehydration, weakness, hunched posture, anorexia, vomiting, abortion, hypothermia, nystagmus, pale mucous membranes, weight loss or failure to gain weight, and occasionally, death (5, 13). Clinical disease is more often observed in infants, but even acutely infected adult monkeys may develop serious clinical disease. Severe cytoarchitectural damage to the large intestinal mucosa allows for occurrence of secondary bacterial infections, which themselves are accompanied by a variety of clinical manifestations. Septicemia is a particular danger. Lastly, nonenteric infections with *S. flexneri* occur uncommonly, and include gingivitis and periodontal disease, and intrauterine infection resulting in abortion (11).

Pathology
Following ingestion, *S. flexneri* invades intestinal M cells (16), or is taken up by macropinocytosis. Specific bacterial virulence factors promote attachment, invasion, and ultimately, destruction of the phagosome, allowing for intracytoplasmic replication and spread. In this regard, *S. flexneri* produces several virulence factors, including O-polysaccharide (21), Pic, sigA, and dksA gene products (1, 7, 12), invasion plasmid antigen B (IpaB) (6) and IpaC (14). Each of these facilitate some aspect of bacterial pathogenesis. In addition, release of the proinflammatory cytokine IL-1 triggers the inflammatory reaction which is characteristic of invasive shigellosis (17). Enteric dysfunction is manifested as both a colonic fluid and electrolyte transport defect, as well as fluid hypersecretion (15). Gross lesions include a reddened, thickened, and edematous cecum and colon. Lumenal contents are watery, and frequently contain mucus, blood, and pieces of sloughed intestinal mucosa. On occasion, intussusception of the small intestine and rectal prolapse occur. The latter is likely due to straining during defecation, a common feature of large intestinal diarrheal diseases. Splenic enlargement with subcapsular petechial hemorrhages has been reported occasionally (13). Mesenteric lymph nodes are often enlarged, congested, and edematous (5). Microscopic lesions include cecal inflammation (typhlitis) and colitis, with multifocal ulceration, hemorrhaging, and excessive mucus production (5, 8, 18). The latter, along with bacteria and sloughed epithelial and inflammatory cells, often gives rise to pseudomembrane formation.

Clinicopathologic changes include electrolyte imbalances, intestinal malabsorption, increased white blood cell numbers (leukocytosis), and anemia (5). Humoral immunity develops and is directed at the membrane-associated proteins of *S. flexneri*. Actively acquired immunity protects against development of disease caused by homologous, but not heterologous challenge (3).

Interference with research
Typical of many diseases of higher laboratory animals, surprisingly little is known of the physiologic effects of *S. flexneri*, other than those directly related to enteric pathology. Known effects include electrolyte imbalances, malabsorption, leukocytosis, anemia, acid-base abnormalities, and apoptosis coupled with release of proinflammatory cytokines (6). In other species, the *Shigella* sp. causes CNS dysfunction, renal failure, and respiratory manifestations, in addition to enteritis and problems associated with malnutrition (19). While some of these have been reported in primates infected with *S. flexneri*, it is uncertain whether they were caused by the bacteria, by concurrent infection with another pathogen, or were due to an indirectly related noninfectious cause. Clearly, natural infection of laboratory primates with *S. flexneri* will interfere with studies involving the enterohepatic, hematopoietic, lymphoreticular, and reproductive systems, and may interfere with studies involving the musculoskeletal, nervous, and urinary systems. Studies in which food intake, body weight or weight gains, or behavior are measured will also be compromised. It is likely that asymptomatically infected carrier animals will continue to serve as useful research subjects, if one can consider an animal that serves as a reservoir of infection for others as useful. However, in cases where animals have recovered from clinically significant infections, it should be noted that it is currently unknown what, if any, long-term effects may arise following recovery from clinical disease.

Diagnosis and control
Shigellosis should be suspected when monkeys develop acute diarrhea. However, since other pathogens such as *Yersinia* spp., *Salmonella enterica* serotype Enteritidis, and *Campylobacter jejuni*, may cause similar signs, laboratory confirmation is necessary. This has traditionally been accomplished by colonoscopy with biopsy and immunohistochemical staining (9), fecal or rectal swab culture, and biochemical testing. Sample collection and transport should be discussed with the diagnostic laboratory prior to sample collection to ensure proper handling and maximal potential for pathogen recovery. It is likely that newly developed PCR assays will assume an increasingly important role in diagnosis (4). If treatment of affected animals is elected, it should consist of supportive therapy to replace lost fluid and electrolytes, restoration of acid-base balance, provision of supplemental heat, and nutritional supplementation. Antimicrobial therapy should be based on sensitivity testing where practical. However, enrofloxacin (5 mg/kg orally, once per day) has generally proven efficacious, as has neomycin, trimethoprim sulfamethoxazole, erythromycin, and tetracycline (5). Generally effective strategies for eradication of *S. flexneri* from the animal colony have been published (5). These include the essential components of thorough disinfection of the premises, treatment of all known, or potential carrier animals, and establishment of a test-and-cull system. Testing has traditionally been by bacterial culture. It is anticipated that PCR assay will replace bacterial culture as a first-line test (4). While effective vaccines have been developed for protection against various *Shigella* spp. in experimental applications (20), their widespread use represents a poor substitute for adequate prevention and control strategies undergirded by excellent hygiene. That said, there may be circumstances where it is impossible to eradicate all *Shigella* spp. from the animal environment, and an alternative control strategy is required. Prevention of infection is based on quarantine, testing, and treatment of incoming animals. *S. flexneri* is zoonotic and can cause serious illness, including death, in humans. Therefore, personnel working around potentially infected animals should exercise caution, and strictly adhere to

hygienic practices and standard operating procedures (10).

Streptococcus pneumoniae

Agent
Primates are susceptible to several species of streptococci. Most important among them is *Streptococcus pneumoniae,* an encapsulated, gram-positive, α-hemolytic coccus that frequently occurs in pairs (diplococci). More than 80 serotypes have been identified. Pathogenic streptococci produce M protein, an antiphagocytic protein that interferes with deposition of complement components necessary for opsonization (3). Other, less common streptococcal infections of primates are caused by *Streptococcus zooepidemicus,* and by members of Lancefield groups A, B, and C (6).

Epidemiology
Typical of the α-hemolytic streptococci, *S. pneumoniae* is a common commensal in the upper respiratory tracts of many species of primates, as well as humans (1). There is a paucity of prevalence surveys of primates. However, it is thought that asymptomatic carriers are common. In contrast, the incidence of clinical disease is low, but compared with other causes of disease, can be significant, especially in infant monkeys (10). Transmission is by aerosol contamination.

Clinical signs
As noted above, many primates live as asymptomatic carriers of *S. pneumoniae*. Clinical disease results when immunologic protection is compromised by concurrent viral infection or waning maternal immunity in infants; or when animals experience significant stress, including that associated with capture, transportation, and quarantine (6). Typical clinical signs have been best described in macaques, and are associated with acute and fulminating onset of CNS disease, specifically, meningoencephalitis. Signs include depression, head pressing, incoordination, circling, seizures, constricted and poorly responsive pupils, nystagmus, slowed reflexes, muscle tremors, flaccid paralysis of the legs, rigidity of the neck (typical of meningeal disease), coma, and frequently, death within 1 to 3 days (6). However, other clinical presentations have been reported. These often accompany signs of CNS dysfunction, and include respiratory distress secondary to pneumonia, purulent nasal discharge, conjunctivitis, ocular discomfort; and a spectrum of signs associated with septicemia, such as hypothermia, slowed capillary refill time indicative of hypotension, and withdrawal to the back of the cage (6). In some cases, death occurs acutely, without evidence of other signs (7). Chimpanzees and squirrel monkeys present with clinical disease somewhat differently, and first present with fever, coughing, head tilt secondary to purulent otitis interna, tonsillitis, and seromucoid to mucopurulent nasal discharge. These cases often rapidly progress to include CNS signs similar to those described above (2, 11). Animals that recover generally do so within a few days to two weeks.

Pathology
Following inhalation exposure, bacterial cell wall components facilitate adherence and invasion of mucosal surfaces. Hematogenous spread disseminates *S. pneumoniae,* which preferentially colonizes the cerebral and/or cerebellar meninges. Gross lesions include accentuated meningeal vasculature, meningeal petechiae, and the presence of variously colored exudates on the brain surface and within the ventricles. Microscopically, meningoencephalitis is apparent as severe fibrinopurulent leptomeningitis, necrotizing vasculitis, thrombosis, and ischemic necrosis. Lesions may extend to the spinal cord (6). In addition to these lesions, animals may experience pneumonia; panophthalmitis; septicemia; disseminated intravascular coagulation; and suppurative arthritis, peritonitis, nephritis, lymphadenitis, and myocarditis. These lesions are all indicative of septicemic spread (6, 8). The streptococcal toxin pneumolysin is largely responsible for promoting inflammation and neutrophil activation, a hallmark of streptococcal disease

(4). Pulmonary lesions are particularly common, and consist primarily of congestion, edema, and purulent bronchopneumonia. Clinicopathologic changes include leukocytosis and increased protein in the cerebrospinal fluid (6). Production of anti-M-protein antibodies facilitate opsonization and destruction of *S. pneumoniae,* allowing clearing of infection. Recovered animals are at least temporarily immune to reinfection.

Interference with research
Little has been reported of the effects of *S. pneumoniae* on primate physiology, beyond what should be obvious on the basis of disease presentations. *S. pneumoniae* has been shown to increase glucose utilization and circulating levels of phenylalanine, the latter indicative of skeletal muscle catabolism (12). In other species, *S. pneumoniae* has cytotoxic effects within the auditory system (5), and stimulates neutrophils to produce an oxidative burst, increase expression of CD-18 (9) and increase release of IL-8 (4). At the least, natural infection of laboratory primates with *S. pneumoniae* may preclude use of animals in research involving the cardiovascular, nervous, and respiratory systems. Septicemic spread may result in primates being completely unusable for any research studies, but certainly those involving the hematopoietic, lymphoreticular, musculoskeletal, and urinary systems. Asymptomatic carrier animals remain useful research subjects.

Diagnosis and control
Infection with *S. pneumoniae* may be suspected with acute onset of CNS signs. Of course there are other bacteria capable of causing similar signs, including *Klebsiella pneumoniae, Pasteurella multocida, Haemophilus influenzae,* and *Neisseria meningitidis* (6). Therefore, laboratory confirmation is necessary. Unfortunately, given the rapid course of the disease, and the generally unfavorable response to antibiotic therapy, a diagnosis is often made postmortem. However, antimortem diagnosis may be accomplished by recovery of the organism in CSF, blood, or respiratory secretions. Demonstration of the organism in tissues, or following growth on blood agar, are confirmatory. It should be noted that streptococci may lose their gram-positive staining when removed from lesions. As noted above, individual animal treatment is often unrewarding. The antibiotics most likely to affect recovery are penicillin and ceftriaxone (6). Antibiotic treatment should be augmented by supportive therapies, including control of seizure activity, and maintenance of fluid and electrolyte balance, and body temperature in cases of hypothermia. It is likely not practical to eliminate all *S. pneumoniae* carriers from the animal colony. Prevention of clinical disease is through reduction of stress among colony animals, and by maintaining high standards of facility cleanliness. *S. pneumoniae* is commonly carried in the mouths of humans, particularly where oral hygiene is neglected (1). Caretakers and others handling primates should practice good oral hygiene to minimize exposure of animals during periods of high stress, such as experimental procedures.

PARASITES

Balantidium coli

Agent
Balantidium coli is a protozoan parasite and member of the Class *Ciliophora*. Most members of the Class are free living and nonparasitic, or are parasitic and symbiotic. In contrast, *B. coli* occasionally causes disease in a wide range of host species, including nonhuman and human primates, pigs, dogs, and experimentally, in others (3).

Epidemiology
Infection of primates with *B. coli* is extremely common (3). *B. coli* infection has been reported in both New and Old World primates, as well as in the great apes (5), and has historically been cited as the most common parasitism diagnosed in the latter (1). As the name suggests, the *Ciliophora* possess cilia for locomotion. They also have two nuclei: a large, kidney-shaped macronucleus and an adjacent and smaller micronucleus. The former is re-

sponsible for cytoplasmic activities while the latter is responsible for asexual reproduction. Trophozoites are oval, and measure 50 to 60 μm in length, although larger forms up to 150 μm in length occasionally occur. Cilia are arranged longitudinally over the trophozoite, and a mouth, or peristome is situated near the anterior end. Cysts are ovoid to spherical, generally measure 40 to 60 μm in length, and are passed in the feces (4). While transmission usually occurs orally by infectious cysts, trophozoites survive up to 3 days in optimal conditions, and are likewise infective.

Clinical signs
The majority of infections with *B. coli* are asymptomatic. Infection of the great apes, however, can lead to severe enteric disease. Clinical signs include weight loss, anorexia, muscle weakness, lethargy, watery diarrhea, straining to defecate, and occasionally along with the latter, rectal prolapse (2, 5).

Pathology
B. coli colonizes the large intestine where it usually causes no pathologic changes. In great apes, however, infection may result in ulcerative enterocolitis, with ulcers extending to the muscularis mucosae. Lymphocytes infiltrate around the lesions. Lesions may be hemorrhagic and coagulation necrosis present (5). Trophozoites are easily recognized within the lesions. It should be noted that *B. coli* may be associated with disease, but secondary to other, primary causes of enterocolitis. In humans, *B. coli* has in addition, rarely been reported in association with pulmonary, peritoneal, urogenital, or hepatic lesions. It remains unknown whether similar aberrant infections occur in laboratory primates.

Interference with research
It is probable that asymptomatic infections with *B. coli* will not compromise the usefulness of affected animals. This is likely to be the case in Old and New World primates. However, definitive data on the subject are lacking. Certainly, natural and clinical infection of great apes will compromise their usefulness as research subjects in studies involving the enterohepatic and musculoskeletal systems, as well as in studies where body weight or activity levels are assessed. Because *B. coli* is sometimes associated with intestinal hemorrhaging, severe infection may also affect studies involving the hematopoietic system. In this regard, some humans infected with *B. coli* experience bloodloss anemia in addition to nutrient malabsorption.

Diagnosis and control
Balantidiasis may be diagnosed by finding the rapidly moving trophozoites in fresh fecal wet mounts. Similarly, trophozoites are readily identified in histologic section. Asymptomatic infections may also be detected using fecal wet mounts and stained fecal preparations, although trophozoite numbers will be lower. It should be noted that simply finding *B. coli* in the feces of primates with diarrhea does not affirm causality. A diligent search should be made for other infectious and noninfectious causes of diarrhea. Clinical balantidiasis should be treated with metronidazole, tetracycline, or diiodohydroxyquin (1, 5). It is unrealistic to expect that primates can be obtained, or remain free of infection with *B. coli*. Preventive efforts should be directed toward sanitation, which will minimize the environmental burden of *B. coli* and of other pathogens. *B. coli* cysts are relatively environmentally resistant, and survive for several days under optimal conditions of moisture and cool temperatures, while the trophozoites are more readily destroyed. Because *B. coli* is capable of causing disease in humans, personnel working with laboratory primates of all kinds, but especially with clinically affected apes, should practice personal protection.

Entamoeba histolytica

Agent
Laboratory primates are susceptible to several species of amoebae, including *Entamoeba histolytica, E. hartmanii, E. coli, E. dispar, E. chattoni, Iodamoeba buetschlii, I. wallacei, Endolimax nana,* and others (15, 16). Most of these are

considered nonpathogenic and will not be discussed further. In contrast, *E. histolytica* is known to cause disease in several species of primates. For a more thorough discussion of *E. histolytica* amebiasis, including an extensive list of references, the interested reader is referred elsewhere (16).

Epidemiology
On a worldwide basis, amoebic infection is quite common in Old World laboratory primates (15). The majority of infections are asymptomatic. In contrast, infections of New World primates are less common but more often clinically significant. *E. histolytica* trophozoites live on the lumenal surface of the large intestine, principally the cecum and colon. Trophozoites represent the feeding form. Trophozoites are 10 to 60 μm in diameter, contain a single spherical nucleus 4 to 7 μm in diameter that contains a distinct central endosome about 0.5 μm in diameter. The endosome is surrounded by a clear zone and the nuclear membrane is lined with fine chromatin granules, so that it appears that the nucleus is lined by a ring of beads. The nuclear morphology is characteristic of the species, and is a very useful diagnostic indicator. Trophozoites may contain food vacuoles containing ingested red blood cells. While the latter feature is commonly cited for differentiating *E. histolytica* from similarly appearing nonpathogenic species, it is often difficult to observe, and requires examination of many trophozoites. It should also be noted that mixed infections are common, so that a diagnosis should not rest on examination of just a few amoebae. Cysts are round, and smaller than trophozoites, roughly 5 to 20 μm in diameter. Immature cysts contain glycogen vacuoles that stain brown with iodine. Glycogen vacuoles disappear as the cyst matures. Cysts form in the large intestine and contain up to four nuclei when fully mature. Once again, the number of nuclei is diagnostically important. Cysts also contain rod-shaped, deeply staining chromatoid bodies. Cysts may mature while in the large intestine, or may pass in the feces and mature to become infectious outside the body. Ingestion of infectious cysts is followed by release of daughter trophozoites, thereby establishing the infection (14). Transmission is only by the fecal-oral route. This may occur through direct ingestion of contaminated feces, or by exposure to contaminated fomites. In addition, flies and cockroaches may serve as mechanical vectors for *E. histolytica*. Infant macaques acquire infection from their mothers between 5 and 10 weeks of age (12).

Clinical signs
As noted above, most infections with *E. histolytica* are asymptomatic in adult Old World primates (1). Factors responsible for mucosal invasion, which leads to clinical disease, are incompletely known. It is thought that potential factors include host species, nutritional status, and the resident intestinal bacterial flora; parasite virulence which varies by strain; and environmental factors (7, 8, 16). In contrast, infant Old World primates, as well as all New World primates, are more likely to develop primary disease. In all cases, clinical disease results in amebic dysentery, which by traditional definition includes abdominal pain, straining during defecation or attempts at defecation, and frequent stools containing blood and mucus. In addition to these, affected monkeys are lethargic and apathetic, weak, dehydrated, lose weight, vomit, and have diarrhea (16).

Pathology
Following ingestion, *E. histolytica* becomes established in the cecum and colon. So long as amoebae do not penetrate the mucosal epithelium, no pathology occurs. However, mucosal invasion results in pathologic changes. Invasion appears to be facilitated by enteric bacteria (9). Lesions include necro-ulcerative colitis and typhlitis, with characteristic flask-shaped mucosal lesions that extend to the muscularis mucosae. There may be hemorrhages with neutrophilic and mononuclear infiltrates. Secondary bacterial enteritis may further exacerbate inflammatory lesions. In se-

vere cases, ulceration may extend through the full thickness of the intestinal wall, resulting in peritonitis. In rare cases, trophozoites gain access to the lymphatic and/or vascular systems, and disseminate hematogenously. In these cases, amebic abscesses may develop in virtually any organ. Most commonly, abscesses occur in the liver, lung, and brain (16). However, there are human case reports of amebic salpingitis (3) and pericarditis (6), cutaneous amebiasis (2), and others. *E. histolytica* elicits a cellular immune response that limits disease but only partially protects against reinfection (17).

Interference with research
There is little information published on the physiologic effects of *E. histolytica* in laboratory primates. In other species, *E. histolytica* elevates liver enzymes when hepatic abscesses are present (13), indirectly causes suppression of host T- and B-cell lymphoproliferation (4) and class II MHC antigen expression (19), modulates macrophage activation (20) and locomotion (10), is cytopathic (8), stimulates IL-8 release from colonic epithelial cells (22), retards fetal growth even in asymptomatic infections (21), and causes lymphoreticular changes (5). Because lesions develop in some asymptomatic monkeys, all natural infections of laboratory primates with *E. histolytica* are likely to affect host physiology to some degree. In asymptomatic animals, effects may be limited to the intestinal tract. In more severe cases, the lymphoreticular system will be affected. In cases of amebic abscess formation, physiologic effects will depend on abscess distribution, but could include physiologic alterations that alter studies involving the enterohepatic, nervous, and respiratory systems. However, because trophozoites may disseminate hematogenously, virtually any body system may be involved.

Diagnosis and control
A diagnosis of amoebic dysentery may be suspected on the basis of clinical signs. Confirmation is obtained by recovery of motile trophozoites in wet mounts prepared from fresh, warm stool samples or large intestinal mucosal scrapings. Additionally, trophozoites in feces or tissues may be identified using a number of stains, including Lugol's iodine, periodic acid-Schiff, trichrome, Giemsa, and iron hematoxylin (16). Examination for morphologic features listed above is essential. In this regard, postmortem invasion of cecal mucosa occurs within an hour of death, by nonpathogenic *E. chattoni,* and may falsely suggest infection by *E. histolytica* (18). PCR assays have been developed to facilitate differentiation between *E. histolytica* and the morphologically similar but nonpathogenic *E. dispar* (11). It should be noted that the finding of amoebae in the stool of animals with enteritis does not by itself confer causality. A thorough search should be conducted for other causes of large intestinal disease (16). Generally effective therapies have been developed for treatment of affected animals (16). These are essentially similar to treatments used to eliminate infection from humans. Personnel working with laboratory primates, particularly New World primates, should know that asymptomatic human infections are common. Special attention needs to be paid toward personal hygiene, especially when handling primate food. Conversely, personnel should be careful to avoid inadvertent exposure to potentially contaminated primate feces, as amebic dysentery and/or amebic abscesses can occur in humans. Prevention of infection of both humans and laboratory primates therefore rests on sanitation practices, including vermin control. *E. histolytica* trophozoites are inactivated by common disinfectants, but cysts are more environmentally resistant, and require hot water or steam for inactivation (16).

Strongyloides spp.

Agent
Primates are susceptible to infection with several species of nematodes in the genus *Strongyloides*. These include *S. cebus, S. fulleborni, S. stercoralis,* and others (12). Among these, in-

fection in the laboratory animal setting is probably most commonly due to *S. fulleborni* in macaques and great apes, and *S. stercoralis* in chimpanzees. Members of the genus live in the environment as nonparasitic, male or female saprophytic worms that reproduce sexually, or as parasitic, parthenogenetic females in the host small intestine. Species parasitizing primates are small, delicate worms generally only a few millimeters in length.

Epidemiology
Infection of primates, including New and Old World monkeys, as well as great apes, is quite common (6, 12). This is especially true where animals are housed on the ground, or where sanitation is inadequate. In the host, parthenogenetic female worms are found buried in the mucosa of the small intestine. There, they release embryonated eggs. For *S. stercoralis*, these hatch nearly immediately, so that first-stage larvae are passed in the feces. Otherwise, eggs hatch in the environment, releasing larvae. Depending on local environmental conditions, larvae develop into either nonparasitic male and female worms, or infectious larvae destined to develop into parasitic female worms. Development to the infectious stage is rapid, requiring as little as 24 h (11). Infection of the host occurs by direct penetration of the oral or esophageal mucous membranes, or compromised skin. Skin conditions are suitably unhealthy when animals are chronically housed in warm, wet, and/or filthy environments. Larvae that penetrate the skin are carried in the blood to the lungs, are coughed up and swallowed, and thereafter end up in the intestine. The prepatent period is 5 to 7 days. In *S. stercoralis* of humans, hyperinfection or autoinfection occur. The former occurs when first-stage larvae rapidly mature to infective third-stage larvae prior to evacuation with the feces. The third-stage larvae are able to penetrate the intestinal mucosa, and undergo systemic migration. Autoinfection occurs when third-stage larvae penetrate the skin of the perineum and undergo systemic migration. It is uncertain whether similar events occur in laboratory primates (11). It is assumed that intrauterine and/or transmammary transmission may occur in primates infected with *Strongyloides* spp. (10). However, the extent to which this occurs has not been determined.

Clinical signs
In most cases, infection with *Strongyloides* spp. is subclinical. In some cases, however, particularly in macaques and the great apes, clinical disease develops. In other host species, infection with *Strongyloides* spp. is more severe in males due to the physiologic effects of testosterone (5). It has yet to be determined whether similar sex differences occur in primate infections. Clinical signs include focal dermatitis, urticaria, hemorrhagic or mucoid diarrhea, anorexia, depression, listlessness, debilitation, vomiting, weight loss or failure to gain weight, dehydration, constipation, labored breathing, coughing, prostration, and occasionally, death (4, 9, 12).

Pathology
Infection with *Strongyloides* spp. proceeds through three phases, namely, invasion, migration, and the intestinal phase (9). During the intestinal phase, worms bury in the intestinal mucosa, where they and their products elicit a profound inflammatory response consisting predominantly of neutrophils and monocytes. Their presence results in severe necrotizing enteritis, occasionally with secondary peritonitis. Intestinal lesions are characterized by focal erosion, ulceration, and hemorrhaging. Intestinal villi are blunted and the normal villous architecture is lost. Larval penetration of the large intestine during hyperinfection results in similar inflammatory changes in that organ. Larval invasion of regional lymphatics results in granulomatous lymphangitis, which may lead to development of regional edema and/or lymphatic fibrosis. The larval migratory phase also causes pulmonary lesions consisting of focal hemorrhages, with granuloma formation (4, 12). Aberrant migration of larvae may result in granulomatous lesions in numerous visceral

TABLE 11-1. Body systems known or likely to be affected by pathogen indicated

Pathogen	Cardio-vascular	Dermal	Endocrine	Entero-hepatic	Hema-topoietic	Lympho-reticular	Musculo-skeletal	Nervous	Reproductive	Respiratory	Urinary
Hepatitis B virus				×		×					
Herpesvirus		×	×	×		×				×	
Respiratory syncytial virus						×				×	
Rotavirus				×							
Simian hemorrhagic fever virus	×	×		×	×	×		×	×	×	×
Simian immunodeficiency virus	×	×		×	×	×		×	×	×	×
Simian retrovirus type D				×	×	×		×	×		
Simian T-cell leukemia virus	×	×		×	×	×				×	
Simian virus 40								×		×	×
Campylobacter spp.				×		×					
Shigella flexneri				×	×	×	×	×	×		×
Streptococcus pneumoniae	×						×	×		×	×
Balantidium coli				×	×		×				
Entamoeba histolytica				×		×		×		×	
Strongyloides spp.		×		×	×	×				×	

organs, most commonly, the liver (8). Immunity involves both cellular and humoral components, as well as nonimmune mechanisms within the small intestine (1, 3).

Interference with research

The point at which worm burdens affect host physiology is, as in so many cases, completely unknown. It is likely that extremely mild infections will not compromise the usefulness of primate research subjects. However, there is certainly a point at which the parasite burden ceases to be truly "subclinical," and affects host physiology. In addition to the obvious effects of clinical strongyloidiasis on the dermal, enterohepatic, lymphoreticular, and respiratory systems, infections of laboratory primates with *Strongyloides* spp. are known to affect the hematopoietic system by causing anemia, basophilia, and eosinophilia (4). Concerning the latter, human infection with *S. stercoralis* induces eosinophilia. In combination, the two appear to affect survival of patients with adult T-cell leukemia (7), suggesting that natural infection of primates with *Strongyloides* spp. might influence studies on STLV-1 infections. In addition to these, natural infection may influence studies in which activity levels are measured. Aberrant infection of visceral organs could compromise research efforts involving those organ systems.

Diagnosis and control

Diagnosis of strongyloidiasis is based on finding large numbers of characteristic, embryonated eggs in the feces. It should be noted that the fecal egg count indicates the level of infection but is not prognostic of clinical outcome (4). Cutaneous lesions may also suggest infection. Clinical cases should be treated supportively as needed, and should receive anthelmintics. Currently, anthelmintic treatment most commonly consists of ivermectin (200 μg/kg i.m.), repeated after 3 weeks as needed (12). It is the routine use of ivermectin that has decreased the incidence of infection in laboratory-housed primates. Other anthelmintics, particularly the benzimidazoles, are also effective (12). Incoming animals should be examined for infection with *Strongyloides* spp., and infected animals likewise treated. Prevention of clinical disease centers around an excellent sanitation program and the provision of dry resting areas. It should be recalled that under optimal conditions infective larvae develop in as little as 24 h, necessitating daily removal of feces. Humans are susceptible to infection with *S. fulleborni, S. stercoralis,* and probably others (2). Therefore, caretakers and others working closely with laboratory primates should use caution, although transmission to humans is unlikely so long as personnel do not have areas of compromised skin that comes in contact with contaminated feces.

REFERENCES

INTRODUCTION

1. **Adams, S. R., E. Muchmore, and J. H. Richardson.** 1995. Biosafety, p. 375–420. *In* B. T. Bennett, C. R. Abee, and R. Henrickson (ed.), *Nonhuman Primates in Biomedical Research. Biology and Management.* Academic Press, Inc., San Diego, Calif.
2. **Gibson, S. V.** 1998. Bacterial and mycotic diseases, p. 59–110. *In* B. T. Bennett, C. R. Abee, and R. Henrickson (ed.), *Nonhuman Primates in iomedical Research. Diseases.* Academic Press, Inc., San Diego, Calif.
3. **Mansfield, K., and N. King.** 1998. Viral diseases, p. 1–57. *In* B. T. Bennett, C. R. Abee, and R. Henrickson (ed.), *Nonhuman Primates in Biomedical Research. Diseases.* Academic Press, Inc., San Diego, Calif.
4. **Toft, J. D., II, and M. L. Eberhard.** 1998. Parasitic diseases, p. 111–205. *In* B. T. Bennett, C. R. Abee, and R. Henrickson (ed.), *Nonhuman Primates in Biomedical Research. Diseases.* Academic Press, Inc., San Diego, Calif.

VIRUSES

Hepatitis B virus
1. **Bancroft, W. H., R. Snitbhan, R. M. Scott, M. Tingpalonpong, W. T. Watson, P. Tanticharoenyos, J. J. Karwacki, and S. Srimarut.** 1977. Transmission of hepatitis B virus to gibbons by exposure to human saliva containing hepatitis B surface antigen. *J. Infect. Dis.* **135:**79–85.
2. **Dienstag, J. L., H. Popper, and R. H. Purcell.** 1976. The pathology of viral hepatitis types

A and B in chimpanzees. *Am. J. Pathol.* **85:**131–148.
3. **Guidotti, L. G., R. Rochford, J. Chung, M. Shapiro, R. Purcell, and F. V. Chisari.** 1999. Viral clearance without destruction of infected cells during acute HBV infection. *Science.* **284:**825–829.
4. **Hu, X., A. Javadian, P. Gagneux, and B. H. Robertson.** 2001. Paired chimpanzee hepatitis B virus (ChHBV) and mtDNA sequences suggest different ChHBV genetic variants are found in geographically distinct chimpanzee subspecies. *Virus Res.* **79:**103–108.
5. **Karasawa, T., T. Shikata, K. Abe, R. Kondo, M. Noro, and T. Oda.** 1985. Ultrastructural studies on liver cell necrosis and lymphocytes in experimental hepatitis B. *Acta. Pathol. Jpn.* **35:**1359–1374.
6. **Kornegay, R. W., W. E. Giddens, Jr., G. L. Van Hoosier, Jr., and W. R. Morton.** 1985. Subacute nonsuppurative hepatitis associated with hepatitis B infection in two cynomolgus monkeys. *Lab. Anim. Sci.* **35:**400–404.
7. **Lafrado, L. J., M. A. Javadian, J. M. Marr, K. A. Wright, J. C. Kelliher, C. S. Dezzutti, L. Cummins, and R. G. Olsen.** 1991. Lymphocyte and neutrophil dysfunction associated with hepatitis B virus and hepatitis non-A, non-B virus infection in the chimpanzee. *J. Med. Primatol.* **20:**302–307.
8. **Lieberman, H. M., W. W. Tung, and D. A. Shafritz.** 1987. Splenic replication of hepatitis B virus in the chimpanzee chronic carrier. *J. Med. Virol.* **21:**347–359.
9. **Mansfield, K., and N. King.** 1998. Viral diseases, p. 1–57. *In* B. T. Bennett, C. R. Abee, and R. Henrickson (ed.), *Nonhuman Primates in Biomedical Research. Diseases.* Academic Press, Inc., San Diego, Calif.
10. **Prince, A. M., R. Whalen, and B. Brotman.** 1997. Successful nucleic acid based immunization of newborn chimpanzees against hepatitis B virus. *Vaccine* **15:**916–919.
11. **Scalise, G., M. R. Mazaheri, J. Kremastinou, C. R. Howard, K. Sorensen, and A. J. Zuckerman.** 1978. Transmission of hepatitis B to the rhesus monkey. Studies on the humoral and cell-mediated immune response. *J. Med. Primatol.* **7:**114–118.
12. **Scott, R. M., R. Snitbhan, W. H. Bancroft, H. J. Alter, and M. Tingpalapong.** 1980. Experimental transmission of hepatitis B virus by semen and saliva. *J. Infect. Dis.* **142:**67–71.
13. **Sly, D. L., W. T. London, and R. H. Purcell.** 1979. Illness in a chimpanzee inoculated with hepatitis B virus. *J. Am. Vet. Med. Assoc.* **175:**987–988.

Herpesvirus
1. **Carlson, C. S., M. G. O'Sullivan, M. J. Jayo, D. K. Anderson, E. S. Harber, W. G. Jerome, B. C. Bullock, and R. L. Heberling.** 1997. Fatal disseminated cercopithecine herpesvirus 1 (herpes B) infection in cynomolgus monkeys (*Macaca fascicularis*). *Vet. Pathol.* **34:**405–414.
2. **Holmes, G. P., L. E. Chapman, J. A. Stewart, S. E. Strauss, J. K. Hilliard, and D. S. Davenport.** 1995. Guidelines for the prevention and treatment of B-virus infections in exposed persons. The B virus Working Group. *Clin. Infect. Dis.* **29:**421–439.
3. **Mansfield, K., and N. King.** 1998. Viral diseases, p. 1–57. *In* B. T. Bennett, C. R. Abee, and R. Henrickson (ed.), *Nonhuman Primates in Biomedical Research. Diseases.* Academic Press, Inc., San Diego, Calif.
4. **Simon, M. A., M. D. Daniel, D. Lee-Parritz, N. W. King, and D. J. Ringler.** 1993. Disseminated B virus infection in a cynomolgus monkey. *Lab. Anim. Sci.* **43:**545–550.
5. **Ward, J. A., and J. K. Hilliard.** 2002. Herpes B virus-specific pathogen-free breeding colonies of macaques: serologic test results and the B-virus status of the macaque. *Contemp. Top. Lab. Anim. Sci.* **41:**36–41.
6. **Weigler, B. J., D. W. Hird, J. K. Hilliard, N. W. Lerche, J. A. Roberts, and L. M. Scott.** 1993. Epidemiology of Cercopithecine herpesvirus 1 (B virus) infection and shedding in a large breeding cohort of rhesus macaques. *J. Infect. Dis.* **167:**257–263.
7. **Weigler, B. J., F. Scinicariello, and J. K. Hilliard.** 1995. Risk of venereal B virus (cercopithecine herpesvirus 1) transmission in rhesus monkeys using molecular epidemiology. *J. Infect. Dis.* **171:**1139–1143.
8. **Weir, E. C., P. N. Bhatt, R. O. Jacoby, J. K. Hilliard, and S. Morgenstern.** 1993. Infrequent shedding and transmission of *Herpesvirus simiae* from seropositive macaques. *Lab. Anim. Sci.* **43:**541.

Repiratory syncytial virus
1. **Belshe, R. B., L. S. Richardson, W. T. London, D. T. Sly, J. H. Lorfeld, E. Camargo, D. A. Prevar, and R. M. Chanock.** 1977. Experimental respiratory syncytial virus infection of four species of primates. *J. Med. Virol.* **1:**157–162.
2. **Brown, G., H. W. Rixon, and R. J. Sugrue.** 2002. Respiratory syncytial virus assembly occurs in GM1-rich regions of the host-cell membrane and alters the cellular distribution of tyrosine phosphorylated caveolin-1. *J. Gen. Virol.* **83:**1841–1850.
3. **Clarke, C. J., N. J. Watt, A. Meredith, N. McIntyre, and S. M. Burns.** 1994. Respiratory

syncytial virus-associated bronchopneumonia in a young chimpanzee. *J. Comp. Pathol.* **110:**207–212.

4. Hickling, T. P., R. Malhotra, H. Bright, W. McDowell, E. D. Blair, and R. B. Sim. 2000. Lung surfactant protein A provides a route of entry for respiratory syncytial virus into host cells. *Viral Immunol.* **13:**125–135.

5. Jaovisidha, P., M. E. Peeples, A. A. Brees, L. R. Carpenter, and J. N. Moy. 1999. Respiratory syncytial virus stimulates neutrophil degranulation and chemokine release. *J. Immunol.* **163:**2816–2820.

6. Johnston, I. D. 1999. Effect of pneumonia in childhood on adult lung function. *J. Pediatr.* **135:**33–37.

7. Mansfield, K., and N. King. 1998. Viral diseases, p. 1–57. *In* B. T. Bennett, C. R. Abee, and R. Henrickson (ed.), *Nonhuman Primates in Biomedical Research. Diseases*. Academic Press, Inc., San Diego, Calif.

8. Mastronarde, J. G., B. He, M. M. Monick, N. Mukaida, K. Matsushima, and G. W. Hunninghake. 1996. Induction of interleukin (IL)-8 gene expression by respiratory syncytial virus involves activation of nuclear factor (NF)-κB and NF-IL-8. *J. Infect. Dis.* **174:**262–267.

9. McArthur-Vaughan, K., and L. J. Gershwin. 2002. A rhesus monkey model of respiratory syncytial virus infection. *J. Med. Primatol.* **31:**61–73.

10. McBride, J. T. 1999. Pulmonary function changes in children after respiratory syncytial virus infection in infancy. *J. Pediatr.* **135:**28–32.

11. Ponnuraj, E. M., A. R. Hayward, A. Raj, H. Wilson, and E. A. Simoes. 2001. Increased replication of respiratory syncytial virus (RSV) in pulmonary infiltrates is associated with enhanced histopathological disease in bonnet monkeys (*Macaca radiata*) pre-immunized with a formalin-inactivated RSV vaccine. *J. Gen. Virol.* **82:**2663–2674.

12. Raza, M. W., C. C. Blackwell, R. A. Elton, and D. M. Weir. 2000. Bactericidal activity of a monocytic cell line (THP-1) against common respiratory tract bacterial pathogens is depressed after infection with respiratory syncytial virus. *J. Med. Microbiol..* **49:**227–233.

13. Schlender, J., G. Walliser, J. Fricke, and K. K. Conzelmann. 2002. Respiratory syncytial virus fusion protein mediates inhibition of mitogen-induced T-cell proliferation by contact. *J. Virol.* **76:**1163–1170.

14. Simoes, E. A., A. R. Hayward, E. A. Ponnuraj, J. P. Straumanis, K. R. Stenmark, H. L. Wilson, and P. G. Babu. 1999. Respiratory syncytial virus infects the Bonnet monkey, *Macaca radiata*. *Pediatr. Dev. Pathol.* **2:**316–326.

15. Smee, D. F., and T. R. Matthews. 1986. Metabolism of ribavirin in respiratory syncytial virus-infected and uninfected cells. *Antimicrob. Agents Chemother.* **30:**117–121.

16. Tripp, R. A., D. Moore, J. Winter, and L. J. Anderson. 2000. Respiratory syncytial virus infection and G and/or SH protein expression contribute to substance P, which mediates inflammation and enhanced pulmonary disease in BALB/c mice. *J. Virol.* **74:**1614–1622.

17. Weltzin, R., V. Traina-Dorge, K. Soike, J. Y. Zhang, P. Mack, G. Soman, G. Drabik, and T. P. Monath. 1996. Intranasal monoclonal IgA antibody to respiratory syncytial virus protects rhesus monkeys against upper and lower respiratory tract infection. *J. Infect. Dis.* **174:**256–261.

Rotavirus

1. Halaihel, N., V. Lievin, J. M. Ball, M. K. Estes, F. Alvarado, and M. Vasseur. 2000. Direct inhibitory effect of rotavirus NSP4 (114-135) peptide on the Na^+-D-glucose symporter of rabbit intestinal brush border membrane. *J. Virol.* **74:**9464–9470.

2. Hjelt, K., P. C. Grauballe, A. Paerregaard, O. H. Nielsen, and P. A. Krasilnikoff. 1987. Protective effect of preexisting rotavirus-specific immunoglobulin A against naturally acquired rotavirus infection in children. *J. Med. Virol.* **21:**39–47.

3. Katyal, R., S. V. Rana, K. Vaiphei, S. Ohja, K. Singh, and V. Singh. 1999. Effect of rotavirus infection on small gut pathophysiology in a mouse model. *J. Gastroenterol. Hepatol.* **14:**779–784.

4. Katyal, R., S. Rana, K. Vaiphei, S. Ojha, V. Singh, and K. Singh. 2001. Effect of rotavirus infection on lipid composition and glucose uptake in infant mouse intestine. *Indian J. Gastroenterol.* **20:**18–21.

5. Mansfield, K., and N. King. 1998. Viral diseases, p. 1–57. *In* B. T. Bennett, C. R. Abee, and R. Henrickson (ed.), *Nonhuman Primates in Biomedical Research. Diseases*. Academic Press, Inc., San Diego, Calif.

6. Michelangeli, F., M. C. Ruiz, J. R. del Castillo, J. E. Ludert, and F. Liprandi. 1991. Effect of rotavirus infection on intracellular calcium homeostasis in cultured cells. *Virology* **181:**520–527.

7. Mitchell, J. D., L. A. Lambeth, L. Sosula, A. Murphy, and M. Albrey. 1977. Transmission of rotavirus gastroenteritis from children to a monkey. *Gut* **18:**156–160.

8. Moe, K., and G. J. Harper. 1983. The effect of relative humidity and temperature on the sur-

vival of bovine rotavirus in aerosol. *Arch. Virol.* **76:**211–216.
9. **Ojeh, C. K., T. M. Cusack, and R. H. Yolken.** 1995. Evaluation of the effects of disinfectants on rotavirus RNA and infectivity by the polymerase chain reaction and cell-culture methods. *Mol. Cell. Probes* **9:**341–346.
10. **Soike, K. F., G. W. Gary, and S. Gibson.** 1980. Susceptibility of nonhuman primate species to infection by simian rotavirus SA-11. *Am. J. Vet. Res.* **41:**1098–1103.
11. **Thouless, M. E., R. F. DiGiacomo, and B. J. Deeb.** 1996. The effect of combined rotavirus and *Escherichia coli* infections in rabbits. *Lab. Anim. Sci.* **46:**381–385.
12. **Unicomb, L. E., S. M. Faruque, M. A. Malek, A. S. Faruque, and M. J. Albert.** 1996. Demonstration of a lack of synergistic effect of rotavirus with other diarrheal pathogens on severity of diarrhea in children. *J. Clin. Microbiol.* **34:**1340–1342.
13. **Weclewicz, K., K. Kristensson, and L. Svensson.** 1994. Rotavirus causes selective vimentin reorganization in monkey kidney CV-1 cells. *J. Gen. Virol.* **75:**3267–3271.
14. **Winiarczyk, S., and Z. Gradzki.** 1999. Comparison of polymerase chain reaction and dot hybridization with enzyme-linked immunoassay, virological examination and polyacrylamide gel electrophoresis for the detection of porcine rotavirus in faecal specimens. *Zentbl. Vetmed. Reihe B* **46:**623–634.
15. **Wyatt, R. G., D. L. Sly, W. T. London, A. E. Palmer, A. R. Kalica, D. H. Kirk, R. M. Chanock, and A. Z. Kapikian.** 1976. Induction of diarrhea in colostrum deprived newborn rhesus monkeys with the human reovirus-like agent in infantile gastroenteritis. *Arch. Virol.* **50:**17–27.
16. **Zhang, M., C. Q. Zeng, A. P. Morris, and M. K. Estes.** 2000. A functional NSP4 enterotoxin peptide secreted from rotavirus-infected cells. *J. Virol.* **74:**11663–11670.

Simian hemorrhagic fever virus
1. **Allen, A. M., A. E. Palmer, N. M. Tauraso, and A. Shelokov.** 1968. Simian hemorrhagic fever. II. Studies in pathology. *Am. J. Trop. Med. Hyg.* **17:**413–421.
2. **Godeny, E. K.** 2002. Enzyme-linked immunosorbent assay for detection of antibodies against simian hemorrhagic fever virus. *Comp. Med.* **52:**229–232.
3. **Gravell, M., W. T. London, M. Leon, A. E. Palmer, and R. W. Hamilton.** 1986. Elimination of persistent simian hemorrhagic fever (SHF) virus infection in patas monkeys. *Proc. Soc. Exp. Biol. Med.* **181:**219–225.
4. **Gravell, M., A. E. Palmer, M. Rodriguez, W. T. London, and R. S. Hamilton.** 1980. Method to detect asymptomatic carriers of simian hemorrhagic fever virus. *Lab. Anim. Sci.* **30:**988–991.
5. **London, W. T.** 1977. Epizootology, transmission and approach to prevention of fatal simian hemorrhagic fever virus in rhesus monkeys. *Nature (London)* **268:**344–345.
6. **Mansfield, K., and N. King.** 1998. Viral diseases, p. 1–57. *In* B. T. Bennett, C. R. Abee, and R. Henrickson (ed.), *Nonhuman Primates in Biomedical Research. Diseases.* Academic Press, Inc., San Diego, Calif.
7. **Palmer, A. E., A. M. Allen, N. M. Tauraso, and S. Shelokov.** 1968. Simian hemorrhagic fever. I. Clinical and epizootiologic aspects of an outbreak among quarantined monkeys. *Am. J. Trop. Med. Hyg.* **17:**404–412.
8. **Renquist, D.** 1990. Outbreak of simian hemorrhagic fever. *J. Med. Primatol.* **19:**77–80.
9. **Weiland, E., and F. Weiland.** 2002. Autoantibodies against golgi apparatus induced by arteriviruses. *Cell. Mol. Biol.* **48:**279–284.

Simian immunodeficiency viruses
1. **Alpers, C. E., C. C. Tsai, K. L. Hudkins, Y. Cui, L. Kuller, R. E. Benveniste, J. M. Ward, and W. R. Morton.** 1997. Focal segmental glomerulosclerosis in primates infected with a simian immunodeficiency virus. *AIDS Res. Hum. Retrovir.* 13:413–424.
2. **Baskerville, A., A. D. Ramsay, B. J. Addis, M. J. Dennis, R. W. Cook, M. P. Cranage, and P. J. Greenaway.** 1992. Interstitial pneumonia in simian immunodeficiency virus infection. *J. Pathol.* **167:**241–247.
3. **Baskin, G. B., M. Murphey-Corb, L. N. Martin, B. Davison-Fairburn, F. S. Hu, and D. Kuebler.** 1991. Thymus in simian immunodeficiency virus-infected rhesus monkeys. *Lab. Investig.* **65:**400–407.
4. **Chalifoux, L. V., M. A. Simon, D. R. Pauley, J. J. MacKey, M. S. Wyand, and D. J. Ringler.** 1992. Arteriopathy in macaques infected with simian immunodeficiency virus. *Lab. Investig.* **67:**338–349.
5. **Chen, Z., P. Zhou, D. D. Ho, N. R. Landau, and P. A. Marx.** 1997. Genetically divergent strains of simian immunodeficiency virus use CCR5 as a coreceptor for entry. *J. Virol.* **71:**2705–2714.
6. **Desrosiers, R. C.** 1990. HIV-1 origins, a finger on the missing link. *Nature* **345:**288–289.
7. **Gerber, M. A., M. L. Chen, F. S. Hu, G. B. Baskin, and L. Petrovich.** 1991. Liver disease in rhesus monkeys infected with simian immu-

nodeficiency virus. *Am. J. Pathol.* **139:**1081–1088.

8. Gold, L. H., H. S. Fox, S. J. Henriksen, M. J. Buchmeier, M. R. Weed, M. S. Taffe, S. Huitron-Resendiz, T. F. Horn, and F. E. Bloom. 1998. Longitudinal analysis of behavioral, neurophysiological, viral and immunological effects of SIV infection in rhesus monkeys. *J. Med. Primatol.* **27:**104–112.

9. Hayami, M., E. Ido, and T. Miura. 1994. Survey of simian immunodeficiency virus among nonhuman primate populations. *Curr. Top. Microbiol. Immunol.* **188:**1–20.

10. Heise, C., P. Vogel, C. J. Miller, C. H. Halsted, and S. Dandekar. 1993. Simian immunodeficiency virus infection of the gastrointestinal tract of rhesus macaques. Functional, pathological, and morphological changes. *Am. J. Pathol.* **142:**1759–1771.

11. Kestens, L., J. Vingerhoets, M. Peeters, G. Vanham, C. Vereecken, G. Penne, H. Niphuis, P. van Eerd, G. van der Groen, P. Gigase, and J. Heeney. 1995. Phenotypic and functional parameters of cellular immunity in a chimpanzee with a naturally acquired simian immunodeficiency virus infection. *J. Infect. Dis.* **172:**957–963.

12. Kewenig, S., T. Schneider, K. Hohloch, K. Lampe-Dreyer, R. Ullrich, N. Stolte, C. Stahl-Hennig, F. J. Kaup, A. Stallmach, and M. Zeitz. 1999. Rapid mucosal CD4$^+$ T-cell depletion and enteropathy in simian immunodeficiency virus-infected rhesus macaques. *Gastroenterology* **116:**1115–1123.

13. Lackner, A. A. 1994. Pathology of simian immunodeficiency virus induced disease. *Curr. Top. Microbiol. Immunol.* **188:**35–64.

14. Larimore, M. D., J. E. Kaplan, M. D. Daniel, N. W. Lerche, P. L. Nara, H. M. McClure, J. W. McVivar, R. W. McKinney, M. Hendry, P. Gerone, M. Rayfield, J. Allan, J. L. Ribas, H. J. Klein, P. B. Jahrling, and B. Brown. 1989. Guidelines for the prevention of simian immunodeficiency virus infection in laboratory workers and handlers. *J. Med. Primatol.* **18:**167–174.

15. Lerche, N. W., J. L. Yee, and M. B. Jennings. 1994. Establishing specific retrovirus-free breeding colonies of macaques: An aproach to primary screening and surveillance. *Lab. Anim. Sci.* **44:**217–221.

16. Mansfield, K., and N. King. 1998. Viral diseases, p. 1–57. *In* B. T. Bennett, C. R. Abee, and R. Henrickson (ed.), *NonhumanPrimates in Biomedical Research. Diseases.* Academic Press, Inc., San Diego, Calif.

17. Mansfield, K. G., K. C. Lin, J. Newman, D. Schauer, J. MacKey, A. A. Lackner, and A. Carville. 2001. Identification of enteropathogenic *Escherichia coli* in simian immunodeficiency virus-infected infant and adult rhesus macaques. *J. Clin. Microbiol.* **39:**971–976.

18. McClure, M. O., T. F. Schulz, R. S. Tedder, J. Gow, J. A. McKeating, R. A. Weiss, and A. Baskerville. 1989. Inoculation of new world primates with human immunodeficiency virus. *J. Med. Primatol.* **18:**329–335.

19. Miller, C. J., P. Vogel, N. J. Alexander, S. Dandekar, A. G. Hendrickx, and P. A. Marx. 1994. Pathology and localization of simian immunodeficiency virus in the reproductive tract of chronically infected male rhesus macaques. *Lab. Investig.* **70:**255–262.

20. Montgomery, M. M., A. F. Dean, F. Taffs, E. J. Stott, P. L. Lantos, and P. J. Luthert. 1999. Progressive dendritic pathology in cynomolgus macaques infected with simian immunodeficiency virus. *Neuropathol. Appl. Neurobiol.* **25:**11–19.

21. Munch, J., N. Stolte, D. Fuchs, C. Stahl-Hennig, and F. Kirchhoff. 2001. Efficient class I major histocompatibility complex downregulation by simian immunodeficiency virus Nef is associated with a strong selective advantage in infected rhesus macaques. *J. Virol.* **75:**10532–10536.

22. Nadler, R. D., A. D. Manocha, and H. M. McClure. 1993. Spermatogenesis and hormone levels in rhesus macaques inoculated with simian immunodeficiency virus. *J. Med. Primatol.* **22:**325–329.

23. Poaty-Mavoungou, V., F. S. Toure, C. Tevi-Benissan, and E. Mavoungou. 2002. Enhancement of natural killer cell activation and antibody-dependent cellular cytotoxicity by interferon-alpha and interleukin-12 in vaginal mucosae SIVmac251-infected *Macaca fascicularis*. *Viral Immunol.* **15:**197–212.

24. Pope, T. W., L. Raymond, L. Foresman, D. Pinson, S. V. Joag, J. Marcario, N. E. Berman, R. Raghavan, P. D. Cheney, O. Narayan, S. Wilkinson, and M. A. Gordon. 1997. Texture analysis of cerebral white matter in SIV-infected macaque monkeys. *J. Neurosci. Methods* **74:**53–64.

25. Shannon, R. P., M. A. Simon, M. A. Mathier, Y. J. Geng, S. Mankad, and A. A. Lackner. 2000. Dilated cardiomyopathy associated with simian AIDS in nonhuman primates. *Circulation* **101:**185–193.

26. Sopper, S., M. Demuth, C. Stahl-Hennig, G. Hunsmann, R. Plesker, C. Coulibaly, S. Czub, M. Ceska, E. Koutsilieri, P. Riederer,

R. Brinkmann, M. Katz, and V. ter Meulen. 1996. The effect of simian immunodeficiency virus infection in vitro and in vivo on the cytokine production of isolated microglia and peripheral macrophages from rhesus monkey. *Virology* **220**:320–329.
27. Westmoreland, S. V., E. Halpern, and A. A. Lackner. 1998. Simian immunodeficiency virus encephalitis in rhesus macaques is associated with rapid disease progression. *J. Neurovirol.* **4**:260–268.
28. Zimmer, M. I., A. T. Larregina, C. M. Castillo, S. Capuano III, L. D. Falo, Jr., M. Murphey-Corb, T. A. Reinhart, and S. M. Barratt-Boyes. 2002. Disrupted homeostasis of Langerhans cells and interdigitating dendritic cells in monkeys with AIDS. *Blood* **99**:2859–2868.

Simian retrovirus type D
1. Cheung, A. T., and M. B. Gardner. 1991. Functional deficiency of polymorphonuclear leukocytes in simian acquired immunodeficiency syndrome. *Am. J. Vet. Res.* **52**:1523–1526.
2. Fikes, J. D., and M. G. O'Sullivan. 1995. Localized retroperitoneal fibromatosis causing intestinal obstruction in a cynomolgus monkey (*Macaca fascicularis*). *Vet. Pathol.* **32**:713–716.
3. Guzman, R. E., R. L. Kerlin, and T. E. Zimmerman. 1999. Histologic lesions in cynomolgus monkeys (*Macaca fascicularis*) naturally infected with simian retrovirus type D: comparison of seropositive, virus-positive, and uninfected animals. *Toxicol. Pathol.* **27**:672–677.
4. Heyes, M. P., M. Gravell, W. T. London, M. Eckhaus, J. H. Vickers, J. A. Yergey, M. April, D. Blackmore, and S. P. Markey. 1990. Sustained increases in cerbrospinal fluid quinolinic acid concentrations in rhesus macaques (*Macaca mulatta*) naturally infected with simian retrovirus type-D. *Brain Res.* **531**:148–158.
5. Kwang, H. S., N. C. Pedersen, N. W. Lerche, K. G. Osborn, P. A. Marx, and M. B. Gardner. 1987. Viremia, antigenemia, and serum antibodies in rhesus macaques infected with simian retrovirus type 1 and their relationship to disease course. *Lab. Investig.* **56**:591–597.
6. Lackner, A. A., M. Schiodt, G. C. Armitage, P. E. Moore, R. J. Munn, P. A. Marx, M. G. Gardner, and L. J. Lowenstine. 1989. Mucosal epithelial cells and langerhans cells are targets for infection by the immunosuppressive type D retrovirus Simian AIDS retrovirus serotype 1. *J. Med. Primatol.* **18**:195–207.
7. Mansfield, K., and N. King. 1998. Viral diseases, p. 1–57. *In* B. T. Bennett, C. R. Abee, and R. Henrickson (ed.), *Nonhuman Primates in Biomedical Research. Diseases.* Academic Press, Inc., San Diego, Calif.
8. Maul, D. H., C. P. Zaiss, M. R. Mackenzie, S. M. Shigi, P. A. Marx, and M. G. Gardner. 1988. Simian retrovirus D serotype 1 has a broad cellular tropism for lymphoid and nonlymphoid cells. *J. Virol.* **62**:1768–1773.
9. Moazed, T. C., and M. E. Thouless. 1993. Viral persistence of simian type D retrovirus (SRV-2/W) in naturally infected pigtailed macaques (*Macaca nemestrina*). *J. Med. Primatol.* **22**:382–389.
10. Osborn, K. G., S. Prahalada, L. J. Lowenstine, M. B. Gardner, D. H. Maul, and R. V. Henrickson. 1984. The pathology of an epizootic of acquired immunodeficiency in rhesus macaques. *Am. J. Pathol.* **114**:94–103.
11. Paramastri, Y. A., J. M. Wallace, K. J. Salleng, L. M. Wilkinson, D. E. Malarkey, and J. M. Cline. 2002. Intracranial lymphomas in simian retrovirus-positive *Macaca fascicularis*. *Vet. Pathol.* **39**:399–402.
12. Roodman, S. T., M. D. Woon, J. W. Hoffman, P. Theodorakis, C. C. Tsai, H. N. Wu, and C. C. Tsai. 1991. Interleukin-6 and retroperitoneal fibromatosis from SRV-2-infected macaques with simian AIDS. *J. Med. Primatol.* **20**:201–205.
13. Schroder, M. A., S. K. Fisk, and N. W. Lerche. 2000. Eradication of simian retrovirus type D from a colony of cynomolgus, rhesus, and stump-tailed macaques by using serial testing and removal. *Contemp. Top. Lab. Anim. Sci.* **39**:16–23.
14. Tsai, C. C., K. E. Follis, K. Snyder, S. Windsor, M. E. Thouless, L. Kuller, and W. R. Morton. 1990. Maternal transmission of type D simian retrovirus (SRV-2) in pigtailed macaques. *J. Med. Primatol.* **19**:203–216.
15. Wang, Y., and M. E. Thouless. 1996. Use of polymerase chain reaction for diagnosis of type D retrovirus infection in macaque blood. *Lab. Anim. Sci.* **46**:187–192.
16. Wilson, B. J., S. M. Shiigi, J. L. Zeigler, L. C. Olson, A. Malley, and C. F. Howard, Jr. 1986. Transmission of simian acquired immunodeficiency syndrome with a type D retrovirus: immunological aspects. *Clin. Immunol. Immunopathol.* **41**:453–460.

Simian T-cell leukemia virus
1. Dezzutti, C. S., D. E. Frazier, and R. G. Olsen. 1990. Efficacy of an HTLV-1 subunit vaccine in prevention of a STLV-1 infection in pig-tailed macaques. *Dev. Biol. Stand.* **72**:287–296.
2. Gessain, A., and R. Mahieux. 2000. Epidemiology, origin and genetic diversity of HTLV-1 retroviruses and STLV-1 simian affiliated retroviruses. *Bull. Soc. Pathol. Exot.* **93**:163–171.

3. Hubbard, G. B., J. P. Moné, J. S. Allan, K. J. Davis III, M. M. Leland, P. M. Banks, and B. Smir. 1993. Spontaneously generated non-Hodgkin's lymphoma in twenty-seven simian T-cell leukemia virus type 1 antibody-positive baboons (*Papio* species). *Lab. Anim. Sci.* **43:**301–309.
4. Lerche, N. W., J. L. Yee, and M. B. Jennings. 1994. Establishing specific retrovirus-free breeding colonies of macaques: An aproach to primary screening and surveillance. *Lab. Anim. Sci.* **44:**217–221.
5. Liska, V., P. N. Fultz, L. Su, and R. M. Ruprecht. 1997. Detection of simian T-cell leukemia virus type 1 infection in seronegative macaques. *AIDS Res. Hum. Retrovir.* **13:**1147–1153.
6. Mahieux, R., C. Chapey, M. C. Georges-Courbot, G. Dubreuil, P. Mauclere, A. Georges, and A. Gessain. 1998. Simian T-cell lymphotropic virus type 1 from *Mandrillus sphinx* as a simian counterpart of human T-cell lymphotropic virus type 1 subtype D. *J. Virol.* **72:**10316–10322.
7. Mansfield, K., and N. King. 1998. Viral diseases, p. 1–57. *In* B. T. Bennett, C. R. Abee, and R. Henrickson (ed.), *Nonhuman Primates in Biomedical Research. Diseases*. Academic Press, Inc., San Diego, Calif.
8. McCarthy, T. J., J. L. Kennedy, J. R. Blakeslee, and B. T. Bennett. 1990. Spontaneous malignant lymphoma and leukemia in a simian T-lymphotropic virus type 1 (STLV-1) antibody positive olive baboon. *Lab. Anim. Sci.* **40:**79–81.
9. Noda, Y., K. Ishikawa, A. Sasagawa, S. Honjo, S. Mori, H. Tsujimoto, and M. Hayami. 1986. Hematologic abnormalities similar to the preleukemic state of adult T-cell leukemia in African green monkeys naturally infected with simian T-cell leukemia virus. *Jpn. J. Cancer Res.* **77:**1227–1234.
10. Takemura, T., M. Yamashita, M. K. Shimada, S. Ohkura, T. Shotake, M. Ikeda, T. Miura, and M. Hayami. 2002. High prevalence of simian T-lymphotropic virus type L in wild ethiopian baboons. *J. Virol.* **76:**1642–1648.
11. Voevodin, A., E. Samilchuk, H. Schatzl, E. Boeri, and G. Franchini. 1996. Interspecies transmission of macaque simian T-cell leukemia/lymphoma virus type 1 in baboons resulted in an outbreak of malignant lymphoma. *J. Virol.* **70:**1633–1639.

Simian virus 40
1. Andrei, G., R. Snoeck, M. Vandeputte, and E. De Clercq. 1997. Activities of various compounds against murine and primate polyomaviruses. *Antimicrob. Agents Chemother.* **41:**587–593.
2. Horvath, C. J., M. A. Simon, D. J. Bergsagel, D. R. Pauley, N. W. King, R. L. Garcea, and D. J. Ringler. 1992. Simian virus 40-induced disease in rhesus monkeys with simian acquired immunodeficiency syndrome. *Am. J. Pathol.* **140:**1431–1440.
3. Hurley, J. P., P. O. Ilyinskii, C. J. Horvath, and M. A. Simon. 1997. A malignant astrocytoma containing simian virus 40 DNA in a macaque infected with simian immunodeficiency virus. *J. Med. Primatol.* **26:**172–180.
4. Mansfield, K., and N. King. 1998. Viral diseases, p. 1–57. *In* B. T. Bennett, C. R. Abee, and R. Henrickson (ed.), *Nonhuman Primates in Biomedical Research. Diseases*. Academic Press, Inc., San Diego, Calif.
5. Newman, J. S., G. B. Baskin, and R. J. Frisque. 1998. Identification of SV40 in brain, kidney and urine of healthy and SIV-infected rhesus macaques. *J. Neurovirol.* **4:**394–406.
6. Simon, M. A., P. O. Ilyinskii, G. B. Baskin, H. Y. Knight, D. R. Pauley, and A. A. Lackner. 1999. Association of simian virus 40 with a central nervous system lesion distinct from progressive multifocal leukoencephalopathy in macaques with AIDS. *Am. J. Pathol.* **154:**437–446.

BACTERIA

Campylobacter spp.
1. Baqar, S., A. L. Bourgeois, P. J. Schultheiss, R. I. Walker, D. M. Rollins, R. L. Haberberger, and O. R. Pavlovskis. 1995. Safety and immunogenicity of a prototype oral whole-cell killed *Campylobacter* vaccine administered with a mucosal adjuvant in non-human primates. *Vaccine* **13:**22–28.
2. Englen, M. D., and L. C. Kelley. 2000. A rapid DNA isolation procedure for the identification of *Campylobacter jejuni* by the polymerase chain reaction. *Lett. Appl. Microbiol.* **31:**421–426.
3. Everest, P. H., A. T. Cole, C. J. Hawkey, S. Knutton, H. Goossens, J. P. Butzler, J. M. Ketley, and P. H. Williams. 1993. Roles of leukotrienes B_4, prostaglandin E_2, and cyclic AMP in *Campylobacter jejuni*-induced intestinal fluid secretion. *Infect. Immun.* **61:**4885–4887.
4. Fitzgeorge, R. B., A. Baskerville, and K. P. Lander. 1981. Experimental infection of rhesus monkeys with a human strain of *Campylobacter jejuni*. *J. Hyg.* **86:**343–351.
5. George, J. W., and N. W. Lerche. 1990. Electrolyte abnormalities associated with diarrhea in rhesus monkeys: 100 cases (1986-1987). *J. Am. Vet. Med. Assoc.* **196:**1654–1658.
6. Gibson, S. V. 1998. Bacterial and mycotic diseases, p. 59–110. *In* B. T. Bennett, C. R. Abee, and R. Henrickson (ed.), *Nonhuman Primates in*

Biomedical Research. Diseases. Academic Press, Inc., San Diego, Calif.

7. **Klipstein, F. A., R. F. Engert, H. Short, and E. A. Schenk.** 1985. Pathogenic properties of *Campylobacter jejuni*: Assay and correlation with clinical manifestations. *Infect. Immun.* **50:**43–49.
8. **Lyte, M., J. J. Varcoe, and M. T. Bailey.** 1998. Anxiogenic effect of subclinical bacterial infection in mice in the absence of overt immune activation. *Physiol. Behav.* **65:**63–68.
9. **O'Sullivan, A. M., C. J. Dore, S. Boyle, C. R. Coid, and A. P. Johnson.** 1988. The effect of *Campylobacter* lipopolysaccharide on fetal development in the mouse. *J. Med. Microbiol.* **26:**101–105.
10. **Pancorbo, P. L., M. A. de Pablo, E. Ortega, A. M. Gallego, C. Alvarez, and G. Alvarez de Cienfuegos.** 1999. Evaluation of cytokine production and phagocytic activity in mice infected with *Campylobacter jejuni*. *Curr. Microbiol.* **39:**129–133.
11. **Russell, R. G., M. J. Blaser, J. I. Sarmiento, and J. Fox.** 1989. Experimental *Campylobacter jejuni* infection in *Macaca nemestrina*. *Infect. Immun.* **57:**1438–1444.
12. **Russell, R. G., M. O'Donnoghue, D. C. Blake, Jr., J. Zulty, and L. J. DeTolla.** 1993. Early colonic damage and invasion of *Campylobacter jejuni* in experimentally challenged infant *Macaca mulatta*. *J. Infect. Dis.* **168:**210–215.
13. **Russell, R. G., S. L. Rosenkranz, L. A. Lee, H. Howard, R. F. DiGiacomo, M. A. Bronsdon, G. A. Blakley, C. C. Tsai, and W. R. Morton.** 1987. Epidemiology and etiology of diarrhea in colony-born *Macaca nemestrina*. *Lab. Anim. Sci.* **37:**309–316.
14. **Torres, O., and J. R. Cruz.** 1993. Protection against *Campylobacter* diarrhea: role of milk IgA antibodies against bacterial surface antigens. *Acta Paediatr.* **82:**835–838.

Shigella flexneri

1. **Al-Hasani, K., I. R. Henderson, H. Sakellaris, K. Rajakumar, T. Grant, J. P. Nataro, R. Robins-Browne, and B. Adler.** 2000. The sigA gene which is borne on the she pathogenicity island of *Shigella flexneri* 2a encodes an exported cytopathic protease involved in intestinal fluid accumulation. *Infect. Immun.* **68:**2457–2463.
2. **Banish, L. D., R. Sims, D. Sack, R. J. Montali, L. Phillips, Jr., and M. Bush.** 1993. Prevalence of shigellosis and other enteric pathogens in a zoologic collection of primates. *J. Am. Vet. Med. Assoc.* **203:**126–132.
3. **Formal, S. B., E. V. Oaks, F. E. Olsen, M. Wingfield-Eggleston, P. J. Snoy, and J. P. Cogan.** 1991. Effect of prior infection with virulent *Shigella flexneri* 2a on the resistance of monkeys to subsequent infection with *Shigella sonnei*. *J. Infect. Dis.* **164:**533–537.
4. **Frankel, G., L. Riley, J. A. Giron, J. Valmassoi, A. Friedmann, N. Strockbine, S. Falkow, and G. K. Schoolnik.** 1990. Detection of *Shigella* in feces using DNA amplification. *J. Infect. Dis.* **161:**1252–1256.
5. **Gibson, S. V.** 1998. Bacterial and mycotic diseases, p. 59–110. *In* B. T. Bennett, C. R. Abee, and R. Henrickson (ed.), *Nonhuman Primates in Biomedical Research. Diseases.* Academic Press, Inc., San Diego, Calif.
6. **Guichon, A., D. Hersh, M. R. Smith, and A. Zychlinsky.** 2001. Structure-function analysis of the *Shigella* virulence factor IpaB. *J. Bacteriol.* **183:**1269–1276.
7. **Henderson, I. R., J. Czeczulin, C. Eslava, F. Noriega, and J. P. Nataro.** 1999. Characterization of pic, a secreted protease of *Shigella flexneri* and enteroaggregative *Escherichia coli*. *Infect. Immun.* **67:**5587–5596.
8. **Karnell, A., F. P. Reinholt, S. Katakura, and A. A. Lindberg.** 1991. *Shigella flexneri* infection: a histopathologic study of colonic biopsies in monkeys infected with virulent and attenuated bacterial strains. *APMIS* **99:**787–796.
9. **Katakura, S., F. P. Reinholt, A. Karnell, P. T. Huan, D. D. Trach, and A. A. Lindberg.** 1990. The pathology of *Shigella flexneri* infection in rhesus monkeys: an endoscopic and histopathological study of colonic lesions. *APMIS* **98:**313–319.
10. **Kennedy, F. M., J. Astbury, J. R. Needham, and T. Cheasty.** 1993. Shigellosis due to occupational contact with non-human primates. *Epidemiol. Infect.* **110:**247–251.
11. **McClure, H. M., P. Alford, and B. Swenson.** 1976. Nonenteric *Shigella* infections in nonhuman primates. *J. Am. Vet. Med. Assoc.* **169:**938–939.
12. **Mogull, S. A., L. J. Runyen-Janecky, M. Hong, and S. M. Payne.** 2001. dksA is required for intercellular spread of *Shigella flexneri* via an RpoS-independent mechanism. *Infect. Immun.* **69:**5742–5751.
13. **Mulder, J. B.** 1971. Shigellosis in nonhuman primates: A review. *Lab. Anim. Sci.* **21:**734–738.
14. **Picking, W. L., L. Coye, J. C. Osiecki, A. Barnoski Serfis, E. Schaper, and W. D. Picking.** 2001. Identification of functional regions within invasion plasmid antigen C (IpaC) of *Shigella flexneri*. *Mol. Microbiol.* **39:**100–111.
15. **Rout, W. R., S. B. Formal, R. A. Giannella, and G. J. Dammin.** 1975. Pathophysiology of *Shigella* diarrhea in the rhesus monkey: intestinal

transport, morphological, and bacteriological studies. *Gastroenterology* **68**:270–278.
16. **Sansonetti, P. J., J. Arondel, J. R. Cantey, M. C. Prevost, and M. Huerre.** 1996. Infection of rabbit Peyer's patches by *Shigella flexneri*: effect of adhesive or invasive bacterial phenotypes on follicle-associated epithelium. *Infect. Immun.* **64**:2752–2764.
17. **Sansonetti, P. J., J. Arondel, J. M. Cavaillon, and M. Huerre.** 1995. Role of interleukin-1 in pathogenesis of experimental shigellosis. *J. Clin. Invest.* **96**:884–892.
18. **Takeuchi, A.** 1982. Early colonic lesions in experimental *Shigella* infection in rhesus monkeys: revisited. *Vet. Pathol. Suppl.* **7**:1–8.
19. **Thapa, B. R., K. Ventkateswarlu, A. K. Malik, and D. Panigrahi.** 1995. Shigellosis in children from north India: a clinicopathological study. *J. Trop. Pediatr.* **41**:303–307.
20. **Venkatesan, M. M., A. B. Hartman, J. W. Newland, V. S. Ivanova, T. L. Hale, M. McDonough, and J. Butterton.** 2002. Construction, characterization, and animal testing of WRSd1, an *Shigella dysenteriae* 1 vaccine. *Infect. Immun.* **70**:2950–2958.
21. **Zhong, Q. P.** 1999. Pathogenic effects of O-polysaccharide from *Shigella flexneri* strain. *World J. Gastroenterol.* **5**:245–248.

Streptococcus pneumoniae
1. **Abe, S., K. Ishihara, and K. Okuda.** 2001. Prevalence of potential respiratory pathogens in the mouths of elderly patients and effects of professional oral care. *Arch. Gerontol. Geriatr.* **32**:45–55.
2. **Berendt, R. F., G. C. Long, and J. S. Walker.** 1975. Influenza alone and in sequence with pneumonia due to *Streptococcus pneumoniae* in the squirrel monkey. *J. Infect. Dis.* **132**:689–693.
3. **Biberstein, E. L., and D. C. Hirsh** 1999. Streptococci, p. 120–126. *In* D. C. Hirsh and Y. C. Zee (ed.), *Veterinary Microbiology*. Blackwell Science, Inc., Malden, Mass.
4. **Cockeran, R., C. Durandt, C. Feldman, T. J. Mitchell, and R. Anderson.** 2002. Pneumolysin activates the synthesis and release of interleukin-8 by human neutrophils in vitro. *J. Infect. Dis.* **186**:562–565.
5. **Comis, S. D., M. P. Osborne, J. Stephen, M. J. Tarlow, T. L. Hayward, T. J. Mitchell, P. W. Andrew, and G. J. Boulnois.** 1993. Cytotoxic effects on hair cells of guinea pig cochlea produced by pneumolysin, the thiol activated toxin of *Streptococcus pneumoniae*. *Acta Otolaryngol.* **113**:152–159.
6. **Gibson, S. V.** 1998. Bacterial and mycotic diseases, p. 59–110. *In* B. T. Bennett, C. R. Abee, and R. Henrickson (ed.), *Nonhuman Primates in Biomedical Research. Diseases*. Academic Press, Inc., San Diego, Calif.
7. **Graczyk, T. K., M. R. Cranfield, S. E. Kempske, and M. A. Eckhaus.** 1995. Fulminant *Streptococcus pneumoniae* meningitis in a lion-tailed macaque (*Macaca silenus*) without detected signs. *J. Wildl. Dis.* **31**:75–78.
8. **Hawley, H. B., T. Yamada, D. F. Mosher, D. P. Fine, and R. F. Berendt.** 1977. Disseminated intravascular coagulopathy during experimental pneumococcal sepsis: studies in normal and asplenic rhesus monkeys. *J. Med. Primatol.* **6**:203–218.
9. **Kragsbjerg, P., and H. Fredlund.** 2001. The effects of live *Streptococcus pneumoniae* and tumor necrosis factor-alpha on neutrophil oxidative burst and beta 2-integrin expression. *Clin. Microbiol. Infect.* **7**:125–129.
10. **Padovan, D., and C. Cantrell.** 1980. Causes of death of infant rhesus and squirrel monkeys. *J. Am. Vet. Med. Assoc.* **183**:1182–1184.
11. **Solleveld, H. A., M. J. van Zwieten, P. J. Heidt, and P. M. van Eerd.** 1984. Clinicopathologic study of six cases of meningitis and meningoencephalitis in chimpanzees (*Pan troglodytes*). *Lab. Anim. Sci.* **34**:86–90.
12. **Wannemacher, R. W., Jr., F. A. Beall, P. G. Canonico, R. E. Dinterman, C. L. Hadick, and H. A. Neufeld.** 1980. Glucose and alanine metabolism during bacterial infections in rats and rhesus monkeys. *Metabolism.* **29**:201–212.

PARASITES

Balantidium coli
1. **Cummins, L. B., M. E. Keeling, and H. M. McClure.** 1973. Preventive medicine in anthropoids: parasite control. *Lab. Anim. Sci.* **23**:819–822.
2. **Lee, R. V., A. W. Prowten, S. Anthone, S. K. Satchidanand, J. E. Fisher, and R. Anthone.** 1990. Typhlitis due to *Balantidium coli* in captive lowland gorillas. *Rev. Infect. Dis.* **12**:1052–1059.
3. **Nakauchi, K.** 1999. The prevalence of *Balantidium coli* infection in fifty-six mammalian species. *J. Vet. Med. Sci.* **61**:63–65.
4. **Soulsby, E. J. L.** 1982. *Helminths, Arthropods and Protozoa of Domesticated Animals*, 7th ed., p. 660–661. Lea & Febiger, Philadelphia, Pa.
5. **Toft, J. D., II, and M. L. Eberhard.** 1998. Parasitic diseases, p. 111–205. *In* B. T. Bennett, C. R. Abee, and R. Henrickson (ed.), *Nonhuman Primates in Biomedical Research. Diseases*. Academic Press, Inc., San Diego, Calif.

Entamoeba histolytica
1. **Beaver, P. C., J. L. Blanchard, and H. R. Seibold.** 1988. Invasive amebiasis in naturally in-

fected New World and Old World monkeys with and without clinical disease. *Am. J. Trop. Med. Hyg.* **39:**343–352.
2. **Beaver, P. C., A. L. Villegas, C. Cuello, and A. D'Allessandro.** 1978. Cutaneous amebiasis of the eyelid with extension into the orbit. *Am. J. Trop. Med. Hyg.* **27:**1133–1136.
3. **Calore, E. E., N. M. Calore, and M. J. Cavaliere.** 2002. Salpingitis due to *Entamoeba histolytica*. *Braz. J. Infect. Dis.* **6:**97–99.
4. **Campbell, D., D. Gaucher, and K. Chadee.** 1999. Serum from *Entamoeba histolytica*-infected gerbils selectively suppresses T cell proliferation by inhibiting interleukin-2 production. *J. Infect. Dis.* **179:**1495–1501.
5. **Chadee, K., and E. Meerovitch.** 1985. *Entamoeba histolytica:* lymphoreticular changes in gerbils (*Meriones unguiculatus*) with experimentally induced cecal amebiasis. *J. Parasitol.* **71:**566–575.
6. **Chao, T. H., Y. H. Li, L. M. Tsai, J. K. Teng, L. J. Lin, and J. H. Chen.** 1998. Amebic liver abscess complicated with cardiac tamponade and mediastinal abscess. *J. Formos. Med. Assoc.* **97:**214–216.
7. **Ghosh, P. K., S. Gupta, S. Naik, A. Ayyagari, and S. R. Naik.** 1998. Effect of bacterial association on virulence of *Entamoeba histolytica* to baby hamster kidney cell monolayers. *Indian J. Exp. Biol.* **36:**911–915.
8. **Gomes, M. A., M. N. Melo, G. P. Pena, and E. F. Silva.** 1997. Virulence parameters in the characterization of strains of *Entamoeba histolytica*. *Rev. Inst. Med. Trop. Sao Paulo* **39:**65–69.
9. **Leroy, A., G. De Bruyne, A. Verspeelt, T. Lauwaet, H. Nelis, and M. Mareel.** 1997. Bacterium-assisted invasion of *Entamoeba histolytica* through human enteric epithelia in two-compartment chambers. *Invasion Metastasis* **17:**138–148.
10. **Rico, G., O. Diaz-Guerra, and R. R. Kretschmer.** 1995. Cyclic nucleotide changes induced in human leukocytes by a product of axenically grown *Entamoeba histolytica* that inhibits human monocyte locomotion. *Parasitol. Res.* **81:**158–162.
11. **Rivera, W. L., and H. Kanbara.** 1999. Detection of *Entamoeba dispar* DNA in macaque feces by polymerase chain reaction. *Parasitol. Res.* **85:**493–495.
12. **Sakakibara, I., Y. Sugimoto, T. Koyama, and S. Honjo.** 1982. Natural transmission of *Entamoeba histolytica* from mother cynomolgus monkeys (*Macaca fascicularis*) to their newborn infants under indoor rearing conditions. *Jikken Dobutsu* **31:**135–138.
13. **Sanchez-Ramirez, B., S. Mata-Gonzalez, A. Valdez, E. Ramos-Martinez, and P. Talamas-Rohana.** 2001. Liver function tests during amoebic liver abscess formation in indomethacin-treated hamsters. *J. Exp. Zool.* **290:**201–206.
14. **Soulsby, E. J. L.** 1982. *Helminths, Arthropods and Protozoa of Domesticated Animals,* 7th ed., p. 660–661. Lea & Febiger, Philadelphia, Pa.
15. **Tachibana, H., X. J. Cheng, S. Kobayashi, N. Matsubayashi, S. Gotoh, and K. Matsubayashi.** 2001. High prevalence of infection with *Entamoeba diapar*, but not *E. histolytica*, in captive macaques. *Parasitol. Res.* **87:**14–17.
16. **Toft, J. D., II, and M. L. Eberhard.** 1998. Parasitic diseases, p. 111–205. *In* B. T. Bennett, C. R. Abee, and R. Henrickson (ed.), *Nonhuman Primates in Biomedical Research. Diseases.* Academic Press, Inc., San Diego, Calif.
17. **Trissl, D.** 1982. Immunology of *Entamoeba histolytica* in human and animal hosts. *Rev. Infect. Dis.* **4:**1154–1184.
18. **Vogel, P., G. Zaucha, S. D. Goodwin, K. Kuehl, and D. Fritz.** 1996. Rapid postmortem invasion of cecal mucosa of macaques by nonpathogenic *Entamoeba chattoni*. *Am. J. Trop. Med. Hyg.* **55:**595–602.
19. **Wang, W., and K. Chadee.** 1995. *Entamoeba histolytica* suppresses gamma interferon-induced macrophage class II major histocompatibility complex Ia molecule and I-Aβ mRNA expression by a prostaglandin E$_2$-dependent mechanism. *Infect. Immun.* **63:**1089–1094.
20. **Wang, W., K. Keller, and K. Chadee.** 1992. Modulation of tumor necrosis factor production by macrophages in *Entamoeba histolytica* infection. *Infect. Immun.* **60:**3169–3174.
21. **Weigel, M. M., A. Calle, R. X. Armijos, I. P. Vega, B. V. Bayas, and C. E. Montenegro.** 1996. The effect of chronic intestinal parasitic infection on maternal and perinatal outcome. *Int. J. Gynaecol. Obstet.* **52:**9–17.
22. **Yu, Y., and K. Chadee.** 1997. *Entamoeba histolytica* stimulates interleukin 8 from human colonic epithelial cells without parasite-enterocyte contact. *Gastroenterology* **112:**1536–1547.

Strongyloides spp.
1. **Barrett, K. E., F. A. Neva, A. A. Gam, J. Cicmanec, W. T. London, J. M. Phillips, and D. D. Metcalfe.** 1988. The immune response to nematode parasites: modulation of mast cell numbers and function during *Strongyloides stercoralis* infections in nonhuman primates. *Am. J. Trop. Med. Hyg.* **38:**574–581.
2. **Freedman, D. O.** 1991. Experimental infection of human subject with *Strongyloides* species. *Rev. Infect. Dis.* **13:**1221–1226.
3. **Genta, R. M., J. S. Harper III, A. A. Gam, W. I. London, and F. A. Neva.** 1984. Exper-

imental disseminated strongyloidiasis in *Erythrocebus patas*. II. Immunology. *Am. J. Trop. Med. Hyg.* **33:**444–450.
4. **Harper, J. S., III, R. M. Genta, A. Gam, W. T. London, and F. A. Neva.** 1984. Experimental disseminated strongyloidiasis in *Erythrocebus patas*. I. Pathology. *Am. J. Trop. Med. Hyg.* **33:**431–443.
5. **Kiyota, M., M. Korenaga, Y. Nawa, and M. Kotani.** 1984. Effect of androgen on the expression of the sex differences in susceptibility to infection with *Strongyloides ratti* in C57BL/6 mice. *Aust. J. Exp. Biol. Med. Sci.* **62:**607–618.
6. **Muriuki, S. M., R. K. Murugu, E. Munene, G. M. Karere, and D. C. Chai.** 1998. Some gastro-intestinal parasites of zoonotic (public health) importance commonly observed in old world non-human primates in Kenya. *Acta Trop.* **71:**73–82.
7. **Plumelle, Y., C. Gonin, A. Edouard, B. J. Bucher, L. Thomas, A. Brebion, and G. Panelatti.** 1997. Effect of *Strongyloides stercoralis* infection and eosinophilia on age at onset and prognosis of adult T-cell leukemia. *Am. J. Clin. Pathol.* **107:**81–87.
8. **Rawat, B., and M. E. Simons.** 1993. *Strongyloides stercoralis* hyperinfestation. Another cause of focal hepatic lesions. *Clin. Imaging* **17:**274–275.
9. **Remfry, J.** 1978. The incidence, pathogenesis, and treatment of helminth infections in rhesus monkeys (*Macaca mulatta*). *Lab. Anim.* **12:**213–218.
10. **Rutherford, A. M.** 1981. Reflections on the passage of *Strongyloides fulleborni* to human infants in mothers milk. *Trop. Doct.* **11:**184–185.
11. **Soulsby, E. J. L.** 1982. *Helminths, Arthropods and Protozoa of Domesticated Animals,* 7th ed., p. 660–661. Lea & Febiger, Philadelphia, Pa.
12. **Toft, J. D., II, and M. L. Eberhard.** 1998. Parasitic diseases, p. 111–205. *In* B. T. Bennett, C. R. Abee, and R. Henrickson (ed.), *Nonhuman Primates in Biomedical Research. Diseases.* Academic Press, Inc., San Diego, Calif.

INDEX

Acariasis
  mice, 57–58, 63
  rabbits, 169–170
  rats, 57–58, 63
Actinobacillus pleuropneumoniae, swine, 299–300, 319
Adenovirus
  canine, 240–242, 265
  MAd-1, 19–21
  MAd-2, 19–21
  mice, 19–21, 62
  rabbits, 147–148, 171
  rats, 19–21, 62
Aleutian disease of mustelids, 197–198
Amebiasis, nonhuman primates, 361–363
Ancylostoma braziliense
  cats, 222–224
  dogs, 261–263
Ancylostoma caninum, dogs, 261–263
Ancylostoma tubaeforme, cats, 222–224
Animal Biosafety Levels, 7
Animal housing, *see* Housing systems
Animal husbandry, historical perspective, 1–2
Antibody production tests, 13
Apes, *see* Nonhuman primates
Ascaris suum, swine, 315–317, 319
Aspiculuris tetraptera, mice, 60–61

Baboons, *see* Nonhuman primates
Bacillus piliformis, see Clostridium piliforme
Bacterial pathogens
  cats, 217–219
  dogs, 248–252
  ferrets, 198–200
  gerbils, 109–111
  guinea pigs, 131–135
  hamsters, 118–121
  mice, 40–56
  nonhuman primates, 355–360
  rabbits, 155–163
  rats, 40–56
  swine, 299–315
Balantidium coli, nonhuman primates, 360–361, 365
Barrier housing, 5–6
Biological safety cabinets, 10
Bordetella bronchiseptica
  dogs, 248–249, 265
  guinea pigs, 131–132, 138
  rabbits, 155, 171
  swine, 300–302, 319
Brucella canis, dogs, 249–250, 265

Caging, *see* Housing systems
Calicivirus, feline, 207–209, 224
Campylobacter, nonhuman primates, 355–356, 365
Campylobacter coli
  dogs, 251
  nonhuman primates, 355
Campylobacter fetus, nonhuman primates, 355
Campylobacter helveticus, dogs, 251
Campylobacter hyointestinalis, nonhuman primates, 355
Campylobacter jejuni
  dogs, 251–252, 265
  nonhuman primates, 355
Campylobacter lari, dogs, 251
Campylobacter laridis, nonhuman primates, 355
Campylobacter sputorum, nonhuman primates, 355

Campylobacter upsaliensis, dogs, 251
Canine adenovirus, 240–242, 265
Canine coronavirus, 242–243, 265
Canine distemper virus
   dogs, 243–244, 265
   ferrets, 196–197, 202
Canis familiaris, see Dogs
Cardiomyopathy virus, see Pleural effusion disease virus
Cardiovascular diseases
   cats, 224
   dogs, 265
   ferrets, 202
   gerbils, 112
   guinea pigs, 138
   hamsters, 122
   mice, 62–63
   nonhuman primates, 365
   rabbits, 171
   rats, 62–63
   swine, 319
Cats, 207–237
   C. felis, 217–219, 224
   dermatomycosis, 219–221, 224
   feline calicivirus, 207–209, 224
   feline coronavirus, 209–210, 224
   feline herpesvirus type 1, 210–212, 224
   feline immunodeficiency virus, 212–214, 224
   feline leukemia virus, 214–216, 224
   feline parvovirus, 216–217, 224
   fleas, 221–222, 224
   housing, 11
   intestinal nematodes, 222–224
Cavia porcellus, see Guinea pigs
Cercopithecine herpesvirus-1, nonhuman primates, 343–345
Cesarean rederivation, 1
Cheyletiella parasitivorax, rabbits, 164, 171
Chimpanzee coryza, 345
Chimpanzees, see Nonhuman primates
Chinese hamster cells, 115
Chlamydia psittaci var. *felis*, see *Chlamydophila felis*
Chlamydophila felis, cats, 217–219, 224
Chlamydophila psittaci, guinea pigs, 132–133, 138
Chronic proliferative enteropathy, swine, 307
Cilia-associated respiratory bacillus
   mice, 40–41, 62
   rabbits, 155–156, 171
   rats, 40–41, 62
Circovirus, porcine, 284–286, 319
Citrobacter rodentium, mice, 41–42, 62
Clostridium perfringens type C, swine, 302–304, 319
Clostridium piliforme
   gerbils, 109–110, 112
   hamsters, 118–119, 122
   mice, 42–43, 63

   rabbits, 156–157, 171
   rats, 42–43, 63
Clostridium spiroforme, rabbits, 157–158, 171
Coccidiosis
   rabbits
      hepatic, 167–168, 171
      intestinal, 168–169, 171
   swine, 317–318
Colonic hyperplasia, murine, 41–42
Commensals, 2
Containment housing, 6–7
Conventional housing, 5
Coronavirus
   canine, 242–243, 265
   feline, 209–210, 224
   porcine respiratory, 298–299, 319
   rabbit enteric, 151–152, 171
Corynebacterium, athymic mice, 44–45, 63
Corynebacterium bovis, mice, 44
Corynebacterium kutscheri
   mice, 43–44, 63
   rats, 43–44, 63
Corynebacterium pseudodiphtheriticum, mice, 44
Coryza, chimpanzee, 345
Cottontail rabbit papillomavirus, 148–149, 171
Cryptosporidium parvum, rabbits, 164–165, 171
Cryptosporidium wrairi, guinea pigs, 135–136, 138
Ctenocephalides, ferrets, 200
Ctenocephalides canis, dogs, 259
Ctenocephalides felis
   cats, 221
   dogs, 259
Cubicle (housing), 7–10
   built-in, 7–8
   freestanding, 9–10
Cytomegalovirus
   guinea pigs, 129–130, 138
   mice, 21–22, 62
   rats, 21–22, 62

Demodex, Syrian hamsters, 121–123
Demodex canis, dogs, 255–257, 265
Demodex cricetuli, hamsters, 121
Demodex sinocricetuli, hamsters, 121
Demyelination, mice, 39–40
Dentostomella translucida, gerbils, 111
Dermatomycosis
   cats, 219–221, 224
   dogs, 252–254, 265
   rabbits, 163–164, 171
Diagnostic laboratory, 13
Dirofilaria immitis
   dogs, 257–259, 265
   ferrets, 201–202
Diseases, infection vs., 2
Distemper virus, canine
   dogs, 243–244, 265
   ferrets, 196–197, 202

Dogs, 239–279
  B. bronchiseptica, 248–249, 265
  B. canis, 249–250, 265
  C. jejuni, 251–252, 265
  canine adenovirus, 240–242, 265
  canine coronavirus, 242–243
  canine distemper virus, 243–244, 265
  D. canis, 255–257, 265
  D. immitis, 257–259, 265
  dermatomycosis, 252–254, 265
  fleas, 259–260, 265
  housing, 11
  intestinal nematodes, 260–263, 265
  intestinal protozoa, 263–266
  M. pachydermatis, 254–255, 265
  parainfluenza virus type 2, 244–246, 265
  parvovirus, 246–248, 265

Echidnophaga gallinacea
  cats, 221
  dogs, 259
Ectromelia virus
  mice, 22–23, 62
  rats, 22–23, 62
Eimeria, swine, 317
Eimeria caviae, guinea pigs, 136–138
Eimeria flavescens, rabbits, 168–169
Eimeria intestinalis, rabbits, 168–169
Eimeria irresidua, rabbits, 168–169
Eimeria magna, rabbits, 168–169
Eimeria media, rabbits, 168–169
Eimeria neoleporis, rabbits, 168–169
Eimeria perforans, rabbits, 168–169
Eimeria piriformis, rabbits, 168–169
Eimeria stiedai, rabbits, 167–168
Encephalitozoon cuniculi
  mice, 58–59, 63
  rabbits, 165–167, 171
  rats, 58–59, 63
Encephalomyelitis virus, Theiler's murine, 39–40, 62
Encephalomyocarditis virus, swine, 282–283, 319
Endocrine diseases
  cats, 224
  dogs, 265
  ferrets, 202
  guinea pigs, 138
  mice, 62–63
  nonhuman primates, 365
  rabbits, 171
  rats, 62–63
  swine, 319
Endolimax nana, nonhuman primates, 361
Entamoeba chattoni, nonhuman primates, 361
Entamoeba coli, nonhuman primates, 361
Entamoeba dispar, nonhuman primates, 361
Entamoeba hartmanii, nonhuman primates, 361

Entamoeba histolytica, nonhuman primates, 361–363, 365
Enteric coronavirus, rabbit, 151–152, 171
Enterohepatic diseases
  cats, 224
  dogs, 265
  ferrets, 202
  gerbils, 112
  guinea pigs, 138
  hamsters, 122
  mice, 62–63
  nonhuman primates, 365
  rabbits, 171
  rats, 62–63
  swine, 319
Enterovirus, porcine, 286–287, 319
Epidermophyton, cats, 219
Epizootic diarrhea of infant mice, see Mouse rotavirus
Erysipeloid, 304
Erysipelothrix rhusiopathiae, swine, 304–305, 319

Feline calicivirus, 207–209, 224
Feline coronavirus, 209–210, 224
Feline herpesvirus type 1, 210–212, 224
Feline immunodeficiency virus, 212–214, 224
Feline leukemia virus, 214–216, 224
Feline parvovirus, 216–217, 224
Felis sylvestris catus, see Cats
Ferrets, 193–206
  canine distemper virus, 196–197, 202
  D. immitis, 201–202
  fleas, 200–202
  H. mustelae, 198–199, 202
  human influenza virus, 193–194, 202
  L. intracellularis, 199–200, 202
  parvovirus, 197–198, 202
  rabies virus, 195–196, 202
  rotavirus, 194–195, 202
Flavobacterium ferrugineum, 40
Fleas
  cats, 221–222, 224
  dogs, 259–260, 265
  ferrets, 200–202
Flexibacter sancti, 40
"Flexispira rappini," mice, 45
Francisella tularensis, rabbits, 158–159, 171
Fungal pathogens
  cats, 219–221
  dogs, 252–255
  mice, 56–57
  rabbits, 163–164
  rats, 56–57

Gerbils, 109–114
  C. piliforme, 109–110, 112
  oxyurids, 111–113
  S. aureus, 110–112

Germ-free isolator, 9, 11
Giardia duodenalis, dogs, 263
Giardia muris
    mice, 59–60, 63
    rats, 59–60, 63
Gnotobiotic derivation, 1
Guinea pigs, 129–146
    B. bronchiseptica, 131–132, 138
    C. psittaci, 132–133, 138
    C. wrairi, 135–136, 138
    cytomegalovirus, 129–130, 138
    E. caviae, 136–138
    inclusion conjunctivitis, 132–133
    lymphocytic choriomeningitis virus, 130–131, 138
    R. caviae, 137–138
    S. pneumoniae, 133–134, 138
    S. zooepidemicus, 134–135, 138

H-1 virus
    mice, 23–24, 62
    rats, 23–24, 62
Haemophilus parasuis, swine, 305–307, 319
Hamsters, 115–127
    C. piliforme, 118–119, 122
    Demodex, 121–123
    L. intracellularis, 119–120, 122
    lymphocytic choriomeningitis virus, 116–117, 122
    oxyurids, 122–123
    pneumonia virus of mice, 117, 122
    S. aureus, 120–122
    Sendai virus, 117–118, 122
    species used in research, 115
Health records, 14
Heartworm, *see Dirofilaria immitis*
Heating, ventilation, and air-conditioning (HVAC) system, 9
Helicobacter
    mice, 45–47, 63
    rats, 45–47, 63
Helicobacter bilis, mice, 45–46
Helicobacter ganmani, mice, 45
Helicobacter hepaticus, mice, 45–46
Helicobacter muridarum
    mice, 45–46
    rats, 45–46
Helicobacter mustelae, ferrets, 198–199, 202
Helicobacter rodentium, mice, 45
Helicobacter trogontum, rats, 45
Helicobacter typhlonius, mice, 45
Hemagglutinating encephalomyelitis virus, swine, 283–284, 319
Hematopoietic diseases
    cats, 224
    dogs, 265
    ferrets, 202
    guinea pigs, 138
    hamsters, 122

mice, 62–63
nonhuman primates, 365
rabbits, 171
rats, 62–63
swine, 319
Hemorrhagic disease virus, rabbit, 152–153, 171
Hemorrhagic fever virus, simian, 347–348, 365
HEPA filter, 7, 10
Hepatic coccidiosis, rabbits, 167–168, 171
Hepatitis B virus, nonhuman primates, 342–343, 365
Hepatitis virus, mouse, 29–31, 62
Herpesvirus
    nonhuman primates, 343–345, 365
    swine, 293–295, 319
Herpesvirus simiae, nonhuman primates, 343–345
Herpesvirus type 1, feline, 210–212, 224
Hexamita muris, see Spironucleus muris
High-efficiency particulate air filter, 7, 10
Hookworms, dogs, 261–263
Housing systems, 5–12
    barrier, 5–6
    biological safety cabinets, 10
    containment (isolation), 6–7
    conventional, 5
    cubicles, 7–10
    germ-free isolator, 9, 11
    immune-deficient animals, 6
    nonrodent species, 11–12
    rodents, 5–11
Human immunodeficiency virus, 348–350
Human influenza virus
    ferrets, 193–194, 202
    type A, 193
    type B, 193
HVAC system, 9

Immune-deficient animals
    housing, 6
    pathogen surveillance, 13
Immunodeficiency virus
    feline, 212–214, 224
    human, 348–350
    simian, 348–351, 365
IMPACT, 13–14
Inclusion conjunctivitis, guinea pig, 132–133
Infection
    disease vs., 2
    subclinical, 2
Infectious microprobe PCR amplification test (IMPACT), 13–14
Infectious tracheobronchitis, dogs, 240
Influenza virus
    human, ferrets, 193–194, 202
    swine, 295–297, 319
Intestinal coccidiosis, rabbits, 168–169, 171

Intestinal nematodes
  cats, 222–224
  dogs, 260–263, 265
Intestinal protozoa, dogs, 263–266
Iodamoeba buetschlii, nonhuman primates, 361
Iodamoeba wallacei, nonhuman primates, 361
Isolation housing, *see* Containment housing
Isospora canis, dogs, 263
Isospora ohioensis, dogs, 263
Isospora suis, swine, 317–319

Kennel cough, 240
Kilham rat virus, 24–25, 62
Klebsiella pneumoniae
  mice, 47–48, 63
  rats, 47–48, 63

Lactate dehydrogenase-elevating virus, mice, 25–27, 62
Lapine parvovirus, 149, 171
Lawsonia intracellularis
  ferrets, 199–200, 202
  hamsters, 119–120, 122
  swine, 307–308, 319
Leptospira, swine, 308–310, 319
Leptospira bratislava, swine, 309
Leptospira canicola, swine, 309
Leptospira icterohaemorrhagiae, swine, 309
Leptospira muenchen, swine, 309
Leptospira pomona, swine, 309
Leptospira tarassovi, swine, 309
Leukemia virus, feline, 214–216, 224
Listeria monocytogenes, rabbits, 159–160, 171
Listeriosis, 159
Lymphocytic choriomeningitis virus
  guinea pigs, 130–131, 138
  hamsters, 116–117, 122
  mice, 27–28, 62
  rats, 27–28, 62
Lymphoreticular diseases
  cats, 224
  dogs, 265
  ferrets, 202
  gerbils, 112
  guinea pigs, 138
  hamsters, 122
  mice, 62–63
  nonhuman primates, 365
  rabbits, 171
  rats, 62–63
  swine, 319

Macaques, *see* Nonhuman primates
MADC rooms, 10
Malassezia pachydermatis, dogs, 254–255, 265
Mammary tumor virus, mouse, 31–32, 62
Mange, swine, 318–320

Mass air displacement "clean" (MADC) rooms, 10
Meriones unguiculatus, see Mongolian gerbils
Mesocricetus auratus, see Syrian hamsters
Mice, 19–107
  acariasis, 57–58, 63
  adenovirus, 19–21, 62
  athymic, *Corynebacterium,* 44–45, 63
  C. kutscheri, 43–44, 63
  C. piliforme, 42–43, 63
  C. rodentium, 41–42, 62
  cilia-associated respiratory bacillus, 40–41, 62
  cytomegalovirus, 21–22, 62
  E. cuniculi, 58–59, 63
  ectromelia virus, 22–23, 62
  G. muris, 59–60, 63
  H-1 virus, 23–24, 62
  Helicobacter, 45–47, 63
  indigenous viruses, eradication, 1
  K. pneumoniae, 47–48, 63
  lactate dehydrogenase-elevating virus, 25–27, 62
  lymphocytic choriomeningitis virus, 27–28, 62
  M. pulmonis, 48–49, 63
  minute virus of mice, 28–29, 62
  mouse hepatitis virus, 29–31, 62
  mouse mammary tumor virus, 31–32, 62
  mouse parvovirus-1, 32, 62
  mouse rotavirus, 32–34, 62
  mouse thymic virus, 34, 62
  oxyuriasis, 60–61, 63
  P. aeruginosa, 51–52, 63
  P. carinii, 56–57, 63
  P. pneumotropica, 49–50, 63
  pneumonia virus of mice, 34–35, 62
  reovirus-3, 36–37, 62
  S. aureus, 54–55, 63
  S. enterica, 52–54, 63
  S. muris, 61–64
  S. pneumoniae, 55–56, 63
  Sendai virus, 37–38, 62
  sialodacryoadenitis virus, 38–39, 62
  Theiler's murine encephalomyelitis virus, 39–40, 62
Micro-Isolator cage
  static, 7–8
  ventilated, 7–8
Microsporum canis
  cats, 219
  dogs, 252–254
  rabbits, 163
Microsporum gypseum
  dogs, 252–254
  rabbits, 163
Microsporum persicolor, cats, 219
Minute virus of mice, 28–29, 62
Mites
  dogs, 255–257
  guinea pigs, 137–138

Mites (*Continued*)
  hamsters, 121–123
  mice, 57–58
  rabbits, 164, 170–172
  rats, 57–58
  swine, 318–320
Monkeys, *see* Nonhuman primates
Mouse hepatitis virus, 29–31, 62
Mouse mammary tumor virus, 31–32, 62
  MMTV-C4, 31–32
  MMTV-L, 31–32
  MMTV-O, 31–32
  MMTV-P, 31–32
  MMTV-S, 31
  MMTV-SW, 31–32
Mouse parvovirus-1, 32, 62
Mouse rotavirus, 32–34, 62
Mouse thymic virus, 34, 62
Mousepox, 22–23
Mus musculus, see Mice
Musculoskeletal diseases
  cats, 224
  dogs, 265
  ferrets, 202
  guinea pigs, 138
  mice, 62–63
  nonhuman primates, 365
  rabbits, 171
  rats, 62–63
  swine, 319
Mustela putorius furo, see Ferrets
Mustelids, Aleutian disease, 197–198
Mycoplasma flocculare, swine, 310
Mycoplasma hyopharyngis, swine, 310
Mycoplasma hyopneumoniae, swine, 310–311, 319
Mycoplasma hyorhinis, swine, 310
Mycoplasma hyosynoviae, swine, 310
Mycoplasma pulmonis
  mice, 48–49, 63
  rats, 48–49, 63
Mycoplasma sualvi, swine, 310
Myobia musculi
  mice, 57–58
  rats, 57–58
Myocoptes musculinus
  mice, 57–58
  rats, 57–58
Myxoma virus, rabbits, 149–150, 171

Necropsy, 13
Nematodes
  ferrets, 201–202
  intestinal
    cats, 222–224
    dogs, 260–263, 265
  nonhuman primates, 363–366
  rabbits, 169

Neospora caninum, dogs, 263
Nervous system diseases
  cats, 224
  dogs, 265
  ferrets, 202
  gerbils, 112
  guinea pigs, 138
  hamsters, 122
  mice, 62–63
  nonhuman primates, 365
  rabbits, 171
  rats, 62–63
  swine, 319
Nonhuman primates, 341–376
  B. coli, 360–361, 365
  Campylobacter, 355–356, 365
  captive bred, 341
  E. histolytica, 361–363, 365
  hepatitis B virus, 342–343, 365
  herpesvirus, 343–345, 365
  housing, 11–12
  respiratory syncytial virus, 345–346, 365
  rotavirus, 346–347, 365
  S. flexneri, 356–358, 365
  S. pneumoniae, 358–360, 365
  simian hemorrhagic fever virus, 347–348, 365
  simian immunodeficiency virus, 348–351, 365
  simian retrovirus type D, 351–352, 365
  simian T-cell leukemia virus, 352–354, 365
  simian virus 40, 354–355, 365
  Strongyloides, 363–366
  wild-caught, 341

Opportunists, 2
Oral papillomavirus, rabbit, 153–154, 171
Orphan parvovirus, *see* Mouse parvovirus-1
Otoacariasis, rabbits, 169–170
Oxyurids
  mice, 60–61, 63
  gerbils, 111–113
  hamsters, 122–123
  rats, 60–61, 63

Papillomavirus
  cottontail rabbit, 148–149, 171
  rabbit oral, 153–154, 171
Parainfluenza virus type 2, dogs, 244–246, 265
Parasites
  cats, 221–224
  dogs, 255–266
  ferrets, 200–202
  gerbils, 111–113
  guinea pigs, 135–138
  hamsters, 121–123
  mice, 57–64
  nonhuman primates, 360–366
  rabbits, 164–172

rats, 57–64
swine, 315–320
Parasiticides, immune-modulating activity, 2
Parvovirus
   dogs, 246–248, 265
   feline, 216–217, 224
   ferrets, 197–198, 202
   lapine, 149, 171
   porcine, 287–289, 319
Parvovirus-1, mouse, 32, 62
Passalurus ambiguus, rabbits, 169, 171
Pasteurella multocida
   rabbits, 160–161, 171
   swine, 311–313, 319
Pasteurella pneumotropica
   mice, 49–50, 63
   rats, 49–50, 63
Pathogen, 2
Pathogen surveillance, 12–16
   caretaker observation, 13
   diagnostic laboratory, 13
   frequency of testing, 15–16
   prevalence-based sampling principles, 15
   principal animals, 14
   sampling strategies, 14
   sentinel animals, 14–15
PCR assay technology, 13–15
Pigs, *see* Swine
Pinworm, *see* Oxyuriasis
Pityrosporum canis, see Malassezia pachydermatis
Pityrosporum pachydermatis, see Malassezia pachydermatis
Pleural effusion disease virus, rabbits, 151, 171
Pleuropneumonia, porcine, 299
Pneumocystis carinii, 50
   mice, 56–57, 63
   rats, 56–57, 63
Pneumonia virus of mice
   mice, 34–35, 62
   Syrian hamsters, 117, 122
Polioencephalomyelitis, mice, 39–40
Porcine circovirus, 284–286, 319
Porcine enterovirus, 286–287, 319
Porcine intestinal adenomatosis, 307
Porcine parvovirus, 287–289, 319
Porcine proliferative enteropathies, 307
Porcine reproductive and respiratory syndrome virus, 289–291, 319
Porcine respiratory coronavirus, 298–299, 319
Porcine rotavirus, 291–293, 319
Primates, nonhuman, *see* Nonhuman primates
Protozoan pathogens
   dogs, 263–266
   nonhuman primates, 360–363
   swine, 317–318
Pseudomonas aeruginosa
   mice, 51–52, 63
   rats, 51–52, 63

Pseudorabies virus, *see* Swine herpesvirus
Psoroptes cuniculi, rabbits, 169–171

Quarantine, 7, 14–15

Rabbits, 147–192
   adenovirus, 147–148, 171
   B. bronchiseptica, 155, 171
   breeds used in research, 147
   C. parasitivorax, 164, 171
   C. parvum, 164–165, 171
   C. piliforme, 156–157, 171
   C. spiroforme, 157–158, 171
   cilia-associated respiratory bacillus, 155–156, 171
   coccidiosis
      hepatic, 167–168, 171
      intestinal, 168–169, 171
   cottontail rabbit papillomavirus, 148–149, 171
   dermatomycosis, 163–164, 171
   E. cuniculi, 165–167, 171
   enteric coronavirus, 151–152, 171
   F. tularensis, 158–159, 171
   hemorrhagic disease virus, 152–153, 171
   L. monocytogenes, 159–160, 171
   lapine parvovirus, 149, 171
   myxoma virus, 149–150, 171
   oral papillomavirus, 153–154, 171
   P. ambiguus, 169, 171
   P. cuniculi, 169–171
   P. multocida, 160–161, 171
   pleural effusion disease virus, 151, 171
   rotavirus, 154–155, 171
   S. aureus, 161–162, 171
   S. scabiei, 170–172
   T. paraluis-cuniculi, 162–163, 171
Rabies, 195–196
Rabies virus, ferrets, 195–196, 202
Radfordia ensifera, rats, 57–58
Rat rotavirus-like agent, 35–36, 62
Rats, 19–107
   acariasis, 57–58, 63
   adenovirus, 19–21, 62
   C. kutscheri, 43–44, 63
   C. piliforme, 42–43, 63
   cilia-associated respiratory bacillus, 40–41, 62
   cytomegalovirus, 21–22, 62
   E. cuniculi, 58–59, 63
   ectromelia virus, 22–23, 62
   G. muris, 59–60, 63
   H-1 virus, 23–24, 62
   Helicobacter, 45–47, 63
   K. pneumoniae, 47–48, 63
   Kilham rat virus, 24–25, 62
   lymphocytic choriomeningitis virus, 27–28, 62
   M. pulmonis, 48–49, 63
   mouse hepatitis virus, 29–31
   oxyuriasis, 60–61, 63

Rats (*Continued*)
  P. aeruginosa, 51–52, 63
  P. carinii, 56–57, 63
  P. pneumotropica, 49–50, 63
  reovirus-3, 36–37, 62
  rotavirus-like agent, 35–36, 62
  S. aureus, 54–55, 63
  S. enterica, 52–54, 63
  S. muris, 61–64
  S. pneumoniae, 55–56, 63
  Sendai virus, 37–38, 62
  sialodacryoadenitis virus, 38–39, 62
  Theiler's murine encephalomyelitis virus, 39–40, 62
Reovirus-3
  mice, 36–37, 62
  rats, 36–37, 62
Reproductive and respiratory syndrome virus, porcine, 289–291, 319
Reproductive system diseases
  cats, 224
  dogs, 265
  guinea pigs, 138
  mice, 62–63
  nonhuman primates, 365
  rabbits, 171
  rats, 62–63
  swine, 319
Respirator suits, 10–11
Respiratory syncytial virus, nonhuman primates, 345–346, 365
Respiratory system diseases
  cats, 224
  dogs, 265
  ferrets, 202
  guinea pigs, 138
  hamsters, 122
  mice, 62–63
  nonhuman primates, 365
  rabbits, 171
  rats, 62–63
  swine, 319
Retrovirus type D, simian, 351–352, 365
Rhinotracheitis, feline viral, 210–212
Rotavirus
  atypical, 194
  ferrets, 194–195, 202
  mouse, 32–34, 62
  nonhuman primates, 346–347, 365
  porcine, 291–293, 319
  rabbits, 154–155, 171
  simian, 346–347, 365
Rotavirus-like agent, rat, 35–36, 62
Roundworms
  dogs, 261–263
  swine, 315–317

Salmonella enterica
  mice, 52–54, 63
  rats, 52–54, 63
Sarcoptes scabiei
  rabbits, 170–172
  swine, 318–320
Sendai virus
  hamsters, 117–118, 122
  mice, 37–38, 62
  rats, 37–38, 62
Sentinel animals, 14–15
Shigella flexneri, nonhuman primates, 356–358, 365
Sialodacryoadenitis virus
  mice, 38–39, 62
  rats, 38–39, 62
Simian hemorrhagic fever virus, 347–348, 365
Simian immunodeficiency virus, 348–351, 365
Simian retrovirus type D, 351–352, 365
Simian rotavirus, 346–347, 365
Simian T-cell leukemia virus, 352–354, 365
Simian virus 40, nonhuman primates, 354–355, 365
Skin diseases
  cats, 224
  dogs, 265
  ferrets, 202
  gerbils, 112
  guinea pigs, 138
  hamsters, 122
  mice, 62–63
  nonhuman primates, 365
  rabbits, 171
  rats, 62–63
  swine, 319
Specific-pathogen-free (SPF) animals, 6–7
SPF animals, *see* Specific-pathogen-free animals
Spironucleus muris
  mice, 61–64
  rats, 61–64
Staphylococcus aureus
  gerbils, 110–112
  hamsters, 120–122
  mice, 54–55, 63
  rabbits, 161–162, 171
  rats, 54–55, 63
Streptococcus alactolyticus, swine, 313
Streptococcus bovis, swine, 313
Streptococcus dysgalactiae, swine, 313
Streptococcus hyointestinalis, swine, 313
Streptococcus intestinalis, swine, 313
Streptococcus pneumoniae
  guinea pigs, 133–134, 138
  mice, 55–56, 63
  nonhuman primates, 358–360, 365
  rats, 55–56, 63
Streptococcus porcinus, swine, 313
Streptococcus suis, swine, 313–315, 319

Streptococcus zooepidemicus
  guinea pigs, 134–135, 138
  nonhuman primates, 359
Strongyloides, nonhuman primates, 363–366
Strongyloides cebus, nonhuman primates, 363
Strongyloides fulleborni, nonhuman primates, 363, 366
Strongyloides stercoralis, nonhuman primates, 363–366
Subclinical infection, 2
Sus scrofa domestica, see Swine
Swine, 281–339
  A. pleuropneumoniae, 299–300, 319
  A. suum, 315–317, 319
  B. bronchiseptica, 300–302, 319
  C. perfringens type C, 302–304, 319
  E. rhusiopathiae, 304–305, 319
  encephalomyocarditis virus, 282–283, 319
  H. parasuis, 305–307, 319
  hemagglutinating encephalomyelitis virus, 283–284, 319
  I. suis, 317–319
  intestinal adenomatosis, 307
  L. intracellularis, 307–308, 319
  Leptospira, 308–310, 319
  M. hyopneumoniae, 310–311, 319
  P. multocida, 311–313, 319
  porcine circovirus, 284–286, 319
  porcine enterovirus, 286–287, 319
  porcine parvovirus, 287–289, 319
  porcine reproductive and respiratory syndrome virus, 289–291, 319
  porcine respiratory coronavirus, 298–299, 319
  porcine rotavirus, 291–293, 319
  proliferative enteropathies, 307
  S. scabiei, 318–320
  S. suis, 313–315, 319
  swine herpesvirus, 293–295, 319
  swine influenza virus, 295–297, 319
  transmissible gastroenteritis virus, 297–298, 319
Swine herpesvirus, 293–295, 319
Swine influenza virus, 295–297, 319
Swine vesicular disease, 286–287
Syphacia mesocriceti, hamsters, 123
Syphacia muris
  hamsters, 123
  mice, 60–61, 111
  rats, 60–61, 111
Syphacia obvelata
  hamsters, 123
  mice, 60–61, 111
  rats, 60–61, 111

T-cell leukemia virus, simian, 352–354, 365
Teschen / Talfan disease, 286–287

Theiler's murine encephalomyelitis virus
  mice, 39–40, 62
  rats, 39–40, 62
Toolan's H-1 virus, *see* H-1 virus
Toxascaris leonina
  cats, 222–224
  dogs, 261–263
Toxocara canis
  cats, 222
  dogs, 261–263
Toxocara cati, cats, 222–224
Tracheobronchitis, dogs, 240
Transmissible gastroenteritis virus, swine, 297–298, 319
Transmissible murine colonic hyperplasia, 41–42
Treponema paraluis-cuniculi, rabbits, 162–163, 171
Trichophyton mentagrophytes
  cats, 219
  dogs, 252–254
  rabbits, 163
Trichuris vulpis, dogs, 261–263
Trixacarus caviae, guinea pigs, 137–138
Tularemia, 158
Tyvek suits, 10–11
Tyzzer's disease, 42–43, 109, 118, 156

Uncinaria stenocephala
  cats, 222–224
  dogs, 261
Urinary tract diseases
  cats, 224
  dogs, 265
  ferrets, 202
  guinea pigs, 138
  hamsters, 122
  mice, 62–63
  nonhuman primates, 365
  rabbits, 171
  rats, 62–63
  swine, 319

Viral pathogens
  cats, 207–217
  dogs, 240–248
  ferrets, 193–198
  guinea pigs, 129–131
  hamsters, 116–118
  mice, 19–40
  nonhuman primates, 342–355
  rabbits, 147–155
  rats, 19–40
  swine, 282–299

Whipworms, dogs, 261–263